Health Care Administration:

A Managerial Perspective

Health Care Administration:
A Managerial Perspective

SAMUEL LEVEY, *Ph.D.*
Professor and Director, Graduate Program in Health Care Administration, Baruch College —Mount Sinai School of Medicine, City University of New York

N. PAUL LOOMBA, *Ph.D.*
Professor and Chairman, Department of Management, Baruch College, City University of New York

J. B. Lippincott Company
Philadelphia · Toronto

ISBN-0-397-52059-X

Library of Congress Catalog Card Number: 72–10830

Printed in the United States of America

8 7 6 5

Library of Congress Cataloging in Publication Data
Levey, Samuel.
  Health care administration: a managerial perspective.

  Includes bibliographical references.
  1. Public health administration.   2. Hospitals—
Administration.   I. Loomba, Narendra Paul, 1927–
joint author.   II. Title.

RA393.L4   658′.91′3621   72-10830
ISBN 0-397-52059-X

To
Linda, Eric, Andrea, Sara
Bibiji, Mahinder, Raj, Ravi

Preface

This volume is directed to two principal audiences: managers of health care organizations, and college students enrolled in various health-related programs. It has been written for the managers and administrators of hospitals, long-term-care facilities, public health programs, and voluntary health agencies. It is also designed as a text for management-oriented courses in graduate and undergraduate programs in hospital and health care administration and health planning, and in schools of allied health professions, dentistry, medicine, nursing, public health and social work. The broad range of topics covered should also make it a useful reference work for non-administrative health professionals who are committed to improving the organization and delivery of health care. The contents of the book represent our efforts leading toward a synthesis of many vital aspects of the various branches of management for a pragmatic approach to the solution of managerial problems in health organizations.

The necessity for designing an effective system of health care is near the top of the priority list of our domestic problems. As is evident from various publications and newspaper editorials across the country, a national debate continues to rage regarding the desirable financial and organizational aspects of legislative proposals for the health care system. The health endeavor is frequently viewed as a system facing a "massive crisis." One indicator of the magnitude, and the potential impact, of the problem is the size of the health care enterprise. Employment in health occupations is projected by the United States Public Health Service to exceed 5,000,000 by 1980. In terms of its economic importance, the health care sector will soon become the largest industry in the United States. Furthermore, our social, political, and economic values are evolving along directions which will place the highest premium on upgrading the "quality of life." Health care, therefore, is increasingly considered as a "right" for everyone—rather than a privilege for those who can afford it. Social forces have already created an environment in which we must contend with two undeniable factors. On the one hand, rising expectations for the level and quality of health care have greatly increased and continue to affect the demand for health services. On the other hand, institutionalized rigidities, and the lack of proper planning in the past, have imposed severe constraints on the supply side. There is a limit to the rate at which inputs (health manpower, biomedical knowledge, and facilities and equipment) to the health delivery system can be increased: especially in the short run. What, then, are the most realistic responses to the crucial problem of improving the quality of our health care system even as we continue to modify the current practices in the search of stated goals and objectives? We are convinced that great potential lies in tapping the knowledge made available by the various branches of modern management, and applying it to the strategic, administrative, and operational problems of health care organizations.

The overall objective of this book, therefore, is to present health administrators with a "set" of management concepts, tools, and techniques which will assist them in the efficient and effective *management* of health organizations. In order to achieve this objective, we will focus our attention on those subsets of the intersections of the various branches of management literature which are conducive to a systems view of health care organizations. We reject the approach of specialization in any one area as being too narrow; we aim instead for the general and conceptual problems of health care management. Accordingly, we have attempted to "synthesize" the diverse and yet related elements from such areas as organization theory, systems, decision-making, planning, control, management science models, and their applications to health problems.

We have designed the book with the conviction that managers of health organizations need to know both the theoretical foundations and practical applications of modern management. Hence, the book integrates our exposition of several management topics with a set of carefully selected articles. Since we have attempted to cover in one volume a very broad spectrum of modern management, the chapters were of necessity not written with the degree of detail that one would find in books devoted exclusively to management. However, we have made a conscious effort to be "substantive," and have attempted to provide a foundation for the reader so that further study can be fruitfully pursued. In addition, we have compiled a thorough bibliography for each chapter so that the reader can readily pursue his areas of interest by going directly to the wealth of knowledge in these sources. The bibliography was the result of an exhaustive search of the literature and has been published separately.

The articles selected cover (in terms of theory, concepts, and specific applications) long-run strategies, as well as day-to-day decision-making and implementational tasks of health administrators. The following criteria were applied in the selection process.

1. Degree of technical content

2. Relevancy to current problems
3. Quality of communication
4. Degree of theoretical content
5. Degree of potential applications
6. Degree of current use
7. Degree of innovation

Exhibit A is a schematic presentation of the organization of the book which is divided into five parts and fourteen chapters.

Exhibit A: **<u>ORGANIZATION OF THE BOOK</u>**

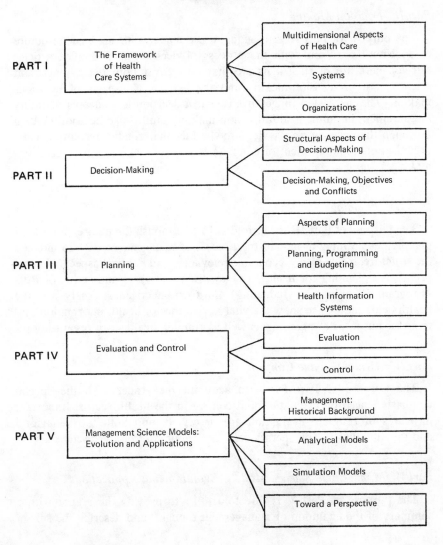

Part I. The Framework of Health Care Systems

The purpose of Part I is threefold: (1) to acquaint the reader with the nature, structure, facts, problems, and some policy issues of health care systems; (2) to establish the concepts of "systems" and "systems approach" in general and as they relate to various aspects of health care administration; and (3) to examine aspects of modern organization theory since health services are rendered in the setting of social, goal-seeking, and adaptive organizations.

Part II. Decision-Making

The purpose of Part II is to acquaint the reader with the basic structure of decision-theory and with the process of decision-making. The articles selected here are of such a nature that they cover both the management science view of decision-making and the behavioral aspects of decision-making. The discussion ranges from what a decision is, concepts of utility measurement in public health decision-making, multi-stage decision-making (through the decision-tree device) to the fact that conflict resolution (i.e., organizational management of conflict) is an essential element in decision-making.

Part III. Planning

The purpose of Part III is fourfold: (1) to establish the nature and role of planning as an integral part of the process of management, (2) to indicate the structure, mechanisms, economic relevance, and political aspects of comprehensive planning for health, (3) to discuss the role and status of PPB (Program, Planning and Budgeting) and Cost-effectiveness Analysis in the health field, and (4) to show the vital importance of health information systems for purposes of planning as well as running health care organizations.

Part IV. Evaluation and Control

The purpose of Part IV is to acquaint the reader with the special emphasis placed on evaluation and control in the health sector. Important measures of program evaluation are described, and both the behavioral and the quantitative (or operational) aspects of control are discussed.

Part V. Management Science Models: Evolution and Applications

The purpose of Part V is threefold: (1) to provide the reader with a summary of the evolution of management thought, and describe the salient characteristics of various "schools" of management, (2) to discuss a selected set of management science models (analytical and simulation) and cite their present and potential applications to problems of health administration, and (3) to offer some thoughts on the future of the health system and its management.

This book, and its accompanying bibliographic volume could not have been completed without the generous assistance and counsel of our students, research assistants, colleagues, and friends in health care. We acknowledge with thanks, the support, encouragement, and helpful suggestions made by S. David Pomrinse, M.D., Director, The Mount Sinai Hospital and Chairman, Department of Administrative Medicine, Mount Sinai School of Medicine, City University of New York; Mr. Jack H. Engelmohr, Executive Director, White Plains Hospital; Dr. Walter Kahoe and Mr. Stuart Freeman of J. B. Lippincott Company.

We are especially indebted to Mr. Harjinder Singh of Computer Design Corporation, Mrs. Lynette Robinson, and Miss Lynn Wasserman, Administrative Assistant in the Graduate Program in Health Care Administration. Mr. Singh coordinated the bibliography project. Mrs. Robinson not only typed the entire manuscript through its several revisions, but also served as a research associate and a general source of encouragement. We are grateful for the permission of the authors of the articles included in this book, and to the publishers of the journals and books in which they originally appeared. Lastly, and most importantly, we would like to acknowledge the perseverance and encouragement of our families. They were selfless in their support throughout the preparation of this book and its accompanying bibliography.

SAMUEL LEVEY
N. PAUL LOOMBA

New York, N.Y.

Contents

Part II
DECISION-MAKING

CHAPTER 4
Structural Aspects of Decision-Making 169

CHAPTER 5
Decision-Making, Objectives and Conflict 229

Part III
PLANNING

CHAPTER 6
Aspects of Planning 269

Part V
MANAGEMENT SCIENCE MODELS:
EVOLUTION AND APPLICATION

Part I

The Framework of Health Care Systems

Chapter 1

Multidimensional Aspects of Health Care

Each and every member of our society is concerned with the subject and concept of "health"—directly or indirectly, individually or collectively, consciously or unconsciously. A "state of good health" is the *most basic* prerequisite for performing the multiple sets of tasks and duties associated with the diverse roles that individuals assume at different stages in their lives. The concept of "health" is intimately related to the idea of "quality of life," and is used to refer to the functioning abilities of not only individuals, but also of organizations, societies, and nations. It is an extremely important and complex concept because it is multidimensional*; it permeates all human activities†; and yet the development of an operational definition of health has been elusive.‡ In a very real sense, the topics of health, health services, health care systems, and health care administration are *intersections* of different but interrelated sets of factors: biological, physical, economic, social, legal, technical, cultural, political and public. The scope of the health field is so wide, and its impact so far-reaching, that some boundary lines must be drawn before we can proceed to discuss any of its multidimensional aspects. Accordingly, it should be stated that we do not propose to present an in-depth analysis of the different com-

---

* For example, it has personal, professional, social, economic, political, and technical components. For an elaboration, see Myers [1965, pp. 41–65]. Also, see Hilleboe [1972].
† "Today, 'health problem' is virtually synonymous with the 'problem of human existence.' Industrialization, urbanization, education, environmental pollution, war, crime, racial problems, housing, city planning or the lack of it: all of these and many additional factors bear importantly on the health of people." [A. Somers, 1971, p. 4].
‡ How to measure "health" and to put a quantitative value on the output of health services are questions of vital interest to physicians, health administrators, and consumers. For a review of the progress made in this direction, see Fanshel and Bush [1970], Packard and Shellard [1970], Kerr and Trantow [1969].

3

ponents, problems, and issues of health care systems in this chapter. Instead, we will identify those aspects that are of the utmost importance to managers and administrators of health institutions, programs, and projects. We will introduce definitions of health, health services, health care systems; distinguish between health care and medical care; and present supplementary schematic diagrams to identify the varieties of problems and issues* that are important to the managers of health care systems. Subsequent chapters are devoted to selected topics of modern management and their present and potential applications to the health field.

1.1 DEFINITIONS

The term "health" can be examined at the individual, the community or public level. For individuals, the term "health" refers to the optimal functioning of the individual; absence of disease, illness, impairment, or injury. In the community or public context, various measures of incidence and prevalence of disease are applied to a defined segment of population. Objective measures of health (health status or health indices) are difficult to construct and operationalize.† *Health services*‡ are all personal and public services performed by individuals or institutions for the purpose of maintaining (e.g., educational and preventive programs) or restoring health. The health care system is the term frequently employed to designate the totality of resources a population or society distributes in the organization and delivery of health services.

A *health care system*§ implies an organized effort at the community state, or national level, to deliver health services in order to attain a set of predetermined health-related goals. Fanshel and Bush [1970, p. 1022] explain:

> To conceive of health services as a system is an analytical tool useful for rational planning. Thus, we say that the health system has a structure in which people and other resources are grouped together into subsystems (programs, institutions, etc.) for the purpose of delivering all types of health services (environmental, educational, financial, etc.). The health system also has a functional relation to the environment about it (such as nonhealth

---

* See *Fortune* (January 1970 issue) for an excellent discussion of several pressing problems in health care.
† See, for example, Rogers [1960, p. 159], Rutstein [1967], Wylie [1970, p. 102]. Goldsmith [1972] presents a review of general health status indicators.
‡ For a pictorial representation of dimensions and strata of some factors relevant to quality of life, quality or level of health of the individual, and quality of health services, see Figures 1, 2, and 3 in Kerr and Trantow [1969].
§ See, for example, Field, Mark G., "The Medical System and Industrial Society," in Alan Sheldon, et al., *Systems and Medical Care,* The MIT Press, Cambridge, Mass., 1970, p. 151. For an analysis of the problem of comparing health care systems, see Yerby [1970].

governmental agencies and organized consumers). The performance of the system relates the output to the input and to the activities performed by the various structural elements.

The major function of any health care system is to achieve an optimal level of health, for a defined population, through comprehensive health services. Health care, the product of health services, is delivered through two primary vehicles: personal health services and public health services. Various terms have been employed in the health field to describe the broad structural-functional characteristics of health care. "Medical care" is the generic term currently used to emphasize the organization, financing and delivery of personal health services. It includes the services of physicians, dentists, nurses, the provision of drugs, orthopedic appliances, hospitals, nursing homes, mental health institutions, and other health resources. "Medical care," therefore, is a subset of the subject of health-care.* However, we will use the two terms interchangeably, and the management concepts to be discussed in this book are equally useful in the organization and delivery of both personal and public health services.

1.2 FACTS, ISSUES AND PROBLEMS OF HEALTH CARE MANAGEMENT

An overall picture of the main data components, facts, issues, and problems of health care can be gleaned from an examination of Table 1.1 and Figures 1.1 through 1.3.

Table 1.1 shows a breakdown of national health expenditures by type of expenditure, and includes data on the relative support provided by various sources of funds, public and private. There are numerous other sources† of data from which health managers can obtain basic facts and statistical data on various components of the health care industry.

Figure 1.1 portrays the vast scope and multidimensional nature of the medical (health) care complex. Three main components with which any health system must deal are shown: consumers of health care, providers of health care, and organizational mechanisms for the delivery of health. The factors relevant to each component are identified.

---

* Arrow [1963] draws a similar distinction between medical-care industry and health-care industry, and presents a survey of the special characteristics of the medical-care market.

† See, U.S. House of Representatives, Committee on Ways and Means: *Basic Facts on the Health Industry,* Washington, D.C., U.S. Government Printing Office, [1971]. Also, see Todd [1972], Rice and Cooper [1972], Klarman et al. [1970], *Statistical Abstract of United States* [1971, pp. 48–60], Somers [1971], *Medical Care Costs and Prices: Background Book* [1972], *Health Resources Statistics* [1971], *Federal Role in Health* [1970], *Reference Data on Socioeconomic Issues of Health* [1971], *New York Times* [June 4, 1972, p. 24] and other references given at the end of Chapter 1.

Table 1.1 NATIONAL HEALTH EXPENDITURES, BY TYPE OF EXPENDITURE AND SOURCE OF FUNDS, FISCAL YEARS, 1970-71

(In Millions) 1970-71

Type of expenditure	Total	Private			Public		
		Total	Consumers	Other	Total	Federal	State and local
Total	$75,012	$46,548	$42,477	$4,071	$28,463	$18,767	$9,696
Health services and supplies	69,479	43,873	42,477	1,396	25,605	16,471	9,134
Hospital care	29,628	14,871	14,472	399	14,757	9,510	5,246
Physicians' services	14,245	10,700	10,688	12	3,545	2,522	1,022
Dentists' services	4,660	4,400	4,400	—	260	154	106
Other professional services	1,475	1,253	1,224	29	222	173	49
Drugs and drug sundries [1]	7,470	6,930	6,930	—	540	271	269
Eyeglasses and appliances	1,915	1,849	1,849	—	66	37	30
Nursing-home care	3,365	1,338	1,314	24	2,027	1,174	853
Expenses for prepayment and administration	2,296	1,600	1,600	—	696	565	131
Government public health activities	1,618	—	—	—	1,618	799	819
Other health services	2,807	932	—	932	1,875	1,266	609
Research and medical-facilities construction	5,533	2,675	—	2,675	2,858	2,296	562
Research [1]	2,019	200	—	200	1,819	1,742	77
Construction	3,514	2,475	—	2,475	1,039	554	485
Publicly owned facilities	875	—	—	—	875	404	471
Privately owned facilities	2,639	2,475	—	2,475	164	150	14

Source: [Rice and Cooper, 1972, p. 7].

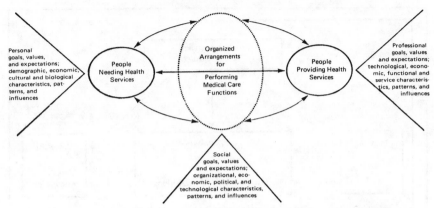

Fig. 1.1. The Medical Care Complex: Boundaries. Source: [Myers, 1965, p. 15]

Figure 1.2 treats the health care system from a different perspective. It provides a conceptual description of the flow of money, services, and information among various components of the health care system. In addition, it points up the roles of funding agencies, educational institutions, and planning function within the framework of an overall system of health care.

Figure 1.3 provides an enumeration of a selected set of hospital problems and health care issues. An examination of Figure 1.3 reveals that the problems and issues of health care are related to managerial knowledge and skills in the areas of "systems," "organizations," "planning," "evaluation," and "control." These are precisely some of the topics to which we have addressed ourselves in subsequent chapters.

There are obviously several other ways of slicing the health care system and presenting different sets of statistical data related to health care. However, most of the important health care problems, issues, factors, considerations, and their interrelationships are covered in Figures 1.1, 1.2, and 1.3.

The health care complex is subject to such strong forces of change from so many directions that health care managers must maintain an active awareness of the important facts, data, and emerging trends in various components and sectors of the health care system. Only in this manner can they discharge their duties toward, and play an active role in, the formulation of those health policies relating to various issues surrounding the organization, management, financing, and delivery of health care. Rather than provide an exhaustive set of health care statistics and an indepth analysis of health care problems and issues, we present below four

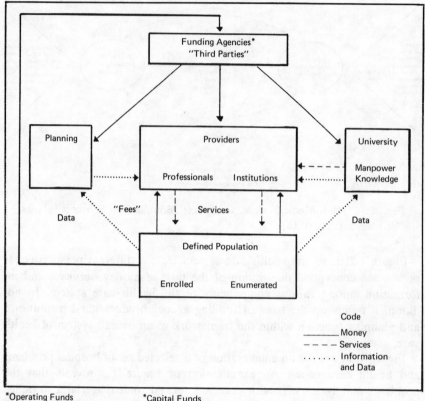

Operating Funds
Governmental: Titles XVIII
and XIX, special grants
Private: Blue Cross-Blue Shield,
commercial insurance, etc.

Capital Funds
Governmental: Hill-Burton,
state, county, municipal
Private: Philanthropy,
borrowing, etc.

Fig. 1.2.   Major pathways for the flow of money, services and information within the medical care system. Source: [Huntley, 1970, p. 19]

interrelated categories under which most of the important problems in health care can be subsumed.*

1. *Basic Facts and Data on the Health Care Industry.* The data shown in Table 1.1, and the wealth of information in the recent report issued by the House Ways and Means Committee (see footnote on page 5) point up two important developments. First, the total health bill stood at $75 billion in fiscal 1971, and it will probably surpass the $80 billion mark in fiscal 1972. Having more than doubled during the last seven years, the

* For a similar view, see Falk [1971, p. 2]. Also, see Somers [1972, p. 85] for a classification of health issues in 9 categories.

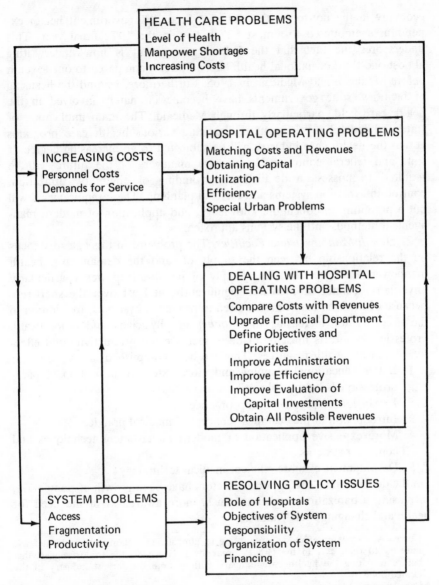

Fig. 1.3. Hospital Problems and Health Care Issues. Source: [Bettauer, 1971, p. 63]

total yearly health expenditures in the United States now accounts for more than 7 percent of our Gross National Product. All available evidence indicates that the health care industry will become the largest sector of the economy in the not-too-distant future.* Secondly, government health expenditures amounted to almost $27 billion in the 1972 fiscal year. This underscores the fact that the federal government is now underwriting almost one-third of national health expenditures—compared to one-seventh before Medicare and Medicaid in 1965. Furthermore, beyond the licensing of facilities, state governments have become intimately involved in the health care field, particularly through Medicaid. The main implication of state and federal involvement in financing various health care programs is that the health care industry will be subjected to an increasing degree of state and federal control.† Health care managers of the future will be required to possess a detailed understanding of eligibility, utilization, control, information systems and regional planning. These requirements will put a premium on education, knowledge, and application of modern management methods and the systems approach.

2. *Health Manpower and Facilities.* The problems in this category focus on the relationship between the supply of, and the demand for, health manpower‡ and facilities. The supply of health manpower (particularly physicians) cannot be increased significantly, at least over the short-run, because of the long lead-time required to produce physicians. In addition to the necessity for increasing the *number* of physicians and other health professionals, efforts must be made to increase the productivity and effectiveness of all health resources. This can be accomplished in several ways:

1. Better educational planning and more extensive utilization of para-professionals§ (e.g., physician's assistants)
2. Expansion of prepaid group practice
3. Introduction of the "campus" concept of medical practice‖
4. More extensive application of modern management techniques and computer systems
5. Development of more efficient medical technology

On the demand side, the important factors have been growth of population, increasing urbanization, higher incomes, more awareness of the need for health and changing social values.♯

---

* Currently, the defense budget amounting to almost $85 billion pushes the defense industry to rank # 1 in the G.N.P. breakdown. However, the trends suggest that before too long the health care industry will become the largest industry in the United States.

† For example, Medicare requires utilization reports from any health care organization providing services to Medicare patients.

‡ For relevant statistics on various categories of health manpower, see, *Health Manpower Perspective* [1967], *Health Resources Statistics* [1970], Losee et al., [1970], *Guide Issue to Hospitals* [1972], *Nursing Home Fact Book* [1971]. See Schwartz [1971] for a view which maintains that the reason for health care "crisis" is not "too few doctors," but poor allocation and use of resources.

§ Letourneau [1968], Coye and Hansen [1969].

‖ Brown [19767, p. 146].

♯ For an amplification of this discussion, see Somers [1971, Chapter 2].

3. *Financing Mechanisms.* Issues involved under this category relate to the question of how the costs of providing health care should be distributed in society. Currently, payments are made either directly by the patient, or through some form of private insurance, or through the channels provided by federal- and state-supported programs. Because of rapidly rising health care costs, problems of access, fragmentation, and lack of a coordinated system of health care, national opinion is rapidly moving towards some national health insurance and delivery network. The question is not whether to institute a national health insurance scheme, but rather when, how much and for whom. [Elling 1971, p. 1.] National health insurance proposals vary widely in terms of eligibility, benefit pattern, financing, administration, effect on health system organization, quality, health manpower, methods of utilization review, audit and fiscal control.*

4. *Lack of Control.* Rising prices and costs† are only one indication that the health care field faces some problems of control. Another serious reason for lack of control is rooted in the very unique nature of health care management. The technical (i.e., medical) skills reside with the doctors; the control for allocating financial resources is usually in the hands of a Board of Directors‡; while the responsibility of running the organization (e.g., a hospital) falls on the shoulders of the health administrator. It is obvious, therefore, that in order to make effective control possible, both structural and operating changes must be introduced in the practice of health care management. In terms of structural changes, we feel that the administrators of the health institutions must be given the authority to formulate policies and *manage* them—not simply administer policies. In terms of operating changes, improvements will have to be made in admission systems, medical records, utilization, controls, and communication channels between different units of the health organization.

We propose that the environment created by structural changes which recognize the crucial role of the health manager will make it viable to introduce the necessary operating changes.§ The health care manager must familiarize himself with modern methods and concepts of management.

---

* For a discussion of major proposals, issues, and goals of national health insurance, see Somers [1971, Chapter 8]. For further analysis of the national health insurance issue, see Berki [1971], Burns [1971], Feldstein [1971], Somers [1972]. For a view opposing the idea of national health insurance, see Garfield [1970].

† *Medical Care Costs and Prices: Background Book* [1972]. Feldstein [1971]. *Research and Statistic Note, No. 4* [1972].

‡ A majority of the Board members is usually drawn from influential citizens of the community who, although deeply interested in the hospital, must devote time to their own business or personal interests.

§ We fully endorse the statement ". . . the committee believes there is no element of health manpower whose impact on hospital effectiveness is more important than the hospital administrator's." [Secretary's Advisory Committee on Hospital Effectiveness, 1968, p, 26.]

A conscious use of management concepts, skills, and techniques will have to be made in order to cope with the rapid changes and complexities of the health field. And it is to this task that this book is devoted.

The selection of articles for Chapter 1 was particularly difficult because of the vast scope of what could be considered important in developing a framework for health care, and within which subsequent management-oriented material must be examined. We selected three articles; each touching on what we think is an important area of consideration.

1.3 CONCLUDING REMARKS*

Sheps' article (Selection 1) surveys the emerging requirements and trends in the role of hospitals as one part of the total health delivery system. Measures adopted to bring structural changes in hospital functions are even more important than the improvements in internal support systems that involve automation and other technical developments. Because of changing social values, increasing financial support from tax dollars, and heightened appreciation of community needs and pressures, the hospital is becoming the nerve center of many of the vital health activities of the community. A partnership involving hospitals and consumers of health care is emerging. This partnership would feed community needs and aspirations as inputs to the hospital decision-making process and help focus the administration's attention on the objectives of effectiveness and economy. Community involvement is a step towards regionalization in health services. Sheps lists a series of crucial issues and major considerations in the development of regional health programs. The trend towards mergers of hospitals or selected services is noted. New requirements arising from comprehensive community health planning programs are emphasized. Finally, the author suggests that social forces will make health institutions more responsive to community health needs and more accountable to the community for their performance.

The purpose of Glaser's article (Selection 2) is to emphasize the need for developing new patterns of health care through an active program of interdisciplinary research at university medical centers. Teaching, research, and patient care are identified as the three classical pursuits of the medical school. The problem of the competing demands for the resources of the medical school imposed by research and teaching requirements on the one hand, and community responsibilities on the other, is explained. While the need for creating new knowledge and educating tomorrow's physicians

---

* We recommend to our readers McNerney [1970] (which analyzes reasons for high costs of medical care) and Kissick [1970] (which reviews the evolution of the role of government in health affairs, and suggests future policy directions).

cannot be ignored, the teaching hospital must meet its social obligations to provide adequate medical care on a community as well as a national level. Glaser believes that the solution does not lie in producing more physicians, but defining and developing new models of health care under carefully organized university programs which lend themselves to experimentation and evaluation. Interdisciplinary teams consisting of systems engineers, computer technologists, political scientists, economists, sociologists, and psychologists should organize studies to develop medical care systems that are more effective for large numbers of patients.

Bailey's article (Selection 3) presents an analysis of how an economist might view the health services industry. The production of medical services is shaped by tradition so that the physician-patient relationship may be more properly seen as agent-principal rather than producer-consumer. Consumer demand for medical services is classified by order of urgency in three categories of health services: (1) emergency or life-saving, (2) curative, and (3) preventive. Income and price effects on the demand for these services are stated. Emergency care is not very responsive to income or price, while the demand for curative services is quite responsive to purely economic factors. Demand for preventive services shows some relationship to income and price, but to generate any substantial increase in demand, educational efforts coupled with price changes would be required. The demand response of these services suggests that health services are not like other goods and services. Hence, reliance upon market processes to generate an optimal level and mix of health services demand can lead to some undesirable resource allocations. Economists, unlike many physicians, are quite inclined to downgrade the free competition explanation of medical practice and to describe the industry as a distinct form of monopoly. Reasons are listed to support this statement. For the market place to act as an efficient allocator of resources, it is important that producers be highly competitive and that consumers be sufficiently knowledgeable to properly evaluate relative worth of goods and services. This implies that the best interests of the society are serviced when producers maximize their own economic interests. But, if producers of medical services, the physicians, maximize their economic interests, this cannot benefit the consumers. Hence the need for government intervention in the medical market place. Economists believe there are three justifiable reasons any time the government intervenes in the market place. One reason occurs whenever services fall into the category of "essential" and quasi-public goods, and when these services possess externalities—benefits that occur to many individuals without their paying directly. A second reason is to affect income distribution. The third area of government intervention is in purchasing goods and services where the market place operates less than full time.

Defining medical care as a right and not as a privilege implies a number of long-term and serious changes in the organization of our delivery system for health services. There are several options open to the government. One is to set itself up as a major producer of medical services. As a second option, government might shun the production route and become a large consumer, acting in the consumer interest both for services purchased directly and for production of medical services in general. Government seems to have selected this option and is now moving rapidly and forcefully to enlarge its role as a consumer of health services. In addition, government is creating positive financial incentives to encourage private producers of health services. As a collective consumer, government in time will become a countervailing power to the monopolistic powers of the physicians in the medical market place.

REFERENCES

Arrow, K. J., "Uncertainty and the Welfare Economics of Medical Care,"
1963   *The American Economic Review,* vol. LIII, no. 5, December, pp.
941–973.

Berki, Sylvester E., "National Health Insurance: An Idea Whose Time Has
1972   Come?" *The Annals of the American Academy of Political and Social
Science,* vol. 399, January, pp. 125–144.

Brown, Ray E., "The Hospital: Proper Portal to All Health Care," *Hospital
1969   Physician,* vol. 5, May, pp. 143, 146, 147.

Burns, E. M., "Health Insurance: Not If, or When, But What Kind?" *American
1971   Journal of Public Health,* vol. 61, November, pp. 2164–2175.

Coye, R. D. and M. F. Hansen, "The Doctor's Assistant," *Journal of the
1969   American Medical Association,* vol. 209, July 28, pp. 529–533.

Falk, I. S., "National Policies and Programs for the Financing of Medical
1971   Care," The 1971 Michael M. Davis Lecture, The University of
Chicago.

Fanshel, S. and J. W. Bush, "A Health-Status Index and Its Application to
1970   Health Services Outcomes," *Operations Research,* vol. 18, November-
December, pp. 1021–1066.

Federal Role in Health, United States Senate, Report of the Committee on
1970   Government Operations, April 30, U.S. Government Printing Office,
Washington, D.C.

Feldstein, M. S., "The Health Care Muddle: A New Approach to National
1971   Health Insurance," *The Public Interest,* vol. 23, Spring, pp. 93–105.

Field, M. G., "The Medical System and Industrial Society," in A. Sheldon,
1970   et al., *Systems and Medical Care,* MIT Press, Cambridge, Mass., p.
151.

Garfield, S. R., "The Delivery of Medical Care," *Scientific American,* vol. 22,
1970   April, pp. 15–23.

Goldsmith, S. B., "The Status of Health Status Indicators," *Health Services
1972   Reports,* vol. 87, March, pp. 212–221.

Guide Issue, Hospitals, Part Two, vol. 46, no. 15, August 1.
1972

Health Manpower, National Advisory Commission Report, volumes I and II
1967 Washington, D.C.
Health Resources Statistics, 1970, Public Health Service, U.S. Department of
1971 Health, Education, and Welfare, U.S. Government Printing Office.
Hilleboe, H. E., "Preventing Future Shock: Health Developments in the
1972 1960's and Imperatives for the 1970's," *American Journal of Public
Health,* vol. 72, no. 2, February, pp. 136–145.
Huntley, R. R., "Improving the Health Services System Through Research and
1970 Development," *Inquiry,* vol. VII, no. 1, March, pp. 15–21.
Kerr, M. and D. J. Trantow, "Defining, Measuring, and Assessing the Quality
1969 of Health Services," *Public Health Reports,* vol. 84, May, pp. 415–
424.
Kissick, W. L., "Health-Policy Directions for the 1970's" *New Journal of
1970 Medicine,* vol. 282, no. 24, June 11, pp. 1343–1354.
Klarman, Herbert E., et al., "Accounting for the Rise in Selected Medical Care
1970 Expenditures," *American Journal of Public Health,* vol. 60, no. 6,
June 1970, pp. 1023–1039.
Letourneau, Charles U., "The Assistant Physician," *Hospital Management,*
1968 April, pp. 55–57.
Losee, G. J. and M. E. Altenderfer, *Health Manpower in Hospitals,* U.S. De-
1970 partment of Health, Education, and Welfare, U.S. Government Printing Office, pp. 2–3.
Medical Care Costs and Prices: Background Book, U.S. Department of Health,
1972 Education and Welfare, Social Security Administration.
McNerney, Walter J., "Does America Need a New Health System," *Blue Cross
1969 News,* March, pp. 353–358.
McNerney, Walter J., "Why Does Medical Care Cost So Much?", *New England
1970 Journal of Medicine,* vol. 282, no. 26, June 25, pp. 1458–1465.
Myers, B. A., "A Guide to Medical Care Administration, Vol. I," American
1965 Public Health Association, Inc.
New York Times, June 4, p. 24.
1972
Nursing Home Fact Book 1970–1971, American Nursing Home Association,
1971 Washington, D.C., July, p. 1.
Packer, A. H. and G. D. Shellard, "Measures of Health-System Effectiveness,"
1970 *Operations Research,* vol. 18, no. 6, November–December, pp.
1067–1070.
Reference Data on Socioeconomic Issues of Health, American Medical As-
1971 sociation (edited by K. E. Monroe).
Research and Statistics Note, No. 4, Social Security Administration, U.S. De-
1972 partment of Health, Education, and Welfare.
Rice, D. P. and B. Cooper, "National Health Expenditures, 1929–71," *Social
1972 Security Bulletin,* January, pp. 3–18.
Rogers, E. S., *Human Ecology and Health,* New York: The Macmillan Co
1960
Rutstein, D. D., *The Coming Revolution in Medicine,* Cambridge, Mass.,
1967 The MIT Press.
Secretary's Advisory Committee on Hospital Effectiveness—Report U.S. De-
1968 partment of Health, Education, and Welfare, Washington, D.C.;
U.S. Government Printing Office.
Somers, A. R., *Health Care in Transition: Directions for the Future,* Hos-
1971 pital Research and Educational Trust, Chicago, Illinois.

Somers, H. M., "National Health Insurance Strategy and Standards," *Medical*
1972   *Care,* vol. X, no. 1, January–February, pp. 85–86.
Schwartz, H., "Too Few Doctors," *New York Times,* June 28.
1971
Statistical Abstract of the United States, Bureau of the Census, U.S. Depart-
1971   ment of Commerce, U.S. Government Printing Office.
Todd, M. C., "Vital Statistics Reporting," *American Journal of Public Health,*
1972   vol. 62, no. 2, February, p. 133.
Wylie, C., "The Definition and Measurement of Health and Disease," *Public*
1970   *Health Reports,* vol. 85, no. 2, February, pp. 100–104.
Yerby, A. S., "What Happens When Ivan, Geoffrey, and John Need a
1970   Doctor?" *Technology Review,* vol. 72, no. 6, April, pp. 24–27.

SELECTION 1

Trends in Hospital Care*

Cecil G. Sheps, M.D., M.P.H.

In discussing developments in our health delivery system, as reflected in trends in hospital care, I am not reporting on a specific research activity. Instead, I shall make a series of observations which reflect my experience as a hospital administrator and an academic student in this field. I shall not discuss the steps, actual or proposed, intended to improve the operating efficiency of hospitals in terms of internal support systems that involve automation and other technical developments. I shall only remark that such measures, important though they may be, offer less hope for improved effectiveness and efficiency than do the measures that modify the role of the hospital in the total system of health services. My concern is with the ways in which hospitals in this country have had to re-think the framework and the manner in which they select the scope of their services in response to community health needs. In other words, I shall be discussing the hospital as a social institution responding to the opportunities provided by scientific progress on the one hand and to social forces on the other.

Historical Development of Hospitals

From its origins of well over a thousand years ago, and for many centuries thereafter, the hospital was generally a shelter for the socially unfit—due to severe physical disability, mental illness, or pauperism. The early hospitals of the past were usually a rather unsavory type, designated for the "sick and suffering poor." Since these institutions were developed, as Benjamin Franklin reports, by those who "did charitably consult together" to relieve the stress of the "distemper'd poor," it is not surprising that they were considered as an activity set apart from the mainstream of medical care of the community as a whole. It is important to note that such old hospitals as the Massachusetts General Hospital and the New York Hospital did not provide care for private patients until the turn of this century.

Scientific developments and the changes in our society have produced the concept of the modern hospital. Hospitals have now become essential to the proper care of a broad spectrum of health problems. If they are not

* *Inquiry*, vol. 8, no. 1, 1971.

yet health centers of the community, certainly hospitals do constitute an integral element in the mainstream of medical care—an essential condition for effective practice for virtually all physicians. In addition to providing care for patients confined to bed with a wide variety of illnesses, the hospital has taken on such other functions as complicated diagnostic procedures and the treatment of ambulatory patients. Gradually the hospital has become the nerve center of many of the vital health activities of the community. Therefore, hospitals have more than beds "plus something." Rather, they are complex organizations with special facilities and highly trained personnel diagnosing and treating a wide variety of human disease.

Hospitals generally describe themselves as community health centers. The opening sentence of a public relations booklet developed a few years ago for hospitals, entitled, "What Everybody Should Know About Hospitals —And How They Keep You Healthy," says, "A modern hospital is part of today's living standard—a health center that serves all!" Such sentiments are usually acceptable to the public and the health professions as general objectives. However, there are real questions about the extent to which hospitals are indeed developing their programs with that objective in mind. There is serious public questioning now, much of it of a turgid nature, regarding this whole matter. In fact, this picture of the modern hospital reflects the programs of very few institutions at best. There is evidence, however, that these true-sounding statements now are being taken very seriously in some quarters.

Most of my comments will be directed at the nonprofit general hospital. This category encompasses approximately 70 percent of the total of over 800,000 general hospital beds in the country. The others are accounted for by government hospitals (24 percent of the beds), and proprietary institutions (six percent).

THE NONPROFIT GENERAL HOSPITAL

The general hospital is the focus of frustrated, anguished attention in the United States today. It is the most salient manifestation of the problems and deficiencies of our health services delivery system. General hospitals represent a major capital investment in the provision of personal health services. They provide a service considered essential to modern community living. The cost of operating them has risen very sharply in recent years at a rate which, thus far, shows no signs of slowing down. At the same time that governmental agencies, such as New York City's, are divesting themselves of the direct operation of the hospitals they own, there are mounting pressures for public control and regulation at the Federal, state, and local community levels.

It has been customary, until very recently, to describe the hospital as a facility. It has been thought of in terms of the physical facility which provides equipment and supporting services. Most of the medical profession has thought of it largely as a workshop for physicians—a place where the physician can obtain the services he orders for his patients. Social trends in recent years have made this concept increasingly unacceptable. Voluntary general hospitals, as a rule, have extended and modified the scope of care they provide almost solely as a function of the perceptions of the members of the medical staff, perceptions which arose out of their individual practice —a foundation which is not necessarily responsive to the health needs of the community, as a *community*.

Twenty years ago, tax funds paid for 25 percent of all expenditures for health and medical care. By 1966, this had increased only to 26 percent. By 1969, however, it had risen to 37 percent. The proportion of the cost of hospital care that is provided through tax funds and quasi-public agencies is very much greater. In the voluntary hospitals of New York City, for example, well over two-thirds of all collections for hospital care now comes from tax funds or Blue Cross. This has heightened the appreciation, on all sides, of the need for greater accountability to the public. The public wants to know what is being done to provide health services that meet the twin objectives of effectiveness and economy.

Decisions about the range, use, and availability of the concentration of equipment and skills in our general hospitals are, on the whole, made with very little direct reference to the health needs of the people living in the areas surrounding the hospital. On all sides, there is more and more evidence that the public will want to be certain that the needs of our underprivileged are being met. In the ghetto areas of large cities of our nation, neighborhood people, alienated by the lack of interest in the health problems that plague them the most and frustrated by the lack of services, have learned to exert public pressure in order to force the hospitals in their community to modify their services appropriately—for example, to provide prenatal care, to develop adequate emergency room services, to find and treat lead poisoning and to treat narcotic addiction. The protest in our cities, the pickets, the demonstrations and the sit-ins have highlighted this need and heightened the appreciation of those who now control these services that effective accommodations must be made to the perceptions, interests and needs of the people. Dramatic demonstrations of social action of this type range from the prolonged sit-in of neighborhood residents in the Harlem Municipal Hospital in New York to demand an enlargement of its heroin addiction treatment activities to the law suit filed by the residents in internal medicine at the Los Angeles-University of Southern California Medical Center, challenging inferior quality of care in their institution because of overcrowding and insufficient supporting services. Incidentally, these actions brought about changes desired by the protestors.

Hospital-Consumer Partnership

I believe the recognition is emerging that a new kind of partnership is needed in the development and operation of our health services. This partnership would bring the needs and interests of consumers into the decision-making structure—not to interfere with professional and technical matters, but rather to help focus their emphasis and maximize their effectiveness in terms of community needs. The people whose lives and welfare are dependent upon local institutions and local programs need to control the policies of these institutions. This creates a new situation for the health professions. They must learn how to work in this new framework enthusiastically, confidently, and well.

Though it is clear that hospitals need to play a central role in the delivery of health services for a community and in planning for health services at the community level, most voluntary hospitals nevertheless remain seriously deficient in their capacity to do this. The health needs of the community, as a community, represent a set of goals which they are not accustomed to face directly. To suddenly confront the fact that what an institution has been doing, though it has been doing some good, is simply not good enough and that there needs to be a radical rearrangement of priorities is very disturbing to those involved.

As central as hospitals are to the provision of health services, most of them are characterized by important deficiencies in terms of their functional connections with the chronic care system and with ambulatory care. Both of these linkages need to be developed much more strongly as continuous programs.

Beginnings are being made. In various parts of the country, general hospitals have merged with or developed extended care facilities and rehabilitation programs, in addition, of course, to the more substantial, though still very inadequate, development of home care programs. The development of some 65 neighborhood health centers and comprehensive community care programs is bringing about increasingly effective functional working relationships with general hospitals which provide special services needed by such centers. Many centers are independent and have worked out arrangements with one or more hospitals. In other instances, the hospitals have sponsored and are administering the center. In all cases, the hospitals and the centers are continuing to learn about the implications of this type of partnership.

Regionalization in Health Services

The need for regionalization in health services has been recognized in the United States and abroad for half a century. In recent years, more and more attention is being given to this approach. The concept of the "medical trading area" or the "problem shed" is fundamental to the recommendations of the National Commission on Community Health Services. It is the underlying framework for the Regional Medical Program, which was set up in the last three years by the Department of Health, Education, and Welfare. Comprehensive Health Planning legislation now taking effect also invokes the concept of regionalization. However, medical schools, hospitals, and physicians have little experience in developing service programs that are aimed at meeting clearly delineated regional needs for health services.

Past experience with the problems faced by agencies attempting to develop effective regional programs indicates that there are a series of crucial issues and major considerations which need hard-headed imaginative exploration. These include:

1 Mechanisms for assuring adequate representation of the public interest; that is, effective and realistic community representation in policy-making.
2 Ways of assuring adequate representation of professional and technical skills and interests.
3 Methods of reconciling the multiplicity of professional and institutional interests with each other and for community service.
4 Mechanisms which will hold promise to stimulate the pooling of resources.

Can these be done by consensus or must there be a franchising authority?

A number of states have adopted the method of franchising as a governmental responsibility. In New York State, for five years now, approval of the State Health Department is required before any hospital can expand its facilities to any significant degree. Recently, the Illinois State Hospital Licensing Board approved regulations for the planned pooling of hospital emergency care resources. More states will follow this lead.

Mergers of Institutions

A recent editorial in *Medical Care* starts with the statement, "In the field of health care, the decade of the seventies and the last quarter of the century will be the era of the merger. Virtually every health institution will be involved in one or more mergers."[1] During the past decade, there have been a number of communities in which corporate combinations have been developed involving two or more voluntary hospitals. This has been more than a response to the logic of developing an appropriate size in the interest of efficiency and economy; it is generally characteristic of these changes that they take place at a time when two or more hospitals in a community find themselves with out-moded physical plants and face the problems of capital funds for new facilities. It is then that the leadership in the community recognizes more readily the need to combine these institutions. Generally, this is not done in order to expand the total bed supply in the community, but rather to provide for these needs in a more economical fashion. Hospital construction costs are rising very rapidly, while the availability of resources to supply these capital requirements is not expanding as quickly. This process of merger is a very complicated one, but useful experience is accumulating.

Another type of merger has been developing in recent years. This is the agreement between one or more hospitals to concentrate specialized services in one of these institutions. The most recent example of this is the plan approved by the Regional Health Planning Council of Seattle. Under this plan, six downtown Seattle hospitals will cooperate in the development of a single obstetric center to handle the maternity cases for which each of them is now providing services. This program, for 8,000–9,000 births a year, certainly holds promise to provide care of a very high standard in the most effective and efficient manner—objectives which could not be reached by the current system of care in Seattle.

Radical changes have been taking place in this past decade in the relationship of hospitals to collective bargaining. The defense that hospitals have used in the past, the fact that they were charitable institutions or public government institutions, has broken down almost completely on a *de facto* and *de jure* basis. For example, the Pennsylvania State Legislature has just extended collective bargaining rights to all public employees, including the employees of any "non-profit organization or any charitable, religious, scientific, literary, recreational, health, educational, or welfare institution receiving grants or appropriations from local, state, or Federal governments." This trend is but another example of the way in which hospitals are being forced out of their institutional isolation from the mainstream of community life.

Until a decade ago, the term "hospital planning" generally meant the way in which a hospital plans for its own physical facilities. In the early 1960s, we saw the development of areawide hospital planning councils. The annual reports of most of these councils revealed that their primary purpose was to prevent the construction of unnecessary hospitals and unnecessary beds. Since then, with the sharpening of the concept of comprehensive community health planning, hospitals have been expected to participate in the larger process of planning health services and health facilities for the total spectrum of health care for the total community. Doing this calls for a radical redefinition of the role of the hospital. In some ways, one could say that the hospital needs to learn how, by linking up with a total system of health care, to occupy a more modest but more important place.

SUMMARY

In summary, I think one can conclude that the social forces which have produced these trends in hospital care will not disappear. They will, instead, grow stronger. They will seriously affect the type of autonomy that hospitals have had in the past, and will develop new ways of making these institutions more responsive to community health needs and more accountable to the community for their performance. This will be as difficult and agonizing as it is inevitable and desirable.

REFERENCE

1 Sieverts, S. and Sigmond, R. "On the Question of Mergers" *Medical Care* 8:261–263. (July–August, 1970)

SELECTION 2

The University Medical Center and Its Responsibility to the Community*

Robert J. Glaser, M.D.

All of us concerned with medical education, and particularly those of us who are involved in medical education on a full-time basis, are painfully aware of the community's increasing expectations regarding the role of university medical centers in many areas relating to patient care. Until the Second World War, the public seemed quite satisfied with the relatively limited activity on the part of our medical schools, at least in the sphere of patient care. Indeed, in some parts of the country a major stimulus to town-gown strife was any move by a medical school faculty to broaden its involvement in patient care beyond the teaching hospital, where teaching was confined primarily to the indigent wards. I am not naïve enough to believe that town-gown problems have disappeared. They continue to exist in a few areas, especially where new schools have come or are coming into being; but this fact notwithstanding, in most areas today our medical schools are expected to broaden rather than to restrict their relationships with the community.

Of the 3 classical pursuits of the medical school (teaching, research, and patient care), in times past the community seemed least concerned with research. First, it was a relatively small endeavor; and second, it seemed rather esoteric—an ivory-tower function. And although teaching occasioned a bit more interest and provoked a bit more criticism, at least within the medical profession, it too was not of major import to the community.

Since the end of World War II, much has changed in our society; and medicine and medical education have been intimately caught up in the changes. The public, through its elected representatives, has provided funds in ever increasing amounts for the support of biomedical research. As new knowledge flowed from the research laboratories, there was heightened interest in the advances reported. Such dramatic alterations as were effected in the course and prognosis of many common infectious diseases by antimicrobial agents like penicillin only sharpened both the

* *Journal of Medical Education,* vol. 43, July 1968.

public's awareness of the potential benefits that modern therapy could bring and its concern with assuring ready access to these benefits. Open heart surgery, transplantation, and other new therapeutic modalities have accentuated the demand.

Meanwhile, the broad social change taking place was exemplified by the growth of health insurance programs, the improvement in the financial capabilities of an increasingly large segment of the population, and the rapid urbanization of this country. In turn, the existing health care system became overtaxed, and the public began to appraise critically the educational system that produced physicians. There followed a call for more physicians and paramedical personnel and for more rapid application of new knowledge to the treatment of disease. Inevitably, it was to the university medical centers that the public's attention was directed; and, as has been noted, these centers were asked and expected to assume a more meaningful and active relationship with their communities.

The situation I have described, though well known to all of us, has developed with great rapidity. Much as Minerva is said to have sprung full grown from the brow of Zeus, so has the demand that the university medical center extend significantly its role in the community come upon us full blown and in a very short span of time.

I would suggest that by and large it is unfair to hold the medical school faculties responsible for the present state of affairs. Perhaps our faculties were somewhat slow to sense the changes occurring about them, and on this basis some criticism may be warranted. But for the most part medical school faculties have been so occupied with the tremendous growth in the scope of their educational and research programs in the past two decades that they have had little time to devote to the consideration of medical care problems on a broad scale. The inadequate support for education and for the development of modern clinical facilities (in contrast to the funds which have been poured into research) has been a heavy burden for our medical schools, has limited long-term planning in critical areas, and has brought many of our schools dangerously close to financial failure.

HISTORICAL BACKGROUND

It is widely recognized that almost all American medical schools, in their present form, have developed since 1910 when Flexner (1) published his famous report on American medical education. True, in the last quarter of the nineteenth century several respectable ventures in university medical education were under way, and the founding of The Johns Hopkins University School of Medicine in 1893 constituted a major landmark in that Hopkins was able to serve as a model for modern university medical education to which Flexner could point. Nonetheless, medical education became a university discipline in fact as well as in name primarily after 1910. And for a goodly number of the following years the university medical center was so limited in its clinical programs that there simply was no question of community involvement. One of the concomitants of the development of modern medical education was, of course, the introduction of the student to the bedside, that is, the institution of clinical clerkships; and with this major advance, pioneered by Osler and a few of his contemporaries, the teaching hospital came into its own and patient care became an integral part of medical education. Yet, as I have pointed out, until World War II most of the teaching of medical students in the United States took place on the indigent wards of publicly supported hospitals and a few major private institutions. During this period, internship and residency programs were small; and although teaching did involve in-hospital medical care and some ambulatory care of the indigent sick, the volume of such patients was relatively small and limited to a single social stratum. Gradually there evolved an increasing number of internship and residency programs in teaching hospitals; and as medical schools developed affiliations with other hospitals in connection with the expansion of their teaching programs, the school-community relationship slowly broadened. Nonetheless, one can support the statement that until the years after World War II, university medical education was to a large degree a relatively isolated phenomenon, isolated in the sense that except in a few special instances, the university medical schools were neither expected to nor did they become responsible in a major way for the health care of large numbers of our citizens. Only recently has social change significantly broadened the exposure of the more affluent to health care in universities.

BALANCE OF ROLES

Since World War II, medicine has become one of the nation's largest industries, and it seems likely that sometime in the next decade it may take the lead. However, the growth history of the health industry differs in one critical area from that of any commercial enterprise. Whereas in general the growth of an industry brings benefits to everyone concerned—both those who provide the product and those who consume it—this has not been the case with respect to the health care industry. For despite the tremendous advances that have been made since World War II in medical research and in our knowledge of disease processes, we have fallen behind in bringing at least some of these advances to an ever more eager and ever increasing body of public consumers. We are thus beginning to see a paradox in that at least in certain areas of health progress there appears to be a leveling off that does not augur well for the future. Specifically, one can point to data for life expectancy to demonstrate that our efforts to lengthen life span have not kept pace with those of a number of other countries; similarly, analysis of the rates for infant mortality shows that between 1959 and 1965 the United States fell from eleventh in the world to eighteenth. It was examination of data such as these that led David Rutstein (2) to state in *The Coming Revolution in Medicine,* an interesting and stimulating monograph: "This enormous expansion in our national medical research programs, together with our lagging national health picture, is the paradox of modern medicine."

We cannot deny that we face a very difficult problem in this country in trying to devise ways in which to provide effectively the quantity and quality of health care that our fellow citizens are demanding and that they deserve. And inasmuch as the source of most biomedical knowledge and almost all biomedical personnel is the university medical center, we must confront the question of the role of these centers in the years ahead.

Very few individuals today would take the position that the university medical center must remain a relatively isolated enclave, aloof from the tremendously pressing problems everywhere about it. On the other hand, many thoughtful individuals are concerned lest the university, in responding to pressures from the community, cease to fulfill its primary obligations to create new knowledge through research and to transmit such knowledge to its students through the teaching process.

Kerr White (3), Professor of Medical Care and Hospitals at Johns Hopkins, very succinctly defined the problem in an issue of the *Yale Journal of Biology and Medicine* honoring Vernon Lippard. White points out that Abraham Flexner in fact initiated a revolution in 1910 when he stimulated the introduction of the physical and biological sciences into medical education and the concepts of the scientific method into medical practice. He suggests that it was Flexner's efforts which in large part underlay the spectacular scientific advances that have been made, particularly in the past few decades. At the same time, he believes, and in my view with good reason, that the social accomplishments of medicine have been much more modest and that, as a result, we have passed from the scientific revolution to what might be called the social revolution. White goes on as follows:

In the post-Flexner era, the politicians and popular press are asking the medical establishment, "What have you done for the community lately?" The statesmen and the scholars are asking, "How can the university and its medical school accelerate the application of medical science in medical service?" Can the medical school concern itself with the medical problems *in* the community without being engulfed by the problems *of* the community? This is the dilemma facing contemporary medical schools; it was clearly foreseen by Flexner in a volume, less celebrated by medical academicians than the "Report," but more enduring as wise counsel for academic administrators.

White is referring to Flexner's book, *Universities—American, English, German,* published in 1930 (4). In this work Flexner set forth as his thesis the postulate that the university must safeguard its primary purposes of teaching and research by avoiding unnecessary service and responsibility for operational programs created not for their intellectual value per se but in response to community pressure. It is a thesis with which many of us are in agreement. The question is, is it a viable one in 1968? How, on the one hand, do we preserve our proper role as a university enterprise—dedicated to teaching and research—and, on the other hand, contribute to the community in an effective and meaningful way? Of all the parts of the university, the medical school is unique. It was appropriately described some years ago by Vernon Lippard, in his Presidential Address before this Association, as the Janus of the university (5). Like Janus—that ancient Roman deity with 2 faces looking in opposite directions, presumably symbolizing the 2 sides of a door—the medical school is expected to look 2 ways, to the inner university, where teaching and research are the objectives, and to the community, where service is the major consideration. How, in these times, can the university medical school carry on its functions in a balanced way? What should its posture be with respect to service?

This question has been examined repeatedly. Fifteen years ago, in their study of American medical schools at mid-century, Deitrick and Berson (6) had this to say:

> The university medical school must guard its staff and faculty members from unduly large service responsibilities. As the number of patients increases the faculty must be expanded or its members will have insufficient time for research and for the instruction of students. This principle was clearly understood by physicians interested in medical education and was put into effect in many instances when funds became available early in the century for the construction of university-owned hospitals. In recent years, such institutions have at times deprecatingly been called ivory towers because they did not attempt to serve all or a large part of the immediate needs of the community. Actually these institutions have been leaders of progress in medical knowledge and the study of diseases. They developed investigations bringing the basic sciences to bear directly on the problems of illness. The residency system of training which has produced the faculties of our medical schools was born and has flourished in such "ivory towers."

In my view, the principle enunciated by Deitrick and Berson is still as important today as it was when it was written. If a medical school faculty is to discharge its obligations in the areas of creating new knowledge and of educating tomorrow's physicians, it cannot be overburdened with patient care. We in teaching hospitals should not be expected to provide all of the medical care that is needed in a large urban setting. Yet, we cannot simply close our eyes to the problems about us. We must recognize our distinct responsibility to the community, particularly in terms of developing models of quality patient care that subsequently can be adopted broadly, especially by physicians and hospitals whose primary function is not the teaching of medical students and house officers but rather the provision of care for large numbers of people.

NEW PATTERNS OF HEALTH CARE

As I view the current scene, it seems to me that in the next decade dramatic changes in the health care system in this country must be brought about or the needs of our populace almost certainly cannot be met. Let us focus, for example, on a relatively simple factor: the number of doctors needed to provide medical care for the American people. No one knows what the ideal physician–population ratio ought to be. In this country it has averaged about 133 per 100,000 people, but the geographical variation is tremendous. In certain urban areas such as Manhattan, the San Francisco Bay Area, and Los Angeles the ratio of physicians to population is much more favorable; yet even for subgroups within these areas and for other parts of the country (rural areas and the South) there are far fewer physicians per population unit. In the late 1950's a national study was carried out to determine how to maintain the then-extant physician–population ratio; it was suggested that 15 to 20 new medical schools, with average class sizes of 100, would have to be established to achieve the goal (7). Considering the great cost of establishing a new medical school, there was real question on the part of many as to whether so many new schools could be developed. Yet since that time 16 new schools have or are soon to open their doors; and we will, therefore, increase significantly the number of physicians graduated in this country by 1975. This fact notwithstanding, there is very little reason to be optimistic about the impact of this increase in physician production on the health care needs of the country. First, there is nothing to suggest that distribution patterns will greatly differ in the next decade from those which have existed for the past twenty years. Second, even if we maintain the present physician-patient ratio and improve distribution, we cannot hope to provide all the medical care being demanded, at least on a broad scale, unless we are able greatly to enhance physician productivity.

If one thinks about the serious lack of physicians in many slum areas of our large cities and in many rural areas, particularly in the South, one cannot help but be concerned. Whereas one can understand the factors that lead physicians to move out of such areas and deter nonindigenous physicians from settling there, the fact remains that huge numbers of patients are without even minimal medical care; and an increase in the number of physicians graduated from the medical schools of this country will in itself do very little to abate this particular problem. During the past year, I had the opportunity to serve as a member of one of the panels of the President's Health Manpower Commission; I believe it is fair to say that all of us who were involved in examining the question of the supply of medical and paramedical personnel soon concluded that numbers per se, although of some import, were not the answer. Inevitably, what is needed is a new approach to the pattern of medical care.

As we develop models for the delivery of health care, attention must also be directed to the problems of financing these services. We are all painfully familiar with what has been happening to hospital rates; these, in turn, reflect the ever rising spiral of salaries for paramedical and nonprofessional personnel that account for more than two thirds of the hospital budget, and the cost of the ever more complex technology that characterizes medical care today.

CONCLUSIONS

The demands are clear and pressing. The question which we must answer is how the university medical center can help to solve these problems that face the national community. Is there a single role? Must we assume that each center will discharge its responsibilities in a fashion identical with every other one? I think it is obvious that such is not the case. We have profited greatly from the diversity that characterizes our medical schools and their teaching hospitals. Just as the various curricula instituted since 1947 by Western Reserve, Johns Hopkins, Stanford, and most recently Duke, all have added to the strength of medical education in our times, so have contributions been made through a variety of clinical efforts across the country. For example, the Boston University home care program and the Tufts' Columbia Point enterprise have been valuable demonstrations of university medical center involvement in patient care outside the university teaching hospital.

The university medical center is inevitably a key community resource; it is a referral center with unique programs that complement those of the community at large. It is or should be the locus for pilot programs directed toward the demonstration of better ways to administer health care to our fellow citizens—programs that can be organized so as to permit observations to be made that, in turn, can validate and refute hypotheses in the field of medical care research. But, as Flexner (4) warned, if and when the university medical center gets so involved in service loads that these become an end in themselves, efforts in education and research will suffer.

In the last analysis, I believe that the demand for more medical service by our citizens will only be met when the pattern by which medical care is distributed is modified. There are many areas in this country where there are no medical schools and no teaching hospitals. Yet quality care must be provided in the hospitals which will serve these areas just as it is in the teaching hospitals. I have already noted that the maldistribution of physicians is one of our major problems. But the solution to this problem awaits the design of new approaches to medical care, perhaps the organization of small centers where groups of doctors, whether formally associated or not, can join in offering comprehensive care, utilizing a hospital and ambulatory care facility as a base. Coupled with such centers, there would have to be devised a system for transporting patients to the doctor; for it is clear that, in many instances, both the patient and the physician fare better when laboratory and other ancillary services are immediately available.

Our university medical centers cannot undertake the job of staffing a multitude of such centers. But they can, in their own facilities, define under controlled conditions the pattern that such regional centers might emulate; and they can also undertake studies, carefully designed, to evaluate the role of paramedical personnel, and especially of nurses, in expanding patient care in rural areas. The current study in progress at the University of Colorado under the imaginative leadership of Silver and Kempe is just one example of the kind of role the university medical center can properly play in the medical care field.

The opportunities are virtually unlimited; for example, now under way at the Harvard Medical School under the direction of Ebert and Pollack is a project aimed at the development of a comprehensive care plan for a defined group of families. Such an undertaking has 2 distinct values; first, it affords a university medical center a basis for providing comprehensive care on a controlled scale that lends itself to experimentation and evaluation; and second, it provides a meaningful way for students and house officers to be introduced to what will undoubtedly be a common approach to medical care, at least in urban areas, in the years ahead.

Thus, as I have noted, the contribution of the university medical center lies predominantly in the area of developing new models of health care. The faculties of our medical schools were expanded over the past two decades to include basic scientists with a variety of skills in order to permit an effective attack on biological problems; the application of the interdisciplinary approach has given us a better understanding of the mechanisms of health and disease than we have ever had before. Similarly, we should mobilize the appropriate expertise within our universities in order to define new models of health care. There are in many of our academic centers scholars who are knowledgeable in subject areas that are pertinent to the pressing problems that medicine faces in these times. I refer to systems engineers, computer technologists, political scientists, economists, sociologists, and psychologists. If in the university medical center we can bring together the talents of these scholars in the organization of studies addressed to the problems of medical care systems, we will almost certainly acquire new knowledge that can be translated into more effective health care for large numbers of patients. Not all such studies will be done or need be done in university medical centers. For example, the current study on multiphasic screening techniques being conducted at the Kaiser Foundation under Collens' direction is, in my view, a most important one. Carried forward as an experimental approach, the Kaiser investigation gives promise of providing a means for evaluating the effectiveness with which automated modern technology can be applied to patient care on a large scale.

STANFORD STUDY

A study in progress at the Stanford University School of Medicine will also provide information that could facilitate the restructuring of the health care system. The study, supported by a grant from the Commonwealth Fund, is directed toward the development of plans for a new Stanford University Hospital. Because we are concerned about our role in the solution of medical care problems in the community, we believe we must have an administrative and physical organization in our teaching hospital that will permit us to carry out on a continuing basis experiments in patient care, the results of which may be used to benefit the community.

Following are 4 of the most important aspects of the study:

1. Emphasis has been placed on an analysis of the reasons for the ever increasing cost of medical care, particularly with respect to hospitalized patients, and on the development of new approaches that might at least control the spiraling costs.

2. Studies have been directed toward the ways in which the largest possible proportion of patients can be cared for on an ambulatory or semi-ambulatory basis.

3. Analysis has been made of the ways in which modern technology, for example, monitoring, can be applied on the broadest possible scale to patient care.

4. Development of plans has been directed toward definition of a physical structure that will incorporate maximum flexibility and thus permit alterations in ongoing programs as such alterations are indicated.

At the outset of the study, we decided that the talents of individuals who traditionally have not been involved in planning hospital facilities and hospital care units should be enlisted. Thus, we have brought together in our Stanford University Hospital Planning Study systems engineers, management experts, skilled computer technologists, and a spectrum of other consultants from disciplines that we believe are germane to our undertaking. Our primary objectives are as follows:

1. To create a modern facility to support with maximum efficiency teaching, research, and patient care.

2. To structure a health care plan that will permit rigid control of costs.

3. To provide new approaches to teaching and training of physicians, including family physicians.

ADEQUATE FUNDING

Without denigrating the dedicated efforts of many individuals who are trying to move medical care research into a position of respect and parity with that of molecular biology, let me suggest that at this point we still have much to do. Specifically, in addition to mobilizing the necessary talents, we must have funds to carry forward our endeavor. We are all familiar with the statement that money isn't everything—but it will do till something better comes along. To date, we are without adequate support to forward our investigations of new patient care methods and without funds to modernize our facilities so that they can accommodate new systems. These funds will of necessity have to come primarily from federal sources. Only with the provision of substantial grants can we hope to achieve success in this difficult area. With such grants we can be expected to contribute to the development of new knowledge and new techniques that will do for patient care in this country what past support of biologic research has done for the expansion of our knowledge of disease. It is in this way that the university medical centers can most effectively serve the national community while preserving their vital role as university enterprises.

REFERENCES

1. FLEXNER, A. *Medical Education in the United States and Canada.* A Report to the Carnegie Foundation for the Advancement of Teaching. Bulletin No. 4. Boston: Updyke, 1910.
2. RUTSTEIN, D. D. *The Coming Revolution in Medicine.* Cambridge, Massachusetts: The Massachusetts Institute of Technology Press, 1967.
3. WHITE, K. L. The Medical School and the Community. *Yale J. Biol. Med.,* **39:** 383–394, 1967.
4. FLEXNER, A. *Universities—American, English, German.* New York: Oxford University Press, 1930.

5. LIPPARD, V. The Medical School—Janus of the University. *J. Med. Educ.*, **30:** 698–706, 1955.
6. DEITRICK, J. E., and BERSON, R. C. *Medical Schools in the United States at Mid-Century.* New York: McGraw-Hill Book Co., Inc., 1953.
7. BANE, F. *Physicians for a Growing America.* Report of the Surgeon General's Consultant Group on Medical Education. U.S. Department of Health, Education, and Welfare, Public Health Service Publication No. 709. Washington, D.C.: U.S. Government Printing Office, 1959.

SELECTION 3

An Economist's View of the Health Services Industry*

Richard M. Bailey

An economist's perspective on developments in the field of health may be compared with analyses that economists make of business organizations and other industries in our society. The rationale of the economist for viewing the production of health services as an industry is based largely on the observation that medical services are produced and sold in our society in a manner not very different from the way in which other goods and services are sold. Specifically, though health professionals like to talk about the "need" for medical care, by and large our health organizations and institutions are structured to respond only to an expressed demand. "Need" is a nice professional concept, but the kinds of health services traditionally produced are those which can be sold in the marketplace. They are medical services which meet the test of the marketplace: services which the public is willing to pay for because of a reasonable expectation that these will be visibly beneficial to them.[1]

THE PRODUCTION OF MEDICAL SERVICES

Historically, medical services have generally been produced by relatively small scale medical practices or, to make the business analogy even stronger, medical firms, where the physician has been the key factor in the production of all health services. Traditionally, these services have been highly personalized and have led to many discussions about the sacred and close physician-patient relationship. These physician services have been tailored to what the physician interprets as the patient's requirements, that is, what kind of care he may require. To put a little more perspective on this analysis by backtracking 40 or 50 years to a time when medical knowledge was much more limited than it is today, we would probably have to admit that much of the physician's service contained a large component of tender, loving care and human concern, and a relatively small amount of scientific information. Usually the physician saw the patient only when the patient was quite ill and suffering from obvious physical dis-

* *Inquiry*, vol. 6, no. 1, 1969.

comfort. This pattern of seeking medical care remains prevalent today. Most patients do not buy services from the physician unless they feel some real discomfort or otherwise sense a problem. Problems defined as minor by the patient are cared for in a multitude of ways: with home remedies, neglect, or what have you. The important point is that the patient comes to the physician only when he is concerned or ill.

Role of the Physician

How, then, has the physician responded to the patient? It should be recognized that the physician is cast in a role somewhat different from that of most producers: the physician-patient relationship may be more properly conceived of as agent-principal rather than producer-consumer. The patient is analogous to the principal in law. He employs an agent, the physician, to act in his best interest. So, the transaction between patient and physician can hardly be regarded as a straight across-the-table bargaining activity in which the patient asks about which services will be produced and what price will be charged. Rather, the patient asks the physician to provide services that the physician believes will contribute to the patient's well-being. Because the physician has taken on this kind of agent or trustee responsibility, the medical profession has, over time, conceived of the process of medical services production as unique. It has opposed the idea that the delivery of medical services can involve a common production process. Much emphasis has been placed upon the "tailor-made" aspects of the transaction. To use commercial terms, we might say that the services typically produced by the physician have been of a job-order type. They have been specially packaged to meet a particular patient requirement for services; they are not mass-produced. Medical services are simply not discussed in terms that refer to a high volume, standardized way of production as is done in most goods and service industries.

Another interesting observation is that those medical services typically produced are primarily only those deliberately sought by the patient. There has been no great promotional effort by the medical profession to sell *more* or *different* kinds of medical services. In fact, a whole body of medical ethics has prevented advertising to create a demand and encourage people to seek more medical services. Indeed, the emphasis has often been placed on discouraging more demand.[2] It is also apparent that the services made available by physicians have been largely curative. Curative services can be sold.[3] Curative services derive from a felt need on the part of the patient. When the patient is ill, the encounter with the physician holds forth some real prospect of being beneficial to him. In this instance, it becomes rational for the patient to go to the physician and buy medical services. This is the way our health service system is largely organized today—on the basis of providing those services that can be sold in a free market setting. But note that this is a limited bundle of services. It may not begin to cover the spectrum of services that should be made available.

Distribution of Medical Services

Concern is expressed today about the distribution of medical services. This problem is closely related to the traditional way of selling medical care. In areas where demand is strong, incomes are high, and people are educated sufficiently to have high expectations from medical services, there we find most of the physicians. Of course, an adequate population base is necessary, but even within a community such as San Francisco, or New York, or Atlanta, the density of physicians and the quantity of services provided are definitely centered in a few geographic areas. Physicians are located where the demand for their services is strong. We likewise find other medical facilities grouping around these sources of strong demand—hospitals, convalescent homes, and related establishments.

CONSUMER DEMAND FOR HEALTH SERVICES[4]

Given that the purchase of most medical services has been in a market setting wherein the consumer has selected and paid for these services as he has when buying other goods, attention now turns to the way in which this market has functioned. A fundamental point to be made in this context is that the consumer has demanded only those medical services which have appeared to be rational for him to buy—services from which he might reasonably expect to receive a visible payoff. We might classify these demands for medical services by order of urgency and, hence, the priority in which medical care has been sought. They are:

1 Demand arising from an emergency/serious situation, where life or death are the alternatives.
2 Demand for treatment of not-so-serious conditions, such as an acute illness where life is not threatened, or a chronic illness where management of the problem is needed. In these cases, it is likely that physical and/or mental discomfort are present.
3 Demand for medical services to detect developing medical problems early, which may make proper management of the condition more efficacious.

Consumer Demand for Life-Sustaining Health Services

Economists refer to the concept of utility as meaning the value that the consumer expects he will receive from his purchase of this or that good or service. Applying this concept to the three types of demand for medical care, one might say that the consumer could expect the greatest utility to be derived from a medical service that is life-saving in nature; less utility from the alleviation of an acute or chronic condition; and, perhaps, to exhibit an ambivalent attitude of either very small or even negative utility regarding the purchase of preventive medical services.

As concerns the prevention of death or serious disabilities, is there any doubt why consumer demand has been strongest (and public expression of urgency greatest) for services that prevent quick death or serious disabling consequences? The great majority of people have a strong desire for services of this type; few have a fervent death wish or like to see others die or be in great pain. We see evidence of this demand expressed in the supply of the many acute-care hospitals which dot the countryside and in the large number of hospital-oriented medical and surgical specialists who are concerned with repairing bodies broken either physically or by damaging disease. Moreover, we even see this expression of demand in the predominant types of health insurance policies that are marketed in this country; these place principal emphasis upon hospital care for acute conditions, with payment being for quite limited duration and the illnesses or accidents covered being those requiring surgery or intensive medical treatment to avoid death or permanent disability.

Consumer Demand for Health Services to Alleviate Acute or Chronic Conditions

The demand for medical services intended to alleviate acute problems that are not life-threatening has been growing rapidly in recent years as the result of numerous factors. Among these are increased patient awareness of the physician's ability to treat such problems (largely related to better drugs and medicines), higher incomes, availability of services, and so on. Patients visiting physicians for such complaints often make up what is known in the trade as the "bread and butter" work of medical practice. These are medical services with which the physician has become quite familiar, and though he personally may not receive as much psychic satisfaction from producing such services as he would from participating in the more dramatic act of saving lives, he is comfortable within this productive role. Thus, as demand for medical care has grown in the aggregate, and many of the earlier killer diseases such as smallpox and polio have been brought under control by vaccination, most physicians have found demand for this type of service growing more markedly than any other.

Economists frequently engage in sharp debates over the nature of certain goods and services in their attempts to classify them as investment or consumption goods. Investment goods are often regarded as those which generate a payoff to the individual or society over a comparatively long period of time and may, in fact, be necessary prerequisites to further productive work. Consumption goods are assumed to yield short-run benefits to the purchaser and, in one way or another, produce some pleasure for the user while being consumed. Applying these investment/consumption criteria to medical services is fraught with problems, but a gross example might be to say that the purchase of an appendectomy for a 14-year-old boy could be called an investment expenditure, while the purchase of an office visit to a dermatologist for removal of a wart on his hand could be called a consumption expenditure. The former may be essential to the preservation of life; the latter to make one's hands more beautiful. It is quite probable that the utility of the first operation exceeds by a wide margin that of the second. Yet, it is this latter type of demand for medical services that is growing rapidly in our generally affluent economy, a type of demand that seems to be more influenced by the income level of the patient than anything else.

As noted above, insurance companies have found the demand for health insurance coverage greatest in those instances where life is at stake. Barring a major catastrophe, demands for medical services of this type are reasonably predictable; they are not services that are willingly sought and thus subject to the personal fancy of the patient. The demand for medical services to alleviate relatively minor problems or self-limiting conditions, however, is subject to widely different and highly unpredictable influences. It is for this reason that insurance companies are reluctant to write policies covering such services unless there is a substantial self-insurance clause in the contract requiring the patient to pay the first $100 or $200 of claims each year. (Both Title XVIII and Title XIX of the Social Security Amendments of 1965 recognize this problem and require that initial costs be borne by the patient each year, normally the first $50.) Since demand by consumers for these services is high and growing, we find physicians and medical institutions organized to produce these services in large quantity. However, just as we find individual patients according lesser priority to these services than to those of a life-threatening type, so also we find hospitals and physicians ranking these services similarly. They are, in a sense, less important. They are more likely to be consumption goods than investment goods.

Consumer Demand for Preventive Health Services

Turning finally to the demand for medical services which emphasize early detection or the prevention of illness, we confront a situation which illustrates most clearly the problems created by consumer ignorance. Economic theory grants that the consumer is rational in making purchases. He considers the various products and services that his tastes dictate; he weighs the expected utility of possessing one or another of the goods or services, taking into account his income and the relative prices of each alternative; and then he makes his decision with the view of maximizing total utility. All of these decision-making activities presuppose that the consumer is well-informed about the choices at hand. Now we find him presented with a new medical service—a service which may detect a disease in its incipient stages or prevent future illness. How is he to evaluate its utility? How can he express a level of effective demand that will lead to the production of the service? If the consumer is rational, he will not buy preventive health services unless he can be convinced that the marginal utility of the service will exceed the marginal utility derived from purchasing some other goods or services. But who can be so convinced? Perhaps a person who is aware that he is in a high risk group. Perhaps a preventive service can be urged upon a patient who is already in the physician's office or hospital for some other reason. In such a case, the marginal cost of the preventive service may appear to be low (or even zero if the service can be disguised as part of the total bill which is covered by insurance). But how can the demand for preventive services be self-generated when the consumer is so often unaware of their existence or, if aware, finds it literally impossible to evaluate how beneficial they may be to him personally? In decision-theory terms, the potential consumer is being asked to evaluate a purchase decision problem which is filled with uncertainty. There is little opportunity to measure the size of the risk that is undertaken by failure to purchase the service. The data do not exist in most instances. Thus, the purchase of preventive services presents a case of consumption under a high degree of uncertainty leading to what appears to be a rational decision on the part of most consumers: a decision *not* to purchase such services.[5]

EFFECT OF INCOME ON DEMAND FOR HEALTH SERVICES

Since our focus is upon consumption theory, let us now discuss the influence that purely economic factors—income and prices—may have upon the decision to purchase various kinds of medical services. Since hard data are not available, we will use graphs to present such relationships. In a sense, these are the author's hypotheses about the effect of income and price upon aggregate medical demand—the way that the population as a whole may behave in its demand for health services.

Income and Demand for Life-Sustaining Services

The effect of income on the demand for medical services to treat serious illnesses falls along a spectrum ranging from high to low. We say that the income effect is high if an aggregate increase in income leads to a more than proportional increase in the demand for these services. Conversely, if there is only a slight increase in demand with an increase in income, the income effect is low. Using a chart whose vertical axis measures income (Y) and whose horizontal axis measures the quantity of these services demanded (Q), the demand curve for life-sustaining health services probably looks like this:

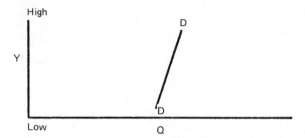

Fig. 1.4.   Consumer demand for life-sustaining health services as a function of income

The demand curve DD reflects a relatively slight effect of income on the demand for services to treat emergency/serious illnesses. That is, level of income may not play a major role in the quantity of such services demanded, except in the sense that the higher one's income the greater may be one's access to the institutions and personnel producing such services. However, heart attacks, cancer, automobile accidents, strokes, and appendicitis strike the rich as well as the poor with approximately equal frequency. Moreover, the health care delivery system rarely closes its doors to people who need such services even though they may not have the income with which to pay for the services. People with emergency or life-threatening medical problems are usually able to enter the medical care delivery system in one way or another without first considering if they have the means to pay. They have a vital and immediate need; they are accepted for treatment; their income is considered later. This opportunity to receive some care coincides with the section of medical ethics which says that no patient will be denied access to medical care if he is in real need. Surely, the care that the poor receive may not be of equal quality with that received by the more affluent patient, but generally some care is available. Of course, as time passes and the population grows, we may see an increase in demand for treatment of emergencies or serious illnesses. But such demand is not usually a direct function of individual income at any particular point in time. Demand for these services, then, is not seen as being particularly sensitive to income of the patient.

Income and Demand for Other Curative Services

Turning to the effect of income level upon the demand for curative services to treat problems that are not life-threatening, we might see a set of relationships as follows:

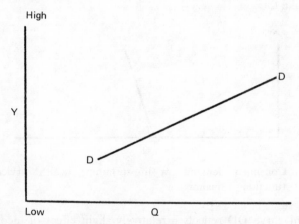

Fig. 1.5. Consumer demand for health services to alleviate minor health problems as a function of income.

The demand curve DD reflects a strong income effect on the demand for these services. The explanation advanced for this relationship is based on two points: 1) the superior nature of medical services vis-à-vis most other goods and services and, 2) the fact that, with higher incomes, the marginal utility of other goods or services which might have been very high when incomes were low now diminishes rapidly, and medical services yield relatively higher utility. Of course, we also find the linkage between education and income level to be very strong. Hence, other factors explaining the increased demand for services to alleviate these acute but not death-inducing illnesses may be related to a different set of values, or to the possession of more information which leads to greater rationality in the allocation of one's income.[6]

It bears note that coverage of these services under either public programs or private insurance contracts results in a subtle increase in the individual's income, an increase, however, that can be spent in only one manner, for the purchase of medical services. Small wonder why third party payment for such services is viewed as a "bottomless pit" into which a very substantial amount of expenditures may rapidly be absorbed.

Income and Demand for Preventive Services

Our final concern is with the effect of income level on the demand for preventive health services. Conceptually, this demand might be pictured thusly:

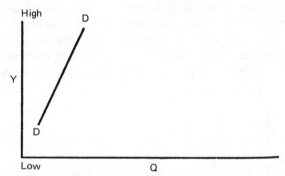

Fig. 1.6   Consumer demand for preventive health services as a function of income.

In this case, we find the total quantity of such services demanded to be low at all income levels (the curve is close to the vertical axis), with perhaps some slight increased propensity to consume these services at the highest income levels. Here, we return to the issue of consumer rationality: Why does the demand for these services appear to be so small? The apparent answer is found in the very uncertain knowledge that the consumer possesses about the value of such services from a medical viewpoint and, accordingly, their dollar value. Spending $100 for a series of tests that are interpreted by the physician as indicating that the patient is in good health may merely confirm what the person already believed to be true. With higher incomes, $100 may seem to be a small price to pay for such assurances; however, greater utility may be attached to the purchase of other goods or services that provide more immediate gratification.

EFFECT OF PRICE ON THE DEMAND FOR HEALTH SERVICES

In the three diagrams that follow, we picture the effect of price (P) upon the aggregate quantity demanded (Q) of certain health services. These diagrams are shaped like the more traditional demand curves found in economics textbooks, whereas the prior diagrams relating income to demand are seldom used quite this way. Again, remember that these are hypotheses of the author.

Price and Demand for Life-Sustaining Services

Applying this concept to the demand for emergency/serious services results in the graph shown in Figure 1.7.

Here, we find the quantity demanded relatively insensitive to price of the service. The reason, again, is that these services are generally not consumed under what might be called "pleasant circumstances." Hence, price may neither act much as a deterrent nor incentive to use. It would be wrong, of course, to assume that there is no effect of price on the demand for these services: witness the effect of hospitalization insurance coverage

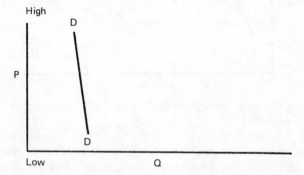

Fig. 1.7. Consumer demand for life-sustaining health services as a function of price.

on the use of hospitals. Insurance, in this case, acts to reduce the out-of-pocket cost of the medical and hospital services to the patient below the going market price. A lower price may then result in a shifting of marginal utilities among various alternative goods or services. But confusion abounds here too. If the medical problem is truly serious, the possession of hospital insurance may merely accelerate the use of the service—the transaction may not be delayed until there is no alternative but hospitalization. It may also be true that many of the medical reasons for hospitalization are not for the treatment of emergency/serious conditions. Some misclassification of the medical problem may arise so that the cost of care can be shifted from the patient to the insurance company. In summary, casual observation of the effect of price on the demand for emergency medical services may indicate a rather close relationship, but if one examines more closely the nature of these services and what they are for, it becomes doubtful if price is as important a factor as assumed.

Price and Demand for Other Curative Services

The effect of price upon the demand for nonserious, curative medical services probably is quite strong, as shown in Figure 1.8.

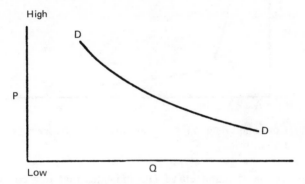

Fig. 1.8.   Consumer demand for health services to alleviate minor health problems as a function of price.

The lowering of price in this instance results in a substantial increase in demand. Several explanations can be offered:
1 A lower price makes a given service more attractive vis-à-vis other alternative purchases. There are many substitute products that compete with medical services when the consumer seeks alleviation of a non-serious problem: various proprietary drugs and medicines, home reme-dies, alcohol, nonprofessional advice, and so on. Lowering the price of medical services makes these alternatives less desirable and hence more medical services are demanded.
2 Insurance coverage may, in essence, lower the price of a given service literally to zero, which removes any economic barrier to use.
3 Lowering price makes the service available to a broader market so that consumers who would never have considered the service as a possible purchase now enter the market, expanding total demand.
As mentioned above, some of these services may be provided to the patient while in a hospital, although options generally exist for producing the services in an outpatient setting.

Price and Demand for Preventive Services

Finally, we consider the effect of price on the demand for preventive medical services. Figure 1.9 illustrates this.

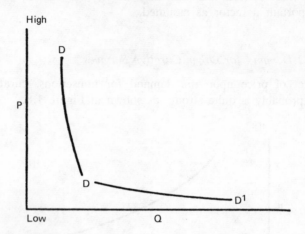

Fig. 1.9. Consumer demand for preventive health service as a function of price.

The segment of the demand curve DD indicates that few consumers buy these services at high prices and only a somewhat larger number buy these services as price decreases. In the aggregate, there is a relatively small amount of demand. As with our explanation of the effect of income on the demand for these services, it appears that if the price of preventive services is high, very few consumers will find the purchase rational; uncertainty of benefit or perhaps even fear of learning something one does not care to know, will serve to make the high cost a deterrent to use. With lower prices, a somewhat larger demand for preventive services may be generated as the price of uncertainty decreases. But, unless the price is lowered almost to (or at) zero, it is doubtful if demand for these services can be stimulated much through regular market (price) incentives. Rather, a problem may still exist in increasing the consumption of such services because in addition to monetary cost, some inconvenience and certainly the expenditure of several hours of patient time is inevitable, and time has value. To shift the demand for these services even further to the right (to increase total consumption), as represented by the DD¹ segment of the demand curve, would probably require a substantial educational effort and improvements in the techniques of practice to reduce the uncertainty attached to the value of such services. Reducing prices substantially (moving down the DD curve) might bring a one-shot increase in demand by people whose tastes incline in this direction. Beyond that, special efforts to increase consumption would probably be needed (DD[1] curve)—but, of course, any efforts that could be made to lower the price of such services closer to zero should prove a great inducement to additional consumption.

Demand Responsive to Economic Factors

To summarize this section on consumer demand for medical services, it should be emphasized that with the exception of demand for emergency, life-saving care—which is not very responsive to either price or income— the demand for other curative services is quite responsive to purely economic factors. Demand for preventive services shows some relationship to income and price levels but to generate any substantial increases in demand, educational efforts coupled with price changes would be required. Accepting the thesis that consumers are basically rational in their decision-making about prospective expenditures (limited primarily by their knowledge of benefits to be derived from various medical services), we may better understand why some services are widely sought even though they may not be highly regarded by physicians, and other services are not purchased although health professionals might give high priority to such consumption. Uncertainty is a very important element in consumer decision-making and when it is present, individual calculations of utility to be derived from a given expenditure may result in purchases that do not optimize the person's best interests. But can the consumer be blamed for such lack of knowledge? It may be that many health services are not like other goods and services. Hence, reliance upon market processes to generate an optimal level and mix of demand can lead to some undesirable resource allocations.

THE MEDICAL MARKET PLACE

The prior discussions of the traditional market for medical services and what seem to be the major economic factors influencing the demand for various kinds of services leads us now to focus upon some private market strengths and weaknesses. Specifically, where does the private market do a good job of allocating resources and where may it be inadequate? In our country, the underlying concept of the value of producing goods and services in a free market setting is based upon the belief that the market is an efficient allocator of resources. By this it is meant that if one accepts as given the income distribution existing among various groups in society —or within any given group, for that matter—then if a good or a service is demanded by an individual who is willing and able to pay for it, producers will respond to provide these services. In this context, we believe that the market is an efficient allocator for it provides the individual with the opportunity to spend his income to attain maximum satisfaction. But this opportunity to spend is always subject to his ability to spend *his* income. If one person has an income of $20,000 a year, he may spend that income differently from the way I might spend $20,000 a year—and that is well and good. We further believe that having this freedom to spend and to select from a wide variety of goods and services in the market is very important to maintaining other individual freedoms. A quite different pattern of expenditures may also be expected when consumers have vastly different levels of income, say, $20,000 per year and $2,000 per year. Even here, economic theory posits that each consumer will have the greatest opportunity to satisfy his desires if markets are free and consumer choice is broad.

The point that needs to be stressed is that for this market to work effectively and to distribute goods and services to various consumers at low prices, it is important that the producers be highly competitive. It is important that the consumer have many options to buy various kinds of goods or services at various prices, at various levels of quality, and in a variety of combinations. If the market is to work effectively, the consumer also must be sufficiently knowledgeable to discriminate in his choices, to know what he is buying, and to be able to discern the relative value of particular goods or services. If we find that producers are competing, and if the consumer is informed, then we can take another step. We can say that in this kind of market setting, consumer well-being will be maximized by encouraging producers to organize their activities to maximize their own best interests.[7] Consumer and producer interests harmonize in a competitive marketplace because strong competition among producers leads to providing a variety of services at low prices. Another way to say this is that the self-interest both of consumers and of producers is served when producers are highly competitive. This leads to the rationalization of profit maximization among producers because, in a competitive market, the producer is able to maximize his profits only by offering services at low prices. If consumers are not satisfied with the producer's prices or services, they will refuse to buy his output and will soon put him out of business. Someone else who responds to the consumers' demands will get the business.

Competition in Medicine

The purpose of this discussion about the marketplace is to lead to a focus on the health services industry. In the field of health, many physicians have traditionally held somewhat fallacious beliefs about the degree of competition existing in medicine. One of these beliefs is that medicine is highly competitive. Economists, on the other hand, are quite inclined to downgrade the free competition explanation of medical practice and to describe the industry as a distinct form of monopoly. The reasons given by economists are:

1 In a highly competitive industry, prices are set by the forces of supply and demand as they interact in the marketplace. In the case of medical practice, prices are set by individual producers who have a high degree of discretion to discriminate in pricing as they see fit.

2 In a competitive industry, price competition is used between producers as a means of attracting a greater number of consumers. In medical practice, the use of price as a competitive instrument is frowned upon and declared to be unethical.

3 In a competitive industry, the product or service that is offered for sale generally is homogeneous. In medical practice, the service offered is conventionally treated as heterogeneous ("individual health care"), with considerable differentiation occurring both in the mix and number and quality of services produced.

4 In a competitive industry, the consumer has the opportunity to be well informed and is able to bargain among the producers to obtain the best terms of sale. In the market for medical services, the consumer is not well informed. He selects his physician on the basis of highly subjective criteria and, after the selection is made, is in a relatively weak position to bargain on price, other services to be purchased, or to whom referral for additional attention will be made, since advertising is unethical.

5 In a competitive industry, there is ready ease of entry into the industry. In medical practice, there are numerous barriers to entry. Nationally, these barriers are erected through the educational process. At the state level, the barriers are maintained by the licensing of physicians. At the local level, medical societies and hospital staffs act as barriers to entry into practice.[8]

By the very way in which medical services are provided, we are saying implicitly that these services are no different from other goods and services. Those who want to buy medical services and have the income to purchase them can do so (subject to being informed as to what is purchased). We have assumed that there is competition and, therefore, as the consumer enters this marketplace to buy medical services, he does so in a setting where the resources supposedly are allocated effectively. Many statements in medical publications are based upon these ideas. Accordingly, physicians are encouraged to act in their own best economic interest, feeling that consumer well-being also will be served well.

I do not believe we can say that if the physician acts in his own economic interest this will benefit the consumer. Of course, there is much conflict in the language here, even within the medical profession. What needs to be recognized, though, is that if one accepts the statements about problems of competition in medicine and about the lack of consumer information or education concerning medical services, it becomes almost impossible to say that the typical market setting for the provision of medical services can solve all the problems in this field today. Some services are not bought because of lack of income; some services are not purchased because the price is too high; some services are not even produced because physicians do not see much of a market for them. Overriding all these matters is the lack of competition in the industry.

Physician-Producers in Strong Position

In summary, an overview of the medical practice industry reveals that the producers are in a very strong bargaining position relative to the consumers. Over the last 20 to 25 years, as demand for medical care has grown for a variety of reasons, the power of the physician-producers in the marketplace has been strongly evident. Because consumers have not been in a good bargaining position, the physician-producers have not been subjected to pressures to be more efficient in their productive activities. The strong demand, moreover, has made it easier for physicians to raise their prices rather than to increase efficiency. If the industry were more competitive, such price increases would not be possible because the competitive incentives to increase efficiency and to reorganize the production process would work to the consumers' advantage, not to the advantage of the producer.

GOVERNMENT'S ROLE IN THE MEDICAL MARKETPLACE

Recently, the medical profession has felt itself besieged by all sorts of pressures from the federal government. Why does government intervene in the marketplace to change certain ground rules? Economists hold that there are three justifiable reasons.[9] One reason is to supply services— often called pure public goods—that simply cannot be provided in the normal market setting. We could not maintain a very good army if different persons decided to buy one day per month of a soldier's time, or one tread for a tank, or one life preserver for some ship, and so on. Market transactions are also inadequate for the purchase of police and fire protection and a number of other goods or services where we know that production would not occur if they were sold only in a market setting. Economists say that these goods possess externalities—benefits that accrue to many individuals without their paying directly. As an example, if I hired my own army to help protect the city in which I live, all other people would get a free ride on my army, they would receive benefits without sharing the costs. Moreover, there probably would be an under-purchase of defense services. To provide adequate "essential" services we recognize that they must be purchased by the public so that everyone shares in the cost who benefits from the externalities. A second reason why government intervenes in economic affairs is to affect the income distribution. Typically, in this country, such intervention is designed to benefit only those persons who suffer the grossest inequalities of income. Hence, we have social security and welfare programs which tax the more affluent and redistribute resources to the poor.

The third area of government intervention is in purchasing goods and services where the market operates less than full time. Examples of some quasi-public goods are such things as highways and research. Certainly, highways and bridges could be private ventures and we could pay each time we drive over them. Research also could be purchased privately. There is the general feeling, however, because of externalities, that not enough research or highways or bridges would be produced to meet the public need. Therefore, government intervenes and produces, or pays to have produced, some of these goods and services.

Market Setting Inadequate for Health Services

I submit that many of the activities of the health services industry fall into the category of quasi-public goods. There is a belief in the public sphere that the market does not work part of the time and does not provide an adequate quantity of medical services. For various reasons, medical services are considered important—more important than certain other kinds of services and goods whose production is left purely in the private market. There is the feeling that these services should be made available to more people—that medical care is a right, not a privilege. The statement implies that medical services should not be denied because of income considerations. Moreover, we are recognizing that the many externalities of medical care make this a unique service. We have witnessed actions by government to stamp out communicable diseases. Here the idea of externalities comes across very strongly. That is, if in trying to eliminate a highly communicable disease we left it solely up to each individual to purchase a vaccine, we would soon have some difficult medical problems on our hands. This could occur because some people would purchase the services and get some benefits, and others would not. Those not able to purchase the services for a variety of reasons (poverty, ignorance, because they are children, and so forth) would be exposed to the disease, and the problem of externalities would be evident. Thus, public policy indicates that problems of communicable disease and sanitation are so important to large numbers of people that they must be dealt with outside of the market setting.

Health Services Rationale Changing

Another point needs brief mention: The rationale regarding health services has changed over time. Part of today's basis is the new concept of the significance of human beings in matters of economic growth. In the past, most growth in the economy was attributed to an increasing abundance of material capital. Now we find the balance has shifted and human capital turns out to be relatively more important—and more scarce.[10] Increasingly, we look at health expenditures in part as investment and in part as consumption. From a national economic policy point of view, it is a wise investment to pay today to obviate some medical problems tomorrow. Prevention now may keep the recipient from becoming totally dependent on society in 10, 20, or 30 years. These public expenditures for specific kinds of personal health services may be viewed as part of a national investment policy.[11] Justification for public investment in personal health is that healthy people are more productive in the long run.

The concept that considers health services to be consumption goods fits in nicely with the various demands for health services mentioned earlier. We usually fail to consider that if a youngster does not get adequate medical care (either because his family neglects his physical needs or has inadequate income to pay for medical services) this neglect may impose a burden on society at some later date if he suffers a serious disabling illness. For all of these reasons—problems of the market setting and of the nonavailability of certain services—government has found a rationale to enter the marketplace and to say that medical care is a right, not a privilege.

Defining medical care as a right and not as a privilege implies a number of long-term and serious changes in the organization of our delivery system for health services. Assuming government is serious in its purpose, there are several options opened for action. The first is for government to set itself up as a major producer of medical services. The rationale to be employed is that there is something wrong with the way these services are provided today: there are not enough of them; they are not adequately distributed; or there is not enough variety. The government could then move in and become a new, large producer of these services.

As a second option, government might shun the production route and become a large consumer, acting in the consumer interest both for services purchased directly and for production of medical services in general. Government seems to have selected this option and is now moving rapidly and forcefully to enlarge its role as a consumer of health services. In fact, government seems to be anxious to be rid of the producer role that it has had, in part, in the past. Public production of health services traditionally has occurred in city health departments, county hospitals, city clinics and VA hospitals. The passage of various pieces of legislation in the last few years has literally worked to destroy many of these governmental health services producing institutions, and government now is oriented to creating incentives for private producers to replace some of these public organizations.

Incentives for Private Production

Let us consider some of these incentives for private production. First, we have the establishment of the Regional Medical Programs. This is a direct governmental attempt to affect the production of medical services at the regional level. Three years ago the Group Practice Facilities Act was passed, based upon public reasoning that there should be more large, comprehensive group medical practices. Incentives—subsidies, if you will—are provided to private physicians to encourage them to form new kinds of organizations for the production of medical services. In 1966, Comprehensive Health Planning legislation was passed by Congress. The focus of this legislation is very broad, but its intent is clear: to place the responsibility for careful planning and organization of the health care delivery system at the local level. All parts of the community are encouraged to consider what is desirable and necessary to make health services broadly available. The Federal government views its role largely as offering seed money to assist the planning process.

Government as a Collective Consumer

Government acts as a major consumer in the sense that it specifically purchases services for some population groups under both Medicare and Medicaid legislation. The major point here is that government is concerned with the market setting, the distribution, and the availability of various kinds of medical services. Government is concerned that the market cannot resolve these problems by itself, especially if we define access to health services as a right. In this way, government behaves like a collective consumer—either creating incentives for production of new services or providing funds for people to buy services where and as they will.

Not only is government thus defined as a collective consumer, it is a considerably better-informed consumer than the average person, in part because it employs many professionals. And, as an informed consumer, government is now asking many new questions about the whole organization of the health care industry: questions about the kinds of services being produced; whether they really accomplish anything; whether they improve health.

These questions have a great bearing on the mix of medical demands. As an economist, I see an interesting situation developing. Within the medical profession specifically, and within the whole industry generally, there are many monopoly powers: monopoly powers with which the individual consumer has been unable to cope in the past. But now, government is entering the scene in its new role of collective consumer and, in the process, is starting to behave like a monopsonist—a very powerful purchaser. Some conflict is inevitable. It is a natural result when any powerful producer meets any powerful consumer head-on. The situation developing in the health field today is analogous to Sears, Roebuck's treatment of its suppliers: "Meet certain standards, or we will buy elsewhere." Government, as an informed consumer with many dollars to spend, is beginning to ask questions not only about the availability of services but about their application at a point in time in the development of a disease when the services will be most effective. In so doing, government's attitude is to create positive financial incentives to encourage private producers to make these services available.

As an example, let us take a given disease—measles. For many years, the treatment of measles was largely in the private sector. People who had the disease, or who sought to purchase an effective vaccine when it became available, were the ones who received care. Parents subconsciously or consciously made decisions for their children—either to let them catch measles and then seek treatment, or to take the child for a vaccination and effectively eliminate the problem. In this setting, measles continued to be a large problem nationally, even after the vaccines were developed because many people did not have their children vaccinated. Now, government as a collective consumer is looking not only at measles but at many other kinds of diseases with one question in mind: What is the best point in time to confront this disease? And, it may well be, as with the measles example, best to say: Eliminate it at its source. Make sure that vaccines are provided for everyone, and back up the availability with strong efforts to get everyone vaccinated.

Government Questions Past Approach

The focus and organization of our medical system in the past has been to deal with problems after the patient has contracted an illness, to deal with problems when the individual sees it directly beneficial for him or his child to see the doctor; or to repair damage that has already occurred. As an informed consumer, government has questioned this approach and accordingly has conducted a number of studies in recent years on cancer, heart, kidney disease, automobile accidents, and so on.[12] The answers that keep coming to the fore would warm an epidemiologist's heart: to be effective in caring for most of these problems, intervention must come early.

If government continues with these analyses and concludes—as an effective, informed consumer—that the best way to obtain these services, or to have these illnesses or diseases treated properly, is to tackle them early, then several actions are likely to follow. One, government may begin to create financial incentives to encourage the private production of these medical services—many of which are barely produced today and many of which are not produced at all because they have not been salable in the private market. This may mean simply that we are going to see an increasing emphasis placed upon the production of preventive services, not only preventive services in the form of annual examinations, but preventive services which carry many implications in terms of changing the whole nature of the medical services production process. Physicians have been reluctant to talk about mass production. All medical services are seen as job-ordered, tailored to the individual patient. In looking after the individual patient, though, physicians too often neglect society. But if instead of the individual buying services at the moment he feels a "real" need, you start asking questions about buying services at the time when they will be most effective for large groups of people, it may mean that physician involvement ultimately will be minimal, or that the production process will be markedly different from that which we now experience.

SUMMARY

The economist's approach is to ask the direct question: How does one get goods or services produced that are in line with society's needs? Generally, the economist does *not* say, "Go start a new governmental firm to produce these services." Rather, he encourages the private production of these services by making it profitable. The analyses that we have covered, which deal with attacking diseases early in their development, can be transferred into specific goals. If government wants to achieve these goals, it may do so by rewarding those producers who respond to these goals. Conversely, the public attitude may make it financially difficult for those who do not respond to meet this kind of demand.

The implications of these changes—for the medical profession, for all the health professions, and for the traditional production process—are great. It means taking a new look at what needs to be done; what services need to be produced in the future. We are saying that individual market demand criteria are not the *only* existing criteria. Increasingly, government seems ready to funnel funds into areas where the payoff to society seems higher. This may be in producing services in ways quite different from those we are accustomed to today. It may mean the complete reorganization of many of the institutions of health. But I do not see government anxious to use force to bring change. Rather, I see government using financial (economic) incentives to effect changes that have seemed only idealistic before. As a society, we are searching for objectives; then exploring ways to make them financially attractive for producers to respond accordingly. The changes that are occurring in the health field need to be viewed in this overall context. The simple phrase that medical care is a right and not a privilege implies tremendous changes in the kinds of medical services that need to be produced, how they will be distributed, how the professions will interact with one another, and how various organizations will respond to meet the needs.

If the marketplace were really adequate, if consumers were really informed, and if there were not powerful professional interests, then we could say, let the market solve the problem. But, I think we must admit that none of these conditions holds today. As we focus more on the problem of the provision of health services, where they are most effective, and how they can be produced, it is to be expected that government will increasingly create incentives for physicians to change, to respond to these new markets. And they will be *new* markets. This must be kept in mind. By so doing, we may be able to surmount any philosophical bugaboos that are carryovers from the days of pure laissez-faire medicine and realize that both health personnel and institutions now need to respond to a new set of market demands in our society.

REFERENCES AND NOTES

1. An interesting discussion of the "need" versus "demand" controversy as applied to the health field may be found in Boulding, Kenneth E. "The Concept of Need for Health Services," *Milbank Memorial Fund Quarterly,* Vol. 44, No. 4, Part 2 (October, 1966), pp. 202–223.
2. The reasons for these professional constraints are not clear-cut. Many positive and negative viewpoints are found in the literature, which reflect the values, self-interest, and/or discipline of the respective authors.
3. A number of the factors affecting patient demand for medical care are included in Feldstein, Paul J. "Research on the Demand for Health Services," *Milbank Memorial Fund Quarterly,* Vol. 44, No. 3, Part 2 (July, 1966), pp. 128–165.
4. The following sections discussing consumer demand for health services draw heavily upon materials published recently by the author in Chapter 10, "The Microeconomics of Health," included in *Notes on Comprehensive Planning for Health,* Henrik L. Blum and Associates, Western Regional Office, A.P.H.A., San Francisco, California, 1968.
5. It should be added that the level of uncertainty which the physician encounters in the production of preventive medical services may also be high. An obvious

reason is because the field of preventive medicine has been relegated to a very low status position within medical education and the profession in general.

6. Economists frequently classify goods and services as "superior" or "inferior." By this we mean that the share of one's income spent to purchase a given good or service will increase more than proportional to increases in total income if it is superior; or the share will decrease if the good is inferior.

7. Quick, James, and Saposnik, Rubin. *Introduction to General Equilibrium Theory and Welfare Economics* (New York: McGraw-Hill Book Company, 1968), p. 137.

8. One of the best articles documenting the market power of organized medicine is Hyde, D. R. *et al.* "The American Medical Association: Power, Purpose and Politics in Organized Medicine," *Yale Law J.,* Vol. 63 (1954), pp. 938–1022.

9. Dorfman, Robert (ed.). *Measuring Benefits of Government Investments* (Washington, D.C.: The Brookings Institution, 1965), p. 4.

10. See such studies as: Denison, Edward F. *The Sources of Economic Growth in the United States,* Supplementary Paper No. 13 (New York: Committee for Economic Development, 1962); Schultz, Theodore W. "Investment in Human Capital," *Amer. Economic Review,* Vol. 51 (1961), or Becker, Gary S. *Human Capital* (New York: Columbia University Press, 1964).

11. This view is the fundamental theme of U. S. Public Health Service. *Estimating the Cost of Illness,* USPHS Pub. No. 947-6 (Washington D.C.: GPO 1966).

12. These studies have emanated from the Department of Health, Education, and Welfare, Office of the Assistant Secretary for Program Coordination, and are titled *Program Analysis: Disease Control Programs.* Several of these have been published.

Chapter 2

Systems

2.1 INTRODUCTION

Systems, systems approach, systems analysis, systems design, and other systems related terms and concepts are being increasingly used in management, engineering, health, social sciences and many other disciplines. Any student of health care should certainly be aware of these concepts and the way of thinking that is represented by the systems approach to the solution of problems. A systemic view which examines each problem at the global level and attempts to discern patterns of underlying causes is the only way of coping with the ever increasing rate of change in our highly complex and technologically oriented society. The very nature and size of the health field compels a rational and systems approach to the management of health services. The total framework of health providers, payers, consumers, and manpower for delivering health care is increasingly being referred to as the health care system. In this chapter, we will define and discuss the term "system"; give a behavioral classification of systems; describe what is meant by systems approach, systems analysis, and systems design; and note some actual systems applications which have been recently cited.

2.2 WHAT IS A SYSTEM?

A *system* is a set of interrelated and interdependent parts designed to achieve a set of goals. This definition of the term "system," although brief, has widespread and far-reaching implications. Not many entities, be they concrete or abstract, consist of less than two parts.* As such anything that is the focus of our attention can be viewed as a system. All human activities relate to and deal with systems. There are social systems, business systems, political systems, health care systems, hospital systems, and

---

* Obviously not all entities have delineated, specified, desired goals. Nor are all entities capable of achieving their goals—because of internal conflicts and external disturbances. Accordingly, in real life, both systems and non-systems coexist simultaneously.

so on. Within a hospital there are patient care systems, information systems, financial systems and other related systems. A hierarchy of systems can thus be created, depending upon the nature, scope, and purpose of the systems study. This means that if a system can be divided into subsystems, then each subsystem can be viewed as a system. Alternatively we can build systems of systems, and systems of systems of systems. However, application of the hierarchical concept cannot be accomplished in a haphazard manner, and it must result in sets of elements and goals which conform to the definition of the system. Selecting an arbitrary subset of the elements of a system will probably not result in a subsystem, merely a random collection of elements without any unifying principle. The point to emphasize is that both the boundaries and the links of a system are determined by the purpose of the study. Those elements and relationships that are not relevant to our purpose are ignored in the systems study.

A system has a structure and a set of goals, properties, functions, inputs, outputs, and in many cases feedback mechanisms. A system connotes order as opposed to chaos; implies a logical as opposed to a haphazard attack on problems; and a global rather than a local point of view. The essence of a system is that its parts are "supposed" to work for the overall objective of the whole. If the components of a system have diametrically conflicting goals, then such a system cannot long survive; even though each part may be operating efficiently in advancing its own individual objective.

2.2.1 Levels of Treatment

The term "system" leads to two different but *related* levels of thought and direction. The first is the philosophical question of a "systemic" view of things. It represents a *way of thinking* about problems and is referred to in the management literature as the "systems approach." It is a "macro" view of the system. The area of research and the body of knowledge known as General Systems Theory* is the foundation stone of this aspect of systems. General systems theory attempts to develop general relationships of the empirical world. Two contemporary approaches to the organization of general systems theory have been suggested [Boulding, 1956, p. 200]. One approach seeks to develop general theoretical models relevant to those phenomena which are found in a number of varied disciplines. Models of inventory control, search models, queuing models, and allocation models are examples of this approach. These models identify problems (or systems) by their structure and then derive general solutions. Models of inventory control (with specified structures) are accordingly useful in hospitals or related health delivery enterprises, and in business firms and government

---

* See, for example, [von Bertalanffy, 1951], [Boulding, 1956], [Johnson et al., 1963].

organizations. A second approach of general systems theory is to structure a hierarchy of complexity for the basic "individual" or unit of behavior, and develop corresponding levels of abstraction for representing systems of different types. Boulding [1956, p. 202] suggests a 9-level hierarchy of complexity, designed to explain several phenomena including the concept of the organization as an "open system."* The significance of constructing such an hierarchy is that it provides an overview of the present gaps in both theoretical and empirical knowledge, and hence is useful for directing research efforts [Boulding, 1956, p. 205]. Because of the influence of systems theory, the managerial processes of planning, organizing, control, and communication have been explained in terms of the systems concept. A relationship between the overall view of the systems approach, and actual applications and implementation at the micro level has also been explored in the literature.†

The second level of conceptualization concerns itself with the design and operation of the system (micro level), subsequent to analysis from the "macro" point of view. At this level, we are concerned with actual information flows (e.g., medical records, payroll records, purchasing records, etc.) within an organization, design of forms, data processing requirements, selection of computer hardware and software, and so on. The essential requirement at the micro level (commonly known as the systems work), is to view the system as a *means* to accomplish operational goals. The emphasis here is on *what* and *how* activities are to be performed. Systems analysis and design are the salient aspects of this level.

2.2.2 Description and Representation

In order to understand a system, we must be able to *describe* and *represent* it. A full description of any system will require specifications on: (1) objectives to which the system addresses itself; (2) the nature of the system (e.g., open or closed; static or dynamic)‡; (3) elements of the system; (4) relationships between system elements, and (5) procedures and mechanisms through which the system will operate. The set of attributes chosen to describe the system of interest depends on the reasons for that description. More importantly, it may depend on the individuals composing the description, a fact which underscores the need for multi-disciplinary teams to conduct the systems effort. For the hospital administrator, the

---

* An "open" system is one that interacts with its environment. For several important definitions relating to systems, see [Ackoff, 1971].

† See, for example, [Johnson et al., 1963], [Emshoff, 1971], [Beckett, 1971] and other references at the end of Chapter 2.

‡ For an excellent discussion of systems and the relationships between a system and its parts, see [Ackoff, 1971].

clinical laboratory or outpatient department is a subsystem; for the regional planner, the individual hospital or extended care facility is a subsystem.

Depending upon the purpose of the system's study, different means can be employed to represent complex systems (e.g., block diagram, flow graphs, mathematical models, etc.). Block diagrams, for example, use the basic building blocks of transformation block, decision block, and feedback operation to construct complex systems.*

Block diagrams show: (1) the input to the system, (2) the output from the system, (3) the exact sequence of operations that take place between these terminals, and (4) the transformation of variables that takes place at each element, or operation [Hare, 1967, p. 34].

It is apparent that any system requires analysis, design, implementation, and management. These activities are continuing and overlapping, since present systems must be improved and new systems developed. In general, three stages exist in the life cycle of a system. These stages and a list of typical activities within each stage are shown in Figure 2.1.

FIG. 2.1
THE THREE STAGES IN THE LIFE CYCLE OF A SYSTEM

Stage 1	Stage 2	Stage 3
Study and Design	*Implement and Install*	*Operate, Evaluate and Modify*
Problem Recognition.	Detail System Design.	Operation.
Determination of Objectives.	File Design.	Efficiency Analysis.
Study Present System.	Develop Programs.	System Modification and Maintenance.
Determine System Requirements.	Develop Test Criteria and Data.	
Design New System.	System Test.	
Propose Solution.	Conversion.	

Source: [Glans et al., 1968, p. 4].

2.3   A BEHAVIORAL CLASSIFICATION OF SYSTEMS

Systems can be classified in a variety of ways depending upon the specified criterion of classification which, in turn, is selected by the purpose of the systems study. For example, we can classify systems (as well as models)†

---

* See Figure 2.1 in [Hare, 1967, p. 28].

† A "system" is some part of reality, and a "model" is an attempt to represent a sytem. Both are perceptions of reality. The relationship between a system and its model is

according to time dependency (static versus dynamic), subject matter (economic, social, political, etc.), content (production, finance, marketing, personnel, etc.), form (transportation, inventory, search, etc.), existence or nonexistence of a property (concrete versus abstract); and area of activity (health, education, welfare). Human and machine systems, physical and behavioral systems, open and closed systems, represent additional classifications of systems. A behavioral classification of systems that reveals the nature of response characteristics of systems has been outlined by Ackoff [1971, p. 665]. This classification is reproduced in Figure 2.2.

FIG. 2.2
A BEHAVIORAL CLASSIFICATION OF SYSTEMS

Type of System	Behavior of System	Outcome of Behavior
State-Maintaining	Variable but determined (reactive)	Fixed
Goal-Seeking	Variable and chosen (responsive)	Fixed
Multi-Goal-Seeking and Purposive	Variable and chosen	Variable but determined
Purposeful	Variable and chosen	Variable and chosen

Source: [Ackoff, 1971, p. 665].

The classification in Figure 2.2 is significant because implicit in it is the need for improving all systems to the level of "purposeful" systems.*

The preceding discussion of the term "system" implies a level of rationality not generally found in practice. Whereas the label of "system" may theoretically be reserved for cases which exhibit requisite characteristics, the term is ordinarily applied whether or not the collection of elements of interest is even remotely capable of achieving desired goals. The conventional practice is to employ the term to refer to results rather than intentions or goals. Thus, the statement that "the system does not work" is often posited when "a system does not exist" would be more accurate. It is of vital importance to understand the distinction between a system and a non-system in order to implement pragmatic solutions to real problems.

2.4 SYSTEMS APPROACH

In the *systems approach* to problem solving, the point of reference is the "whole" rather than the individual parts. As previously implied, the systems

one of definition. Model building and decision models are discussed in Part II of this book. Two classes of management science models are presented in Chapter 12 and 13.
* A purposeful system is one which selects ends as well as means and thus displays *will*. [Ackoff 1971, p, 666.]

approach is founded in the construct that prior to the implementation of any decision, at any level, or concerning any segment of the organization (or system), one must examine its ultimate impact upon the objective(s) of the system. The systems approach is a way of thinking; it represents a conscious attempt to analyze the problem from a global vantage point, and then determining a solution to maximize the system's measure of performance. This can be accomplished only if a careful analysis of the system is conducted, with particular attention to the nature of relationships that exist among measures of effectiveness of the system and its various parts or subsystems.* Certain major differences between *systems approaches* and *traditional organization approaches* are compared by McDonough and Garrett as follows [1965, p. 17].

a) *Organization* emphasizes the design of organization structure, and then thinks of the communications needed for this structure. (*Systems* emphasizes the design of communication structure, and then thinks of the organization needed to complement this structure.)

b) *Organization* stresses chains of command, authority, and responsibility. (*Systems* stresses channels of communication, information flow, and decisions.)

c) *Organization* provides compartments of authority and responsibility. (*Systems* provides network between question and answer points.)

2.5   SYSTEMS ANALYSIS

Systems analysis refers to the process of discovering relevant and dependable relationships between various parts of a system.† Systems analysis requires three steps: the definition of the system, the analysis of the system's properties, and the improvement or correction of the system [Hertz & Eddison, 1964, p. 125]. To define a system means the selection of *relevant* parts (e.g., medical staff, patient admissions, reimbursement structures), relevant connections between parts, and methods of data collection. The analysis of system's properties is made to gain knowledge about the system's response characteristics (e.g., the effect of additional registered nurses on costs and service) and for examining its structure for completeness, con-

---

* See [Churchman, 1968] for an excellent discussion of "the systems approach." Churchman concludes that *the* systems approach really consists of a continuing debate between various attitudes of mind with respect to society.

† The literature offers a multitude of definitions for systems analysis. The reader is referred to [Steiner 1969, pp. 392–412] for a discussion of the various definitions. In some definitions the term systems analysis is used to imply cost-effectiveness analysis while in others it is used synonymously with operations research. We have focused our discussion on the informational and data processing aspects of systems analysis. Cost-effectiveness analysis is presented in Chapter 7. Operations research (management science) is the focus of Part V.

sistency, and correctness of transformation at each element.* The improvement or correction of the system requires either changing the definition of the system (e.g., solo versus group practice of medicine) or changing its structure (e.g., single versus shared services) or a change in the transformation properties of its elements (e.g., introducing new technology). Simulation methods, heuristic methods,† learning programs, and programs or mechanisms that introduce goal and value changing abilities into the system can be used for effecting systems improvement [Hertz & Eddison, 1964, pp. 143–155].

In operational terms, systems analysis means: (1) describing basic system flows which trace inputs into and outputs from each system element, (2) listing processing requirements at each step, (3) devising the improved system and testing it for feasibility, viability, costs, and effectiveness, (4) specifying a schedule of tasks to be performed by user and system personnel (*who* will do *what* and *when*);‡ and (5) implementation and control of the new system.

Systems analysis is meant to be the precursor of systems design. Its purpose is to specify goals and to determine the importance and nature of the factors or conditions which might have a bearing on achieving the desired goals. In this type of analysis one does not accept that extant goals, elements or linkages are acceptable, only that knowledge of them may be useful in devising the desired system. For example, an analysis undertaken to improve a blood-bank inventory service should not merely focus on improving the control procedures; it must instead start with an evaluation of the overall objectives of the entire question of various types of inventories and their relationships to other service sectors. The reason for adopting such an attitude is to avoid filling gaps in a basically unsound structure which may have ill-defined goals. The focus must instead be on specifying more relevant objectives and goals.

The techniques most commonly identified with systems analysis are those which fall under the headings of cost-effectiveness studies, management science, and operations research. However, the techniques of systems analysis need not be esoteric in order to be valid and "common sense" is

---

* For a set of *outside response tests* and *inside structural tests,* see [Hertz & Eddison, 1964, p. 136]. They classify methods of systems analysis into "*outside* and *inside* tests, where the boundary defined for the system makes the distinction. The outside tests treat the system itself as a *black box.* The inside tests probe within the system mainly to ask questions about structure, malfunction, and improvement."

† See Chapter 13 of this book for a discussion of simulation and heuristic models.

‡ Systems development or analysis is a continuing task. [McDonough and Garrett, 1964, p. 201] discuss in detail seven phases of "systems development and the management of change": (1) Problem definition (priority setting), (2) written information requirements, (3) systems design, (4) programming, (5) operating, (6) format and display, and (7) feedback and evaluation.

often the most important tool. Systems analysis is not limited to employing a set of narrow techniques, but rather draws on the knowledge embodied in such fields as accounting, management, engineering, medicine and the social and physical sciences. The techniques used should be dictated by the purpose of the analysis and the nature of the entity which is to be examined, rather than the analysis being made to conform to a particular set of techniques.

2.6 SYSTEMS DESIGN

Systems design is the process whereby information developed through systems analysis is synthesized with related knowledge in order to establish a system capable of achieving desired goals. It requires the selection of elements and linkages, with the recognition that alternative configurations are capable, with varying degrees of success, of goal achievement. It is a practical process which is constrained by the availability of time, money and manpower, and inherently limited by the "state-of-the-art."

Systems design concentrates on the configuration of system's elements and on choosing and describing the method by which information requirements are met. It is the vehicle for implementing decisions based on the results of systems analysis. Systems design means that alternative arrangements of systems components must be evaluated in terms of their impact on the system's measure of effectiveness.* It involves using established methods and techniques, applying new procedures, and devising new arrangements. The final choice of a specific system design is made by testing different designs against a set of criteria (e.g., viability, measurability, reliability). Systems design is both an art and a science and is the key stage in systems work.

It is clear from the previous discussion that the central thread of any system is information, and the flow of information between various links of the communication network that represents a system. Hence, the importance of hospital or health information systems. How the various pieces of systems analysis fit together is illustrated in Figure 2.3.

2.7 SYSTEMS APPLICATIONS

Organizations are increasingly being analyzed from a systems point of view in both a descriptive and normative context.† The emphasis here is

---

* A simulation procedure for systems design is illustrated schematically in [McMillan and Gonzalez, 1965, p. 19].
† Young, in [Cleland and King, 1969, p. 51].

Fig. 2.3
Summary Diagram For Management Systems

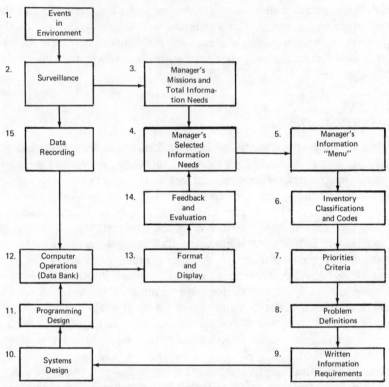

Source: [McDonough & Garrett, 1965, p. 203].

not on the traditional structure or authority relationships, but on the flow of information, energy, material, and behavior. Young asserts that "only when the organization is designed (organizational planning) from a systems orientation will it be able to take full advantage of the new and emerging managerial technologies which include quantitative methods, the computer, information sciences, and the behavior sciences." That a systems view of health care organizations is gaining acceptance is evident from several case studies* of systems research reported in the health care literature (e.g., a total system's design for hospital materials movement, the development of analytical decision models for shared services, a systems simulation of the resource requirements for health care facilities). We cite below some specific examples.

William Horvath [1966, p. 391] has stressed the importance of systems analysis in health problems by suggesting that for "the medical system to

---

* See, for example, Spring 1970 issue of *Health Services Research.*

function effectively in the face of increasing technical advances, the medical profession will have to draw on the resources of systems analysis." As a first step he proposes the use of gaming and simulation procedures (professional health care workers serving as the players) to investigate such areas as government actions and their consequences, hospitalization versus home care, various public health and sanitation programs, the costs of medical care, and the role of medical schools in the health system. Horvath also contends that "this is the only way in which the interrelationships of the different parts of the system can be understood, hopefully to the point where it will be possible to predict the effects of any particular part of the system of changes made in other parts" [1966, p. 391].

Flagle [1962, p. 591] formulates some important problems of health services (providing adequate care, maintaining hospital staff and facilities, preserving financial stability) on the basis of the system's concept in which demand for health services is matched by flow of specialized human and physical resources. Franklin [1971] has investigated the necessary conditions, political and economic aspects, and the negotiation and bargaining process involved in the formation of a multi-hospital system.

A systems analysis study for improving the effectiveness of the hospital medication system by observing its present performance has been reported by Conley [1971]. Osterhaus [1969] has presented a model of a hospital system in which the flows of materials information, and patients are traced along with the controls exercised on these flows by two decision centers (i.e., the Physician and the Hospital).

Young [1968, pp. 79–95] has described a conceptual framework for hospital administrative decision systems. The hospital is viewed as a communication network whose nodes are functional components such as pharmacy, radiology, accounting, supply services and laboratories. Methods of building decision rules at various nodes of the system are described by considering decisions on allocation of nurses and logistic resources, utilization of facilities (e.g., bed occupancy) and medical decisions (e.g., diagnosis and therapy). According to Young, "such a dynamic decision system, based on analysis of constantly changing current data and integrated with the overall objectives of the organization, will permit an effective and timely response to the variable demands that characterize the hospital" [1968, p. 79]. We present Young's article as selection 5.

An approach to the analysis of the health care system (with the patient as the focal point) has recently been suggested by Smallwood et al. [1971, pp. 1300–1322]. Figure 2.4 shows the four-cell matrix formed by two columns representing problem areas (decisions) and the two rows indicating whether the problem relates to an individual or to a group or society. It is suggested that the tools and concepts of systems analysis can be applied to any or all problems relating to topics contained in the four cells.

FIG. 2.4
FOUR HEALTH-CARE PROBLEM AREAS

	Decision: To select a medical action in response to a need.	Decision: To design a system to provide necessary health services.
Individual	Medical Diagnosis and Treatment.	Individual Facility Design.
Society	Health Services Program.	Regional Health System Design.

Source: [Smallwood et al. 1971, p. 1302].

2.8 CONCLUDING REMARKS

Divergent opinions exist concerning the appropriateness of designating an entity as a system. For example, those who believe that present methods for providing health care services are sorely deficient (and are based on ill-conceived priorities), skeptically refer to the "non-system of health care." On the other hand, those who are more optimistic about the current state of affairs consider that a "health care system" does indeed exist, although they concede that numerous imperfections are evident. An equally important determinant which accounts for the lack of consensus is that conceptualization of a system requires placing boundaries or restrictions upon goals—and the boundaries selected by individuals or groups are not always uniform or congruent, even when they ought to be. For example, consideration of programs for providing comprehensive health services to the medically indigent involves elements and goals that are not necessarily contemplated when similar benefits are designed for enrollees of a group insurance plan.

It is apparent from the preceding discussion that the term system is more readily defined abstractly than concretely. However, the systems approach is the only realistic way for managing health care institutions which are now subject to complex and increasing pressures from all sectors of society.

In this introductory section, we have attempted to give a brief survey of the main aspects of the concept of a system. A brief discussion on the classification of systems was provided. What is a system? How can a system be described and represented? At what levels can systems be treated? What is the essence of the "systems approach"? What is the core of systems analysis and systems design? These are some of the questions to which we addressed ourselves. In addition, we have cited several applications of the concept of systems approach to health related problems.

The substance of the two readings selected for this chapter can more meaningfully be absorbed when one is armed with the information woven into the introductory section.

Modern literature in arts as well as in sciences discusses the need for a systems approach in solving problems. Yet, not very many attempts have been as successful as Churchman's discussion of what is meant by systems and the "systems approach." Churchman (selection 4) defines a system as a set of parts coordinated to accomplish a set of goals. Five basic considerations are identified as being essential in thinking about the meaning of a system: (1) the total system objectives, (2) the system's environment, (3) the resources of the system, (4) the components of the systems, and (5) the management of the system. Churchman cautions us regarding the difficulty of identifying *real* objectives as compared with *stated* objectives. Similarly, a great deal of care is required before the true *measure of performance* (real objective) of the system can be distinguished from the *obvious* objectives of the system. The important point is that we must find as many relevant consequences of the system activities as we can, and *explicitly* enter these aspects of the system into building measures of system performance. "Environment" of the system is made up of things and people that are "fixed" or "given" from the system's point of view. Whether something is to be classified as environment of the system is decided by two criteria: (1) Is it relevant to our objective? and (2) Can we do anything about it? Churchman makes a very important point by observing that "often systems fail to perform properly simply because their managers have come to believe that some aspect of the world is outside the system and not subject to any control." In contrast to the environment, the "resources" of the system are the things the system can change and use to its own advantage. The resources exist *inside* the system. They are used to shape specific actions (taken by system's components or parts) of the system. Another important consideration for the administrator is that the expanding technology may enormously enhance the capabilities of the available resources. Computer utilization is cited as a case in point. Systems objectives, environment, and resources interact within the framework of the system structure consisting of *components* of the system. "The ultimate aim of component thinking is to discover those components (missions) whose measures of performance are truly related to the measures of performance of the overall system." Components should be designed with a mission-oriented view. That is, the components should encompass categories of basic "jobs" or "activities" which surface from a rational breakdown of the tasks that the system must perform. Churchman warns us that due to rigidities which systems exhibit as a result of political and historical reasons, there is bound to be a lot of resistance to a mission-oriented view of the components of a system. Yet, only by analyzing missions can the worth of an activity for the total system be evaluated.

The last item in the basic considerations regarding a system is its management. The management of the system involves setting its objectives, making plans in order to achieve these objectives, allocating resources, implementing the plan and controlling the system performance. Here, the lesson for the administrator is that control "does not only mean the examination of whether plans are being carried out correctly; it also implies an evaluation of the plans and consequently a change of plans."

Young (Selection 5) suggests that the hospital information system must always be considered in the context of the decision-making framework within which it is to operate. A viable system must be capable of control as well as communication; the flow of data in itself is of limited usefulness as a management tool unless it is synthesized into a form that prescribes the action to be taken. Considering the hospital as a communications network, with its functional components as information network nodes, Young describes methods of building decision rules into the system at every node, using as examples the allocation of nursing and logistic resources, the utilization of facilities, and medical decisions. Such a dynamic decision system, based on analysis of constantly changing current data and integrated with the overall objectives of the organization, will permit an effective and timely response to the variable demands that characterize the hospital.

The two readings in this section were selected for two reasons. First, they provide a clear insight into the concepts of systems, systems approach, and related terms. Secondly, they indicate the potential for applying these concepts for solving health related problems.

REFERENCES

Ackoff, R. L., "Toward a System of Systems Concept," *Management Science,*
1971   vol. 17, no. 11, July, pp. 661–671.
Beckett, J. A., *Management Dynamics: The New Synthesis,* New York:
1971   McGraw-Hill.
Bertalanffy, von L., "General Systems Theory: A New Approach to Unity of
1951   Science," *Human Biology,* vol. 23, December, pp. 303–361.
Boulding, K. E., "General Systems Theory—The Skeleton of Science," *Man-
1956   agement Science,* vol. 2, no. 3, April, pp. 197–208.
Churchman, C. W., *The Systems Approach,* New York: Delacorte Press.
1968

Conley, D., "A Management Team Approach to Hospital Systems Analysis,"
1971   *Hospital Administration,* Winter, pp. 58–78.
Emshoff, J. R., *Analysis of Behavioral Systems,* New York: The Macmillan
1971   Company.
Flagle, C. D., "Operations Research in the Health Services," *Operations Re-*
1962   *search,* September–October, pp. 591–603.
Franklin, C. L., "The Urban Multi-Hospital System: Necessary Conditions,"
1971   *Hospital Administration,* Winter, pp. 25–34.
Glans, T. B., et al., *Management Systems,* New York: Holt, Rinehart & Winston.
1968
Greenwood, F., *Managing the Systems Analysis Function,* New York: Ameri-
1968   can Management Association.
Hare, van C., Jr., *Systems Analysis: A Diagnostic Approach,* New York: Har-
1967   court, Brace and World.
Hertz, D. B., and R. T. Eddison (eds.), *Progress in Operations Research,*
1964   *Volume II,* New York: John Wiley & Sons.
Horvath, W. J., "The Systems Approach to the National Health Problem,"
1966   *Management Science,* vol. 12, no. 10, June, pp. B391–B395.
Johnson, R., F. E. Kast, and J. E. Rosenzweig, *The Theory and Management*
1963   *of Systems,* New York: McGraw-Hill.
McDonough, A. M., and L. J. Garrett, *Management Systems,* Homewood, Ill.:
1965   Richard D. Irwin.
McMillan, C., and R. F. Gonzalez, *Systems Analysis: A Computer Approach to*
1965   *Decision Models,* Homewood, Ill.: Richard D. Irwin.
Osterhaus, L. B., "Systems Concepts for Hospitals," *Hospital Administration,*
1969   Summer, pp. 57–66.
Smallwood, R. D., Edward J. Sondik, and Fred L. Offensend, "Toward an
1971   Integrated Methodology for the Analysis of Health-Care Systems,"
        Operations Research, vol. 19, no. 6, October, pp. 1300–1322.
Steiner, G. A., *Top Management Planning,* New York: Macmillan.
1969
Young, J. P., "A Conceptual Framework for Hospital Administrative Decision
1968   System," *Health Services Research,* Summer, pp. 79–95.
Young, S., "Organization as a Total System," in *Systems, Organizations, Analy-*
1969   *sis, Management: A Book of Readings* by D. I. Cleland, and W. R.
        King, New York: McGraw-Hill.

SELECTION 4

Systems*

*C. West Churchman**

There is a story often told in logic texts about a group of blind men who are assigned the task of describing an elephant. Because each blind man was located at a different part of the body, a horrendous argument arose in which each claimed to have a complete understanding of the total elephantine system.

What is interesting about this story is not so much the fate of the blind men but the magnificent role that the teller had given himself—namely, the ability to see the whole elephant and consequently observe the ridiculous behavior of the blind systems describers. The story is in fact a piece of arrogance. It assumes that a very logically astute wise man can always get on top of a situation, so to speak, and look at the foolishness of people who are incapable of seeing the whole. This piece of arrogance is what I called "management science" in the last chapter.

The arrogance cannot be allowed to remain unchallenged. Only if we could be sure that the objectives of the management scientist were pure and really in line with those of the total system, and only if we could be sure that he had the observational powers comparable to those of the observer of the blind men could we feel that the scientist had the ability to see the whole.

But in the spirit of the debate, let's allow the management scientist to describe how he climbs to the vantage point from which he can view the whole system. His method is one of defining carefully what he's talking about. He begins with the term "system." Although, he says, the word "system" has been defined in many ways, all definers will agree that a system is a set of parts coordinated to accomplish a set of goals. An animal, for example, is a system, a marvelously contrived one, with many different parts which contribute in various ways to the sustaining of its life, to its reproductive pattern, and to its play.

In order to make this definition more precise and also more useful, we have to say what we mean by "parts" and their coordination. Specifically, the management scientist's aim is to spell out in detail what the whole

* From: C. West Churchman, *The Systems Approach,* New York, Delacorte Press, 1968, pp. 38–47.

system is, the environment in which it lives, what its objective is, and how this is supported by the activities of the parts.

To develop this thinking further, we shall have to lay out a series of thinking steps, much as any manual of logic or rhetoric attempts to do. The readers should bear in mind, however, that these steps are by no means steps that must be taken in sequence. Rather, as one proceeds in thinking about the system, in all likelihood it will be necessary to reexamine the thoughts one has already had in some previous steps. Logic is essentially a process of checking and rechecking one's reasoning.

With this in mind, we can outline five basic considerations that the scientist believes must be kept in mind when thinking about the meaning of a system:

1. the total system objectives and, more specifically, the performance measures of the whole system;

2. the system's environment: the fixed constraints;

3. the resources of the system;

4. the components of the system, their activities, goals and measures of performance;

5. the management of the system.

It goes without saying that there are other ways of thinking about systems, but this list is both minimal and informative.

The objectives of the overall system are a logical place to begin, because, as we have seen, so many mistakes may be made in subsequent thinking about the system once one has ignored the true objectives of the whole.

At the outset, however, we must beware of a confusion about the word "objective." The inhabitants of systems dearly love to state what their objectives are, and the statements they issue have a number of purposes that are quite independent of the performance of the system. The president of a university wishes to attain as large a budget as possible for the university's operations. As a consequence, he must appear before a number of legislative committees and before the public, and in these appearances he must state the objectives of the university in as attractive a manner as possible. His aim is to attain as much prestige and as much political power as he can in order to obtain for his university the largest possible budget for its operation. Hence, he speaks of quality of education, eminence of faculty, public service, and the like. Similarly, the head of a large business firm in his public appearance must present a glowing picture of the objectives of his firm. He does this not only to attract customers but also to attract satisfactory investment funds.

In many firms and government agencies, these vague statements are often called *the* objectives, but from the scientist's point of view they are obviously too vague and also somewhat misleading. For example, if we take the public statements too seriously, we may be misled in identifying the real as compared with the stated objectives of the system. The president of a university is apt to make us think that the sole objective of the university is the creation of new knowledge and the teaching of knowledge to eligible students. The head of the business firm is apt to make us think the sole objective of his firm is the maximization of net profit subject to considerations of public service.

Now the scientist's test of the objective of a system is the determination of whether the system will knowingly sacrifice other goals in order to attain the objective. If a person says that his real objective in life is public service and yet occasionally he seems quite willing to spend time in private service in order to maximize his income, then the scientist would say that his *stated* objective is not his *real* objective. He has been willing to sacrifice his stated objective at some time in order to attain some other goal.

A common fallacy in stating objectives is to emphasize the obvious. For example, consider a medical laboratory that tests specimens which doctors send in. What is the objective of the laboratory? One obvious answer is to say that the objective is to make as accurate a test as possible. But the real objective is not "accuracy" but what accuracy is good for: improving the doctor's diagnosis. Once we look ahead to the desired, concrete outcome, says the scientist, then we can ask ourselves how important the objective really is. In some cases, improved accuracy may not be worth the cost, i.e., the sacrifice of other objectives.

Of course, it is no easy matter to determine the real objectives of a system, any more than it is an easy matter to determine the real objectives of an individual person. We all hide our real objectives because in some cases they are hardly satisfactory ones from the point of view of other people; if they are widely publicized they may be harmful in terms of our prospects of attaining various kinds of support in our lives.

In order to clarify the matter, the scientist needs to move from the vague statement of objectives to some precise and specific measures of performance of the overall system. The measure of performance of the system is a score, so to speak, that tells us how well the system is doing. The higher the score, the better the performance. A student in class often comes to think of his objective as the attaining of as high a grade as possible. In this case the measure of performance becomes quite clear, and it's interesting to many a teacher to note that students seek to attain a high grade even at the sacrifice of a real understanding of the content of the course. They seek the high grade because they believe that high grades will lead to scholarships and other opportunities in the future. Their *stated* purpose is to learn, but their *real* measure of performance is the grade.

In the same manner, if we look very carefully at certain cities we may come to expect that the real objective of the government of the city is to sustain the opportunities of the high-income citizens by providing them with satisfactory areas for living and satisfactory resources and space for their work. Thus the claims that the city is trying to serve *all* the citizens are refuted by the city supervisor's willingness to sacrifice these aims in favor of sustaining the opportunities of the higher-income bracket. The *real* measure of performance, then, is the city's capability of keeping large industries within the city boundaries and keeping the level of income of the high-income group as high as possible.

Similarly, in the case of certain firms, some economists believe that the objective of the firm is not net profit but growth of personnel or gross profit, these two measures representing the size of the empire, so to speak. The point is that, in these firms, the managers are willing to sacrifice a certain amount of net profit in order to increase the size of the firm, in terms of either personnel or gross earnings or assets.

It will come as no surprise that a careful study of certain colleges and universities indicates that the true measure of their performance is not in terms of education but in terms of the number of students graduated.

These remarks give us some clue about the character of the management scientist. He wishes to strip away all the folderol nonsense about "my heart is pure and I'm out to serve mankind, or motherhood." He wants to see what this beast called the system is really up to, and he can do so only by carefully watching what it actually does, not what it says it does. Furthermore, he thinks he can strip away enough of the noise of confusion and uncertainty to see a central "measure" or "score" for the system.

We can already begin to hear a rumble of complaint from his opponents. Some of them will want to point out that an additional distinction must be made between the *real* objectives and the *legitimate* objectives of the system. The legitimate objectives of the system have to do with the morality of the system objectives. For example, the management scientist may define the objective of a highway system in terms of what he calls "thru-put," meaning by this the number of cars that are able to pass over specified segments of the highway within a given period of time. However, the objective itself may not be "legitimate" from a social point of view, not only because of the cost of accidents but also because of the inconvenience that may occur when cars pour off the exits of the freeways, and the ugliness of the freeway system itself.

But to the thorough-thinking management scientist, this objection is not a serious one. In thinking about systems, he replies, we must move from what is often the real objective of the system managers to wider considerations. We may in fact have to begin to consider how to put the cost of accidents and ugliness into our measures. Intangible as these may be, he says, we shall see that the measurement of them is really not so difficult as might appear at first sight. In fact, there are some excellently worked-out cases in which highway engineers, as well as the designers of aircraft, have developed measures of the cost of an accident, in terms of the lost capability of the individual in earning income throughout the rest of his life. To the humanist, this may seem a very crass way of putting a number on the loss of a limb or a head, but to the management scientist it is the only practical way in which we can think about the so-called intangible aspects of the systems. In other words, he says, if we want to *think* about how loss of life or happiness or beauty is related to system performance, we can't simply say that these are so elusive that they cannot be defined, because by saying this we mean that we don't want to think about them at all. In order to think about them satisfactorily, we are going to have to be explicit and make our stand on the way in which these aspects of systems enter into measures of system performance.

The management scientist is turning out to be persistent, at least, though his persistence may leave a number of his listeners uncomfortable. He is not only persistent but also alert. With experience, he becomes convinced that the "obvious" measures of performance are not the real ones.

One example of the fallacy of the obvious has quite an ironic twist. In the field of health, with the advent of vaccines for many "classic" diseases, it seems obvious that the "health system" should eliminate the blights. Recently, for example, steps have been taken to eliminate measles. It looks as though the measure of performance should be the reduction in percentage of children who come down with measles, possibly weighted by the reduction in the seriousness of the cases. A newspaper editorial points out that measles in the Near and Far East often proves fatal; consequently, goes the argument, a "success" of the system according to the above measure will result in reduction in infant mortality, and consequently will produce an "intolerable" increase in population in underdeveloped areas. Here again the character of the "whole systems" thinker becomes apparent: perhaps it is "better" to let measles do its ugly work than to allow the starvation resulting from the population explosion. This is just another example in which costs must be included in the measure of performance.

Thus in the determination of a measure of performance, the scientist will seek to find as many relevant consequences of the system activities as he can. Admittedly, he too will make mistakes and will have to revise his opinion in the light of further evidence. But his persistence and alertness, and his intent to be as objective as possible, will enable him, he believes, to minimize his errors.

Supposing that some success has been attained in determining the system objective ("measure of performance"), the next aspect of the system the management scientist considers is its environment. The environment of the system is what lies "outside" of the system. This also is no easy matter to determine. When we look at an automobile we can make a first stab at estimating what's inside the automobile and what's outside of it. We feel like saying that what lies beyond the paint job is in the environment of the automobile. But is this correct? Is it correct to say, for example, that what lies beyond the paint job of a factory is necessarily outside of the factory as a system? The factory may have agents in all parts of the country who are purchasing raw materials or selling its products. These are surely "part" of the total system of the factory, and yet they are not usually within its walls. In a more subtle case, the managers of the factory may belong to various political organizations through which they are capable of exerting various kinds of political pressures. Their political activities in this case certainly "belong" to the system, although again they hardly take place within the "shell" of the system. And, returning to the automobile and considering what it is used for, we can doubt whether its paint is the real boundary of its system.

Perhaps, after all, the super-observer of the blind men trying to describe the elephant was himself rather blind. Does the skin of the elephant really represent the dividing line between the elephant and its environment? Maybe an understanding of the habitat of the elephant is essential, and perhaps the habitat should be regarded as part of the elephantine system.

Marshall McLuhan has pointed out that in the age of electric technology the telephone has actually become a part of the individual person. Indeed in many cases, it would be hard to differentiate between the ear and the telephone that serves the ear. His point is that we cannot "cut off" the telephone any more than we can cut a person's ear off in any satisfactory way. The telephone is part of the system that we call the individual person.

Hence the scientist has to have a way of thinking about the environment of a system that is richer and more subtle than a mere looking for boundaries. He does this by noting that, when we say that something lies "outside" the system, we mean that the system can do relatively little about its characteristics or its behavior. Environment, in effect, makes up the things and people that are "fixed" or "given," from the system's point of view. For example, if a system operates under a fixed budget that is given to it by some higher agency and the budget cannot be changed by any activities of the system, then we would have to say that the budgetary constraints are in the environment of the system. But if by some organizational change the system could influence the budget, then some of the budgetary process would belong inside the system.

Not only is the environment something that is outside the system's control, but it is also something that determines in part how the system performs. Thus, if the system is operating in a very cold climate so that its equipment must be designed to withstand various kinds of severe temperature change, then we would say that temperature changes are in the environment, because these dictate the given possibilities of the system performance and yet the system can do nothing about the temperature changes.

One of the most important aspects of the environment of the system is the "requirement schedule." In the case of an industrial firm this consists of the sales demands. Of course in some sense the firm can do something about the demands by means of advertising, pricing, and the like. But to the extent that the demand for the firm's products is, so to speak, determined by individual people outside who are the customers of the firm, then the demand lies in the environment of the system, because it is a "given" and because its nature influences system performance.

Here again we get some insight into the character of the management scientist. The environment is not the air we breathe, or the social group we belong to, or the house we live in, no matter how much these may seem to be outside us. In each case, we must ask, "Can I do anything about it?" and "Does it matter relative to my objectives?" If the answer to the first question is "No" but to the second is "Yes," then "it" is in the environment.

The management scientist is normally a very careful person, and he knows how difficult it is to determine the system's environment and that the problems need to be reviewed systematically and continuously. Often systems fail to perform properly simply because their managers have come to believe that some aspect of the world is outside the system and not subject to any control. I was recently watching a television show whose theme was that the poor pay more than the rich for home products. The purpose of the show was to indicate how stores increase prices in poor neighborhoods, and specifically how credit agencies often require the poor to pay far higher interest rates than do the rich. In its thinking about how to overcome this community difficulty, the program urged an education of the poor, so that they would not be duped by salesmen of freezers, television sets, and the like. In its analysis of how it comes to happen that the credit system is so unfair to the lower-income groups, the program described how the credit system is controlled by banks and ultimately by policy makers on Wall Street. But the program designers did not even think it advisable to educate any of the banks and Wall Street with respect to the impact of their policy on the poor communities of cities. In other words, the program designers had taken the policies of the banks and of Wall Street to be in the environment of the credit system, and hence not subject to any change. From the management scientist's point of view, it's clear that some mistake may have been made here. It might in fact be possible, if one were to employ a systems approach to credit policies, to show how the rather rigid policies with respect to low-income groups generate a series of community problems which themselves badly affect the operation of the community and hence increase the costs of operation of large industries and even of the banks themselves.

Next we turn to a consideration of the resources of the system. These are *inside* the system. They are the means that the system uses to do its jobs. Typically when we turn to the measurement of resources we do so in terms of money, of man hours, and of equipment. Resources, as opposed to the environment, are the things the system can change and use to its own advantage. The system can decide which of its men shall work on which jobs, or how its money shall be spent on various activities, or what the time limits will be on various kinds of activity.

Just as it is difficult to think adequately about the environment of the system, it is also quite difficult to think adequately about its real resources. I have already had something to say about this in the illustration of idle time, idle equipment and idle men. Here the manager, overanxious about his resources, may come to believe that idle men and idle equipment imply an unused resource, and if he sets about too energetically to change the idleness into work, he may find that he is actually decreasing his resources.

Within many systems a very careful analysis is made of resources. The traditional company balance sheet in effect is a listing of the various kinds of resources that a firm has available, especially when these resources can be translated into money: buildings, equipment, accounts receivable, cash, etc. But the management scientist has concluded that the traditional balance sheet leaves out many of the important resources of a firm. It does not give a detailed account of the type of personnel that the firm has available in terms of their educational background and personal capabilities, for example. Something like "good will," which is surely a resource, is often represented by a fictitious number on the balance sheet.

But there is an even more serious objection to the income statement of an organization; this statement is supposed to show how resources were used. The management scientist is chiefly interested in learning from experience, since this is always the hallmark of excellence in science. But the typical income statement hides almost all the relevant information that should be collected if one is to learn from an organization's past. The real lessons to be learned are the lessons of lost opportunities, the possibilities that were never actualized because the resources were used elsewhere. These lost opportunities are the cases that should be watched, but they are practically never described in the operating statement of business organizations.

For the management scientist, the systems approach entails the construction of "management information systems" that will record the relevant information for decision-making purposes and specifically will tell the richest story about the use of resources, including lost opportunities. Later on we shall look into the design of such a management-information system in some detail.

There is another aspect of resource determination that is quite important in an age of expanding technology: it is quite essential that firms and government agencies pay special attention to technological advances that may be able to increase their resources enormously. We shall have some things to say, for example, about increasing computer capabilities and how these lead in effect to a "free" increase in a firm's resources. In looking and thinking about a system, the management scientist pays attention not only to existing resources but also to the manner in which resources can be increased, that is, to the manner in which the systems can be used to create better resources in the future, by means of research and development in the case of hardware types of equipment, or by training and education of personnel, and by various kinds of political activities which will increase the budget and investment potential. In fact, for many systems a component that deals with the increase of resources may be the most important component of the system.

Resources are the general reservoir out of which the specific actions of the system can be shaped. The specific actions are taken by the components, or parts, or subsystems (all these terms being used interchangeably in management science). Components is the fourth item in the "thinking" list on page 73. Here again, says our scientist, our thinking is apt to be blurred by tradition. Organizations are often divided into departments, divisions, offices, and groups of men, but careful examination shows that these are not the real *components* of the system even though they carry labels that seem to indicate that they are. For example, in industrial firms a department may be labeled "production"; this should lead us to think that only within this component can one find the manufacture of products. Another department will be labeled "marketing"; one should therefore believe that only in that department would one find the activities dealing with distribution and sales of products. And yet in many firms the distribution function must be conceived as part of the production component simply because it would be quite impossible to determine how the distribution of products should occur independent of the way in which the products are made. And perhaps the production department has a great deal to do with the manner in which products are sold simply because production must deal in many cases directly with the customer in satisfying his orders. If the customer is badly disappointed, then the activities of the production department may decrease sales.

It is for this reason that in thinking about systems the management scientist ignores the traditional lines of division and turns instead to the basic "missions" or "jobs" or "activities," all of these labels being used to describe the same kind of thing, namely, the rational breakdown of the tasks the system must perform. Thus in the case of a city or a state, the basic missions may be defined in terms of health, education, recreation, and the like. If they are so defined, the scientist sees that many different agencies are engaged in the mission of health, even though their labels may not so indicate. For example, the motor-vehicles department of a state may have a good deal to say about the steps that should be taken to identify an individual on the highway who is intoxicated or is overcome by a stroke. The scientist wants to say, therefore, that the motor-vehicles department is actively engaged in the health mission. In the same fashion the educational function of the state takes place not only within the department of education, but in many other departments which are engaged in various kinds of training programs for their own personnel and educational programs for the public by means of brochures, short courses, TV demonstrations, and the like. The overall valuation of the education mission therefore cannot take place within traditional department lines.

There is bound to be a lot of resistance to this mission-oriented view of the "components" of a system. In terms of politics, the head of a department knows that his department is a unit and a distinguishable part of the total organization. He has to do battle for budget and personnel with other "components," and he is judged in terms of how well his "part" has done in supporting the total organization's goals. Furthermore, the people who work in his department identify themselves with the department, not the so-called mission, which merely exists in the head of the management scientist. This is especially the case in universities. It may be that mathematics and philosophy are widely studied and practiced in all the fields of learning, but *the* departments of mathematics, and philosophy define what these subjects "really" mean—i.e., really mean to the true mathematician and philosopher.

The management scientist, however, is not a very sympathetic fellow. He can see that political and personal ambitions influence people into believing that the parts of the system should be as independent as possible. People want to say that "education" should take place in a quite separate department from "health" or "recreation." But the management scientist believes that this is a fallacious way to think about the matter. Normally the educational activity does have a good deal to do with health, and health has a good deal to do with education. The proponents of a clear separation of function may urge, therefore, that we think about other kinds of functions which are more separable and in which separate measures of performance can be generated, thereby preserving the integrity of the department. This idea is frequently carried out in machine design in which each component of a machine has a specific function to perform and the performance of a given part is as independent as possible of the performance of other parts. Even in machine design, however, this may not be a feasible way to approach the problem.

Why is the management scientist so persistent in talking about missions rather than departments? Simply because by analyzing missions he can estimate the worth of an activity for the total system, whereas there is no feasible way of estimating the worth of a department's performance. He needs to know whether one activity of a system component is better than another. But if a department's activity belongs to several larger missions, it may not be possible to distinguish its real contribution. This is why the management scientist is so skeptical about managerial accounting, in any of its various forms. The managerial accountant wants to generate "scores" of departmental performance, or "cost centers" which can be examined for their utilization of resources. But insufficient thinking goes into the identification of these scores and centers in terms of their real contribution to the total system objective.

But why do we need components at all? The management scientist would like to look at each choice of the whole system in a direct way, without having to subdivide the choice. But this is not feasible. Consequently, the real reason for the separation of the system into components is to provide the analyst with the kind of information he needs in order to tell whether the system is operating properly and what should be done next. As we shall see, the management scientist thinks he has succeeded reasonably well in certain cases in identifying the real components (missions) of a system. Unfortunately, to date, in most city and state governments there is no adequate systems analysis of the total system in terms of real components; for historical reasons the state and city governments are divided into departments and divisions that often have no relevance to the true components of the system. As a consequence, says the scientist, the management of our large government systems of states and cities becomes more and more difficult each year. Because the decision making that governs different missions is not centralized, the real missions of the state, e.g., in terms of health, education, recreation, sanitation, and so on, cannot be carried out because there is no management of these missions. One of the greatest dangers in component design is the rigidity which has occurred so frequently in the political designs of the cities and states. The assignment of responsibilities becomes fixed by law and impossible to break. What occurs is a kind of hardening of the communication arteries and the disease that sets in is well known to most administrators. Even the most obvious plans for the various missions of the city and state cannot be carried out simply because there is absolutely no way to break up the rigidities of the system that have occurred because of political history.

It goes without saying that our management scientist is antipolitical, simply because so much of politics thwarts the rationality of his designs.

He goes so far as to say that city, state, and federal governments cannot be regarded as "systems," because in their design there is no rational plan of the components of the system and of their operation. Nevertheless, there are notable exceptions. Some governmental departments, e.g., the Department of Defense and the National Aeronautics and Space Administration, have taken the "system challenge" quite seriously, as have several state governments. In industry, "system thinking" has often infiltrated quite deeply, even though the concepts of the "whole system"—i.e., the whole corporation—are still very difficult to define. The optimistic management scientist looks forward to a "systems era," in which man at last will be able to understand the systems he has created and lives in.

The ultimate aim of component thinking is to discover those components (missions) whose measures of performance are truly related to the measure of performance of the overall system. One obvious desideratum is that as the measure of performance of a component increases (all other things being equal), so should the measure of performance of the total system. Otherwise, the component is not truly contributing to the system performance. For example, in industrial practice if the measure of performance of a component is in terms of its output per unit cost, then it would be essential to show that, as this measure increases, the total performance of the system increases. If, however, drastic cost-reduction methods are imposed on the component that result in decreased quality of its service or product, then it may very well happen that someone has instituted a measure of performance for the component that does not imply an increase in system performance. For example, a production department may institute various kinds of cost-reduction policies resulting in decrease in inventories. Its output per unit of cost may therefore go up, but the performance of the entire firm may go down simply because the cut in inventory leads to unsatisfactory shortages.

As we shall see, this problem of measuring the performance of a component gets to be a very tricky and difficult one as we go deeper into the design of large systems. Although the simple requirement that the measure of performance of the component should go up as the total system performance goes up seems quite obvious, nevertheless it does not follow that a component can simply push its way along its measure of performance and ignore all of the other components of the system. If some other part of the system changes, say because of the technological improvement, then it may become essential to change the measure of performance of the given component. In office procedures, for example, a typical measure of performance of the office is in terms of the number of letters or documents that are typed per man-hour of office staff. But suppose a systems-and-procedures group shows how various kinds of routine letters can be reduced in size while still containing all relevant information. The measure of performance of the office would go up as a result of this activity but would hardly characterize a true increase in performance of the office. Of course, the point here is that the "office" *per se* is not a true component of the system, since in this case the component should include those who study it in order to improve it.

These considerations bring us to the last aspect of the system, its management. The management of a system has to deal with the generation of the plans for the system, i.e., consideration of all of the things we have discussed, the overall goals, the environment, the utilization of resources, and the components. The management sets the component goals, allocates the resources, and controls the system performance.

This description of management, however, creates something of a paradox for the management scientist. After all, it is he who has been scheming and plotting with his models and analyses to determine the goals, environment, resources, and components. Is he, therefore, the manager; does he intend to "take over" with his computer army?

The truth of the matter is that he doesn't want to. He is not a man of action, but a man of ideas. A man of action takes risks, and if he fails, not only does he get fired but his organization may be ruined; the man of action is willing to risk fortunes besides his own. The management scientist is typically a single risk-taker: if he fails, he doesn't have to bear the responsibility of the whole organization's failure.

Hence, we've found one chink in the scientist's armor: he doesn't really understand how he himself is a component of the system he observes. He likes to think that he can stand apart, like the elephant observer, and merely recommend, but not act. How naïve this must appear to the politician is hard to say, but certainly the politician's appreciation of the situation is the more sophisticated one. "Mere" recommendation is a fantasy; in the management scientist's own terminology, it is doubtful whether the study of a system is a separable mission.

For the moment, we'll forget this embarrassment of the management scientist and talk instead of other ways in which he can aid the managers of systems. Not only does the management of a system generate the plans of the system, but it also must make sure that the plans are being carried out in accordance with its original ideas. If they are not, management must determine why they are not. This activity is often called "control," although modern managers hasten to add that the term "control" does not imply strong coercion on the part of management. Indeed, many control procedures operate by exception, so that the management does not interfere with the operations of a component except when the component gives evidence of too great a deviation from plan. However, control does not only mean the examination of whether plans are being carried out correctly; it also implies an evaluation of the plans and consequently a change of plans. As we shall see, one of the critical aspects of the management of systems is the planning for change of plans, because no one can claim to have set down the correct overall objectives, or a correct definition of the environment, or a fully precise definition of resources, or the ultimate definition of the components. Therefore, the management part of the system must receive information that tells it when its concept of the system is erroneous and must include steps that will provide for a change.

The control function of management can be studied by the scientist. The late Norbert Wiener compared this function of the management of the system to the steersman of a ship. The captain of the ship has the responsibility of making sure that the ship goes to its destination within the prescribed time limit of its schedule. This is one version of the overall objective of the ship. The "environment" of the ship is the set of external conditions the ship must face: the weather, the direction the wind blows, the pattern of the waves, etc. From the captain's point of view, the environment also includes the performance characteristics of machinery and men, since these are "givens" on any voyage. The ship's resources are its men and machinery, as these can be deployed in various ways. The components of the ship are the engine-room mission, the maintenance mission, the galley mission, and so on. The captain of the ship as the manager generates the plans for the ship's operations and makes sure of the implementation of his plans. He institutes various kinds of information systems throughout the ship that inform him where a deviation from plan has occurred, and his task is to determine why the deviation has occurred, to evaluate the performance of the ship, and then finally, if necessary, to change his plan if the information indicates the advisability of doing so. This may be called the "cybernetic loop"* of the management function, because it is what the steersman of a ship is supposed to accomplish. A very critical aspect of a cybernetic loop is the determination of how quickly information should be transmitted. Anyone who has tried to steer a rowboat through rough waters will recognize that, if one responds too quickly —or else too slowly—to the pattern of the waves, he is in real trouble. What is required is an information-feedback loop that permits one to react to the pattern of wind and waves in an optimal fashion.

Wiener and his followers developed a theory of cybernetics which has mainly been applied to the design of machinery. But it is only natural for the management scientist to attempt to apply the theory to the management control of large organizations.

Thus far we have stated the preliminary case for the management scientist's approach to systems, with some critical comments from the sidelines. Does the management scientist's approach work? If "work" means

---

* From the Greek word for "steersman."

"use," then it does indeed work. Hundreds of large industrial firms in transportation, power, communication, and materials all use management science under such labels as "operations research," "system science," or "system engineering," "systems analysis," etc. In all cases the avowed purpose of these groups is to approach problems in the spirit outlined in this chapter. Similarly, every section of the military establishment uses management scientists in the design of weapon systems, of information systems (e.g., SAGE and SACCS), of logistics systems, etc. Management science is used extensively in the nonmilitary divisions of the federal government, in public health, in education, in the post office, patent office, National Bureau of Standards, etc. Several states and a number of cities are developing management-science capability as an integral part of their government administration.

It would be wrong to say that all these applications of management science proceed with equal competence or even from exactly the same viewpoint. An illustration may help to enrich the flavor of the approach, however; in the illustration, I'll keep the debate going by allowing the critics their say. The critics often view with alarm, or even disgust, what they regard to be the wholesale and uncritical use of "science" in the important problems of today's government. Some of them want the old tried-and-true method of experience to remain. Some want government to dwindle away. Some are afraid of the inhumane attitude of the scientist. Some think the scientist is simply naïve. They deserve their say, and what they have to say can best be said in the context of an actual illustration, to which we now turn.

SELECTION 5

A Conceptual Framework for Hospital Administrative Decision Systems*

John P. Young

A considerable amount of current research attention in the health services is being directed toward the creation of what are variously called health information systems, hospital information systems, or regional information systems. Associated with ongoing or proposed research efforts is the almost ritualistic assertion that the "systems approach" is being applied to the design of future automated processes for the improvement of the quality of care. Many current efforts reflect a growing, and desirable, interest in the area of information flow; that is, the creation, acquisition, storage, and retrieval of pertinent data within health systems for use in medical and administrative decision making. Although much of the interest has been focused on systems configurations and associated hardware components, significant efforts have also concentrated on computer-aided diagnostic and therapeutic strategies, patient monitoring, medical records, and large-scale community or regional data banks.

A rather disturbing characteristic of contemporary research, however, has been the fragmentary and seemingly uncoordinated approaches to admittedly complex problems of system design and implementation; this has resulted in the duplication of efforts on some aspects of the problem and the neglect of other aspects. Hardware components and systems configurations are being examined for information-processing capabilities without regard for the total medical and administrative decision framework within which they are to operate. Assumptions are being made as to the specific needs of health services that may ultimately lead to unsuitable or incompatible systems.

The purpose of this discussion is to provide a conceptual context for examining the needs of health services relative to the acquisition and utilization of information and to stress at least some of the fundamental requirements for the development of a viable information system. To this end it appears helpful, for the present, to limit attention largely to hospital information systems; here systems bounds are more clearly definable, re-

---

* *Health Services Research,* Summer, 1968.

search has already produced results that can be evaluated, and overall objectives are more easily discernible. Indeed, many of the notions proposed are generalizable, albeit not without some modifications, to larger and more complex systems.

THE HOSPITAL AS A SYSTEM

Traditionally, hospitals have been regarded as deterministic health service systems dealing with care loads that, for both medical and administrative purposes, are viewed as virtually constant. This assertion warrants further elaboration. It is intuitively recognized that the number and kinds of patients moving into and through the hospital facility are, in fact, generated by stochastic phenomena and are therefore subject to considerable fluctuation in time. Nevertheless, the general inability to identify and cope with the underlying natural forces that operate to produce such variation, and the concomitant uncertainty, have usually forced hospital administrators, in frustration, to turn to accumulated historical utilization data for guidance. These data are manipulated so as to provide "averages" as an estimate for predictive purposes, such as average admission rates, average lengths of stay, and average nursing hours per patient day. The administrators then proceed to allocate resources according to constant measures of anticipated peak needs, as a function of the averages and of some tacitly acceptable risk of shortage. Regardless of empirical administrative skill, alternate periods of surplus and shortage are bound to occur.

A growing amount of relatively recent research, however, has made such a conceptualization of the typical hospital organization quite outmoded [1-3] and has clearly indicated the ultimate ineffectiveness of attempting to conduct administrative and medical decision making within such an invariant framework. Rather, as Klarman notes in reviewing the efforts of many kinds of researchers in hospital design and utilization, there is a growing tendency to accept the hospital as a system inevitably dominated by chance [4], that is, a system that must respond rapidly to a highly variable flow of patients and their demands for care with a correspondingly variable matching flow of services and resources. A deterministic, or relatively stable, system demands little and infrequent administrative attention. Decisions are made, based on equilibrium assumptions, that are intended, and may apply, for long-term operation. If the environmental basis does not change, or if changes are small and transient, no further decisions are called for other than those dictated by formulated rules for the routine daily operation of the system. But a system that is confronted with a great deal of change, or variability, must be placed under continuous administrative control if the operation of the system is to be effective. Changes must be detected as soon as they occur or as soon as they can be predicted, and administrative action must be taken, based on sound quantitative information that permits evaluation of the departure of the state of the system from that desired. Under these circumstances, effective decision making must necessarily be a dynamic, never-ending process that accurately anticipates needs, appraises the disparity between indicated needs and their fulfillment, and selects from among many possible courses of action those which will optimally satisfy these needs.

THE HOSPITAL AS A COMMUNICATIONS NETWORK

In order to deal with such a system analytically, and as a basis for the application of the systems approach, it is useful to consider the total hospital organization as a communications network [5]. In essence, a communications network can be depicted simply as a collection of nodes between which information is passed or transmitted. Each of the nodes, of course, is assumed to have capabilities for the creation and utilization of varying amounts of information. Although admittedly oversimplified, the use of such a paradigm permits interesting analogies and extensions.

It can be argued that in a hospital the essential flow of information emanates from the patient [6, 7]. Indications of care needs give rise to a flow of events, usually initiated by the medical and nursing staff, that has far-reaching multiplicative effects on many functional components of the hospital organization: pharmacy, radiology, laboratories, supply services, accounting, and so forth. A considerable amount of information transmission, in written or oral form, is required to assure that appropriate activities take place. But the definition of information flow implied in the concept of a total information system cannot be limited to the standard forms of communication. Rather, it must be extended to include such forms as statistical data, medical records, the flow of resources and services, and so on. In other words, any characteristic of the organization that can be observed and recorded constitutes potential information for a communications network and a basis for decision making. Viewed in this manner, the hospital is an extremely intricate system of communication links through which an enormous amount of largely neglected information is continuously flowing.

It should be emphasized that such information exists as a basis for both administrative and medical action. Information that is not acted upon may be delightful as a historical record, but it serves no useful purpose in helping to determine an effective response of the system to demands made upon it. Yet much of the information available as a guide to action is frequently ignored or incorrectly interpreted. As a result, the system response is often delayed, inappropriate, and ineffectual, even though most hospital organizations, because of their inherent resilience and redundancy, are able to cope with needs, however suboptimally.

Any decision that has been made, good or bad, must necessarily be supplemented by subsequent decisions. As noted earlier, a basic characteristic of a hospital is change, largely induced by chance factors: change in patients, change in needs, and change in required response. Temporal actions must be such that the hospital organization responds rapidly and appropriately to change, however unanticipated. The response, and the decisions directing the response, must be based on instantaneous information that reflects the existing conditions, the predicted trends, and the amount and quality of the resources demanded. Obviously, additional information will be created as a result of the implementation of previous decisions. This information in turn will form part of the basis for determining future action. The information feedback process serves to indicate the state of the system at any instant of time; actions taken to achieve a desired state based on information feedback imply the continuous exertion of management control.

The study of such control systems, called "cybernetics" [8, 9], is a rapidly growing field of research with particular applicability to health services. Howland and McDowell [6], as an example, view the patient as the focus of activities in a nurse-physician-patient triad aimed at restoring him to homeostatic equilibrium; they propose that care needs be determined by studying nursing units as a collection of interdependent cybernetic systems. In a more general sense, "control system" or "cybernetic system" may be used to denote any purposeful grouping of elements to achieve a specific goal. Hence it is not inappropriate to apply the terms, for present purposes, to the notion of a communications network [10]. The goals of the system may be simply the maintenance of specified norms, as in a stable, self-adaptive system, or may be a state of affairs hitherto unattained —a predictive, evolving system. In either case, in order to be viable the system must possess adequate capabilities for communication and control. This implies four somewhat sequential properties:

1. The capacity for sensing departures, or predicting future departures, from norms or objectives—the error signal. In routine repetitive processes, a prediction may avert error and replace the error signal.

2. The capacity to transform the error signal into a prescription for action to reduce the error—a decision or strategy.

3. The capacity to respond to the decision by an appropriate allocation of resources and effort.

4. The capacity to sense the results of the preceding steps and hence continue the process of error correction as necessary.

A rather trivial but nevertheless basic physical analogy is the common household thermostat. The state of the system at any time is the indicated temperature. Control is maintained by means of a temperature setting; if the ambient temperature falls below this level the error is detected, and this information is fed to a heat source. A heat input is then initiated to restore the system to the desired state. In much the same way, the hospital administrator must have available a cybernetic process with corresponding decision rules for control; that is, the organizational mechanisms and procedures for initiating the course of action called for by the information feedback system [11].

THE HOSPITAL ORGANIZATION MEMORY

Effective management control can be exerted only if the necessary information is available in a form carefully structured for decision making. This implies that the information system should provide stimuli in the form of administrative action indicators, based on analytical models of the system and its components and on the appropriate manipulation of the flow of information.

One may then pause for a moment and reflect on the manner in which pertinent quantitative information is, in fact, available. As noted, an enormous amount of information is constantly being created, transmitted, and stored in the communications network. Much of the information that ultimately comes to the administrator for decision making comes to him from some form of storage, however temporary. Every organization has a memory in which data may be stored. The most obvious repositories are files, books, ledgers, proliferating pieces of paper, and recently the computer—all containing varying amounts of recorded and usually redundant information. A secondary store of organizational knowledge and information is in the minds of the persons comprising the organization; such data are drawn upon for a considerable number of decisions that are said to be based on intuition or experience. But in any case the access time required to obtain the stored information is often prohibitively high, the retrieved information is frequently rendered useless by the time lag, and in many instances the nature of the form of storage may result in incomplete or misleading information.

In recent years, computers and computer storage systems have been shown to offer particular advantages for the storage and processing of organizational information and for the manipulation of such information for decision-making purposes. Indeed, there has been a remarkable surge, certainly in industry but also in health organizations, toward utilizing computers as a means for generally improving operational efficiency. But most applications, in the health services especially, have tended to concentrate primarily on handling fiscal data or patient statistics. Although much research is now in progress [12-14], attempts to extend computer-system capabilities to deal with decision processes have been slow and painful and have resulted in only marginal successes. As a matter of fact, there have been instances of disillusionment with computer systems that resulted essentially from inadequate advance study of the organizational context within which the computer was to operate, of existing procedures and the manner in which they needed to be modified or improved, and of the basic role the computer was to assume in dealing with organizational information [15]. It must be recognized that the computer, by itself, remains a piece of hardware that may be of little relative importance in decision making; it is merely an extremely efficient processor of large amounts of data—unless software is provided that permits it to do more. In other words, the computer becomes a vital management decision tool only when the programming on which it relies for its operation has been specifically designed so as to synthesize the flow of information into a form that prescribes the action to be taken. This requires valid, internally programmed, abstracted models of the various functional parts of the organization, focused on the myriad decisions that need to be made and integrated to provide a total hospital decision system based on quantitative information produced by the system components.

COMPONENTS OF THE HOSPITAL SYSTEM

For the purposes of this discussion it may be assumed that an appropriate and adequate time-shared data processing system is available—as it no doubt will be at some time in the future. If the hospital organization is abstracted as a complex cybernetic communications network, as was suggested earlier, the computer necessarily becomes the primary node through which all information must flow. The organization itself may be decomposed analytically in terms of its various functional components; these, as network nodes, then represent interrelated but identifiable information or decision subsets controlling the operation of the components. It is entirely feasible for the computer, upon request, to produce data which accurately reflect conditions within the organization at any instant in time and which indicate the character of the decision subset, or the specific actions to be taken, at every node.

Most current information system proposals, unfortunately, are not so oriented. As a result, the information flowing through and out of the computer, although impressive in volume, may nevertheless be of questionable value to the hospital administrator. What prescriptive action do the output data indicate for the administrator when the decision rules have not been carefully formulated for the operation of each of the system components? To what extent can he make effective decisions when the output data on which they must be based, although abundant, accurate, and timely, are derived from system components whose operational procedures are not optimally designed to integrate with overall organizational objectives?

In other words, the functional subdivisions of the hospital organization must themselves be studied and reorganized for harmonious and effective operation. The decision rules that govern their operation become the decision subsets that must be synthesized to provide a basis for overall organizational decisions. The information flow through the computer will then make it possible for administrative action to be taken and will furnish the necessary feedback for system control.

A considerable amount of administrative decision-theory-oriented research has been, and is being, conducted in many of the functional areas of the hospital organization [16, 17]. Much more needs to be done, particularly with a view to ultimate implementation within a hospital communications network. This implies that no component of the hospital can be studied in isolation or can operate without regard for the needs of the total system; external demands influence the response of the individual components, which in turn affects the remainder of the network. For present purposes, it is sufficient to indicate some of the more important studies and their results and to suggest the manner in which the decision rules that have been developed relate to the management information system envisioned here.

The Allocation of Nursing Resources

It can be argued that to a large extent the therapeutic progress of patients is closely related to the amount and quality of nursing care received. Although diagnostic and prescriptive decisions are made primarily by physicians, decisions concerning the provision of daily bedside care are the ultimate responsibility of the nursing staff. Traditionally, most nursing-unit staffing in short-term hospitals has been guided by rules of thumb that provide fixed amounts of nursing hours per patient day, based on historical measures of peak need as implied by average bed occupancy. Such procedures usually have not attempted to respond directly to the highly variable demand for care; they were frequently based on relatively long-term estimates of the number of patients to be cared for rather than on the actual and immediate aggregate nursing care required by individual patients. A more effective procedure, and one that can be shown to require fewer total nursing hours when confronted by stochastic demand, is to detect and respond cybernetically to increases and decreases in the demand for patient care when and where it occurs within the hospital system.

Information flow as to care needs exists between the patient and the nursing staff. The early work by Connor [18-20] showed that there is a linear relationship between the degree of illness of a patient, as reflected by his degree of self-sufficiency, and the amount of direct nursing care required. Using work-sampling techniques, a quantitative index was formulated that permitted prediction of the nursing personnel requirement from patient-condition information supplied by the nursing unit. Specifically, this index was based on a daily patient-classification system that (1) focused on those aspects of patient care that create large demands on nurse staff time and (2) anticipated the total hours of direct care to be furnished to a patient population categorized as to the number of total-care, partial-care, and self-care patients. Nursing personnel were allocated to the individual units each day according to a predicted care load rather than a somewhat misleading bed count.

Such patient-classification systems and staffing procedures have proved easy to implement as administrative routines and have been warmly accepted by the nursing profession [21]. A number of subsequent studies have extended and refined the procedures for application in pediatric and extended care facilities. Additional work by Wolfe [22] has shown the advantages of applying integer linear programming techniques to construct a multiple-assignment model for matching various nursing skills with the spectrum of specific task complexes demanded by various categories of patients as part of their direct-care needs. The allocation model that has been developed yields information for nursing administration as to the predicted quantitative care needs in particular nursing units and the optimal assignments of staff to satisfy these needs; it also supports the staffing decision with a definitive measure of the relative value of each alternative available. Jelinek, in a more detailed recent study [23], has developed an econometric model of the total patient care system in a nursing unit that provides an increased understanding of the day-to-day operational aspects of nursing care and a method for periodically examining the overall effects of changes in organizational, work-load, and environmental factors on the outcome of patient care. The model is useful not only for daily allocation of nursing staff but also for long-range planning of organizational and staffing policies.

At present the classification of patients, the computation of care loads, and the scheduling and assignment of nursing personnel are in most instances done manually [24]. To implement the more effective multiple-assignment techniques, however, all the procedures must be, and have been, designed for ultimate processing by the computer [25]. Within the conceptual framework of the cybernetic communications network, the information flow on patient condition and needs supplied by the nursing units, acting as nodes in the network, forms the basis for a number of decision subsets in the administration of patient care. Input stations on each unit can furnish not only information concerning the characteristics of the patient population but also data on bed occupancy, doctors' orders, requests for medical and physical therapy, and so forth, much of which is eventually recorded in the medical and fiscal records. This implies that considerable portions of the data can also be manipulated by other nodes in the network as a basis for their own operation. The ramifications inherent in the availability of valid data on hospital operations should be apparent. Obviously the allocation of nursing resources to meet highly variable patient needs is more effectively accomplished; and, as stored information in a computerized communications system, data related to many other aspects of patient care also become available for decision making.

The Allocation of Logistic Resources

It need hardly be stated that effective patient care is inextricably dependent on an efficient logistic flow. Supply items that are not available to a nursing unit at the moment when needed, for example, may create crucial deficiencies in patient care; at the least, unacceptable amounts of time and effort may need to be expended to obtain or find reasonable substitutes for items in which there is a shortage. On the other hand, inventory levels based on traditional rules of thumb derived from some estimate of peak needs inevitably lead to chronic oversupply and excessive storage-space requirements. For critical items, of course, a minimum storage level may be imperative even though demand is rare. But for many commonly used noncritical items it is possible to design resupply procedures and optimum inventory levels that respond to variability in consumption and in physician preference.

Work by Flagle [26], Middelhoven [27], and Hsieh [28] emphasizes the stochastic nature of illness and clearly shows the correlation of demand for supplies with care needs of individual patients. Hsieh was able to implement a linen-resupply system in which daily laundry needs were predicted on the basis of patient condition and the direct-care index discussed earlier. Gue, with Flagle, suggested the feasibility of using the daily patient-classification system to anticipate the consumption of nonpharmaceutical supplies and demonstrated the validity of using well-known "inventory theory" techniques for analytically determining inventory levels sensitive to variations in demands. Middelhoven extended this work by measuring the distribution of usage rates among nursing units and evaluated automatic resupply procedures designed to minimize risk of shortage while providing economic service. Reed and Stanley [29] proposed procedures for improved overall economic control of general hospital inventories, with emphasis placed on optimal reorder points and purchase quantities. Specifically, these studies have shown that it is possible to obtain, for example, indications of present stock levels, future stock levels, replenishments, and expected shortages. Moreover, taking into account time lags in delivery and the advantages of group purchasing, computer data can be utilized to determine economic purchase policies and central storage arrangements.

Specific problems of logistic distribution and flow in such areas as dietary and pharmacy services have received increased attention. Balintfy [30] has employed linear programming techniques to study the economic planning of menus for hospital inpatients. Computer programs are being developed that will provide the dietitian with the proper mix and the purchase quantities of food items, recognizing nutritional constraints, medical restrictions, and the need to minimize the overall costs of food-service operations. Tester [31] and Barker and Heller [32] have studied the flow of pharmacy items and have concentrated their attention on the use of prepackaged unit dosages dispensed by both centralized and decentralized satellite pharmacies within a hospital. Hsieh [33] has extended this work into a study of information flow related to the demand for and use of drugs. He has evaluated computer-based communications systems that establish control over the distribution of medications and maintain surveillance over the effects of drug administration.

A major concern of Bartscht et al. [34] has been the staffing requirements for many logistic functions within a hospital. Decision procedures have been developed for laundry, dietary, and pharmacy operations, for example, that can be used to plan personnel needs in terms of work loads based on daily inpatient bed occupancy. The methodologies used in these studies have extended to analyze the operation and staffing of admissions offices, x-ray departments, messenger services, and many other ancillary services in response to measures of anticipated demands.

It should be clear that the continuous flow of information related to patient condition and therapeutic needs can be utilized to predict consumption of supplies and to provide allocation mechanisms for control of logistic resources. Given current data on usage rates, preference patterns, and anticipated demand, the computer system can be made to assist in the evaluation of alternative logistic procedures and in the derivation of administrative decision rules governing the flow of supplies and the allocation of manpower throughout the hospital system.

Utilization of Facilities

Research on the problems of utilization of facilities has generally been concerned with the administrative decisions required to deal with the demand for inpatient, clinical, and ancillary services. For example, one of the most frequently encountered administrative measures of the utilization of a hospital's resources is the census, a daily physical count of the number of patients occupying beds in the inpatient areas. Statistically averaged census figures are taken as a gross indication of the extent of services to be provided and an approximate determinant of revenue. Nevertheless, a perennial problem for the hospital administrator is the anticipation of future bed occupancy with sufficient accuracy to allocate his resources effectively.

It has long been recognized that daily bed occupancy is subject to large random and seasonal fluctuations; such variability is typical in most short-term hospitals and has made any sort of precise prediction of bed needs difficult and unreliable. But as noted earlier, what has not been widely recognized until recently is the fact that the demand for hospital services is essentially probabilistic in nature—that admissions and length of stay are largely dominated by identifiable underlying chance phenomena [2].

Attempts to deal rationally with this situation have led hospital administrators to resort to planning for levels of peak demand that can be met with reasonable assurance. In 1946 the Commission on Hospital Care [35] suggested that from a theoretical point of view, and on the basis of experience, bed occupancy will rarely exceed or be less than average daily census plus or minus approximately four times the square root of the average daily census. Although this may have been the first definitive recognition of the value inherent in the use of statistical distributions for describing the census, it did not prove to be of much assistance for prediction and planning: obviously, very few chance variables exceed plus or minus four standard deviations. Nevertheless, implicit in this proposed rule of thumb is reliance on the well-known Poisson distribution for statistically describing and predicting bed occupancy. Bailey [36], Blumberg [37], and Thompson et al. [38] recognized this fact and extended the use of such procedures for estimating bed needs and expected occupancy both within communities and within specific service areas in a hospital. Bailey, indeed, showed that the average daily occupancy is essentially the product of the average daily admission rate and the average length of stay, a measure that explicitly assumes a Poisson distribution of occupancy. However, although the Poisson distribution does, indeed, provide the hospital administrator with a means for analytically describing fluctuations in daily census, its very use is an overt admission that little has been done to reduce the effects of chance factors. For the Poisson distribution the variance is equal to the mean; any prediction of average occupancy must necessarily be associated with considerable uncertainty. The results are no more accurate than if one applied what may be called the "straight-edge" technique; that is, plotting a graph of the daily census over time and laying a ruler along peaks to form some estimate of needs.

Unfortunately, most studies of health service systems have been cognitive rather than normative, and the systems have been permitted to retain their inherent variability. Although statistical data are often used to describe existing conditions, and although organizational and procedural changes are often based on deficiencies reflected by the data, few or no attempts are made to deal with fundamental sources of uncertainty through the application of meaningful administrative control. Young [39, 40] has proposed the use of queuing-theory models to describe typical hospital inpatient units and has embedded these models in the framework of an information feedback control system to derive decision rules for administrative control of bed utilization. He has shown that the use of such cybernetic models can lead to higher average occupancy rates with simultaneous improvements in census stability. A major portion of the control is exercised over elective admissions, and decision rules provided to the admissions officer are based on an instantaneous knowledge of the state of the system at any given time.

Additional work by Taylor, using queuing theory and link analysis, focused on the flow of patients through various outpatient clinics of a hospital and provided improved procedures for scheduling patients and guiding their movement through the clinics so as to minimize waiting time while maximizing physician utilization [41]. The Community Systems Foundation [42] has evaluated the effects of various scheduling procedures on operating-room utilization, the allocation of manpower in operating rooms, and bed occupancy. Additional work has included the demand and flow patterns for such ancillary services as x-ray. Resh [43] extended the models proposed by Young into a two-stage sequential decision model for scheduling the flow of patients through the operating room and into the inpatient unit.

The approaches used in these and similar studies are readily applicable to many situations in the hospital involving a flow of patients, elective or emergency, whose care needs must be satisfied by an effective service system. Obviously, this requires a continuous flow of information concerning, for example, unscheduled admissions, the number and kinds of patients occupying beds, operating-room availability, elective-patient waiting lists, discharge patterns, and demand for ancillary services. Also, the models proposed for providing day-to-day administrative decision rules require computer manipulation of input data from many sources. These kinds of data, when stored within the computer system become the information feedback required for the effective control of the hospital system. Within the context of the overall hospital communication network, these data combine with the concurrent flow of data on patient condition and care needs supplied by the individual nursing units. Given the appropriately structured decision rules, the administrator is provided with a quantitative view of the system; he is therefore in a position to effectively anticipate demands and allocate beds, assign nursing staff, schedule services, and regulate the flow of supplies.

Medical Decisions

The fundamental basis for most decisions related to diagnosis and therapy is the information emanating from the patient [44]. Such information, together with the physician's response, is recorded in more or less detail for future reference or study. Traditionally, the primary physical repository of all information about a patient has been the medical history, or record, usually consisting of a folder with miscellaneous paper and film inserts. In the past, these records largely served their purpose and became part of the memory of the organizational information network; now their storage, retrieval, and circulation have become an intolerable burden. For the larger hospitals especially, demands for storage are voracious, access time is inordinately long, and circulation control is difficult to maintain.

A good deal of research has increasingly pointed toward the need for and feasibility of automated systems [45, 46, 12]. It has been advocated that all patient information be stored in computers, in structured or narrative form, even though much of the information does not play a vital role in the current treatment of the patient. Obviously this would require large computer storage capacities and expensive retrieval systems. An alternative is to miniaturize the medical history, using any of the more modern forms of microfilm. Such a system would provide a central inviolate film storage, with complete records readily available in duplicate film or hard copy. Although space requirements would be reduced drastically, problems of retrieval time, updating of information, and reproduction costs detract from the desirability of this kind of system. A logical and perhaps more economical approach is a combination of computer and film storage: the entire medical history may be miniaturized to permanent film storage and retrieved when needed in disposable paper form; at the same time pertinent patient information may be abstracted and maintained in computer storage systems to serve many of the functions of the traditional medical record.

A combined system of this sort offers many obvious advantages beyond a more effective medical-record storage and retrieval system. For example, a problem area that has attracted increasing amounts of study has been the logic of screening and diagnosis and the decisions required for therapy. Walton [47] has examined the relationships between symptom complexes and diseases and has proposed computerized models, based on statistical decision-theory and pattern-recognition methodologies, for use in screening outpatients. These models provide sets of decision rules for specifying, on the basis of diagnostic information, the assignment of a patient to the appropriate outpatient specialty clinic. Lincoln and Parker [48], using Bayesian approaches, developed probabilistic models for the computer-aided prediction of diseases, given the stored results of an array of laboratory tests and physical examinations. Collen [49] has developed automated multiphasic screening procedures, with large amounts of derived patient data being fed into a medical data base. These stored data are used for diagnosis and therapy, while at the same time providing indications of normal values for reference purposes. Flagle [50] has cast the entire process of diagnosis and therapy into the format of a game against nature, recognizing that this kind of approach requires (1) a set of probabilities relating symptoms to a disease, (2) values or costs of outcomes of action, and (3) a rational process for combining probabilities and values to arrive at a decision.

These and other continuing studies point to the rather attractive possibilities that emerge once a computer system has been designed to function as a central node in a hospital communications network. Given information as to the state of the patient via the nurses' station, laboratory reports, medical history, and the like, the computer becomes a medical decision tool for assistance in screening and diagnosis, and the appropriately manipulated quantitative output becomes useful in the selection of therapeutic strategies.

AN INTEGRATED SYSTEM

This discussion has emphasized several of the more important components of the hospital organization that have been the subject of ongoing research and has indicated the manner in which information flow can be utilized in administrative decision making. These decision subsets are, of course, not the only nodes in the synthesized communications network; others are equally important for the effective functioning of the hospital system and must be considered in an integrated information system. As an example, financial data and social data must be processed for billing purposes. Myriad fiscal data are utilized for accounting purposes and for long-range planning. In addition, routine information flow related to maintenance and housekeeping activities forms the basis for many decisions affecting supporting activities within the hospital organization.

Clearly, as was pointed out at the beginning of this discussion, an enormous amount of information is available which is potentially useful but which is left largely untapped because of the complex communication and information flow problems that remain unsolved. Barnett [51], although emphasizing the crucial need for improved information-processing systems in the patient care process, nevertheless issued a caveat concerning claims for what in fact currently exists, what is possible, and what is promised for the future. A considerable amount of systems analysis and engineering is needed before many of the objectives discussed here are realized; to this end it is useful to consider briefly a number of factors that may prove important in the developmental process.

It would appear that initial prospects for the successful development and implementation of an information system might be enhanced if the research were initially focused on specific problem areas such as the development of a medical data base, the computerization of medical histories, or the use of assignment models for staffing. Of course, any research that does not consider the relative position of the functional subcomponent of the system vis-à-vis the objectives of the overall system would ultimately lead to suboptimization, with subsequent inability to link areas in the most effective manner. It would appear that the most viable system can be produced only through the efforts of largely inhouse teams that are thoroughly familiar with needs and objectives of the organization and willing to accept responsibility for the major research program. In addition, substantial support must be provided for the developmental effort over prolonged periods of time, including the periods of seemingly overwhelming discouragement and frustration that are bound to occur. Finally, inevitable questions arise concerning the extent to which the installation of hardware configurations should be delayed until appropriate decision models are provided: can the ultimate system design be completely, or even partially, specified without prior analysis of what decisions need to be made and exactly what the system is to be used for? Indeed, a number of hospital organizations, enamored of the apparent efficiency of modern computers, have obtained contemporary data processing systems that have proved disappointingly ineffective and inadequate in facilitating decisions related to the overall health care process.

The major objective must necessarily be provision of means for assimilating and processing the flow of information in the hospital organization in such a manner that the response to highly variable needs is effective and timely. Decision making, in terms of the choice of a course of action from among many alternatives, must be based on quantitative analysis of data reflecting the state of the system at any node in the network. The computer becomes the central cybernetic processing tool; information created by the flow of patients, and reflecting their demands on the system, is stored and utilized for the control of logistics, manpower, services, and finances—as related to diagnostic and therapeutic patient care. Only in this way can a hospital organization hope to deal effectively with variable demands that defy deterministic treatment.

REFERENCES

1. Flagle, C. D. Operations research in the health services. *Op. Res.* 10:591 September–October 1962.
2. Balintfy, J. L. *Mathematical Models and Analysis of Certain Stochastic Processes in General Hospitals.* Doctoral dissertation, The Johns Hopkins University (Industrial Engineering Department) 1962.
3. Flagle, C. D. and J. P. Young. Application of operations research and industrial engineering to problems of health services, hospitals, and public health. *J. Ind. Eng.* 17:609 November 1966.
4. Klarman, H. E. *The Economics of Health.* New York: Columbia University Press, 1965.
5. Young, J. P. Information nexus guides decision system. *Mod. Hosp.* 106:101 February 1966.
6. Howland, D. and W. E. McDowell. The measurement of patient care: A conceptual framework. *Nurs. Res.* 13:4 Winter 1964.
7. Howland, D. A hospital system model. *Nursing Research* 12:232 Fall 1963.
8. Wiener, N. *Cybernetics.* New York: John Wiley & Sons, 1961.
9. Ashby, W. R. *Introduction to Cybernetics.* New York: John Wiley & Sons, 1957.
10. Flagle, C. D. Unpublished paper presented at Health Services Research Study Section Systems Seminar, Washington, September 1967.
11. Conference on the use of data mechanization and computers in clinical medicine, sessions on The hospital as a cybernetic system and Prospects for automation in the hospital system, New York Academy of Sciences, New York, Jan. 15–17, 1968.
12. Barnett, G. O. *An Annotated Selected Bibliography on the Applications of Computers to Patient Care.* Report from Laboratory of Computer Science, Massachusetts General Hospital, Boston, 1967.
13. Barnett, G. O. and P. A. Castleman. A time-sharing computer system for patient-care activities. *Computers & Biomed. Res.* 1:41 March 1967.
14. Barnett, G. O. and J. J. Baruch. *Hospital Computer Project, Status Report, Memorandum No. 9,* Massachusetts General Hospital, Boston, 1966.
15. Brown, R. E. *Judgment in Administration,* pp. 200–220. New York: McGraw-Hill Book Company, 1966.
16. *Abstracts of Hospital Management Studies,* Vols. I, II, III. Ann Arbor, Mich.: Cooperative Information Center for Hospital Management Studies, University of Michigan, 1967.
17. Smalley, H. E. and J. R. Freeman. *Hospital Industrial Engineering: A Guide to the Improvement of Hospital Management Systems.* New York: Reinhold Publishing Corporation, 1966.
18. Connor, R. J. *A Hospital Inpatient Classification System.* Doctoral dissertation. The Johns Hopkins University (Industrial Engineering Department) 1960.
19. Connor, R. J. A work sampling study of variations in nursing workload. *Hospitals, J.A.H.A.* 35:40 May 1, 1961.
20. Connor, R. J. et al. Effective use of nursing resources: A research report. *Hospitals, J.A.H.A.* 35:30 May 1, 1961.
21. Levine, E. and F. G. Abdellah. *Better Patient Care Through Nursing Research.* New York: The Macmillan Company, 1965.
22. Wolfe, H. *A Multiple Assignment Model for Staffing Nursing Units.* Doctoral dissertation, The Johns Hopkins University (Department of Operations Research and Industrial Engineering) 1964.
23. Jelinek, R. C. A structural model for the patient care operation. *Health Serv. Res.* 2:226 Fall–Winter 1967.
24. Wolfe, H. and J. P. Young. Staffing the nursing unit, Part I: Controlled variable staffing, *Nurs. Res.* 14:236 Summer 1965.

25. Wolfe, H. and J. P. Young. Staffing the nursing unit, Part II: The multiple assignment technique. *Nurs. Res.* 14:299 Fall 1965.
26. Flagle, C. D. Operations Research in Health Services. Progress report, June 1962–October 1962. The Johns Hopkins Hospital, Operations Research Division.
27. Middelhoven, W. *Analysis and Reorganization of a Central Supply Delivery System.* Master's essay, The Johns Hopkins University (Department of Operations Research and Industrial Engineering) 1964.
28. Hsieh, R. K. C. *A Study of Linen Processing and Distribution in a Hospital.* Master's essay, The Johns Hopkins University (Industrial Engineering Department) 1961.
29. Reed, R. J. and W. E. Stanley. Optimizing control of hospital inventories. *J. Ind. Eng.* 16:48 January–February 1965.
30. Balintfy, J. L. and A. Prekopa. Nature of random variation in the nutrient composition of meals. *Health Serv. Res.* 1:148 Fall 1966.
31. Tester, W. W. *A Study of Patient Care Involving a Unit Dose System.* Progress report, June 1964–June 1965, USPHS Research Grant HM-00328, College of Pharmacy, University of Iowa.
32. Barker, K. N. and W. M. Heller. The development of a centralized unit dose dispensing system. *Am. J. Hosp. Pharm.* 20:568 November 1963. (Part I of a six-part article that appeared in subsequent issues.)
33. Hsieh, R. K. C. Evaluation of formal communications systems in a hospital. *Health Serv. Res.* 1:222 Winter 1966.
34. Bartscht, K. G. et al. *The Development of an Effective Methodology for Determining Staffing Requirements in Hospitals.* Project report, Hospital Systems Research Group, University of Michigan, February 1965.
35. Commission on Hospital Care. *Hospital Care in the United States,* Chap. XXI. New York: The Commonwealth Fund, 1947.
36. Bailey, N. T. J. Statistics in hospital planning and design. *J. Applied Statist.* 5:146 November 1956.
37. Blumberg, M. S. DPF concept helps predict bed needs. *Mod. Hosp.* 97:75 December 1961.
38. Thompson, J. D., O. W. Avant, and E. D. Spiker. How queuing theory works for the hospital. *Mod. Hosp.* 94:75 March 1960.
39. Young, J. P. Stabilization of inpatient bed occupancy through control of admissions. *Hospitals, J.A.H.A.* 39:41 Oct. 1, 1965.
40. Young, J. P. Administrative control of multiple channel queuing systems with parallel input streams. *Op. Res.* 14:145 January–February 1966.
41. Flagle, C. D. et al. *Analysis of Congestion in an Outpatient Clinic.* Final report, USPHS Grant W-96, The Johns Hopkins Hospital, Operations Research Division.
42. Community Systems Foundation. *An Analysis of the Surgical Suite of the Wilmer Ophthalmological Institute of The Johns Hopkins Hospital.* Project MDJH 2a, September 1965.
43. Resh, M. *Mathematical Programming of Admissions Scheduling in Hospitals.* Doctoral dissertation, The Johns Hopkins University (Department of Operations Research and Industrial Engineering) 1967.
44. Gue, R. L. *A Stochastic Description of Direct Patient Care and Its Relation to Communication in a Hospital.* Doctoral dissertation, The Johns Hopkins University (Department of Operations Research and Industrial Engineering) 1964.
45. Empey, S. L. Computer applications in medicine and the biological sciences: Bibliography. *Communications ACM* 6:176 April 1963.
46. Empey, S. L. Computer applications in medicine and the biological sciences: Bibliography II. *Ibid.* 7:245 April 1964.
47. Walton, W. W. *Modern Decision Theory Applied to Medical Diagnosis.* Doctoral dissertation, The Johns Hopkins University (Department of Operations Research and Industrial Engineering) 1964.
48. Lincoln, T. L. and R. D. Parker. Medical diagnosis using Bayes theorem. *Health Serv. Res.* 2:34 Spring 1967.

49. Collen, M. F. Periodic health examinations using an automated multitest laboratory. *J.A.M.A.* 195:830 March 7, 1966.
50. Flagle, C. D. A decision theoretical comparison of three methods of screening for a single disease. *Proc. 5th Berkeley Symposium on Mathematical Statistics and Probability, 1965.*
51. Barnett, G. O. Unpublished paper presented at Health Services Research Study Section Systems Seminar, Washington, September 1967.

Chapter 3

Organizations

3.1 INTRODUCTION

Organizations are a dominant fact of life in modern societies. A vast proportion of our life is spent as participants in organizations, formal or informal. At any one point in time, we are simultaneously members of various organizations—health, business, social, political, public, religious, or others. If we want to influence the direction and effectiveness of organizations (as individuals, administrators, members of special interest groups or as plain citizens), it is imperative that we gain an understanding of the nature, structure, and behavior of organizations. Organizational questions are either of the "macro" or "micro" type, depending upon the nature of the problem and the particular vantage point. The macro considerations are particularly important in the sphere of broad social issues, such as health care and education. The health care field must always face the necessity of making decisions on how best to restructure, and thereby improve, the delivery of health services. These are strategic, policy decisions whose impact will be far-reaching on all types of health care organizations. These organizational decisions and their implications for the emerging tasks and responsibilities of health care administrators point up the need for understanding organizations, their functioning and structure, and the behavior of their components (individuals and groups). In this section we will define the terms "organization" and "organization structure"; relate organization to the concept of a system; show the scope of organization theory; and briefly describe a set of concepts required for understanding organization behavior.

3.2 ORGANIZATION AND ORGANIZATIONAL STRUCTURE

"Organization" has been considered in the management literature as one of the main managerial functions.* To organize is "to form as or into a whole consisting of interdependent or coordinated parts, especially for

---

* Other commonly listed functions are: Planning, Leadership, and Control.

harmonious or united action" [Random House Dictionary, 1967]. The term organization can be viewed in a variety of ways. Organization is both a *process* and an *entity*. The process of organization includes all activities necessary for delineating organizational goals, assembling human and other resources, structuring work and authority relationships and adapting organizational responses to internal and external demands. It is an attempt at building and then continuously modifying (in response to organizational climate) the *structure* of the organization.* The result of this dynamic process is the entity called an organization. Formally, we will define an *organization* as a body of two or more persons engaged in the pursuit of common goals.† Organization *structure* refers to the authority-responsibility relationships among various hierarchical levels and persons who perform different organizational tasks. It is designed to formalize work assignments, vertical and horizontal relationships, and other duties. Organization structure is often summarized in organization charts and supplemented by job descriptions, work manuals, and so on. However, an organization chart is a "static" representation and it seldom captures the realities of organizational life which is dynamic; is in a continuous state of flux and finds its expression both in formal and informal groups (which are not shown in organization charts). Organization structure and the flow and direction of information within the organization are obviously related. The impact of personality on structure, and vice-versa, has also been reported in the literature [Argyris, 1957].

3.3 ORGANIZATION AS A "SYSTEM"

An organization is a *system;* because the definition of "organization" fulfills the requirements of what is called a system (it has at least two interrelated elements and a set of goals). Hence, all the concepts and tools of systems analysis can be applied to the analysis, understanding, and management of organizations. It should be emphasized, however, that organizations are primarily human systems and regardless of the mode (and the model) employed to analyze organizations, the role of humans cannot be ignored. Since organizations interact with their environments, organizations are classified as "open" systems. Organizations respond to the changing

---

* See, for example [Lawrence & Lorsch, 1967] for a description of how internal structures and processes of organizations are related to the facts of their environment. The authors advance a contingency theory of organization which, "rather than propounding one best way to organize under all conditions, focuses on the organizational characteristics which lead to effective performance given the specific demands of an organization's environment."

† See [Tannenbaum, et al. 1961, p. 255] for several different but related definitions of organization.

conditions in the environment by the process of adaptation and learning.

From a systems point of view, Ackoff defines organization as a "purposeful system that contains at least two purposeful elements which have common purpose relative to which the system has a functional division of labor; its functionally distinct subsets can respond to each other's behavior through observation and communication; and at least one subset has system-control function" [Ackoff, 1971, p. 670], Ackoff differentiates between "organizations" and "organisms" by noting that although both are purposeful systems, organizations contain purposeful elements while organisms do not. All the elements of an organization can display "will"; while in an organism "only the whole can display 'will,' none of the parts can." An organization thus represents the highest form of behavioral systems.

A systems view of organization implies that organizations can be described and analyzed in terms of those subsystems of the organization which are the focus of study. Each subsystem has its own objectives, attitudes, opinions, role, structure, behavior, activities, processes, and norms. An understanding of the subsystems and their mutual interaction is important for predicting the behavior of organizations.*

Organizations and systems are very closely related, as is shown in Figure 3.1, which draws a parallel between different management functions (management of organization) and various steps of systems analysis.

3.4 ORGANIZATIONAL FORMS

Organizations can be formal or informal, small or large, simple or complex. A distinction can be drawn between formal organizations that are *deliberately* formed and informal organizations that arise through unconscious ordering [Carzo and Yanouzas, 1967, p. 6]. Informal organizations can evolve into formal organizations and in most cases exert significant impact on the behavior of individuals.

Both formal and informal organizations have existed, in one form or the other, since the dawn of history. It is through the device of organization that man has produced the present level of science, technology and productivity. What has changed over the centuries is not the "fact" of organization but the *form* and *characteristics* of organization. For example, we have witnessed in the last decade the "matrix"† organization and

---

* Characteristics of technical, social, and power subsystems are given in [Carzo and Yanouzas, 1967, p. 240].

† The "matrix" organization [see, for example, Mee, 1964] is project-oriented (as opposed to functional- or process-oriented). During the life of the project, the project manager exercises complete authority over the personnel drawn from different functional departments.

FIG. 3.1
RELATED CONCEPTS OF ORGANIZATION AND SYSTEMS

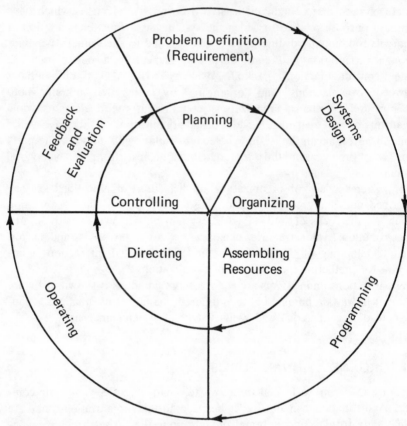

Source: [McDonough and Garrett, 1965, p. 10].

the "free-form"* organization emerge. As to the general form of present and future organizations, the authors subscribe to the view that organizations will continue to be hierarchical in nature, provide the framework for satisfying higher level human needs, and exhibit Simon's three layers of decision processes.†

---

* The essence of "free-form" management [Ways, 1966] is loosely defined responsibilities at top management level. Similar in concept to matrix organization, the "free-form" is a product of the conglomerate movement in the 1960's.

† See [Simon, 1960, p. 49]. Simon predicts that future organizations will continue to be constructed in three layers: "(1) an underlying system of physical production and distribution processes, (2) a layer of programmed (and probably largely automated) decision processes for governing the routine day-to-day operation of the physical system, and (3) a layer of non-programmed decision processes (carried out in a man-machine system) for monitoring the first-level processes, redesigning them, and changing parameter values."

The special characteristics of modern organizations are their large size, an ever-increasing rate of change, complex technology, rapidly changing social values and increased emphasis on integrative skills. As Thompson [1961, p. 6] has pointed out, there is in modern organizations a growing gap between authority (the right to decide) and ability (the power to do). This fact, created by an extremely fast pace of technology, has resulted in increased conflict between hierarchical and specialist roles. The implications of the new characteristics of organizations are that we must gain meaningful insights into organizational behavior and its determinants. What constitutes organizational behavior? What are its basic units of analysis? What types of concepts and conceptual framework can be used to understand organizational behavior? These are the kinds of questions that organization theory attempts to answer.

3.5 ORGANIZATION THEORY

Organization theory is the study of activities and behavior of organizations and their various elements. Organization theory, by its very scope, is an extremely broad area of study. As March has pointed out, "it is not easy to identify the universe of organization theory" [March, 1965, p. x]. The topics covered in the *Handbook of Organizations* range from individual decision-making, group behavior, interpersonal relations, to the description of special organizations (e.g., hospitals, unions, schools, prisons, political parties, and county government). The handbook covers a total of 28 topics including a chapter entitled "Hospitals: Technology, Structure, and Goals."*

3.5.1 *Routes to the Study of Organizations*

There are various routes to the study of organizations. Organizations have been analyzed as communication networks, logistic systems, social systems, political systems, technical systems, economic systems, and as means of problem-solving and decision-making.† A study of organizations can be conducted not only from various perspectives (e.g., social, economic,

---

* The chapter, written by Charles Perrow, is a critical review of sociological studies of mental and general hospitals. Elsewhere [Perrow, 1961] has given an analysis of goals in four different types of hospitals (those dominated by trustees, by the medical staff, by the administration, and by some other form of leadership). Also see [Elling and Halebsky, 1961], for a discussion of relationships between organizational (internal) characteristics of general hospitals and the support received in terms of funds, patients, and community participation.

† See, for example, [McGuire, 1965], [McGuire, (editor), 1962], [March & Simon, 1958], [Cyert & March, 1963], [Latham, in Hampton et al., 1968] and Part II of this book.

political), but also by focusing on different elements as the basic units of analysis. For example, the focus can be on individual behavior, group behavior, intergroup behavior, role behavior (as opposed to jobs or individuals), or the entire organization.

The nature and behavior of organizations is an important area of study and research in management. "Organization theory and human-behavior" is one of the major schools of management thought.* The particular emphasis of the behavioral school is on the analysis and understanding of organizations by relating human behavior to organizational performance. Other schools, particularly the "operational" school is oriented more toward the management (as opposed to analysis and understanding) of organizations. It is clear that the management of organizations cannot be divorced from the analysis and understanding of organizations.

3.5.2 *Concepts for Understanding Organization Behavior*

To understand organizations, and the behavior of individuals and groups within them, we need to learn a set of concepts and tools of analysis including theories of motivation, leadership, social exchange, interaction, functional analysis, and political concepts for organizational analysis [Hampton et al. 1968, p. 12]. Each of these concepts comprises a rich body of published literature [see bibliography at the end of Chapter 3]. Although an extensive discussion of these topics is beyond the scope of this book, the reader is provided with appropriate definitions and specific primary or secondary references.

Theories of motivation attempt to explain individual behavior and guide management in designing and implementing policies to influence individual behavior. They rest on need satisfaction as the central cause of human behavior. A well-known theory of motivation is due to the late A. H. Maslow.† Maslow suggested a hierarchy of five basic and related needs: physiological, safety, social, esteem, and self-actualization.‡ As soon as needs are

---

* Various classifications of schools of management thought exist in the literature. See, for example, [Koontz, 1964], [Newman et al., 1967], and [Starr, 1971]. The most important are: management science, organization theory and human-behavior, and what Starr calls the "operational" school.
† Originally published in "A Theory of Human Motivation," *Psychology Review*, vol. 50, 1943, pp. 370–396. This classic article has since been reprinted in several books including [Hampton et al., 1968].
‡ L. B. Barnes has suggested a modification of these needs and related them to an organization system defined in the dimensions of autonomy, opportunity for interaction and influence [Lawrence and Seiler, 1965, p. 158]. For a schematic diagram of a possible relationship between the concepts of organizational systems and an individual's needs, see [Lawrence and Seiler, 1965, p. 450]. For a brief review of motivation theories we recommend the reader to [Filley and House, 1969, Chapter 15].

satisfied, they no longer act as sources of motivation. Hence, motivation must be directed to unmet, operative needs. Litwin and Stringer [1968] have related three types of motivation (achievement motivation, power motivation, and affiliation motivation) to leadership style and organizational climate.* Personality differences, the manager's strengths and weaknesses, nature of the tasks, and work climate are identified as key elements in "managing motivation." It should be noted that motivation and need satisfaction are the basic ingredients in any human situation. Ericson has summarized responses of noncybernetic and cybernetic organizations to human needs and social values [Ericson, 1969]. His analysis is made with the purpose of illustrating "enhancement potential" of cybernetic† organizations. The idea of need satisfaction is intimately tied to such management practices as decentralization, participative decision-making, job enlargement, incentive systems, and training programs.

Leadership, as we mentioned earlier, is one of the major managerial functions. Leadership involves an attempt on the part of the leader to influence the motivation, attitude, and behavior of another individual or a group. Tannenbaum and Massarik define leadership as "interpersonal influence, exercised in situation and directed, through the communication process, toward the attainment of a specific goal or goals" [Tannenbaum et al., 1961, p. 24]. Theories of leadership have been constructed with focus on: (1) traits of the leader (physical as well as psychological), (2) behavior pattern of the leader (autocratic, supportive, etc.), (3) the situation (demands of the situation determine the type of leader), and (4) the follower (his problems, attitudes, and needs).‡ Research on leadership indicates that "social sensitivity" and "action flexibility" are the two most important variables in leadership effectiveness. A successful and effective leader is the one who can understand through empathy the most relevant forces in each situation *and* adjust his behavior accordingly.

The concept of social exchange views the interaction between persons as exchange of not only material goods, but also non-material goods, such as the symbols of approval or prestige.§ The exchange process tends to move towards a state of equilibrium between the "rewards" of what an individual receives and the "costs" of what he gives. The concept, useful in studying group behavior, considers the manager as a bargainer, and management as a process of brokerage.

---

* The concept of organizational climate (the perceived environmental quality) has been explored by several authors in terms of its nature, determinants, consequences, and its relationship with individual and group behavior. See [Tagiuri and Litwin, 1968].
† Briefly, *cybernetics* is the study of control systems. A general model of the cybernetic organization is given in [Starr, 1971, p. 654]. Also, see [Ashby, 1956].
‡ See [Tannenbaum and Massarik, 1957] and [Filley and House, 1969, Chapter 16].
§ [Homans in Hampton et al., 1968, p. 51].

Interaction theory* conceives of relations between persons as a mutually dependent system involving interactions (interpersonal contacts), activities (physical acts performed by people) and sentiments (how individuals feel). The environment (consisting of economic, technical, legal, social, and cultural forces) can have impact on the social system, directly or indirectly, through the channels of interactions, activities, or sentiments.† The problem for the manager is to create change in sentiments by introducing changes in activities and interactions. In contrast to the bargaining role of the manager, the emphasis is on his role as the designer of systems of interaction, activities and sentiments.

The essence of functional analysis lies in emphasizing that management policies can result in unintended consequences. The functional approach, used to study the behavior of the entire organization, builds on the concepts of "function," "dysfunction," "manifest" consequences and "latent" consequences. *Functions* are defined as "observed consequences which make for the adaptation or adjustment of a given system." *Dysfunctions* are "those observed consequences which lessen the adaptation or adjustment of the system." Intended consequences are called *manifest,* while unintended ones are called *latent.* Functions are performed to meet needs, but the introduction of unintended consequences (dysfunctions) create new problems and needs which, in turn, must be met by changing organizational structure. Functional analysis deals with three major problems [Hampton et al., 1968, p. 648]. (1) "How does the organization maintain itself? How does it encourage contribution from the various parts so that they remain a part of the functioning whole? (2) How does the total organization accomplish its objectives in relation to the external environment? (3) How does the organization modify itself internally in order to respond to environmental changes?"

Political concepts are important in organizational analysis because, whatever else they may be, organizations represent political systems. Power, authority, responsibility, and delegation are variables which can be understood and related to human behavior in the context of a corporation (or organization) as a political system. As Earl Latham‡ has said: "The corporation is a body politic which exhibits describable characteristics common to all bodies politic. In a functional view of all such political systems it can be said that there are five essential elements: (1) an authoritative allocation of principle functions; (2) a symbolic system for the ratification of collective decisions; (3) an operating system of command; (4) a system of rewards and punishments; and (5) institutions for the enforce-

---

* First advanced by Chappel and Arensberg and refined by George Homans. See [Whyte, 1959, pp. 41 and 54–55].
† [Whyte 1959, p. 65].
‡ See [Hampton et al., 1968, pp. 82–97].

ment of the common rules. A system of organized behavior which contains these elements is a political system, whether one calls it the state or the corporation."

3.6 CONCLUDING REMARKS

The purpose of this chapter has been to present some important aspects of organizations and focus on the development, theory, structure, and practice of management in complex organizations. The three articles selected for this chapter treat these areas of organizations: the formation, role, and importance of organizational goals; organizations as political structures; and leadership patterns for organizations of tomorrow.

Herbert Simon's classic paper (Selection 6) is devoted to an examination of how organizational goals are formed. A distinction is made between goals and motives. Goals are defined as value premises that serve as inputs to decisions. Motives are any causes that lead individuals to select some goals rather than others as premises for their decisions. Organizational decision-making takes place in the context of multiple constraints or requirements, and sometimes one of these constraints is chosen as the goal of the action. However, for many purposes it is more meaningful to refer to the whole set of requirements as the (complex) goal of the action. Linear programming is employed to illustrate the relevance of multiple criteria in decision-making. The author emphasizes the dual role of the goals of the action. First, the goals may be used directly to synthesize proposed solutions (alternative generation). Second, the goals may be used to test the satisfactoriness of a proposed solution (alternative testing). Goals can also be subdivided into *personal* and *role defined*. Personal goals motivate the individual to adopt the role, and then the goals and constraints appropriate to the role become a part of the decision-making system. Interpersonal differences in role behavior are described. An organizational decision-making system is described as one in which (1) particular decision-making processes are aimed at finding courses of action that are feasible or satisfactory in the light of multiple goals and constraints, and (2) decisions reached in one part of the organization enter as goals or constraints into the decisions being made in other parts of the organization. The author concludes that organization goal is the constraints, or sets of constraints, imposed by the organizational roles, which have only indirect relation to the motives of the decision-makers.

Zaleznik (Selection 7) notes that the competition for power is characteristic of all political structures. And, whatever else organizations may be (problem-solving instruments, socio-technical systems, reward systems, and so on), they are political structures. They provide both a power base for the development of executive careers and for the expression of individual interests and motives. Organizational life is a dynamic configuration of interest conflicts and power relations existing in an economy of scarcity. Managers form coalitions, compete for the top of the political pyramid, and in so doing often impose their personal defenses into the stage of organizational life. Zaleznik suggests that a frank recognition of the importance of personality factors and a sensitive use of the strengths and limitations of people in decisions on power distributions can improve the quality of organizational life. *Selection of goals* (partial vs. total), and *orientation toward action* are suggested as dimensions of the executives cognitive biases. The author, then, outlines four cognitive management styles in organizational life: (1) bureaucratic, (2) conversion, (3) compliance, and (4) problem-solving.

Bennis (Selection 8) predicts that organizations of the future will be "adaptive, problem-solving, temporary systems of diverse specialists, linked together by coordinating executives in organic flux"—rather than pyramidal bureaucracies. Four factors leading to this direction are identified: rapid and unexpected growth, need for diversification, complex technology and resulting interdependence, and changing managerial values. Leadership of these organizations will become a significant social process, "requiring as much interpersonal competence as substantive competence, if not more." A listing of the main problems confronting modern organization is given, and corresponding tasks of the future leader are enumerated. Organizational problems are: integration, social influence, collaboration, adaptation, identity, and revitalization. The attributes of a new leadership style capable of handling these problems are also described. Bennis, then, proceeds to list five important sets of competencies needed for the new concept of leadership. The author emphasizes the need for understanding such terms as open systems and dynamic systems. We have dwelled on these terms in Chapters 2 and 3.

REFERENCES

Ackoff, R. A., "Towards a System of Systems Concept," *Management Science,* 1971   vol. 17, no. 11, July, pp. 661–671.

Argyris, C., "The Individual and Organization: Some Problems of Mutual 1957   Adjustment," *Administrative Science Quarterly,* vol. 2, June, pp. 1–24.

Ashby, W. R., *An Introduction to Cybernetics,* New York: John Wiley & Sons. 1956

Carzo, R., Jr., and J. N. Yanouzas, *Formal Organization: A Systems Approach,* 1967   Homewood, Ill.: Richard D. Irwin.

Cleland, D. I., and W. R. King (eds.), *Systems, Organizations, Analysis, Man-*
1969 *agement,* New York: McGraw-Hill.
Cyert, R. M., and J. G. March, *A Behavioral Theory of the Firm,* Englewood
1963 Cliffs, N.J.: Prentice-Hall.
Dale, E., *Organization,* New York: American Management Association.
1967
Elling, R. H. and S. Halebsky, "Organizational Differentiation and Support: A
1961 Conceptual Framework," *Administrative Science Quarterly,* vol. 6,
September, pp. 186–209.
Ericson, R. F. "Organizational Cybernetics and Human Values," *Program of*
1969 *Policy Studies in Science and Technology.* George Washington University, Washington, D.C., Monograph No. 4, September.
Filley, A. C., and R. J. House, *Managerial Process and Organizational Be-*
1969 *havior,* Glenview, Ill.: Scott, Foresman and Co.
Hampton, D. R., C. E. Summer, and R. A. Webber (eds.), *Organizational*
1968 *Behavior and the Practice of Management* New York: Scott, Fores-
man and Co.
Hill, W. A., and D. Egan (eds.), *Readings in Organization Theory: A Be-*
1967 *havioral Approach,* Boston, Mass.: Allyn and Bacon.
Koontz, H. (ed.), *Toward a Unified Theory of Management,* New York: Mc-
1964 Graw-Hill.
Lawrence, P. R., and J. W. Lorsch, *Organization and Environment: Managing*
1967 *Differentiation and Integration,* Division of Research, Graduate
School of Business Administration, Harvard University.
Lawrence, P. R., and J. A. Seiler, *Organizational Behavior and Administration,*
1965 *Cases, Concepts, and Research Findings,* (Revised edition), Home-
wood, Ill.: Richard D. Irwin.
Likert, R., *New Patterns of Management,* New York: McGraw-Hill.
1961
Litwin, G. H., and R. A. Stringer, *Motivation and Organizational Climate,*
1968 Boston, Mass.: Division of Research, Graduate School of Business
Administration, Harvard University.
Lorsch, J. W. and P. R. Lawrence (eds.), *Studies in Organization Design,*
1970 Homewood, Ill.: Richard D. Irwin.
March, J. G. (ed.), *Handbook of Organizations,* Chicago: Rand McNally & Co.
1965
March, J. G., and H. A. Simon, *Organizations,* New York: John Wiley &
1958 Sons.
McGuire, J. W., *Theories of Business Behavior,* Englewood Cliffs, N.J.:
1964 Prentice-Hall, Inc.
McGuire, J. W. (ed.), *Interdisciplinary Studies in Business Behavior,* Cin-
1962 cinnati, O.: South-western Publishing Co.
McKeown, T., "Organization of Hospitals for Community Health Services and
1969 Future Patterns of Medical Care," *Johns Hopkins Medical Journal,*
vol. 124, no. 5, May, pp. 272–276.
Mee, J. F., "Matrix Organization," *Business Horizons,* Summer.
1964
Newman, W. H., C. E. Summer, and E. K. Warren, *The Process of Manage-*
1967 *ment,* Englewood Cliffs, N.J.: Prentice-Hall.
Perrow, C., "The Analysis of Goals in Complex Organizations," *American*
1961 *Sociological Review,* July, pp. 854–866.

Porter, D. E., and P. B. Applewhite (eds.), *Studies in Organizational Be-*
1964   *havior and Management,* Scranton, Pa.: International Text Book
        Company.
Simon, H. A., *The New Science of Management Decision,* New York: Harper
1960   & Row.
Solkoff, N., "The Use of Personality and Attitude Tests in Predicting the
1968   Academic Success of Medical and Law Students," Journal of Medical
        Education, vol. 43, December, pp. 1251–53.
Starr, M. K., *Management: A Modern Approach,* New York: Harcourt Brace
1971   Jovanovich.
Tagiuri, R., and G. H. Litwin (eds.), *Organizational Climate: Explorations of*
1968   *a Concept,* Boston: Division of Research, Graduate School of Busi-
        ness Administration, Harvard University.
Tannenbaum, R., and F. Massarik, "Leadership: A Frame of Reference,"
1957   *Management Science,* vol. 4, pp. 1–19.
Tannenbaum, R., I. R. Weschler, and F. Massarik, *Leadership and Organiza-*
1961   *tion: A Behavioral Science Approach,* New York: McGraw-Hill.
Thompson, V. A., *Modern Organization: A General Theory,* New York:
1961   Alfred A. Knopf.
Torgerson, P. E., and I. T. Weinstock, *Management: An Integrated Approach,*
1972   Englewood Cliffs, N.J.: Prentice-Hall.
Ways, M., "Tomorrows Management: A More Adventurous Life in a Free
1966   Form Corporation," *Fortune,* July 1, pp. 84–87, 148–150.
Whyte, W. F., *Man and Organization,* Homewood, Ill.: Richard D. Irwin.
1959
Whyte, W. F., *Organizational Behavior: Theory and Application,* Homewood,
1969   Ill.: Richard D. Irwin.

SELECTION 6

On the Concept
of Organizational Goal*

Herbert A. Simon

Few discussions of organization theory manage to get along without introducing some concept of "organization goal." In the classical economic theory of the firm, where no distinction is made between an organization and a single entrepreneur, the organization's goal—the goal of the firm—is simply identical with the goal of the real or hypothetical entrepreneur. In general, it is thought not to be problematical to postulate that individuals have goals. If it is not, this solution raises no difficulties.

When we are interested in the internal structure of an organization, however, the problem cannot be avoided in this way. Either we must explain organizational behavior in terms of the goals of the individual members of the organization, or we must postulate the existence of one or more organization goals, over and above the goals of the individuals.[2]

The first alternative is an attractive one. It protects us from the danger of reifying the organization, of treating it as a superindividual entity having an existence and behavior independent of the behavior of its members. The difficulty with this alternative is that it is hard to carry off. The usual way it is attempted is by identifying the phrase "organization goals" with "goals of the firm's owners" or, alternatively, "goals of the firm's top management," or "goals of those who hold legitimate authority to direct the organization."

But this solution raises new difficulties, for we often have occasion to observe that the goals that actually underlie the decisions made in an organization do not coincide with the goals of the owners, or of top management, but have been modified by managers and employees at all echelons. Must we conclude, then, that it is the goals of the latter—of subordinate managers and employees—that are governing organizational behavior? Presumably not, because the kinds of behavior taking place are not those we would expect if the managers and employees were consulting only their personal goals. The whole concept of an informal organization, modified by, but not identical with, the goals either of management or of individual employees, becomes hazy and ambiguous if we follow this path.

* *Administrative Science Quarterly,* vol. 4, June, 1964.

Let us see if we can find a way between this Scylla and the Charybdis of reification. The first step toward clarification is to maintain a distinction between goals, on the one hand, and motives, on the other. By *goals* we shall mean value premises that can serve as inputs to decisions. By *motives* we mean the causes, whatever they are, that lead individuals to select some goals rather than others as premises for their decisions. In the next section we shall develop the concept of goal, defined as above. In subsequent sections we shall undertake to explicate the notion of *organization goal* and to clarify the relations between organization goals and personal motives.

Before we can define "organization goals" we shall have to be clear on what we mean by "goals of an individual." We shall begin by considering the latter question.

GOALS AND DECISIONS: MULTIPLE CRITERIA

Our discussion of goals will be much simplified if we have a definite model before us of the situation we are considering. In recent years in the field of management science or operations research, we have learned to build formal models to characterize even quite elaborate and complex decision situations, and to use these models to reach "optimal" decisions. Since many of these models make use of the tool of linear programming, we will employ a linear programming framework to describe the decision situation. No mathematical knowledge will be assumed beyond the ability to read algebraic notation.[3]

The optimal diet problem is a typical simple linear programming problem. We are given a list of foods, and for each item on the list its price, its calory content, and its proportions of each of the minerals and vitamins relevant to nutrition. Then we are given a set of nutritional requirements, which may include statements about minimum daily intake of minerals, vitamins, and calories, and may also put limits on maximum intake of some or all of these components.

The diet problem is to find that sublist of foods and their quantities that will meet the nutritional requirements at least cost. The problem can be formalized as follows:

Let the various foods be numbered from 1 through N, and the various nutritional components from 1 through M. Let x_i be the quantity of the ith food in the diet, y_j be the total quantity of the jth nutritional component in the diet, and p_i the price of the ith food. Let a_{ij} be the amount of the jth nutritional component in a unit quantity of the ith food; let b_j be the minimum requirement of the jth nutritional component, and c_j the maximum allowance. (Some of the b_j's may be zero, and some of the c_j's infinite.) Then:

(1) $\Sigma \, a_{ij} x_i = y_j,$ for $j = 1, \ldots, M;$

i.e., the total consumption of the jth nutritional element is the sum of the quantities of that element for each of the foods consumed. The nutritional requirements can be stated:

(2) $c_j \geqq y_j \geqq b_j,$ for $j = 1, \ldots, M;$

i.e., the total quantity of the jth element must lie between b_j and c_j. The quantity of each food consumed must be non-negative, although it may be zero:

(3) $x_i \geqq 0,$ $i = 1, \ldots, N.$

Finally, the total cost of the diet is to be minimized; we are to find:

(4) $\underset{x}{\text{Min}} \, \underset{i}{\Sigma} \, x_i p_i.$

A diet (the solution is not necessarily unique) that satisfies all the relations (2), (3), (4) is called an *optimal* diet. A diet that satisfies the inequalities (2) and (3) (called *constraints*), but which is not necessarily a minimum cost diet, is called a *feasible* diet.

What is the goal of the diet decision? It would be an appropriate use of ordinary language to say that the goal is to minimize the cost of obtaining an adequate diet, for the condition (4) is the criterion we are minimizing. This criterion puts the emphasis on economy as the goal.

Alternatively, we might direct our attention primarily to the constraints, and in particular to the nutritional requirements (2). Then we might say that the goal is to find a nutritionally satisfactory diet that is economical. Although we still mention costs in this statement, we have clearly shifted the emphasis to the adequacy of the diet from a nutritional standpoint. The primary goal has now become good nutrition.

The relation between the criterion function (4) and the constraints (2) can be made even more symmetrical. Let us replace the criterion (4) with a new constraint:

(5) $\Sigma \, x_i p_i \leqq k,$

that is to say, with the requirement that the total cost of the diet not exceed some constant, k. Now the set of feasible diets has been restricted to those that satisfy (5) as well as (2) and (3). But since the minimization condition has been removed, there is apparently no basis for choosing one of these diets over another.

Under some circumstances, we can, however, restrict the set of diets that deserve consideration to a subset of the feasible set. Suppose that all the nutritional constraints (2) are minimal constraints, and that we would always prefer, *ceteris paribus*, a greater amount of any nutritional factor to a smaller amount. We will say that diet A is dominated by diet B if the cost of diet B is no greater than the cost of diet A, and if diet B contains at least as much of each nutritional factor as does diet A, and more of at least one factor. We will call the set of diets in the feasible set that is undominated by other diets in that set the Pareto optimal set.

Our preference for one or the other of the diets in the Pareto optimal set will depend on the relative importance we assign to cost in comparison with amounts of nutritional factors, and to the amounts of these factors in relation with each other. If cost is the most important factor, then we will again choose the diet that is selected by criterion (4). On the other hand, if we attach great importance to nutritional factor j, we will generally choose a quite different feasible diet—one in which the quantity of factor j is as great as possible. Within the limits set by the constraints, it would be quite reasonable to call whatever criterion led us to select a particular member of the Pareto optimal set our goal. But if the constraints are strong enough, so that the feasible set and, *a fortiori,* the Pareto optimal set is very small, then the constraints will have as much or more influence on what diet we finally select than will the goal, so defined. For example, if we set one or more of the nutritional requirements very high, so that only a narrow range of diets also satisfy the budget constraint (5), then introducing the cost minimization criterion as the final selection rule will have relatively little effect on what diet we choose.

Under such circumstances it might be well to give up the idea that the decision situation can be described in terms of a simple goal. Instead, it would be more reasonable to speak of a whole set of goals—the whole set, in fact, of nutritional and budgetary constraints—that the decision maker is trying to attain. To paraphrase a familiar epigram: "If you allow me to determine the constraints, I don't care who selects the optimization criterion."

MULTIPLE CRITERIA IN ORGANIZATIONS

To show the organizational relevance of our example it is only necessary to suppose that the decision we are discussing has arisen within a business firm that manufactures commercial stock feeds, that the nutritional requirements are requirements for hogs and the prices those of available feed ingredients, and that the finished feed prices facing the firm are fixed. Then minimizing the cost of feed meeting certain nutritional standards is identical with maximizing the profit from selling feed meeting those standards. Cost minimization represents the profit-maximizing goal of the company.

We can equally well say that the goal of the feed company is to provide its customers with the best feed possible, in terms of nutritional standards, at a given price, i.e., to produce feeds that are in the Pareto optimal set. Presumably this is what industry spokesmen mean when they say that the goal of business is not profit but efficient production of goods and services. If we had enlarged our model to give some of the prices that appear in it the status of constraints, instead of fixing them as constants, we could have introduced other goals, for example, the goal of suppliers' profits, or, if there were a labor input, the goal of high wages.[4]

We may summarize the discussion to this point as follows. In the decision-making situations of real life, a course of action, to be acceptable, must satisfy a whole set of requirements, or constraints. Sometimes one of these requirements is singled out and referred to as the goal of the action. But the choice of one of the constraints, from many, is to a large extent arbitrary. For many purposes it is more meaningful to refer to the whole set of requirements as the (complex) goal of the action. This conclusion applies both to individual and organizational decision making.

SEARCH FOR A COURSE OF ACTION

Thus far, we have assumed that the set of possible actions is known in advance to the decision maker. In many, if not most, real-life situations, possible courses of action must be discovered, designed, or synthesized. In the process of searching for a satisfactory solution, the goals of the action—that is, the constraints that must be satisfied by the solution—may play a guiding role in two ways. First, the goals may be used directly to synthesize proposed solutions (*alternative generation*). Second, the goals may be used to test the satisfactoriness of a proposed solution (*alternative testing*).[5]

We may illustrate these possibilities by considering what goes on in the mind of a chess player when he is trying to choose a move in a game. One requirement of a good move is that it put pressure on the opponent by attacking him in some way or by preparing an attack. This requirement suggests possible moves to an experienced player (alternative generation). For example, if the opponent's king is not well protected, the player will search for moves that attack the king, but after a possible move has been generated in this way (and thus automatically satisfies the requirement that it put pressure on the opponent), it must be tested against other requirements (alternative testing). For example, it will not be satisfactory if it permits a counterattack that is more potent than the attack or that can be carried out more quickly.

The decisions of everyday organizational life are similar to these decisions in chess. A bank officer who is investing trust funds in stocks and bonds may, because of the terms of the trust document, take as his goal increasing the capital value of the fund. This will lead him to consider buying common stock in firms in growth industries (alternative generation). But he will check each possible purchase against other requirements: that the firm's financial structure be sound, its past earnings record satisfactory, and so on (alternative testing). All these considerations can be counted among his goals in constructing the portfolio, but some of the goals serve as generators of possible portfolios, others as checks.[6]

The process of designing courses of action provides us, then, with another source of asymmetry between the goals that guide the actual synthesis and the constraints that determine whether possible courses of action are in fact feasible. In general, the search will continue until one decision in the feasible set is found, or, at most, a very few alternatives. Which member of the feasible set is discovered and selected may depend considerably on the search process, that is, on which requirements serve as goals or generators, in the sense just defined, and which as constraints or tests.

In a multiperson situation, one man's goals may be another man's constraints. The feed manufacturer may seek to produce feed as cheaply as possible, searching, for example, for possible new ingredients. The feed, however, has to meet certain nutritional specifications. The hog farmer may seek the best quality of feed, searching, for example, for new manufacturers. The feed, however, cannot cost more than his funds allow; if it is too expensive, he must cut quality or quantity. A sale will be made when a lot of feed is feasible in terms of the requirements of both manufacturer and farmer. Do manufacturer and farmer have the same goals? In one sense, clearly not, for there is a definite conflict of interest between them: the farmer wishes to buy cheap, the manufacturer to sell dear. On the other hand, if a bargain can be struck that meets the requirements of both—if the feasible set that satisfies both sets of constraints is not empty—then there is another sense in which they do have a common goal. In the limiting case of perfect competition, the constraints imposed by the market and the technology actually narrow down the feasible set to a single point, determining uniquely the quantity of goods they will exchange and the price.

The neatness and definiteness of the limiting case of perfect competition should not blind us to the fact that most real-life situations do not fit this case exactly. Typically, the generation of alternatives (e.g., product invention, development, and design) is a laborious, costly process. Typically, also, there is a practically unlimited sea of potential alternatives. A river valley development plan that aims at the generation of electric power, subject to appropriate provision for irrigation, flood control, and recreation will generally look quite different from a plan that aims at flood control, subject to appropriate provision for the other goals mentioned. Even though the plans generated in both cases will be examined for their suitability along the dimensions mentioned, it is almost certain that quite different plans will be devised and proposed for consideration in the two cases, and that the plans finally selected will represent quite distinct points in the feasible set.

In later paragraphs we shall state some reasons for supposing that the total sets of constraints considered by decision makers in different parts of an organization are likely to be quite similar, but that different decision makers are likely to divide the constraints between generators and tests in quite different ways. Under these circumstances, if we use the phrase organization goals broadly to denote the constraint sets, we will conclude that organizations do, indeed, have goals (widely shared constraint sets). If we use the phrase organization goals narrowly to denote the generators, we will conclude that there is little communality of goals among the several parts of large organizations and that subgoal formation and goal conflict are prominent and significant features of organizational life. The distinction we have made between generators and tests helps resolve this ambiguity, but also underlines the importance of always making explicit which sense of goal is intended.

MOTIVATION FOR GOALS

If by motivation we mean whatever it is that causes someone to follow a particular course of action, then every action is motivated—by definition. But in most human behavior the relation between motives and action is not simple; it is mediated by a whole chain of events and surrounding conditions.

We observe a man scratching his arm. His motive (or goal)? To relieve an itch.

We observe a man reaching into a medicine cabinet. His motive (or goal)? To get a bottle of lotion that, his wife has assured him, is very effective in relieving the itch of mosquito bites. Or have we misstated his motive? Is it to apply the lotion to his arm? Or, as before, to relieve the itch? But the connection between action and goal is much more complex in this case than in the previous one. There intervenes between them a means-end chain (get bottle, apply lotion, relieve itch), an expectation (that the lotion will relieve the itch), and a social belief supporting the expectation (that the wife's assurance is a reliable predictor of the lotion's efficacy). The relation between the action and the ultimate goal has become highly indirect and contingent, even in this simple case. Notice that these new complications of indirectness are super-imposed on the complications we have discussed earlier—that the goal is pursued only within limits imposed by numerous side constraints (don't knock over the other bottles in the medicine cabinet, don't brush against the fresh paint, and so on).

Our point is identical with the point of the venerable story of the three bricklayers who were asked what they were doing. "Laying bricks," "Building a wall," "Helping to erect a great cathedral," were their respective answers. The investment trust officer whose behavior we considered earlier could answer in any of these modes, or others. "I am trying to select a stock for this investment portfolio." "I am assembling a portfolio that will provide retirement income for my client." "I am employed as in investment trust officer." Now it is the step of indirectness between the second and third answers that has principal interest for organization theory. The investment trust officer presumably has no "personal" interest in the retirement income of his client, only a "professional" interest in his role as trust officer and bank employee. He does have, on the other hand, a personal interest in maintaining that role and that employment status.

ROLE BEHAVIOR

Of course, in real life the line of demarcation between personal and professional interests is not a sharp one, for personal satisfactions may arise from the competent performance of a professional role, and both personal satisfactions and dissatisfactions may result from innumerable conditions that surround the employment. Nevertheless, it is exceedingly important, as a first approximation, to distinguish between the answers to two questions of motive: "Why do you keep (or take) this job?" and "Why do you make this particular investment decision?" The first question is properly answered in terms of the personal motives or goals of the occupant of the role, the second question in terms of goals that define behavior appropriate to the role itself.

Corresponding to this subdivision of goals into personal and role-defined goals, organization theory is sometimes divided into two subparts: (1) a theory of motivation explaining the decisions of people to participate in and remain in organizations; and (2) a theory of decision making within organizations comprised of such people.[7]

In the motivational theory formulated by Barnard and me, it is postulated that the motives of each group of participants can be divided into *inducements* (aspects of participation that are desired by the participants) and *contributions* (aspects of participation that are inputs to the organization's production function but that generally have negative utility to participants). Each participant is motivated to maximize, or at least increase, his inducements while decreasing his contributions, and this motivation is a crucial consideration in explaining the decision to join (or remain). But "joining" means accepting an organizational role, and hence we do not need any additional motivational assumptions beyond those of inducements-contributions theory to explain the ensuing role-enacting behavior.

I hasten to repeat the caveat, introduced a few paragraphs above, that in thus separating our consideration of organizational role-enacting behavior from our consideration of personal motivation—allowing the decision to join as the only bridge between them—we are proposing an abstraction from the complexities of real life. A good deal of the significant research on human relations and informal organization, which has contributed heavily in the last generation to our understanding of organizational behavior, has been concerned specifically with the phenomena that this abstraction excludes. Thus, desire for power and concern for personal advancement represent an intrusion of personal goals upon organizational role, as do the social and craft satisfactions and dissatisfactions associated with work.

To say that the abstraction is sometimes untenable is not to deny that there may be many situations in which it is highly useful. There are, first of all, many organizational decisions that simply do not affect personal motives at all—where organizational goals and personal goals are orthogonal, so to speak. As a trivial example, the secretary's inducement-contribution balance is generally in no whit affected by the choice between typing a letter to A or a letter to B or by the content of the letter. Second, personal motives may enter the decision process as fixed constraints (only courses of action that satisfy the constraints are considered, but the constraints have no influence on the choice of action within the set). Thus, the terms of the employment contract may limit work to a forty-hour week but may have little to say about what goes on during the forty hours.[8]

The abstraction of organizational role from personal goals turns out to be particularly useful in studying the cognitive aspects of organizational decision making, for the abstraction is consonant with some known facts about human cognitive processes. Of all the knowledge, attitudes, and values stored in a human memory, only a very small fraction are evoked in a given concrete situation. Thus, an individual can assume a wide variety of roles when these are evoked by appropriate circumstances, each of which may interact only weakly with the others. At one time he may be a father, at another a machinist, at another a chess player. Current information processing theories of human cognition postulate that there is only modest overlap of the subsets of memory contents—information and programs—that are evoked by these several roles. Thus, we might postulate that the day-to-day organizational environment evokes quite different associations out of the memory of the participant from those evoked when he is considering a change of jobs. To the extent this is so, it provides a further explanation of why his "personal" system of inducements and contributions, i.e., the utilities that enter into the latter decisions, will have no effect on his "organizational" decisions, i.e., those that are made while the first set is evoked.

The ability of a single individual to shift from one role to another as a function of the environment in which he finds himself thus helps explain the extent to which organizational goals become internalized, that is, are automatically evoked and applied during performance of the role. By whatever means the individual was originally motivated to adopt the role in the first place, the goals and constraints appropriate to the role become a part of the decision-making program, stored in his memory, that defines his role behavior.

INTERPERSONAL DIFFERENCES

Although the considerations introduced in the last section show that the uncoupling of organizational role from personal goals need not be complete, it may be useful to indicate a little more specifically how differences among individuals can affect their behavior in roles that are identical from an organizational standpoint.

A role must be understood not as a specific, stereotyped set of behaviors, but as a *program* (as that word is understood in computer technology) for determining the courses of action to be taken over the range of circumstances that arise. In previous sections we have given examples of such programs and have shown that they can be highly complex; for instance, a single decision may be a function of a large number of program instructions or premises.

Thus, while we may conceive of an ideal type of role that incorporates only organizational goals among its premises, the roles that members of organizations actually enact invariably incorporate both organizational and personal goals. We have already seen how both can be part of the total system of constraints.

But interpersonal differences in the enactment of roles go far beyond the incorporation of personal goals in the role. Role behavior depends on means-end premises as well as goal premises. Thus, particular professional training may provide an individual with specific techniques and knowledge for solving problems (accounting techniques, legal techniques, and so on), which are then drawn upon as part of the program evoked by his role. In this way, a chief executive with an accounting background may find different problem solutions from a chief executive, in the same position, with a legal background.

An individual may incorporate in his role not only a professional style but also a personal style. He may bring to the role, for example, habits and beliefs that provide him with crucial premises for his handling of interpersonal relations. Thus, an authoritarian personality will behave quite differently from a more permissive person when both are in the same organizational role and pursuing the same organizational goals.

The leeway for the expression of individual differences in role behavior is commonly narrowest in the handling of those matters that come to the role occupant at the initiative of others and is commonly broadest in his exercise of initiative and in selecting those discretionary matters to which he will attend and give priority. In terms used in earlier paragraphs, premises supplied by the organizational environment generally control alternative selection more closely than alternative generation.

THE ORGANIZATIONAL DECISION-MAKING SYSTEM

Let us limit ourselves for the present to situations where occupational roles are almost completely divorced from personal goals and pursue the implications of this factoring of the behavior of organizational participants into its personal and organizational components. If we now consider the organizational decision-making programs of all the participants, together with the connecting flow of communication, we can assemble them into a composite description of the organizational decision-making system—a system that has been largely abstracted from the individual motives that determine participation.

In the simplest case, of a small, relatively unspecialized organization, we are back to a decision-making situation not unlike that of the optimal diet problem. The language of "goals," "requirements," "constraints," that we applied there is equally applicable to similarly uncomplicated organizational situations.

In more complicated cases, abstracting out the organizational decision-making system from personal motives does not remove all aspects of interpersonal (more accurately, interrole) difference from the decision-making process. For when many persons in specialized roles participate in making an organization's decisions, the total system is not likely to be monolithic in structure. Individual roles will differ with respect to the number and kinds of communications they receive and the parts of the environment from which they receive them. They will differ with respect to the evaluative communications they receive from other roles. They will differ in their search programs. Hence, even within our abstraction, which neglects personal motives, we can accommodate the phenomena of differential perception and subgoal formation.

To make our discussion more specific, let us again consider a specific example of an organizational decision-making system—in this case a system for controlling inventory and production. We suppose a factory in which decisions have to be made about (1) the aggregate rate of production, that is, the work force that will be employed and the hours employees will work each week, (2) the allocation of aggregate production facilities among the several products the factory makes, and (3) the scheduling of the sequence in which the individual products will be handled on the production facilities. Let us call these the aggregate production decision, item allocation decision, and scheduling decision, respectively. The three sets of decisions may be made by different roles in the organization; in general, we would expect the aggregate decision to be handled at more central levels than the others. The real world situation will always include complications beyond those we have described, for it will involve decisions with respect to shipments to warehouses, decisions as to which products to hold in warehouse inventories, and many others.

Now we could conceive of an omniscient Planner (the entrepreneur of classical economic theory) who, by solving a set of simultaneous equations, would make each and all of these interrelated decisions. Decision problems of this kind have been widely studied during the past decade by management scientists, with the result that we now know a great deal about the mathematical structures of the problems and the magnitude of the computations that would be required to solve them. We know, in particular, that discovery of the optimal solution of a complete problem of this kind is well beyond the powers of existing or prospective computational equipment.

In actual organizational practice, no one attempts to find an optimal solution for the whole problem. Instead, various particular decisions, or groups of decisions, within the whole complex are made by specialized members or units of the organization. In making these particular decisions, the specialized units do not solve the whole problem, but find a "satisfactory" solution for one or more subproblems, where some of the effects of the solution on other parts of the system are incorporated in the definition of "satisfactory."

For example, standard costs may be set as constraints for a manufacturing executive. If he finds that his operations are not meeting those constraints, he will search for ways of lowering his costs. Longer production runs may occur to him as a means for accomplishing this end. He can achieve longer production runs if the number of style variations in product is reduced, so he proposes product standardization as a solution to his cost problem. Presumably he will not implement the solution until he has tested it against constraints introduced by the sales department—

objections that refusal to meet special requirements of customers will lose sales.

Anyone familiar with organizational life can multiply examples of this sort, where different problems will come to attention in different parts of the organization, or where different solutions will be generated for a problem, depending on where it arises in the organization. The important point to be noted here is that we do not have to postulate conflict in personal goals or motivations in order to explain such conflicts or discrepancies. They could, and would, equally well arise if each of the organizational decision-making roles were being enacted by digital computers, where the usual sort of personal limits on the acceptance of organizational roles would be entirely absent. The discrepancies arise out of the cognitive inability of the decision makers to deal with the entire problem as a set of simultaneous relations, each to be treated symmetrically with the others.[9]

An aspect of the division of decision-making labor that is common to virtually all organizations is the distinction between the kinds of general, aggregative decisions that are made at high levels of the organization, and the kinds of specific, item-by-item decisions that are made at low levels. We have already alluded to this distinction in the preceding example of a system for controlling inventory and production. When executives at high levels in such a system make decisions about "aggregate inventory," this mode of factoring the decision-making problem already involves radical simplification and approximation. For example, there is no single, well-defined total cost associated with a given total value of aggregate inventories. There will generally be different costs associated with each of the different kinds of items that make up the inventory (for example, different items may have different spoilage rates or obsolescence rates), and different probabilities and costs associated with stock-outs of each kind of item. Thus, a given aggregate inventory will have different costs depending on its composition in terms of individual items.

To design a system for making decisions about the aggregate work force, production rate, and inventories requires an assumption that the aggregate inventory will never depart very far from a typical composition in terms of individual item types. The assumption is likely to be tolerable because subsidiary decisions are continually being made at other points in the organization about the inventories of individual items. These subsidiary decisions prevent the aggregate inventory from becoming severely unbalanced, hence make averages meaningful for the aggregate.

The assumption required for aggregation is not unlike that made by an engineer when he controls the temperature of a tank of water, with a single thermometer as indicator, knowing that sufficient mixing of the liquid in the tank is going on to maintain a stable pattern of temperature relations among its parts. Without such a stable pattern it would be infeasible to control the process by means of a measurement of the average temperature.

If one set of decisions is made, on this approximate basis, about aggregate work force, production rate, and inventories, then these decisions can be used as constraints in making detailed decisions at subsidiary levels about the inventory or production of particular items. If the aggregate decision has been reached to make one million gallons of paint next month, then other decisions can be reached as to how much paint of each kind to make, subject to the constraint that the production quotas for the individual items should, when added together, total one million gallons.[10]

This simple example serves to elucidate how the whole mass of decisions that are continually being made in a complex organization can be viewed as an organized system. They constitute a system in which (1) particular decision-making processes are aimed at finding courses of action that are feasible or satisfactory in the light of multiple goals and constraints, and (2) decisions reached in any one part of the organization enter as goals or constraints into the decisions being made in other parts of the organization.

There is no guarantee that the decisions reached will be optimal with respect to any over-all organizational goal. The system is a loosely coupled one. Nevertheless, the results of the over-all system can be measured against one or more organizational goals, and changes can be made in the decision-making structure when these results are adjudged unsatisfactory.

Further, if we look at the decision-making structure in an actual organization, we see that it is usually put together in such a way as to insure that the decisions made by specialized units will be made in cognizance of the more general goals. Individual units are linked to the total system by production schedules, systems of rewards and penalties based on cost and profit goals, inventory limits, and so on. The loose coupling among the parts has the positive consequence of permitting specific constraints in great variety to be imposed on subsystems without rendering their decision-making mechanisms inoperative.

THE DECISION-MAKING SYSTEM AND ORGANIZATIONAL BEHAVIOR

In the previous sections great pains were taken to distinguish the goals and constraints (inducements and contributions) that motivate people to accept organizational roles from the goals and constraints that enter into their decision making when they are enacting those organizational roles. On the one hand, the system of personal inducements and contributions imposes constraints that the organization must satisfy if it is to survive. On the other hand, the constraints incorporated in the organizational roles, hence in what I have called here the organizational decision-making system, are the constraints that a course of action must satisfy in order for the organization to adopt it.

There is no necessary *logical* connection between these two sets of constraints. After all, organizations sometimes fail to survive, and their demise can often be attributed to failure to incorporate all the important motivational concerns of participants among the constraints in the organizational decision-making system. For example, a major cause of small business failure is working capital shortage, a result of failure to constrain actions to those that are consistent with creditors' demands for prompt payment. Similarly, new products often fail because incorrect assumptions about the inducements important to consumers are reflected in the constraints that guide product design. (It is widely believed that the troubles of the Chrysler Corporation stemmed from the design premise that car purchasers were primarily interested in buying a good piece of machinery.)

In general, however, there is a strong empirical connection between the two sets of constraints, for the organizations we will usually observe in the real world—those that have succeeded in surviving for some time—will be precisely those which have developed organizational decision-making systems whose constraints guarantee that their actions maintain a favorable balance of inducements to contributions for their participants. The argument, an evolutionary one, is the same one we can apply to biological organisms. There is no logical requirement that the temperatures, oxygen concentrations, and so on, maintained in the tissues of a bird by its physiological processes should lie within the ranges required for its survival. It is simply that we will not often have opportunities for observing birds whose physiological regulators do not reflect these external constraints. Such birds are soon extinct.[11]

Thus, what the sociologists calls the functional requisites for survival can usually give us good clues for predicting organizational goals; however, if the functional requisites resemble the goals, the similarity is empirical, not definitional. What the goals are must be inferred from observation of the organization's decision-making processes, whether these processes be directed toward survival or suicide.

CONCLUSIONS

We can now summarize our answers to the question that introduced this paper: What is the meaning of the phrase "organizational goal"? First, we discovered that it is doubtful whether decisions are generally directed toward achieving *a* goal. It is easier, and clearer, to view decisions as being concerned with discovering courses of action that satisfy a whole set of constraints. It is this set, and not any one of its members, that is most accurately viewed as the goal of the action.

If we select any of the constraints for special attention, it is (a) because of its relation to the motivations of the decision maker, or (b) because of its relation to the search process that is generating or designing particular courses of action. Those constraints that motivate the decision maker and those that guide his search for actions are sometimes regarded as more "goal-like" than those that limit the actions he may consider or those that are used to test whether a potential course of action he has designed is satisfactory. Whether we treat all the constraints symmetrically or refer to some asymmetrically as goals is largely a matter of linguistic or analytic convenience.

When we come to organizational decisions, we observe that many, if not most, of the constraints that define a satisfactory course of action are associated with an organizational role and hence only indirectly with the personal motives of the individual who assumes that role. In this situation it is convenient to use the phrase organization goal to refer to constraints, or sets of constraints, imposed by the organizational role, which has only this indirect relation to the motives of the decision makers.

If we examine the constraint set of an organizational decision-making system, we will generally find that it contains constraints that reflect virtually all the inducements and contributions important to various classes of participants. These constraints tend to remove from consideration possible courses of action that are inimical to survival. They do not, of course, by themselves, often fully determine the course of action.

In view of the hierarchical structure that is typical of most formal organizations, it is a reasonable use of language to employ organizational goal to refer particularly to the constraint sets and criteria of search that define roles at the upper levels. Thus it is reasonable to speak of conservation of forest resources as a principal goal of the U.S. Forest Service, or reducing fire losses as a principal goal of a city fire department. For high-level executives in these organizations will seek out and support actions that advance these goals, and subordinate employees will do the same or will at least tailor their choices to constraints established by the higher echelons with this end in view.

Finally, since there are large elements of decentralization in the decision making in any large organization, different constraints may define the decision problems of different positions or specialized units. For example, "profit" may not enter directly into the decision making of most members of a business organization. Again, this does not mean that it is improper or meaningless to regard profit as a principal goal of the business. It simply means that the decision-making mechanism is a loosely coupled system in which the profit constraint is only one among a number of constraints and enters into most subsystems only in indirect ways. It would be both legitimate and realistic to describe most business firms as directed toward profit making—subject to a number of side constraints—operating through a network of decision-making processes that introduces many gross approximations into the search for profitable courses of action. Further, the goal ascription does not imply that any employee is motivated by the firm's profit goal, although some may be.

This view of the nature of organization goals leaves us with a picture of organizational decision making that is not simple. But it provides us with an entirely operational way of showing, by describing the structure of the organizational decision-making mechanism, how and to what extent overall goals, like "profit" or "conserving forest resources" help to determine the actual courses of action that are chosen.

REFERENCES

2 The present discussion is generally compatible with, but not identical to, that of my colleagues, R. M. Cyert and J. G. March, who discuss organizational goals in ch. iii of *A Behavioral Theory of the Firm* (Englewood Cliffs, N.J., 1963). Their analysis is most germane to the paragraphs of this paper that treat of motivation for goals and organizational survival.

3 There are now a substantial number of elementary discussions of linear programming in the management science literature. For a treatment that develops the point of view proposed here, see A. Charnes and W. W. Cooper, *Management Models and Industrial Applications of Linear Programming* (New York, 1961), ch. i. See also Charnes and Cooper, Deterministic Equivalents for Optimizing and Satisfying under Chance Constraints, *Operations Research,* 11 (1963), 18–39.

4 See "A Comparison of Organization Theories," in my *Models of Man* (New York, 1957), pp. 170–182.

5 For further discussion of the role of generators and tests in decision making and problem solving, see A. Newell and H. A. Simon, "The Processes of Creative Thinking," in H. E. Gruber, G. Terrell, and M. Wertheimer, eds., *Contemporary Approaches to Creative Thinking* (New York, 1962), particularly pp. 77–91.

6 G. P. E. Clarkson, "A Model of Trust Investment Behavior," in Cyert and March, *op. cit.*

7 For further discussion and references, see J. G. March and H. A. Simon, *Organizations* (New York, 1958), ch. iv.

8 See "A Formal Theory of Employment Relation," in *Models of Man,* op. cit.

9 For some empirical evidence, see D. C. Dearborn and H. A. Simon, Selective Perception: A Note on the Departmental Identification of Executives, *Sociometry,* 21 (1958), 140–144.

10 A system of this kind is developed in detail in "Determining Production Quantities under Aggregate Constraints," in C. Holt, F. Modigliani, J. Muth, and H. A. Simon, *Planning Production, Inventories, and Work Force* (Englewood Cliffs, N.J., 1960).

11 The relation between the functional requisites for survival and the actual constraints of the operating system is a central concept in W. R. Ashby's notion of a multistable system. See his *Design for a Brain* (2d ed.; New York, 1960).

SELECTION 7

Power and Politics in Organizational Life*

Abraham Zaleznik

How the limitations of businessmen, in their cognitive and emotional capacities, play a major role in decision making

There are few business activities more prone to a credibility gap than the way in which executives approach organizational life. A sense of disbelief occurs when managers purport to make decisions in rationalistic terms while most observers and participants know that personalities and politics play a significant if not an overriding role. Where does the error lie? In the theory which insists that decisions should be rationalistic and nonpersonal? Or in the practice which treats business organizations as political structures?

Whatever else organizations may be (problem-solving instruments, sociotechnical systems, reward systems, and so on), they are political structures. This means that organizations operate by distributing authority and setting a stage for the exercise of power. It is no wonder, therefore, that individuals who are highly motivated to secure and use power find a familiar and hospitable environment in business.

At the same time, executives are reluctant to acknowledge the place of power both in individual motivation and in organizational relationships. Somehow, power and politics are dirty words. And in linking these words to the play of personalities in organizations, some managers withdraw into the safety of organizational logics.

As I shall suggest in this article, frank recognition of the importance of personality factors and a sensitive use of the strengths and limitations of people in decisions on power distributions can improve the quality of organizational life.

POLITICAL PYRAMID

Organizations provide a power base for individuals. From a purely economic standpoint, organizations exist to create a surplus of income over costs by meeting needs in the marketplace. But organizations also are

* From *Harvard Business Review*, May–June, 1970.

political structures which provide opportunities for people to develop careers and therefore provide platforms for the expression of individual interests and motives. The development of careers, particularly at high managerial and professional levels, depends on accumulation of power as the vehicle for transforming individual interests into activities which influence other people.

Scarcity and Competition

A political pyramid exists when people compete for power in an economy of scarcity. In other words, people cannot get the power they want just for the asking. Instead, they have to enter into the decisions on how to distribute authority in a particular formal organization structure. Scarcity of power arises under two sets of conditions:

1. Where individuals gain power in absolute terms at someone else's expense.

2. Where there is a gain comparatively—not literally at someone else's expense—resulting in a relative shift in the distribution of power. In either case, the psychology of scarcity and comparison takes over. The human being tends to make comparisons as a basis for his sense of self-esteem. He may compare himself with other people, and decide that his absolute loss or the shift in proportional shares of authority reflects an attrition in his power base. He may also compare his position relative to others against a personal standard and feel a sense of loss. This tendency to compare is deeply ingrained in people, especially since they experience early in life the effects of comparisons in the family where—in an absolute sense— time and attention, if not love and affection, go to the most dependent member.

Corporate acquisitions and mergers illustrate the effects of both types of comparisons. In the case of one merger, the president of the acquired company resigned rather than accept the relative displacement in rank which occurred when he no longer could act as a chief executive officer. Two vice presidents vied for the position of executive vice president. Because of their conflicting ambitions, the expedient of making them equals drove the competition underground, but not for long. The vice president with the weaker power base soon resigned in the face of his inability to consolidate a workable definition of his responsibilities. His departure resulted in increased powers for the remaining vice president and the gradual elimination of "rival camps" which had been covertly identified with the main contenders for power.

The fact that organizations are pyramids produces a scarcity of positions the higher one moves in the hierarchy. This scarcity, coupled with inequalities, certainly needs to be recognized. While it may be humane and socially desirable to say that people are different rather than unequal in their potential, nevertheless executive talent is in short supply. The end result should be to move the more able people into the top positions and to accord them the pay, responsibility, and authority to match their potential.

On the other side, the strong desires of equally able people for the few top positions available means that someone will either have to face the realization of unfulfilled ambition or have to shift his interest to another organization.[1]

Constituents and Clients

Besides the conditions of scarcity and competition, politics in organizations grows out of the existence of constituencies. A superior may be content himself with shifts in the allocation of resources and consequently power, but he represents subordinates who, for their own reasons, may be unhappy with the changes. These subordinates affirm and support their boss. They can also withdraw affirmation and support, and consequently isolate the superior with all the painful consequences this entails.

While appointments to positions come from above, affirmation of position comes from below. The only difference between party and organizational politics is in the subtlety of the voting procedure. Consider:

In a large consumer products corporation, one division received almost no capital funds for expansion while another division, which had developed a new marketing approach for products common to both, expanded dramatically. The head of the static division found his power diminished considerably, as reflected in how seriously his subordinates took his efforts at influence (e.g., in programs to increase the profit return from existing volume).

He initiated one program after another with little support from subordinates because he could not make a claim for capital funds. The flow of capital funds in this corporation provided a measure of power gains and losses in both an absolute and a relative sense.

Power and Action

Still another factor which heightens the competition for power that is characteristic of all political structures is the incessant need to use whatever power one possesses. Corporations have an implicit "banking" system in power transactions. The initial "capitalization" which makes up an individual's power base consists of three elements:

1. The quantity of formal authority vested in his position relative to other positions.

2. The authority vested in his expertise and reputation for competence (a factor weighted by how important the expertise is for the growth areas of the corporation as against the historically stable areas of its business).

3. The attractiveness of his personality to others (a combination of respect for him as well as liking, although these two sources of attraction are often in conflict).

This capitalization of power reflects the total esteem with which others regard the individual. By a process which is still not too clear, the individual internalizes all of the sources of power capital in a manner parallel to the way he develops a sense of self-esteem. The individual knows he has power, assesses it realistically, and is willing to risk his personal esteem to influence others.

A critical element here is the risk in the uses of power. The individual must perform *and* get results. If he fails to do either, an attrition occurs in his power base in direct proportion to the doubts other people entertained in their earlier appraisals of him.

What occurs here is an erosion of confidence which ultimately leads the individual to doubt himself and undermines the psychological work which led him in the first place to internalize authority as a prelude to action. (While, as I have suggested, the psychological work that an individual goes through to consolidate his esteem capital is a crucial aspect of power relations, I shall have to reserve careful examination of this problem until a later date. The objective now is to examine from a political framework the problems of organizational life.)

What distinguishes alterations in the authority structure from other types of organizational change is their direct confrontation with the political character of corporate life. Such confrontations are real manipulations of power as compared with the indirect approaches which play on ideologies and attitudes. In the first case, the potency and reality of shifts in authority have an instantaneous effect on what people do, how they interact, and how they think about themselves. In the second case, the shifts in attitude are often based on the willingness of people to respond the way authority figures want them to; ordinarily, however, these shifts in attitude are but temporary expressions of compliance.

One of the most common errors executives make is to confuse compliance with commitment. Compliance is an attitude of acceptance when a directive from an authority figure asks for a change in an individual's position, activities, or ideas. The individual complies or "goes along" usually because he is indifferent to the scope of the directive and the changes it proposes. If compliance occurs out of indifference, then one can predict little difficulty in translating the intent of directives into actual implementation.[2]

Commitment, on the other hand, represents a strong motivation on the part of an individual to adopt or resist the intent of a directive. If the individual commits himself to a change, then he will use his ingenuity to interpret and implement the change in such a way as to assure its success. If he decides to fight or block the change, the individual may act as if he complies but reserve other times and places to negate the effects of directives. For example:

□ In one large company, the top management met regularly for purposes of organizational planning. The executives responsible for implementing planning decisions could usually be counted on to carry them out when they had fought hard and openly in the course of reaching such decisions. When they seemed to accept a decision, giving all signs of compliance, the decision usually ended up as a notation in the minutes. Surface compliance occurred most frequently when problems involved loyalties to subordinates.

In one instance, a division head agreed to accept a highly regarded executive from another division to meet a serious manpower shortage in his organization. When the time came to effect the transfer, however, this division general manager refused, with some justification, on the grounds that bringing someone in from outside would demoralize his staff. He used compliance initially to respond to the problem of "family" loyalties to which he felt committed. Needless to say, the existence of these loyalties was the major problem to be faced in carrying out organizational planning.

Compliance as a tactic to avoid changes and commitment as an expression of strong motivation in dealing with organizational problems are in turn related to how individuals define their interests. In the power relations among executives, the so-called areas of common interest are usually reserved for the banalities of human relationships. The more significant areas of attention usually force conflicts of interest, especially competition for power, to the surface.

INTEREST CONFLICTS

Organizations demand, on the one hand, cooperative endeavor and commitment to common purposes. The realities of experience in organizations, on the other hand, show that conflicts of interest exist among people who ultimately share a common fate and are supposed to work together. What makes business more political and less ideological and rationalistic is the overriding importance of conflicts of interest.

If an individual (or group) is told that his job scope is reduced in either absolute or proportional terms for *the good of the corporation,* he faces a conflict. Should he acquiesce for the idea of common good or fight in the service of his self-interest? Any rational man will fight (how constructively depends on the absence of neurotic conflicts and on ego strength). His willingness to fight increases as he comes to realize the intangible nature of what people think is good for the organization. And, in point of fact, his willingness may serve the interests of corporate purpose by highlighting issues and stimulating careful thinking before the reaching of final decisions.

Secondary Effects

Conflicts of interest in the competition for resources are easily recognized, as for example, in capital budgeting or in allocating money for research and development. But these conflicts can be subjected to bargaining procedures which all parties to the competition validate by their participation.

The secondary effects of bargaining do involve organizational and power issues. However, the fact that these power issues *follow* debate on economic problems rather than *lead* it creates a manifest content which can be objectified much more readily than in areas where the primary considerations are the distributions of authority.

In such cases, which include developing a new formal organization structure, management succession, promotions, corporate mergers, and entry of new executives, the conflicts of interest are severe and direct simply because there are no objective measures of right or wrong courses of action. The critical question which has to be answered in specific actions is: Who gets power and position? This involves particular people with their strengths and weaknesses and a specific historical context in which actions are understood in symbolic as well as rational terms. To illustrate:

A large corporation, General Motors in fact, inadvertently confirmed what every seasoned executive knows: that coalitions of power to overcome feelings of rivalry and the play of personal ambitions are fragile solutions. The appointment of Edward Cole to the presidency followed by Semon Knudsen's resignation shattered the illusion that the rational processes in business stand apart or even dominate the human emotions and ties that bind men to one another. If any corporation prides itself on rationality, General Motors is it. To have to experience so publicly the inference that major corporate life, particularly at the executive levels, is not so rational after all, can be damaging to the sense of security people get from belief in an idea as it is embodied in a corporate image.

The fact that Knudsen subsequently was discharged from the presidency of Ford (an event I shall discuss later in this article) suggests that personalities and the politics of corporations are less aberrations and more conditions of life in large organizations.

But just as General Motors wants to maintain an image, many executives prefer to ignore what this illustration suggests: that organizations are political structures which feed on the psychology of comparison. To know something about the psychology of comparison takes us into the theory of self-esteem in both its conscious manifestations and its unconscious origins. Besides possibly enlightening us in general and giving a more realistic picture of people and organizations, there are some practical benefits in such knowledge. These benefits include:

○ Increased freedom to act more directly; instead of trying to "get around" a problem, one can meet it.

○ Greater objectivity about people's strengths and limitations, and, therefore, the ability to use them more honestly as well as effectively.

○ More effective planning in organizational design and in distribution of authority; instead of searching for the "one best solution" in organization structure, one accepts a range of alternatives and then gives priority to the personal or emotional concerns that inhibit action.

POWER RELATIONS

Organizational life within a political frame is a series of contradictions. It is an exercise in rationality, but its energy comes from the ideas in the minds of power figures the content of which, as well as their origins, are only dimly perceived. It deals with sources of authority and their distribution; yet it depends in the first place on the existence of a balance of power in the hands of an individual who initiates actions and gets results. It has many rituals associated with it, such as participation, democratization, and the sharing of power; yet the real outcome is the consolidation of power around a central figure to whom other individuals make emotional attachments.

Faulty Coalitions

The formal organization structure implements a coalition among key executives. The forms differ, and the psychological significance of various coalitions also differs. But no organization can function without a consolidation of power in the relationship of a central figure with his select group. The coalition need not exist between the chief executive and his immediate subordinates or staff. It may indeed bypass the second level as in the case of Presidents of the United States who do not build confident relationships within their cabinets, but instead rely on members of the executive staff or on selected individuals outside the formal apparatus.

The failure to establish a coalition within the executive structure of an organization can result in severe problems, such as paralysis in the form of inability to make decisions and to evaluate performance, and in-fighting and overt rivalry within the executive group.

When a coalition fails to develop, the first place to look for causes is the chief executive and his problems in creating confident relationships. The causes are many and complex, but they usually hinge around the nature of the chief executive's defenses and what he needs to avoid as a means of alleviating stress. For example:

☐ The "palace revolt," which led to Semon Knudsen's departure from Ford Motor Company, is an illustration of the failure in the formation of a coalition. While it is true that Henry Ford II named Knudsen president of the company, Knudsen's ultimate power as a newcomer to an established power structure depended on forming an alliance. The particular individual with whom an alliance seemed crucial was Lee Iacocca. For some reason, Knudsen and Iacocca competed for power and influence instead of using cooperatively a power base to which both contributed as is the case with most workable coalitions. In the absence of a coalition, the alternate postures of rivalry and battle for control erupted. Ford ultimately responded by weighing his power with one side over the other.

As I have indicated, it is not at all clear why in Knudsen's case the coalition failed to develop. But in any failure the place to look is in the personalities of the main actors and in the nature of their defenses which make certain coalitions improbable no matter how strongly other realities indicate their necessity.

But defensiveness on the part of a chief executive can also result in building an unrealistic and unworkable coalition, with the self-enforced isolation which is its consequence. One of the most frequently encountered defensive maneuvers which leads to the formation of unrealistic coalitions or to the isolation of the chief executive is the fear of rivalry.

A realistic coalition matches formal authority and competence with the emotional commitments necessary to establish and maintain the coalition. The fear of rivals on the part of chief executives, or the jealousy on the part of subordinates of the chief executive's power, can at the extreme result in paranoid distortions. People become suspicious of one another, and through selective perceptions and projections of their own fantasies create a world of plots and counterplots.

The displacement of personal concerns onto substantive material in decision making is potentially the most dangerous form of defensiveness. The need for defenses arises because people become anxious about the significance of evaluations within existing power coalitions. But perhaps even more basic is the fear and the rivalry to which all coalitions are susceptible given the nature of investments people make in power relations. While it is easy to dismiss emotional reactions like these as neurotic distortions, their prevalence and impact deserve careful attention in all phases of organizational life.

Unconscious Collusions

All individuals and consequently groups experience areas of stress which mobilize defenses. The fact that coalitions embody defensive maneuvers on those occasions where stress goes beyond the usual level of tolerance is not surprising. An even more serious problem, however, occurs when the main force that binds men in a structure is the need to defend against or to act out the conflicts which individuals cannot tolerate alone.

Where coalitions represent the aggregation of power with conscious intention of using the abilities of members for constructive purposes, collusions represent predominance of unconscious conflict and defensive behavior. In organizational life, the presence of collusions and their causes often become the knot which has to be unraveled before any changes can be implemented.

The collusion of latent interests among executives can become the central theme and sustaining force of an organization structure of top management. For a collusion to take hold, the conflicts of the "power figure" have to be communicated and sensed by others as an overriding need which seeks active expression in the form of a theme. The themes vary just as do the structures which make a collusion. Thus one common theme is the need to control; another is the need to be admired and idealized; and still another is the need to find a scapegoat to attack in response to frustrations in solving problems.

If people could hold on to and keep within themselves areas of personal conflict, there would be far fewer collusions in organizational life. But it is part of the human condition for conflicts and needs to take over life situations. As a result, we find numerous instances of collusions controlling the behavior of executives. To illustrate:

☐ A multidivisional corporation found itself with a revolution on its hands. The president was sensitive to the opinions of a few outside board members representing important stockholder interests. He was so concerned that he would be criticized by these board members he demanded from vice presidents full information on their activities and complete loyalty to him. Over a period of years, he moved divisional chief executives to corporate headquarters so he could assure himself of their loyalty. Other executives joined in to gratify the president's need for control and loyalty.

The result of this collusion, however, was to create a schism between headquarters and field operations. Some of the staff members in the field managed to inform the board members of the lack of attention to and understanding of field problems. Discontent grew to such an extent that the board placed the president on early retirement.

Subsequently, the new president, with the support of the board, decentralized authority and appointed new division heads who were to make their offices in divisional headquarters with full authority to manage their respective organizations. One of the lingering problems of the new president was to dissolve the collusion at headquarters without wholesale firing of vice presidents.

Just as power distributions are central to the tasks of organizational planning, so the conservation of power is often the underlying function of collusions. Thus:

□ A manufacturing vice president of a medium-sized company witnessed over a period of 15 years a procession of changes in top management and ownership. He had managed to retain his job because he made himself indispensable in the management of the factory.

To each new top management, he stressed the importance of "home rule" as a means of assuring loyalty and performance in the plant. He also tacitly encouraged each supervisor to go along with whatever cliques happened to form and dominate the shop floor.

However, over time a gradual loss of competitive position, coupled with open conflict among cliques in the form of union disputes, led to the dismissal of the vice president. None of his successors could reassert control over the shop, and the company eventually moved or liquidated many of the operations in this plant.

"LIFE DRAMAS"

Faulty coalitions and unconscious collusions, as I have illustrated, can result from the defensive needs of a chief executive. These needs, which often appear as a demand on others to bolster the self-esteem of the chief executive, are tolerated to a remarkable degree and persist for a long time before harmful effects become apparent to outside stockholders, bankers, or boards of directors which ultimately control the distributions of power in organizations. Occasionally, corporations undergo critical conflicts in organizational politics which cannot be ignored in the conscious deliberations which affect how power gets distributed or used.

Intertwined with the various expressions of power conflicts in organizations are three underlying "life dramas" deserving careful attention:

The *first* portrays stripping the powers of a *parental figure*.

The *second* portrays the predominance of *paranoid thinking*, where distortions of reality result from the surfacing of conflicts which formerly had been contained in collusions.

The *third* portrays a *ritualistic ceremonial* in which real power issues are submerged or isolated in compulsive behavior but at the cost of real problem solving and work.

Parental Figure

The chief executive in a business, along with the heads of states, religious bodies, and social movements, becomes an object for other people. The term "object" should be understood, in a psychological sense, as a person who is the recipient of strong emotional attachments from others. It is obvious that a chief executive is the *object* because he controls so many of the levers which ultimately direct the flow of rewards and punishments. But there is something to say beyond this obvious calculation of rewards and punishments as the basis for the emotional attachments between leader and led as *object* and *subject*.

Where a leader displays unusual attributes in his intuitive gifts, cultivated abilities, or deeper personal qualities, his fate as the *object* is governed by powerful emotions. I hesitate to use the word "charismatic" to describe such a leader, partially because it suggests a mystique but also because, in its reference to the "great" man as charismatic leader, it expands to superhuman proportions what really belongs to the psychology of everyday life.

What makes for strong emotional attachments is as much in the need of the *subject* as in the qualities of the *object*. In other words, the personalities of leaders take on proportions which meet what subordinates need and even demand. If leaders in fact respond with the special charisma that is often invested in them at the outset, then they are parties to a self-fulfilling prophecy. Of course, the qualities demanded have to be present in some nascent form ready to emerge as soon as the emotional currents become real in authority relationships.

The emotional attachments I am referring to usually contain mixtures of positive and negative feelings. If the current were only of one kind, such as either admiration or hostility, then the authority relationship would be simpler to describe as well as to manage. All too often, the way positive feelings blend into the negative sets off secondary currents of emotion which intensify the relationships.

On the one side, subordinates cannot help but have fantasies of what they would do if they held the No. 1 position. Such fantasies, besides providing fleeting pleasures and helping one to regulate his ambitions, also provide channels for imaginative and constructive approaches to solving problems. It is only a short step from imagining what one would do as chief executive to explaining to the real chief executive the ideas which have been distilled from this flight into fantasy. If the chief executive senses envy in back of the thoughts, he may become frightened and choke off ideas which can be used quite constructively.

Critical episode: But suppose a situation arises where not one but several subordinates enjoy the same fantasy of being No. 1? Suppose also that subordinates feel deprived in their relationship with the chief executive? Suppose finally that facing the organization there are substantive problems which are more or less out of control. With these three conditions, and depending on the severity of the real problems besetting the enterprise, the stage is set for a collusion which, when acted out, becomes a critical episode of displacing the parental figure. To demonstrate:

☐ In November 1967, the directors of the Interpublic Group, a $700 million complex in advertising and public relations, moved for the resignation of the leader and chief executive officer, Marion Harper, Jr. Briefly, Harper had managed over a period of 18 years to build the world's largest conglomerate in market services, advertising, and information on the base of a personally successful agency career. In expanding from this base, Harper made acquisitions, started new companies, and widened his orbit into international branches and companies.

As often happens, the innovator and creative person is careless in controlling what he has built so that financial problems become evident. In Harper's case, he appeared either unwilling or unable to recognize the seriousness of his financial problems and, in particular, the significance of allowing cash balances to go below the minimum required in agreements with lending institutions.

Harper seemed careless in another, even more telling, way. Instead of developing a strong coalition among his executive group, he relied on individual ties to him in which he clearly dominated the relationship. If any of the executives "crossed" him, Harper would exile the offender to one of the "remote" branches or place him on partial retirement.

When the financial problems became critical, the aggrieved executives who had once been dependent on Harper and then cast out, formed their own coalition, and managed to garner the votes necessary to, in effect, fire the head man. Although little information is available on the aftermath of this palace revolution, the new coalition had its own problems—which, one would reasonably judge, included contentions for power.

A cynic viewing this illustration of the demise of a parental figure could conclude that if one seeks to maintain power by dominance, then one had best go all the way. This means that to take some but not all of the power away from rebellious sons sets the stage for a cabal among the deprived. With a score to settle, they await only the right circumstances to move in and depose the aggressor.

While this cynical view has its own appeal, it ignores the deeper issues of why otherwise brilliant men fail to recognize the realistic needs for coalitions in the relationships of superior and subordinates. To answer this question, we would need to understand how powerful people operate with massive blind spots which limit vision and the ability to maneuver in the face of realistic problems.

The one purpose that coalitions serve is to guard against the effects of blind spots, since it is seldom the case that two people have identical limitations in their vision and ability to respond. The need to control and dominate in a personalistic sense is perhaps the most serious of all possible blind spots which can affect a chief executive, because he makes it difficult for people to help him, while creating grievances which sooner or later lead to attacks on him.

The unseating of a chief executive by a coalition of subordinates seldom reduces the emotional charge built up in the uncertain attachments to the ousted leader. A new head man has to emerge and establish a confident coalition. Until the contentions for power subside and the guilt reactions attached to deposing the leader dissolve, individuals remain vulnerable to their own blind spots and unconscious reactions to striving for power.

The references to a parental figure in the preceding discussion may appear to exaggerate the meaning of power conflicts. In whatever ways it exaggerates, it also condenses a variety of truths about coalitions among executives. The chief executive is the central *object* in a coalition because he occupies a position analogous to parents in the family. He is at the nucleus of a political structure whose prototype is the family in which jealousy, envy, love, and hate find original impetus and expression.

It would be a gross error to assume that in making an analogy between the family and formal organizations the parental role is strictly paternal. There are also characteristics of the mother figure in certain types of chief executives and combinations of mother-father in the formation of executive coalitions.

Chief executives can also suffer from depersonalization in their roles and as a result become emotionally cold and detached. The causes of depersonalization are complex but, in brief, have some connections to the narrow definitions of rationality which exclude the importance of emotions in guiding communication as well as thought.

For the purpose of interpreting how defensive styles affect the behavior of leaders, there is some truth to the suggestion that the neutrality and lack of warmth characteristic of some leaders is a result of an ingrained fear of becoming the *object* for other people—for to become the *object* arouses fears that subordinates will become envious and compete for power.

Paranoid Thinking

This is a form of distortion in ideas and perception to which all human beings are susceptible from time to time. For those individuals who are concerned in their work with the consolidation and uses of power, the experience with suspiciousness, the attribution of bad motives to others, jealousy, and anxiety (characteristics of paranoid thinking), may be more than a passing state of mind.

In fact, such ideas and fantasies may indeed be communicated to others and may even be the main force which binds men into collusions. Organizational life is particularly vulnerable to the effects of paranoid thinking because it stimulates comparisons while it evokes anticipations of added power or fears of diminished power.

To complicate matters even more and to suggest just how ambiguous organizational decisions become, there may be some truth and substance in back of the suspicions, distrust, and jealousies which enflame thinking. Personality conflicts do affect decisions in allocating authority and responsibility, and an individual may not be distorting at all to sense that he had been excluded or denied an ambition based on some undercurrents in his relationships with others. To call these sensitivities paranoid thinking may itself be a gross distortion. But no matter how real the events, the paranoid potential is still high as a fallout of organizational life.

Paranoid thinking goes beyond suspiciousness, distrust, and jealousy. It may take the form of grandiose ideas and overestimation of one's power and control. This form of distortion leads to swings in mood from elation to despair, from a sense of omnipotence to helplessness. Again, when acted out, the search for complete control produces the tragedies which the initial distortions attempt to overcome. The tragedy of Jimmy Hoffa is a good case in point. Consider:

□ From all indications, Hoffa performed brilliantly as president of the teamsters' union. He was a superb organizer and bargainer, and in many ways a highly moral and even prudish man. There is little evidence to support allegations that he used his office to enrich himself.

Hoffa's troubles stemmed from his angry reactions when he could not get his way in managing the union's pension fund and from his relations with the government. In overestimating his power, Hoffa fell victim to the illusion that no controls outside himself could channel his actions. At this writing, Hoffa is serving a sentence in Lewisburg Penitentiary, having been found guilty of tampering with a jury.*

It is interesting to note that Hoffa's successor delegated considerable authority to regional officers, a step that removed him from direct comparisons with Hoffa and served to cement a coalition of top officers in the teamsters.

Executives, too, can be victims of their successes just as much as of their failures. If past sucesses lead to the false sense of omnipotence which goes unchecked in, say, the executive's control of the board of directors, then he and his organization become the victims of changing times and competitive pressures along with the weakening in perception and reasoning which often accompanies aging.

One could speculate with some reason that paranoid distortions are the direct result of senility and the inability to accept the fact of death. While intellectually aware of the inevitability of death, gifted executives can sometimes not accept emotionally the ultimate in the limitations of power. The disintegration of personality in the conflict between the head and the heart is what we come to recognize as the paranoid potential in all forms of our collective relations.

Ritualistic Ceremonial

Any collective experience, such as organizational life with its capacity for charging the atmosphere in the imagery of power conflicts, can fall victim to rigidities. The rigidities I have in mind consist mainly of the formation and elaboration of structures, procedures, and other ceremonials which create the illusion of solving problems but in reality only give people something to act on to discharge valuable energies.

The best example of a ritualistic approach to real problems is the ever-ready solution of bringing people together in a committee on the naive grounds that the exchange of ideas is bound to produce a solution. There are even fads and fashions to ritualism as in the sudden appearance of favorite words like "brainstorming" or "synergism."

It is not that bringing people together to discuss problems is bad. Instead, it is the naive faith which accompanies such proposals, ultimately deflecting attention from where it properly belongs. Thus:

□ In one research organization, professionals faced severe problems arising from personal jealousies as well as differences of opinion on the correct goals and content for the research program. Someone would periodically suggest that the problems could not be solved unless people came

---

* Mr. Hoffa has since been released.

together, preferably for a weekend away from the job, to share ideas and really get down to the "nitty-gritty" of the problem. (It is interesting to note that no one ever defines the "nitty-gritty.") The group would indeed follow such suggestions and typically end the weekend with a feeling of euphoria brought on by considerable drinking and a sumptuous meal.

The most concrete proposal for action was in the idea that the basic problem stemmed from the organization's increased size so that people no longer knew one another and their work. The solution which appeared, only shortly to disappear, was to publish a laboratory newsletter that would keep people abreast of their colleagues' newest ideas.

In a more general vein, ritualism can be invoked to deal with any real or fancied danger, with uncertainty, ambivalent attitudes, or a sense of personal helplessness. Rituals are used even in the attempt to manipulate people. That power relations in organizations should become a fertile field for ritualism should not surprise anyone.

As I have tried to indicate, the problems of organizational life involve the dangers associated with losses of power; the uncertainties are legion especially in the recognition that there is no one best way to organize and distribute power, and yet any individual must make a commitment to some form of organization.

Ambivalent attitudes, such as the simultaneous experience of love and hate, are also associated with authority relationships, particularly in how superior-subordinate become the subject and object for the expression of dependency reactions. In addition, the sense of helplessness is particularly sensitized in the events which project gains and losses in power and status.

Finally, superior and subordinate in any power structure are constantly tempted to manipulate each other as a way of gaining control over one's environment, and the more so when there is a lack of confidence and credibility in the organization's efforts to solve problems in realistic ways.

The negative effects of ritualism are precisely in the expenditure of energy to carry out the rituals and also in the childlike expectation that the magic formulas of organizational life substitute for diagnosing and solving real problems. When the heads of organizations are unsure of the bases for the exercise of power and become defensive, the easy solution is to play for time by invoking rituals which may temporarily relieve anxiety.

Similarly, when executives fail to understand the structure and potential of the power coalitions they establish (either consciously or unconsciously), they increasingly rely on rituals to deflect attention away from their responsibilities. And, when leaders are timid men incapable of initiating or responding, the spontaneous reaction is to use people to act out rituals. Usually, the content and symbolism in the rituals provide important clues about the underlying defensiveness of the executive.

Obsessional leaders: The gravitational pull to ceremonials and magic is irresistible. In positions of power, obsessional leaders use in their public performances the mechanisms of defense which originate in their private conflicts. These defenses include hyper-rationality, the isolation of thought and feeling, reactive behavior in turning anger into moral righteousness, and passive control of other people as well as their own thought processes.

Very frequently, particularly in this day and age of psychologizing conflict, obsessive leaders "get religion" and try to convert others into some new state of mind. The use of sensitivity training with its attachments to "openness" and "leveling" in power relations seems to be the current favorite.

What these leaders do not readily understand is the fallacy of imposing a total solution for the problem of power relations where reality dictates at best the possibility of only partial and transient solutions. To force openness through the use of group pressure in T-groups and to expect to sustain this pressure in everyday life is to be supremely ritualistic. People intelligently resist saying everything they think to other people because they somehow have a deep recognition that this route leads to becoming over-extended emotionally and, ultimately, to sadistic relationships.

Intelligent uses of power: The choice fortunately is not between ritualistic civility and naive openness in human relationships, particularly where power is concerned. In between is the choice of defining those partial problems which can be solved and through which bright people can learn something about the intelligent uses of power.

We should not lose sight of the basic lesson that people in positions of power differ from "ordinary" human beings mainly in their capacity to impose their personal defenses onto the stage of corporate life. Fortunately, the relationships are susceptible to intelligent management, and it is to the nature of this intelligence that I wish to address the conclusion of this article.

COMING FULL CIRCLE

The main job of organizational life, whether it concerns developing a new political pyramid, making new appointments to executive positions, or undergoing management succession at top levels, is to bring talented individuals into location for the legitimate uses of power. This is bound to be a highly charged event in corporate relationships because of the real changes in power distributions and the emotional reactions people experience along with the incremental gains and losses of power.

The demand, on the one hand, is for objectivity in assessing people and needs (as opposed to pseudorationality and rationalizing). This objectivity, on the other hand, has to be salvaged from the impact of psychological stresses which impel people to act out fantasies associated with power conflicts. The stresses of change in power relations tend to increase defensiveness to which counterreactions of rationalizing and of myth-making serve no enduring purpose except perhaps to drive underground the concerns which make people react defensively in the first place.

Stylistic Biases

Thought and action in the politics of organizational life are subject to the two kinds of errors commonly found in practical life: the errors of omission and those of commission. It is both what people do and what they neglect to do that result in the negative effects of action outweighing the positive. But besides the specific errors of omission and commission (the tactical aspects of action), there are also the more strategic aspects which have to be evaluated. The strategic aspects deal both with the corporate aims and objectives and with the style of the leaders who initiate change.

In general, leaders approach change with certain stylistic biases over which they may not have too much control. There is a preferred approach to power problems which derives from the personality of the leader and his defenses as well as from the realities of the situation. Of particular importance as stylistic biases are the preferences for partial, as contrasted with total, approaches and the preferences for substance over form.

Partial vs. total: The partial approaches attempt to define and segregate problems which become amenable to solution by directive, negotiation, consensus, and compromise.

The total approaches usually escalate the issues in power relations so that implicitly people act as though it were necessary to undergo major conversions. The conversions can be directed toward personality structure, ideals, and beliefs, or toward values which are themselves connected to important aspects of personal experience.

When conversions become the end products of change, then one usually finds the sensitization of concerns over such matters as who dominates and who submits, who controls and who is being controlled, who is accepted and who is rejected. The aftermath of these concerns is the heightening of fantasy and defense at the expense of reality.

It may come as something of a disappointment to readers who are favorably disposed to psychology to consider the possibility that while organizations do have an impact on the attitudes of their constituent members, they cannot change personality structures or carry out therapeutic procedures. People may become more effective while working in certain kinds of organizations, but only when effectiveness is not dependent on the solution of neurotic conflict.

The advocates of total approaches seem to miss this point in their eagerness to convert people and organizations from one set of ideals to another. It becomes a good deal wiser, if these propositions are true, to scale down and make concrete the objectives that one is seeking to achieve.

A good illustration is in the attention given to decentralization of authority. Decentralization can be viewed in the image of conversion to certain ideals about who should have power and how this power should be used responsibly, or through an analytical approach to decide selectively where power is ill-placed and ill-used and to work on change at these locations. In other words, the theory of the partial approach to organizations asserts priorities and depends on good diagnostic observation and thought.

Substance vs. form: Leaders can also present a stylistic bias in their preference for substance or form. Substance, in the language of organizations, is the detail of goals and performance—that is, who has to do what with whom to meet specific objectives. Form directs attention to the relationship of "who to whom" and attempts to achieve goals by specifying how the people should act in relation to each other.

There is no way in which matters of form can be divorced from substance. But students of organization should at least be clear that attention to form *ahead* of substance threatens a person's sense of what is reasonable in undertaking actions. Attention to form may also present an implicit attack on one's conception of his independence and freedom from constraint.

Making form secondary to substance has another virtue: it can secure agreement on priorities without the need of predetermining who will have to give way in the ultimate give-and-take of the negotiations that must precede decisions on organization structure.

The two dimensions of bias, shown in the *Exhibit I* matrix, along with the four cells which result, clarify different executive approaches to power.

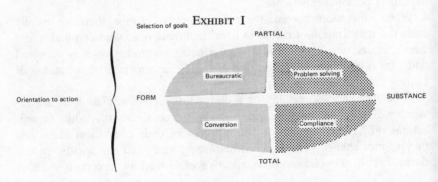

The two dimensions define the executive's cognitive biases in: (1) selection of goals (partial vs total), and (2) orientation toward action (form vs. substance).

In the *bureaucratic* approach—that is, partial goals and attachment to form as a mode of acting—the emphasis is on procedure and the establishment of precedent and rule to control the uses of power.

The appeal of this approach is its promise of certainty in corporate relationships and in the depersonalization of power. The weaknesses of the bureaucratic approach are too familiar to need detailing here. Its major defect, however, is its inability to separate the vital from the trivial. It more easily commands energy over irrelevant issues because the latent function of the bureaucratic approach is to bypass conflict.

My contention here is that few important problems can be attended to without conflict of ideas and interests. Eventually organizations become stagnant because the bureaucratic approaches seldom bring together power and the vital issues which together make organizations dynamic.

The *conversion* approach (total-form) is notable through the human relations and sensitivity training movements as well as ideological programs, such as the Scanlon Plan and other forms of participative management. The popularity of "management by objectives" bears some scrutiny as a conversion movement directed toward power figures.

Another "total" approach which differs from conversion in its emphasis on substance is *compliance* with the directives of the powerful leader. This is the arena of the authoritarian personality (in both the leader, who has the power, and in the led, who seek submission), for whom personal power gets expressed in some higher goal that makes it possible for ends to justify means. The ideals may, for example, be race, as with dictator Adolf Hitler, or religion, as with Father Charles Coughlin, a dictator-type of the depression. In business, the illustrations are of a technological variety as with Frederick Winslow Taylor's "scientific management" and Henry Ford's automobile and assembly line.

Almost any technology can assume the proportions of the total approach if it is advanced by a charismatic leader and has deep emotional appeal. This explains the popularity of "management information systems," "value analysis," and "program planning and budgeting" which lead to a belief that the system itself is based on order, rationality, and control; therefore, the belief in turn helps to counteract the fears of chaos and lack of control which make people willing to demand total dependence and compliance in power relations. The effects of this fear on how people seek to arrange power relations in business, government, and the community cannot be overestimated.

Problem-Solving Approach

It should be perfectly obvious by now that my favored approach to organizational life combines the biases in *Exhibit I* of the partial substantive quadrant which I have designated "problem solving." From observation of competent business executives, we know it is precisely their ability to define problems worthy of thought and action and to use their organization to evolve solutions which characterize their style.

The contrary notion that executives are primarily caretakers, mediators, and seekers of consensus is more a myth than an accurate portrayal of how the competent ones attach themselves to power. To have power and not direct it to some substantive end that can be attained in the real world is to waste energy. The difficulties with the problem-solving approach are in risking power in favor of a substantive goal.

While there are no absolute right answers in problem solving, there are ways of evaluating the correctness of a program and plan. With a favorable average, the executive finds his power base enhanced and his ability to take risks increased.

The problem-solving approach to organization structure operates according to certain premises:

1. That organization structure is an instrument rather than an end. This means that a structure should be established or modified quickly instead of stringing out deliberations as though there actually exists a best and single solution for the problem of allocating power.

2. That organization structure can be changed but should not be tinkered with. This means that members of an executive organization can rely on a structure and can implement it without the uncertainty which comes from the constant modification of the organization chart.

3. That organization structure expresses the working coalition attached to the chief executive. In other words, the coalition has to be established de facto for the structure to mean anything. If the structure is out of line with the coalition, there will be an erosion of power and effectiveness. If no coalition exists in the minds of participants, putting it on paper in the form of an organization chart is nothing more than an academic exercise and a confusing one at that.

4. That organization structure represents a blend of people and job definitions, but the priority is in describing the structure to accommodate competent people. The reason for this priority lies in the fact that competent executives are hard to find. Therefore, as an action principle, one should ensure the effective uses of the scarcest resources rather than conform to some ideal version of power relations.

5. That organization structure is a product of negotiation and compro-

mise among executives who hold semiautonomous power bases. The more the power base of an executive is his demonstrated competence, the greater his autonomy of power and therefore capacity to determine the outcome in the allocations of power. The basic criticism of the problem-solving approach is in the danger of defining issues narrowly and ultimately undermining the moral-ethical basis of leadership. This criticism is valid, but as with so many problems in practical affairs, it can be overcome only by leaders who can see beyond the limits of immediate contingencies. In fact, I have tried to show throughout this article how the limitations of leaders, in both their cognitive and their emotional capacities, become the causes of power problems.

We have therefore come full circle in this analysis: because power problems are the effects of personality on structure, the solutions demand thinking which is free from the disabilities of emotional conflicts. This insight is often the margin between enduring with what exists or taking those modest steps which align competence with institutional authority in the service of human needs.

REFERENCES

[1] See my article, "The Management of Disappointment," HBR November–December 1967, p. 59.

[2] See Chester Barnard, *The Function of the Executive* (Cambridge, Harvard University Press, 1938), p. 167.

SELECTION 8

New Patterns of Leadership for Tomorrow's Organizations*

Warren G. Bennis

Two years ago, I forecast that in the next 25 to 50 years we would participate in the end of bureaucracy as we know it and in the rise of new social systems better suited to the Twentieth Century demands of industrialization (*see* Technology Review, *Apr., 1966, pp. 36 ff.*). This forecast was based on the evolutionary principle that every age develops an organizational form appropriate to its genius and that the prevailing form today—the pyramidal, centralized, functionally specialized, impersonal mechanism known as *bureaucracy*—is out of joint with contemporary realities.

This breakdown of a venerable form of organization so appropriate to Nineteenth Century conditions is caused, I argued, by a number of factors, but chiefly the following four:

1. Rapid and unexpected change.

2. Growth in size where the volume of an organization's traditional product is not enough to sustain growth.

3. Complexity of modern technology, where integration between activities and persons of very diverse, highly specialized competence is required.

4. The psychological threat springing from a change in managerial values toward more humanistic, democratic practices.

Organizations of the future, I predicted, would have some unique characteristics. The key word will be "temporary." There will be adaptive, rapidly changing *temporary systems*. Organization charts will consist of project groups rather than stratified functional groups, which now is the case. Adaptive, problem-solving, temporary systems of diverse specialists, linked together by co-ordinating executives in organic flux—this is the organizational form that will gradually replace bureaucracy.

Ironically, the bold future I was predicting two years ago is now a mundane reality; it can be observed today where the most interesting and advanced practices exist. We live in a time and place where rapid social and technological change is endemic, and so perhaps it should not be too

* *Technology Review,* vol. 70, no. 6, April, 1968.

surprising that a distant future can invade overnight, so to speak— certainly before the forecast is fully comprehended.

New Styles and Tasks of Leadership

The question of the leadership of these new-style organizations was left unanswered in the original article. Are there any guidelines transferable to their management from present managerial practices? Do the behavioral sciences provide any suggestions for leaders of the future? How can these complex, ever-changing, free-form, kaleidoscopic patterns be co-ordinated? There can be no definitive answers to these questions until the future emerges in a more or less unambiguous way. But we clearly need to attempt an evaluation of the leadership requirements for organizations of the future, for without the effort we shall inevitably back into the future instead of managing it effectively.

Developing Rewarding Human Systems

The general direction of these organizational changes—toward more service and professional organizations, toward more educated, younger, and mobile employees, toward more diverse, complex, science-based systems, toward a more turbulent and uncertain environment—forces us to consider new styles of leadership. Leading the enterprise of the future will become a significant social process, requiring as much interpersonal competence as substantive competence, if not more.

One convenient focus for a discussion of leadership is to summarize the main problems confronting modern organizations and to understand the kinds of tasks and strategies linked to the solution of these problems. These are summarized in the chart on the next to last page of the article which also shows some possible executive steps.

A simple way to understand the problem of integration is to compute the ratio between what an individual gives and what he receives in his day-to-day transactions. In organizational terms, we can ask: Are the *contributions* to the organization about equivalent to the *inducements* received? There is nothing startling or new about this formulation. What is interesting is that organizations frequently do not know what is truly rewarding. This is particularly true in the case of the professionals and highly trained workers who will dominate the organizations of the future, with whom conventional policies and practices regarding incentives— never particularly sensitive—tend to be inappropriate.

Most organizations regard economic rewards as the primary incentive to peak performance. These are not unimportant to the professional, but—provided economic rewards are equitable—other incentives become far more potent. Professionals tend to seek such rewards as full utilization of their talent and training; professional status (not necessarily within the organization, but externally with respect to their profession); and opportunities for development and further learning. The "good place to work" resembles a super-graduate school, alive with dialogue and senior colleagues, where the employee will work not only to satisfy organizational demands but, perhaps primarily, to fulfill self-imposed demands of his profession.

How (or even *if*) these needs can be deliberately controlled by the leadership is not at all clear. Company-sponsored courses, T-groups, and other so-called adult education courses may contribute. The idea that education has a terminal point is clearly old-fashioned. A "drop-out" may soon be redefined to mean anyone who has not *returned* to school.

However the problem of professional and personal growth is resolved, it is clear that many of the older forms of incentives will have to be reconstituted. Even more profound will be the blurring of the boundaries between work and play, between affiliative and achievement drives which Nineteenth Century necessities and mores have unsuccessfully attempted to compartmentalize.

Developing Executive Collaboration

It is quaint to think that one man, no matter how omniscient and omnipotent, can comprehend, to say nothing of control, the diversity and complexity of the modern organization. Followers and leaders who think this is possible are entrapped in a false dream, a child's fantasy of absolute power and absolute dependence. As a result, there has been a tendency to move away (tacitly) from a "presidential" form of power to a "cabinet" or team concept. Such a system of an "executive constellation" by no means implies an abdication of responsibility by the chief executive. It is a way of multiplying executive power through a realistic allocation of effort. Despite all the problems inherent in the executive constellation concept—the difficulties of building an effective team, of achieving compatibility, etc.—it is hard to see other valid solutions to the constraints of magnitude and sheer overload of the leader's role.

Not unrelated to the problem of developing an effective executive constellation is another key task of the leader—building a collaborative climate. An effective collaborative climate is easier to experience and harder to achieve than a formal description, but most students of group behavior would agree that it should include the following ingredients: flexible and adaptive structure; utilization of member's talents; clear and agreed-upon goals; norms of openness, trust, and cooperation; interdependence; high intrinsic rewards; and transactional controls—i.e., members of the unit should have a high degree of autonomy and a high degree of participation in making key decisions.

Developing this group "synergy" is difficult. Lack of experience and strong cultural biases against group efforts worsen the problem. Groups, like other highly complicated organisms, need interaction, trust, communication, and commitment, and these ingredients require a period of gestation. But expensive and time-consuming as it is, building synergetic and collaborative cultures will become essential. Modern problems, too complex and diversified for one man or one discipline, require a blending of skills and perspectives, and only effective problem-solving units will be able to master them.

Identification with the Adaptive Process

Man's accommodation to change is generally painful, but characteristically and ironically he continues to seek out new inventions which disorder his serenity and undermine his competence. One striking index of the rapidity of modern change—for me, the most dramatic single index—is the shrinking interval between the time of a discovery and its commercial application. The transistor was discovered in 1948; by 1960 over 50 per cent of *all* electronic equipment utilized transistors in place of conventional vacuum tubes.

The increasing tempo of discovery and its application make modern organizations acutely dependent on their success in responding flexibly and appropriately to new information. How can the leadership create an atmosphere of continuity and stability in this environment of change? Whitehead put the problem well when he said, "The art of society consists first in the maintenance of the symbolic code, and secondly, in the fearlessness of revision . . . Those societies which cannot combine reverence to their symbols with freedom of revision must ultimately decay . . ."

There is no easy solution to the tension between stability and change. We are not yet an emotionally adaptive society, though a remarkable aspect of our generation is its commitment to change in thought and action. Executive leadership must take some responsibility in creating a climate that provides the security to identify with the adaptive process without fear of losing status and its psychological companion, a lowered self-esteem. Creating an environment that increases a tolerance for ambiguity and where one can make a virtue out of contingency, in contrast to an environment which induces hesitancy and its reckless counterpart, expedience, is one of the most challenging tasks for the new leadership.

Supra-Organizational Goals and Commitments

The new organizations we speak of, with their bands of "pseudo-species" coping within a turbulent environment, are particularly allergic to problems of identity. Professional and regional orientations lead frequently to fragmentation, inter-group conflicts and power plays and rigid compartmentalization devoid of any unifying sense of purpose or mission.

The university is a wondrous place for the development of advanced battle techniques between groups which far overshadow their business counterparts in subterfuge and sabotage. Quite often a university becomes a loose collection of competing departments, schools, institutes, committees, centers, and programs, largely noncommunicating because of the multiplicity of specialist jargons and interests and held together, as Robert Hutchins once said, chiefly by a central heating system. Having heard variations of this theme over the years, a number of faculty and administrators at one large university, who thought they could "wear the over-all university hat," formed what later came to be known as "the HATS group." They came from many departments and hierarchical levels, represented a rough microcosm of the entire university, and have become a prototype through the important role they have played in influencing university policy.

There are a number of functions that leadership can perform in addition to encouraging HATS groups. It can identify and support those individuals who can serve as articulating points between various groups and departments. There are many individuals who have a bi-cultural facility, a capacity for psychological and intellectual affinity with different languages and cultures, who can provide articulation between seemingly inimical interests, who can break down the pseudo-species, transcend vested interests, regional ties and professional biases. Leadership can seek out and encourage these people. It can work at the interfaces of the pseudo-species, setting up new programs in the interstitial areas, in order to create more inter-group articulations. This is precisely what Mary Parker Follett had in mind when she discussed leadership in terms of an ability to bring about a "creative synthesis" between differing codes of conduct. Chester Barnard in his classic *Functions of the Executive* recognized this, and he also recognized the cost in personal energy of this kind of synthesis. He wrote, "It seems to me that the struggle to maintain cooperation among men should as surely destroy some men morally as battle destroys some physically."

Revitalization: Controlling Destiny

The issue of revitalization—the organization's taking conscious responsibility for its own evolution—confronts the leader with the penultimate challenge: growth or decay. His urgent problem is to develop a climate of inquiry and enough psychological and employment security for continual re-assessment and renewal. The organizational culture must encourage individuals to participate in social evolution against unknown, uncertain, and implacable forces and to collect valid data and act on limited information without fear of losing control.

The three-step "action-research" model of data-generation, feedback, and action-planning sounds deceptively simple. In fact, it is difficult. Quite often the important data cannot be collected by the leader. Even when the data are known, there are many organizational short circuits and "dithering devices" which distort and prevent the data from reaching the right places at the right time. And even when data-generation and feedback are satisfactorily completed, organizational inhibitions may not lead to implementation. But some progressive organizations are setting up organizational development departments that attempt to reduce the "implementation gap" between information, new ideas and action. These departments become the center for the entire strategic side of the organization, including not only long-run planning but plans for gaining participation and commitment to the plans. This last step is the most crucial for the guarantee of successful implementation.

New Concepts for Leadership

In addition to substantive competence and comprehension of both social and technical systems, the new leader will have to possess interpersonal skills, not the least of which is the ability to defer his own immediate desires and gratifications in order to cultivate the talents of others. Just as salesmen are admonished that "you gotta know the territory," so too the manager must be at home in the "social territory," the complex and dynamic interaction of individuals, roles, groups, and organizational and cultural systems.

Leadership is as much craft as science. Analytical methods, drawn primarily from social psychology and sociology, suffice for business leaders to understand the scientific aspects of their profession, but the main instrument or "tool" for the leader-as-a-craftsman is *himself* and how creatively he can use his own personality. Leaders, like physicians, are "iatrogenic"—that is, capable of spreading as well as curing disease. Unless the leader understands his actions and their effects on others, he may be a "carrier" rather than a solver of problems. Thus he must be willing and able to set up reliable mechanisms of feedback so that he can conceptualize the "social territory" of which he is an important part—and at the same time realize how he influences it.

Another aspect of the "social territory" that has key significance for leadership is the idea of *system*. At least two decades of research have been making this point unsuccessfully. Research has shown that productivity can be modified by group norms, that training effects deteriorate if the training is not compatible with the goals of the social system, that group cohesiveness is a powerful motivator, that inter-group conflict is a major problem facing organizations, that individuals take many of their cues and derive a good deal of their satisfaction from their primary work group, that identification with the small work group turns out to be the only stable predictor of productivity, and so on.

This evidence is often cited and rarely acted upon. It seems that individuals, living amidst complex and subtle organizational conditions, tend to oversimplify and distort complex realities so that "people" rather than conditions embody the problem. This tendency toward personalization can be observed in many situations. We can see it in distorted polarizations such as the "good guy" leader and his "hatchet man" assistant. It is easier to blame heroes and villains than the system. For if the problems are embroidered into the fabric of the system, complex as it is, the system can be changed. But it is hard to change people.

"Other-Directed" Leadership

One famous typology in the social sciences was introduced by David Riesman in his book, *The Lonely Crowd*. He asserted that contemporary man is more "other-directed" than his father—or certainly than his grandfather, who would have been characterized as "inner-directed." These character types refer essentially to the ways individuals are influenced and the forces which shape their perspectives. "Other-directed" man takes his cues from his peer group rather than from his parents; in other words, he takes his relationships more seriously than he does his relatives. His ideology, values, and norms are transmitted to him and accepted by the particular social group with which he associates. He is a "pleaser," cooperative and accommodating. "Inner-directed" man, to extend an exaggeration, responds to some internal gyroscope, typically internalized parental pressures. He responds not to any social grouping but to some inner cues, shadowed reflections of his parents' dictates. "Inner-directed" man is rigid, unyielding, and acts on principles. Studies conducted in industrial settings have consistently shown that organizations tend to reward the aggressive, forceful, decisive "inner-directed" leader rather than the co-operative, adaptable, "other-directed" leader. Now a new study of the leadership in service-oriented organizations by E. E. Lawlor and L. W. Porter shows that "other-directed" leaders tend to be more highly rewarded in this setting than "inner-directed" leaders. In the service-oriented growth industries of education, health, welfare, government, and professional organizations, the prime requisites of a leader are interpersonal competence and "other-directedness."

An Agricultural Model of Leadership

I have not found the right word or phrase that accurately portrays the concept of future leadership I have in mind. The most appropriate metaphor I have found to characterize adaptive leadership is an "agricultural" model: The leader's job is to build a climate where growth and development are culturally induced, conditions where people and ideas and resources can be seeded, cultivated, and integrated to optimum effectiveness and growth. Roy Ash, an astute industrialist who is Chairman of Litton Industries, remarked recently: "If the larger corporations, classically viewed as efficient machines rather than hothouses for fomenting innovation, can become both of these at once, industrial competition will have taken on new dimensions." I think Ash captures exactly the shift in metaphor I am getting at, from a mechanical model to an organic one.

Up until very recent times, the metaphor most commonly used to describe power and leadership in organizations derived from Helmholtz's laws of mechanics, and the language reflects this derivation: social engineering, equilibrium, friction, and resistance are typical of the words we use.

MAIN TASKS AND STRATEGIES OF LEADERSHIP IN CONTEMPORARY ORGANIZATIONS.

Modern organizations are confronted with a series of circumstances and problems which have no true counterparts in corporate history, and these needs require new strategies and impose new tasks upon modern corporate

leadership. The chart attempts to list the new problems, and their conse-
quences, in grossly oversimplified form.

Problem	Tasks of the Leader
Integration The problem of integrating individual needs and organizational goals	Developing rewarding human systems
Social Influence The problem of distributing power	Developing executive constellations
Collaboration The problem of producing mechanisms for the control of conflict	Building a collaborative climate
Adaptation The problem of responding to a turbulent, uncertain environment	Identification with the adaptive process
Identity The problem of clarity, commitment, and consensus to organizational goals	Developing supra-organizational goals
Revitalization The problem of growth and decay	Organizational "self-renewal"

The vocabulary for adaptive organizations requires an organic metaphor, a description of *process*—not of structural arrangements. This description must include such terms as open, dynamic systems, developmental, organic, and adaptive.

The key aspect of the process insofar as leadership is concerned is the ability of the leader to develop a collaborative relationship with his subordinates. This is not to say that the leader should be a "good guy" or seek popularity, but it does mean that he will have to learn to negotiate and collaborate with his associates. Because the leader cannot know everything, his subordinates will have the information and competencies that the leader needs; his access to this information will depend entirely on his ability to collaborate with his employees and colleagues. While Marx argued that power accrues to the man with property, we argue that power accrues to the man who can gather and control information wisely. The psychological "contract," if we may use that term, between leader and led is more satisfying and almost always more productive if the relationship is based on collaboration. Studies of scientists and engineers, for example, show that no unilateral conditions, where scientists decide for themselves or where the director decides for them, ever matched the quality of work under a collaborative relationship where research and development decisions were reached through a collaborative process.

Toward a New Leadership Style

All of these strategic and practical considerations lead to a totally new concept of leadership, the pivotal aspect of which is that the leader depends less on substantive knowledge about a particular topic than on the understanding and possession of skills summarized under the agricultural model. The role of the leader has become infinitely more complex, for he is now at the center of a highly variegated set of pressures and roles. He presides over a complex establishment; his job is to co-ordinate, transact, motivate, and integrate. Simply, he must have the knowledge and competence to produce environments where the most able people can realize their talents, co-ordinate their efforts, remain committed to organizational goals, and integrate their efforts in a manner that no one of them working alone could surpass. Perhaps the most difficult aspect of this style of leadership is to transact (and confront) those recalcitrant parts of the system that are retarded, stunted, or afraid to grow. This will require enormous energy, saintly patience, and a sophisticated optimism in growth (or a high tolerance for disenchantment).

This new concept of leadership embraces five important sets of competencies:

1. Knowledge of large, complex systems, their dynamics and their "tribal customs."

2. Practical theories of intervening and guiding these systems, theories that encompass methods for seeding, nurturing, and integrating individuals and groups.

3. Interpersonal competence. This includes at least three components: (a) the sensitivity to understand the effects of one's own behavior on others and how one's own personality shapes his particular leadership style and value system; (b) a capacity to develop adequate methods for valid feedback; and (c) managing conflict. (There was a time when I believed that consensus was a valid operating procedure. I no longer think this is realistic given the scale and diversity of organizations. In fact, I've come to think that the quest for consensus, except in pre-literate face-to-face cultures where it may be feasible, is a misplaced nostalgia for a folk-society as chimerical, incidentally, as the American adolescent search for "identity.")

4. A set of values and competencies which enables one to know when to confront and attack, if necessary, and when to support and provide the psychological safety so necessary for growth.

5. An ability to develop and use all types of information systems, including high-speed electronic computers. The job of the leader will be to collect, organize, and transmit information.

The role of leadership described here is clearly more demanding and formidable than any historical precedent, including both king and pope. Let us hope that this new role of leadership is not only more potent but also more gratifying.

Part II

Decision-Making

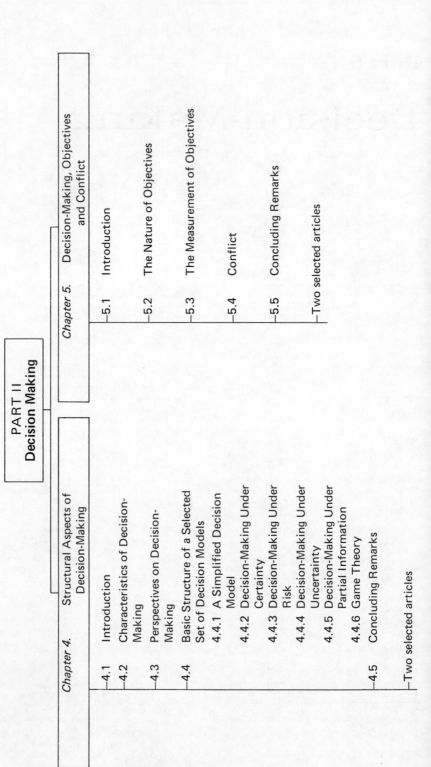

PART II
Decision Making

Chapter 4. Structural Aspects of Decision-Making

4.1 Introduction

4.2 Characteristics of Decision-Making

4.3 Perspectives on Decision-Making

4.4 Basic Structure of a Selected Set of Decision Models

4.4.1 A Simplified Decision Model

4.4.2 Decision-Making Under Certainty

4.4.3 Decision-Making Under Risk

4.4.4 Decision-Making Under Uncertainty

4.4.5 Decision-Making Under Partial Information

4.4.6 Game Theory

4.5 Concluding Remarks

Two selected articles

Chapter 5. Decision-Making, Objectives and Conflict

5.1 Introduction

5.2 The Nature of Objectives

5.3 The Measurement of Objectives

5.4 Conflict

5.5 Concluding Remarks

Two selected articles

Chapter 4

Structural Aspects of Decision-Making

4.1 INTRODUCTION

In Part I we focused our attention on the overall framework of health care systems. The global importance of health care systems was emphasized by noting their social, economic, political, technical, human and even moral components. In order to help the reader develop an insight into the organismic nature of health care organizations, we included in Part I several readings exploring the nature, character, and properties of "systems" and "organizations." The reason for this is obvious. Any health care facility is both a system and an organization. If we understand the structural and behavioral aspects of systems and organizations, we can do a better job of managing them. Management, however, is essentially the process of making decisions for achieving a set of objectives. It is, therefore, desirable that the health care administrator be exposed to some of the most important aspects of decisions and decision-making. In this chapter we introduce the reader to characteristics of decision-making; present a variety of perspectives on decision-making; and give the basic structure of a selected set of decision models.

4.2 CHARACTERISTICS OF DECISION-MAKING

A *decision* is the conclusion of a process by which one chooses among available alternatives for the purpose of achieving a set of desired objectives. Decision-making involves all the thinking and activities that are required to produce a choice among alternative courses of action; it is the central activity of all human beings. The making of decisions is the essence of managing. Planning, organizing, control, leadership, and all other aspects of management are executed through the making and implementation of decisions.

Several characteristics of decisions and decision-making can be noted.

169

Decision-making is a *continuous* activity that occurs in all types of organizations—hospitals and related institutions, political, social, business, military, etc. Since individuals, groups, institutions, organizations—indeed all systems—are goal-seeking* entities, decision-making is *ubiquitous*. Decisions are made with the help of criteria that are deeply rooted in the philosophy and value system of the decision-maker. Decision-making is both an art and a science. As an art decision-making draws heavily on judgment and creativity.† The science of decision-making emphasizes the building of decision models based on deductive, inductive, analytical, or simulation approaches. (See Part V of this book.) Decisions are rarely isolated affairs; they usually reflect the conclusion of one process and at the same time the beginning of another. Decisions, in other words, are *sequential* in nature, and the output from one decision serves as input for one or more subsequent decisions. Decisions are made for the purpose of attaining a desired state of affairs in the future. Thus, the decision problem can be viewed as choosing a path that will move a system from a given state to a desired state.‡

Decisions are to be differentiated from habit and reflex in that decision-making is a *deliberative process*. Decision-making, problem-solving, and creativity are related concepts; distinctions among these may best be made not in terms of process but in terms of product.§

The *pervasive nature* of decision-making becomes evident from the fact that various disciplines (philosophy, economics, statistics, operations research, psychology, sociology, political science) have shown keen interest in developing theories of decision-making.‖ The main concern of economic theory and statistical decision theory, for example, has been with the normative aspects of decision-making. That is, how people *ought* to behave and make decisions; not how they *do* behave. The "economic man"

---

* The distinction between an "objective" and a "goal" is essentially related to time and specificity. Briefly, a goal can be viewed as a short-term target along the dimension of a stated objective. Ansoff [1965, p. 40] describes an objective in terms of three elements: an *attribute* which is chosen as a measure of efficiency; a *yardstick* or scale to measure the objective; and a *goal* which specifies a particular value on the scale. Also see [Ackoff, 1971, pp. 666–667]. Ackoff distinguishes between *goal, objective,* and *ideal*.

† For a discussion of the creative process and its different stages, see [Jones, 1959, pp. 25–52]. The reader is referred to [Brown, 1966] for a discussion of the role and nature of judgment in administration. Brown defines judgment as the matching of facts with values.

‡ A state of system is the values of its relevant properties at a given point in time. See [Ackoff, 1971, p. 662].

§ See [March, 1965, p. 48]. High achievement need, flexibility, a tolerance of ambiguity and uncertainty, habits of searching and exploration; and freedom from conventionalized attitudes have been identified as factors favoring effective problem solving. See [Costello and Zalkind, 1963, p. 382].

‖ In addition to the list given at the end of Part II, the reader should consult [March, 1965, pp. 82–86 and pp. 644–649] for other valuable references. A review of theoretical literature in economics and psychology (the two main disciplines contributing to the theory of decision-making) is given in [Edwards, 1954] and [Simon, 1959].

is assumed to behave *rationally* which requires: (1) the ability to state objectives clearly and to rank them in some order of preference,* and (2) the employment of proper means to maximize (or optimize) the stated objectives. The behavioral sciences have developed theories of how individuals behave and make decisions in organizational settings. [Cyert and March, 1963] and [March and Simon, 1958]. In place of global rationality of the economic man, for example, Simon proposes an "administrative man" who has a choosing organism of limited knowledge and ability [1957, p. 265].

4.3 PERSPECTIVES ON DECISION-MAKING

Decisions and decision-making can be studied and classified from a number of perspectives. For example, depending upon the level of organizational hierarchy, decisions can be classified into strategic, administrative, and operational decisions [Ansoff, 1965, p. 8]. Briefly, strategic decisions refer to defining the organization's relationships with the outside environment. In the health care setting, decisions regarding the design of a national health insurance program; decisions regarding hospital location, mergers, and specialization and decisions relating to major investments in ambulatory care programs, are examples of strategic decisions.† Administrative decisions deal with organization structure (structuring the internal relationships of authority, responsibility, and accountability between and within various units of the organization according to the guidelines set by the strategic decisions), structure of resource conversion and internal services (facilities design, work flows, employment) and resource acquisition and development. The design of a health information system is a clear example of an administrative decision because it sets the framework of who does what—and of the various authority, responsibility and accountability relationships. The acquisition of diagnostic and therapeutic equipment, employment of ward managers, etc. are also examples of administrative decisions.

Lastly, operational decisions are made to handle the routine and day-to-day problems of the organizational units doing the actual work. Scheduling of nursing staff, admission and discharge procedures, control of inventories are examples of operational decisions. This three-way classification is useful not only for understanding the *hierarchical nature* of organizational decisions, it is also important for realizing that the framework of management is a means-end chain where the means selected by higher level

---

* Ordering requires transitivity; i.e., if we prefer A to B, and B to C, then A must be preferred to C. Mathematically, if $A > B$, and $B > C$; then $A > C$.

† Recent proliferation of health planners at the institutional and area-wide level attests to the recognition of the strategic decision-making function. See Chapter 6 of this book.

decisions become the objectives to be achieved by lower level decisions.*

Decisions are required for problems that are either repetitive or novel, static or dynamic, well-structured or ill-structured.† Decisions can also be classified as *programmed* and *nonprogrammed* [Simon, 1960, p. 5]. Decisions are programmed to the extent that they are routine, repetitive, and can be handled with definite procedures. Such decisions can usually be made with the aid of computer programs and the administrator need not devote a large proportion of his time to solving them. Decisions on inventory control, employee benefits, patient scheduling, etc. are typical examples of programmed decisions. Decisions are nonprogrammed to the extent that they are novel and unstructured, and well-defined procedures for handling them do not exist. Strategic decisions on the question of hospital mergers or the creation of neighborhood health centers, etc. are examples of nonprogrammed decisions. The classification of decisions into the *programmed* and *nonprogrammed* varieties with appropriate decision-making techniques is shown in Figure 4.1.

FIG. 4.1
TRADITIONAL AND MODERN TECHNIQUES FOR DECISION-MAKING

Types of Decisions	Decision-Making Techniques Traditional	Modern
Programmed: Routine, repetitive decisions. Organization develops specific processes for handling them.	1. Habit 2. Clerical routine: Standard operating procedures. 3. Organization structure: Common expectations. A system of subgoals. Well-defined informational channels.	1. Operations Research: Mathematical analysis. Models. Computer simulation. 2. Electronic data processing.
Nonprogrammed: One-shot, ill-structured novel, policy decisions. Handled by general problem-solving processes.	1. Judgment, intuition, and creativity. 2. Rules of thumb. 3. Selection and training of executives.	Heuristic problem-solving techniques applied to: (a) training human decision makers. (b) constructing heuristic computer programs.

Source: [Simon, 1960, p. 8].

* [Starr, 1971, pp. 580–582] identifies five decision levels: (1) universal level, (2) global level, (3) strategic level, (4) tactical level, and (5) tool level. This classification has advantages while analyzing multi-national organizations such as United Nations, EEC, etc.

† Well-structured problems are those that have clear-cut, unambiguous objectives and for which straightforward decision processes exist. Ill-structured problems are vaguely defined problems. See [Simon, 1958]

Another classification is that of *individual* versus *managerial* decision-making. The distinction between individual and managerial decision-making relates essentially to the scope, complexity, context, and the length of chain between the decision and its implementation. The more the number of people that are affected by the decision, the greater the complexity, the longer the chain between the decision and its implementation, the higher is its managerial content. The distinction between individual and managerial decision-making is valid more in terms of degree than origin. The basic structure of decisions, the steps involved before the final choice is made, and the logical processes for understanding them are the same. In the modern world of specialization and interdependence, individual decision-making is essentially "managerial" in character. This is certainly the case with respect to health care administrators because many of their decisions affect a large population.

Another approach to the study of decision-making lies in the distinction between *normative* (or prescriptive) versus *descriptive* theories of decision-making. A normative decision model identifies an optimal strategy (course of action) for the decision-maker. It *prescribes* a specific course of action and states what *ought* to be done, by applying a criterion of choice which is part of the model. A descriptive model describes what *is;* not what ought to be—and it does not contain the criterion of choice. Economic theory, operations research, management science, and statistical decision-theory have contributed mainly to the development of normative decision-making. On the other hand, behavioral scientists, psychologists, and sociologists have developed descriptive theories of decision-making.

Decision-making can also be classified into *individual* versus *organizational** decision-making. Both normative and descriptive theories of individual decision-making are of interest to the health care administrator. Normative theories of individual decision-making focus on optimal decision rules under conditions of certainty, risk, uncertainty, and conflict.† Descriptive theories of individual decision-making revolve around the concept of "satisficing" rather than optimizing, "bounded rationality," and the "level of aspiration."‡ Organizational decision-making considers the processes by which individuals, or group of individuals, make decisions (in organizational settings) to pursue their *role defined* goals. Normative as well as descriptive theories of organizational decision-making can be found in the literature [March, 1965, p. 644]. Theories of organizations as a single decision-maker with a single objective, multiple decision-makers

---

* For a schematic of the organizational decision process in an abstract form, see Figure 6.1 in Cyert and March [1963, p. 126].

† See March [1965, Chapter 2].

‡ For a discussion of these concepts and for a formal statement of the principle of bounded rationality, the reader is referred to Simon [1957, p. 198].

with a single goal structure, and multiple decision-makers with multiple goal structures have been advanced to explain organizational decision-making under different assumptions [March, 1965, Chapter 14]. The organizational view of the decision-making process is that actual choices in an organization are determined by the manner in which organizational goals are formed, the organizational alternatives are searched, and their consequences are projected. It is obvious that individual and organizational decision-making are closely related; organizational decision models can in many cases be formed by imposing additional constraints on individual decision-making models.

Decision models can be *static* or *dynamic*. Static models are those in which time is not one of the variables or parameters. The static model is a single state model in which, for a given period of time, only one decision has to be made. A linear programming model, for example, is a static model (see Chapter 12). Dynamic decision models are multi-state models calling for a series of sequential* decisions. Decision-tree analysis and dynamic programming are two examples of dynamic models.† A decision tree is a network of nodes and branches. There are two types of nodes: action nodes and chance nodes. Each node has more than one branch emanating from it and feeding into either another node or a terminal outcome. The tree consists of at least two separate time intervals or decision stages. Each action branch represents a course of action and each chance branch represents a possible outcome. Probability distributions of the branches growing from each chance node are assumed to be known, as are the projected payoffs at the end of each branch. Decision-making involves choosing an optimal path through the decision tree.‡ The decision-tree type of analysis is of special relevance to the health administrator when deciding whether or not to erect new facilities (of different capacities) on the basis of projected need for services.

4.4 BASIC STRUCTURE OF A SELECTED SET OF DECISION MODELS

Decisions are made in the real world inhabited by health care providers, government, labor, entrepreneurs, competitors, consumers, general public, and of course, by other decision-makers. It is to be expected, therefore, that decision models will exhibit a great deal of variability and complexity. It is nevertheless possible to describe, and build, a basic decision model that is common to all decision problems. In order to set up a basic decision

---

* See [Lusted, 1971] and [Magee, 1964].
† Wagner [1969, Chapters 8, 9 and 10].
‡ See [Magee, 1964], [Hespos and Strassman, 1965].

model, all the factors which have a bearing on the problem can be divided into two sets. One set consists of all those factors which are under the control of the decision-maker. A specific combination of these *controllable* factors (for example, manpower and equipment or resources) defines a course of action or a *strategy*. In a given problem, the decision-maker can devise a finite or infinite number of strategies.* The other set consists of the environmental factors, variables or constants, over which the decision-maker has little control (*noncontrollable factors*). A particular configuration of these factors, as faced by the decision-maker, is either a result of the actions of a rational opponent or a result of several random events, or both. If a rational opponent is involved, the decision-maker must consider the opponent's potential actions as part of the decision problem. The opponent's course of action, referred to as a *competitive strategy,* may or may not be known in advance, but it cannot be ignored. How to make rational decisions under specified conditions of conflict (or cooperation) is the domain of game theory. How to make rational decisions under conditions of risk and uncertainty is the domain of decision theory.†

The decision problem can be structured so that the actions of the rational opponents are either ignored or are subsumed under the acts of nature. In such a case, the strategies of the decision-maker interact with some *state of nature*‡ to produce a result, a consequence, or a payoff.§

4.4.1 A Simplified Decision Model

In view of the above discussion, we can build a simplified decision model as:

$$R = f(C_i, U_j) \tag{4.1}$$

where

R = the result or payoff associated with a given strategy or course of action (the payoff is represented by some measure of the outcome or by utility).

C_i = the set of controllable variables.

U_j = the set of variables (and constants) which is not controlled by the decision-maker, but which affects R.

f = the functional relationship between the dependent variable R and the independent variables (and constants) C_i and U_j.

---

* Whether the number of strategies is finite or infinite is determined by whether the variables are "continuous" or "discrete."

† Game theory is considered to be a subset of decision theory. See [Luce and Raiffa, 1958] and [Von Neumann and Morgenstern, 1947].

‡ The term *state of nature* is used to describe a specific combination of noncontrollable factors—emerging from random and natural events. The state of nature, in effect, is the environment of the decision problem.

§ See [Starr, 1971, pp. 118–161]; [Miller and Starr, 1969, pp. 102–127].

In real-life decision problems, the controllable variables can be manipulated only within certain ranges. This fact is made a part of the decision model by specifying a set of inequality constraints.* As far as the non-controllable variables are concerned, the decision-maker attempts to forecast their behavior by building suitable probability distributions. Once the model is complete, the problem can be solved analytically (e.g., by the methods of calculus or by some iterative procedure) or by the techniques of simulation. (See Part V.)

The simplified decision model shown in equation (4.1) can also be represented as a decision matrix, assuming of course, that we have a finite number of strategies, states of nature, and payoffs. Such a matrix is shown in Figure 4.2.

FIG. 4.2
A SIMPLIFIED DECISION MATRIX

	N_1	N_2	N_3
S_1	R_{11}	R_{12}	R_{13}
S_2	R_{21}	R_{22}	R_{23}
S_3	R_{31}	R_{32}	R_{33}

In the decision matrix shown in Figure 4.2 we have 3 strategies, 3 states of nature, and 9 outcomes or results. Each outcome is a result of the interaction of a certain strategy with a specific state of nature. The decision problem is to choose that strategy which yields the best results.

The matrix of Figure 4.2 omits many elements which must be specified before one can proceed to make the "best" choice from among the identified strategies. For example, assumptions regarding the stability or instability of the system and ambiguity or nonambiguity of the environments must be made. Probability distributions for the states of nature could be constructed, and estimates on the magnitude of various possible payoffs must be built.

Since decisions are implemented in the future, some assumptions or statements regarding the future states of nature must be made. This involves the specification of the probability distribution of the states of nature. In other words, the likelihood of the occurrence of a specific state of nature is given by attaching to it a probability measure.† In this manner we can

---

* For example, a linear programming problem consists of three parts: (1) a linear objective function of the form $P = f(x_1, x_2, ...x_n)$; (2) a set of linear constraints (to show the limits on controllable resources, and (3) a set of non-negativity constraints. See [Loomba, 1964].

† The probability measure can be in the "relative frequency" sense so that any new information does not change the decision-maker's degree of belief; or it can be in the "personal belief" sense which admits new information and is subject to change as a result thereof.

identify four types of decision models.* (1) Decision-making under *certainty,* (2) decision-making under *risk,* (3) decision-making under *uncertainty,* and (4) decision-making under *partial information.*†

4.4.2 *Decision-making under Certainty*

Decision-making under *certainty* implies complete information regarding the decision problem. The assumptions are that the decision-maker is able to enumerate and list all possible strategies or courses of action, knows the requirements to carry them out, and can project their respective consequences with complete certainty. This implies that the decision-maker is predicting a single state of nature, and that he attaches a probability of one to it. Under the assumption of certainty, the decision matrix of Figure 4.2 reduces to a single column matrix. This means that the optimal solution can be identified by comparing all the payoffs or results as they appear in the unicolumn matrix. On the surface this appears to be a simple task, but difficulties arise when the number of possible strategies (and "payoffs" associated with them) becomes extremely large: thereby making the search process time consuming and very costly. For example, a linear programming problem generates an infinite number of feasible solutions and, therefore, some extremely efficient method of search must be employed. Management science has developed various efficient methods of search (e.g., simplex, transportation, assignment, and other optimization models).‡

4.4.3 *Decision-making under Risk*

In decision-making under *risk* we assume that: (1) there is more than one state of nature, (2) we can attach a probability measure to each state of nature, (3) strategies can be listed, and (4) the consequence or result of each strategy in conjunction with different states of nature can be projected. These assumptions imply that decision-making under risk can be represented by the decision-matrix of Figure 4.2, provided the probabilities associated with each state of nature are entered into the decision matrix. The *optimal* strategy in decision-making under risk is identified by calculating the *expected value* of each strategy, and then choosing that strategy which has the highest (if it is a profit-type objective) or the lowest (if it is a cost-type objective) value. Two things should be noted in connection

---

* These four models are static decision models. Furthermore, each pits the decision-maker against "nature," and the impact of competitors is either ignored or indirectly reflected in the results. In the "partial information" model, the states of nature are usually the finite alternatives of a competitor.

† See [Luce and Raiffa, 1958, Chapters 2 and 13], [Dantzig, 1963, Chapters 1 and 25].

‡ A very useful classification of various optimization techniques is given in [Connors and Teichrow, 1967, p. 4].

with the application of "expected value" criterion in decision-making under risk. First, no account is being taken of the "quality" of risk. In other words, the choice is being made strictly in terms of "weighted" outcomes, and the "range" of outcomes is not being considered. Secondly, the probabilities attached to different states of nature are objective probabilities which assume the existence of a stable system.

4.4.4 Decision-making under Uncertainty

Decision-making under *uncertainty* assumes that no probability measures can be attached to different states of nature. In all other aspects the "uncertainty" decision matrix is similar to the "risk" decision matrix. Thus, decision-making under uncertainty can also be represented by the decision matrix of Figure 4.2; strategies can be listed, their consequences in conjunction with different states of nature can be projected, but the probability distribution of the states of nature is assumed *not* to be known. How do we identify the optimal strategy in decision-making under uncertainty? By the application of some choice criteria which in real-life situations can be either subjective or one of the "rational" criteria developed by decision theorists.* The importance of the personal value system in decision-making cannot be ignored; it is especially significant for choosing a specific course of action under the uncertainty framework.

4.4.5 Decision-making under Partial Information

Lastly, there is *decision-making under partial information* (or partial ignorance). This category deals with those cases in which the probabilities of various states are arrived at subjectively—as opposed to the case of risk in which the probability distribution is objective and corresponds to the "relative frequency" sense. This category of decision-making is gaining greater importance, as the use of Bayesian statistics becomes more prevalent in decision-making.† The Bayesian approach can convert an "uncertain" decision problem into a "risk" decision problem by attaching "personal" probabilities to different states of nature. These personal probabilities represent the decision-maker's degree of confidence (or doubt) regarding the likelihood of occurrence of each state. Since these probabilities are personal in nature, they are subject to revision as new information becomes available, or is purchased at a cost.‡ The choice of a strategy in decision-making under partial information can be made by the application of the expected

---

* Examples of such criteria include the maximin, the minimax regret, the Hurwicz criterion, the Laplace criterion and so on. See [Luce and Raiffa, 1958, pp. 278–286].
† [Frank and Green, 1967, p. 25] cite several applications.
‡ This aspect raises questions regarding the cost and value of information. See [Bierman et al., 1961, Chapters 12 and 22].

value criterion, or by analyzing additional information if such information is available. The analysis requires posterior probabilities which are calculated by the application of Baye's theorem.*

4.4.6 Game Theory

We mentioned earlier that game theory concerns making rational decisions under conditions of conflict (or cooperation). Game theory models can be classified in a number of ways,† according to the number of players (2 persons or more than 2 persons), sum of the payments (i.e., zero sum or nonzero sum), number of moves (finite or infinite), and the amount of information (complete or partial). Of the various models, the 2-person zero sum game is the most developed, and has been used in the resolution of business, political, and investment problems.‡ In a 2-person zero sum game the assumptions are: (1) the gains of one player equal exactly the losses of the other; (2) the strategies of both the players are known in advance, (3) the payoffs are known in advance; and (4) the game is repetitive. The decision matrix for a zero sum 2-person game contains the strategies of each player and all possible payoffs. Given the strategies of both players and their associated payoffs, the purpose of game theory models is to provide a rational approach for choosing a strategy. The rational choice leads to that strategy which leaves the decision-maker "best off," no matter what strategy is chosen by the opponent. Similarly, the rational choice for the competitor is that strategy which places him in the most preferred position relative to the decision-maker.

The decision-making models discussed above are models of "rational" choice. It is desirable that we understand the limitations of these models. To quote Simon [1957, p. 252]:

> . . . In most global models of rational choice, *all* alternatives are evaluated before a choice is made. In actual human decision-making, alternatives are often examined sequentially. We may, or may not, know the mechanism that determines the order of procedure. When alternatives are examined sequentially, we may regard the first satisfactory alternative that is evaluated as much as the one actually selected.

4.5 CONCLUDING REMARKS

Our discussion on decision-making can be summarized by stating that regardless of the nature or type of decision, these elements of decision-making must be consciously considered:

---

* For an interesting example and calculations. See [Frank and Green, 1967, pp. 10–22].
† [J. C. C. McKinsey, 1952, pp. 3–6].
‡ [Shubik, 1955], [Bennion, 1956].

a) decision-maker and a set of objectives;
b) context and environment of the decision problem;
c) alternative courses of action;
d) assumptions regarding the future;
e) consequences of alternative courses of action;
f) choice according to a decision criterion; and
g) implementation and control.*

These elements are present in every decision problem. In actual practice, the decision-maker identifies the problem and its hierarchical nature, states the objectives for which the problem is being perceived and formulated, scans the environment in light of the stated objectives, identifies relevant variables that in his judgment affect the outcome, develops functional relationships between the dependent and independent variables, specifies the constraints of the problem, and chooses a course of action according to a decision criterion. As decision problems are usually dynamic and sequential in nature, the decision-maker exercises control of implementation of decisions by continually observing the outputs, and making necessary changes in the inputs by utilizing feedback channels.

Archer's article (Selection 9) presents basic concepts of decision-making. The article examines decision-making under conditions of certainty, risk, and uncertainty. The decision problem is formulated in the format of a matrix, with "strategies," "states of nature" and "payoffs" being the basic components of the decision-matrix. Since the same "payoff" can yield varying degrees of satisfaction to different persons, the concepts of utility and utility measurement are discussed. How the technique of "standard gamble" can be used to transform simple rankings to a cardinal utility scale, ranging from 0 to 1, is illustrated. How a decision problem involving two dimensions (e.g., average payoff *and* variance) can be analyzed is illustrated through the device of an indifference curve. The following aspects of decision-making are not explicitly covered by Archer: (1) single versus multiple objectives, under conditions of certainty as well as risk, (2) single stage versus multiple stage decision-making (i.e., static versus dynamic decision problems), and (3) "sensitivity" analysis of decision problems.

The question of how to structure and solve decision problems with multiple objectives will be discussed in Chapter 5. Eilon's article (Selection 10) also presents ways to handle decision problems (under certainty as well as risk) with multiple measures of performance. A distinction between

---

* [Simon, 1960, p. 2] lists three phases of the decision-making process: *Intelligence, Design,* and *Choice.* He defines intelligence as "searching the environment for conditions calling for decision." The design activity consists of "inventing, developing, and analyzing possible courses of action." The choice is "selecting a particular course of action from those available." Most practical problems would also require the fourth phase, namely, *Implementation and Control.*

static and dynamic decisions was made in section 4.3; and we refer the reader to Rappaport [1967], for a discussion of applied sensitivity analysis.*

Eilon's article describes the decision process as a series of eight steps starting with information input and ending with decision "resolution" according to some "choice criteria" operating on the decision model. Various aspects of rationality in decision-making and the relationship of rationality with utility maximization are examined. It is emphasized that the most important aspects of the decision process are the model building and choice of criterion stages. A very important aspect of Eilon's article is that it treats explicitly the question of multiple objectives in decision-making. Eilon suggests the existence of a continuum of informal and formal procedures and the associated control consisting of a mix of "personalistic" and "impersonalistic" characteristics. It is pointed out that the type of control in decision-making is determined essentially by the degree of involvement of the decision-maker in various stages of the decision process. Control (formal or informal) and decision-making are related and crucial points in the decision process are identified.

REFERENCES

Ackoff, R. L., "Towards a System of Systems Concepts," *Management Science,*
1971   vol. 17, no. 11, July, pp. 661–671
Ackoff, R. L., and M. W. Sasieni, *Fundamentals of Operations Research,* New
1968   York: John Wiley & Sons.
Ansoff, H. I., *Corporate Strategy,* New York: McGraw-Hill.
1965
Bennion, E. G., "Capital Budgeting and Game Theory," *Harvard Business*
1956   *Review,* November–December.
Bierman, H., Jr., et al., *Quantitative Analysis for Business Decisions,* Home-
1961   wood, Ill.: Richard D. Irwin.
Brown, R. E., *Judgment in Administration,* New York: McGraw-Hill.
1966
Connors, M. M., and D. Tiechrow, *Optimal Control of Dynamic Operations*
1967   *Research Models,* Scranton, Pa.: International Textbook Company.
Costello, T. W., and S. Zalkind, *Psychology in Administration,* Englewood
1963   Cliffs, N.J.: Prentice-Hall.
Cyert, A. M., and J. G. March, *A Behavioral Theory of the Firm,* Englewood
1963   Cliffs, N.J.: Prentice-Hall, pp. 114–127.
Dantzig, G. B., *Linear Programming and Extensions,* Princeton, N.J.: Prince-
1963   ton University Press.
Edwards, W., "The Theory of Decision-Making," *Psychological Bulletin,* vol.
1954   51, no. 4, pp. 380–411.
Frank, R. E., and P. E. Green, *Quantitative Methods in Marketing,* Engle-
1967   wood Cliffs, N.J.: Prentice-Hall.

---

* Also see Chapter 12, section 12.5.

Green, P. E., and D. S. Tull, *Research for Marketing Decisions,* Englewood
1970   Cliffs, N.J.: Prentice-Hall.
Hammond, J. S., III, "Better Decisions with Preference Theory," *Harvard*
1967   *Business Review,* vol. 45, November–December, pp. 123–141.
Hespos, R. F., and P. A. Strassman, "Stochastic Decision Trees for the Analysis
1965   of Investment Decisions," *Management Science,* vol. 11, August, pp.
      244–259.
Jones, M. H., *Executive Decision Making,* Homewood, Ill.: Richard D. Irwin.
1959
Loomba, N. P., *Linear Programming,* New York: McGraw-Hill.
1964
Luce, R. D., and H. Raiffa, *Games and Decisions,* New York: John Wiley &
1958   Sons.
Lusted, L. B., "Decision-Making Studies in Patient Management," *The New*
1971   *England Journal of Medicine,* vol. 284, February 25, pp. 416–424.
Magee, J. F., "Decision Trees for Decision Making," *Harvard Business Review.*
1964
March, J. G., *Handbook of Organizations,* Chicago, Ill.: Rand McNally.
1965
March, J. G., and H. A. Simon, *Organizations,* New York: John Wiley & Sons.
1958
McKinsey, J. C. C., *Introduction to the Theory of Games,* New York: Mc-
1952   Graw-Hill.
Miller, D. W., and M. K. Starr, *Executive Decisions and Operations Research,*
1969   2nd edition, Englewood Cliffs, N.J.: Prentice-Hall.
Rappaport, A., "Sensitivity Analysis in Decision Making," *The Accounting*
1967   *Review,* vol. 42, July, pp. 441–455.
Shubik, M., "The Uses of Game Theory in Management Science," *Manage-*
1955   *ment Science,* vol. 2, October, pp. 40–54.
Simon, H. A., *Models of Man,* New York: John Wiley & Sons.
1957
Simon, H. A., "Theories of Decision Making in Economics and Behavioral
1959   Science," *The American Economic Review,* vol. XLIX, no. 3, June,
      pp. 253–281.
Simon, H. A., *The New Science of Management Decision,* New York:
1960   Harper & Row.
Simon, H. A., and A. Newel, "Heuristic Problem Solving: The Next Advance
1958   in Operations Research," *Operations Research,* vol. 6, no. 1, January,
      pp. 1–10.
Starr, M. K., *Management: A Modern Approach,* New York: Harcourt Brace
1971   Jovanovich.
Von Neumann, J., and O. Morgenstern, *Theory of Games and Economic Be-*
1947   *havior,* Princeton, N.J.: Princeton University Press.
Wagner, H. M., *Principles of Operations Research,* Englewood Cliffs, N.J.:
1969   Prentice-Hall.

SELECTION 9

The Structure of Management Decision Theory*

Stephen H. Archer

MANAGERIAL ACTIVITY

A considerable amount of managerial activity customarily precedes the actual decision. In large organizations these activities may be carried on in the management structure, or at least in part, by people other than the official decision-maker. Staff people and others in the line organization discover problems, define them, and prepare the alternatives for decision. The decision is only the conclusion of some process. The process in a broad sense includes: (1) the activities of discovering and defining things to decide about; (2) determining the objective of the organization; and, (3) the enumeration and preparation of the alternative ways of making a decision.

After the preparation of alternative plans or strategies, the payoff of each strategy has to be determined. The information required to determine the payoff is secured only at some cost. Management has the difficult task of deciding when the costs of securing additional information are warranted by the nature of the problem (another decision in itself). At some point, the costs of securing additional information are not warranted and the decision-maker must make decisions in the face of some uncertainties.

A manager *must* choose among alternative strategies. Failure of the manager to make a choice will cause certain malfunctioning in the organizational activity; the importance of the decision abstention is dependent upon the significance and nature of the particular managerial "component" in the structure.

The manager elects one strategy over others based on criteria such as minimum cost, greatest rate of return, maximum sales, or some combination of criteria or objectives. A goal or a mix of goals exists that he is striving to attain. The goals are probably not completely personal goals, for his personal objectives become reshaped and modified subject to the pressures of stockholders, employees, other managers, and so on. In the organization, the mix of specific goals that maximizes his utility includes, among other considerations, achieving what he believes others feel should be the organizational goals. If his beliefs as to the organizational goals deviate too far

---

* *Academy of Management Journal,* vol. 7, December, 1964.

from the beliefs of others, his selection of strategies will be criticized. The manager compares the various strategies to find the one (or a mix of several) that comes closest to the attainment of his goal(s); that is, he optimizes.

The mix of specific objectives of the individual are, in effect, only one in his mind—his satisfaction or his utility. The goal of good health, for example, must be weighed by an individual against the goal of respect of his work partners which might be gained by industriousness and achievement. The goal of health restricts complete concentration on the "respect" goal and thus a lesser attainment of this goal is accepted. The resultant compromise of these specific goals is the ultimate single goal of personal maximum utility—one goal. If one can accept the decision-maker's one goal of maximum utility, the difficulty of dealing with the problem of "dimensionality" (many dimensions) of goals disappears.[1]

COMPONENTS OF THE DECISION MATRIX

It is obvious that an outcome of a decision must occur after the decision is made. The time between a decision and its final outcome may vary considerably depending upon the type of decision and the accuracy desired in the measurement of the outcome.

Outcome Measurement

Some outcomes may not be fully measured even in centuries. On the other hand, many outcomes are measurable for practical purposes, within a reasonably short time after the decision has been made. In some cases this time elapse is very short, perhaps less than a second. For example, the decision to turn a door knob to the left instead of to the right will produce an outcome which is known within a very brief period after the decision is made. The decision of a country, on the other hand, to join the European Common Market may produce an outcome that likely would not be known for many years or perhaps centuries in the future.

Rather than waiting indefinitely to measure the outcome of some decision, it is customary to establish an arbitrary cut-off time—say, ten years, in the case of the Common Market. During this period, most of the direct effects of the outcome should have occurred. Nevertheless, some amount of time must pass before an outcome is determined, and the payoff or measured outcome is a function of the length of the measurement period. The payoff predicted depends upon the arbitrary cutoff time selected and the danger of selecting the wrong strategy will be less if the predicted pay-offs reflect the more complete impact of the strategy.

Strategies

The alternatives available in any decision problem are referred to as "strategies." The number of strategies to choose from may vary from two to infinity (if there were only one, there would be no decision). The decision alternatives in the case of opening a door were to turn the door knob to the left or to the right and this involved only two alternatives. The decision to select a text for a particular class may involve numerous, but a finite number, of alternatives. If, however, one were producing ale, the quantity of water to add to the mix may include alternatives of ten gallons, one gallon, and one millionth of a gallon. Although these seem to be a finite number of alternatives, the alternatives are really infinite; the inaccuracy of the measurement system prevents one from measuring infinitesimal quantities or differences in volumes of water that might be added.

In most operating circumstances, however, all possible alternatives are not enumerated or considered, but only a limited range of alternatives. The range may still leave an infinite number from which to select, as in the ale example. But there are enough rules of good beer-making to establish that the water added ought to be within the range of, say, 8 to 8½ gallons to a ten-gallon barrel. This still leaves an infinite number of points between 8 and 8½ gallons, but one might decide to structure the alternatives in only tenths of gallons. In the choice of a textbook, certain rules are also likely to act to circumscribe the number of alternatives which a decision-maker must face. For example, the rules might be that no text more than ten years old will be considered; no text will be considered that was not produced by a publisher of college texts; no text will be considered which is not relevant to the nature of the course being given (some objective measure of relevancy).

Strategies are sometimes innumerable and must be described as an infinite number within a certain range. There are certain techniques for eliminating strategies from further consideration—those which are known not to be considered as successful in achieving the objectives. The elimination of certain strategies from the group to be considered is accomplished using the information of the person enumerating the strategies. He predicts, based upon his knowledge and experience (reflected in the form of "rules" for action), that these strategies could not result in outcomes as satisfactory as those remaining to be considered. The techniques for restricting the number of strategies available may be fairly crude and imperfect. They are practical. It is certainly possible that some of the strategies eliminated might be desirable but, in effect, the person restricting or enumerating strategies considers the probability of their satisfactory payoff to be so extremely small as not to be worth the cost involved in further consideration.

This problem of deciding how many strategies to present the decision-maker and the risks of error involved in elimination of strategies is a very important problem in decision theory.

A rather formalized procedure has been used in some cases for reducing the number of alternatives to be considered. This procedure, referred to as "heuristic programming" consists of successive applications of rules (usually with the aid of a computer) deemed to be appropriate, so that the number of alternatives is reduced to sufficiently few as to be manageable by the decision-maker. If the rules are sufficient, the number of strategies can be reduced to one, and thereby eliminate the decision problem. The models of ways of arriving at a decision under the various conditions that follow in this paper are nothing more than rules to reduce alternative strategies to one—the optimal. Decision theory becomes a case of heuristic programming in a broad sense.

In other cases, the problem of operating management is not to restrict the number of alternatives to a manageable number, but more to be aware of a sufficient range of alternatives. Management may at times benefit by simply attempting to enumerate alternative strategies rather than choosing among only the few traditionally-used strategies.

Payoffs

The selection of any one strategy will result in a payoff or outcome. If we were fortunate enough to know the payoff associated with each strategy we would be able then to simply select the strategy with the largest payoff, assuming maximization. The determination of such a payoff requires a complete understanding of the manner in which the decision and its resultant activities yield a particular payoff. This situation of being able to predict the payoff with certainty would be very unusual for most business situations.

Frequently our prediction is less than perfect; that is, the situation is not one of certainty. Our predictions of payoff are dealt with by such conditional phrases as "assuming certain conditions" or "depending upon the state of the economy" or similar expressions illustrating the lack of complete understanding of the operation of the system with which we are involved. There are so many variables about which we know so little that in most cases we cannot predict the payoff that results from the interaction of these unknown variables with the activities undertaken as a result of the decision. Customarily we know of only a few of the variables that affect the outcome and have less than perfect knowledge of their influence on the outcome. Therefore, the outcome or payoff is predicted with less than complete certainty.

Conditions

More recently, popular decision theory has reduced or eliminated the model constraint of certainty or one state of nature in dealing with decision problems. This permits us to predict outcomes that depend upon particular "states of nature" or conditions that occur.

Under this model, it is not necessary to know what causes these conditions to occur but it is desirable to know the approximate relative frequency with which these different conditions are expected to occur. (However, knowledge of the causes of the occurrence of these states may be very useful in determining their expected relative frequency.) If we can present the relative frequency of the states of nature by some probability distribution, we may then concentrate our efforts on the problem of determining the payoff given a certain state of nature. Presumably, the state of nature describes the conditions within which the activities set in motion by the decision operate.

The conditions or states of nature include the states of variables over which control is limited or non-existent, many of which might be termed environmental variables, as well as others. A state of nature, for example in a particular problem might refer to the state of the economy, weather conditions, inventory levels and so forth. The assumption in this type of model is that after the state of nature has been described, the payoff resulting from the selection of a particular strategy can be precisely determined (or approximated in the sense that measurement systems in practice are limited).

An example of an elementary enumeration of strategies, states of nature and associated payoffs is presented in matrix (tabular) form below.

| | *States of Nature (N)* | | |
Strategies(S)	N_1	N_2	N_3
S_1	P_{11}	P_{12}	P_{13}
S_2	P_{21}	P_{22}	P_{23}
S_3	P_{31}	P_{32}	P_{33}

The strategies are enumerated in the rows and the states of nature in the columns. The payoff associated with a state and the choice of a strategy is given in the body of the table.

In actuality, determination of the payoff, given the state of nature, is not likely to be precise, nor will the enumerations of strategies or states of nature be complete. However, the model exists; the degree of refinement depends upon the particular problem involved and the reliability which one desires to achieve. In most business problems the payoffs, given certain states of nature, are not completely deterministic, but at least the estimates of the payoffs are more accurate (or should be more accurate) than under the assumption of no variability in the state of nature at all (the certainty model).

STATES OF NATURE

The different conditions under which payoffs are determined bear some further consideration and inspection.

Certainty

Under conditions of certainty, the payoff resulting from the selection of a particular strategy is known. It is assumed that the payoff resulting from the decision can be precisely measured; in other words, only one state of nature is assumed to exist. Prediction is involved, but prediction is assumed to be perfect. A substantial amount of knowledge and understanding of the working and behavior of the system is required in order to exert enough control to be able to assume a state of certainty. In probability terms, the probability that a certain state of nature exists is assumed to be one. The assumption of certainty simplifies the decision but ignores variations in conditions which often exist, leading to improper decisions.

For example, our strategies might be the selection of various inventory levels to attain on January 1 of the coming year; the payoffs in this case are stated in terms of profits.

Strategies: Inventory levels	States of Nature
200	$ 50
250	300
300	500
350	200

In this case, the enumeration of strategies has been limited by prior decision and knowledge, to the range of 200 units to 350 units. Additional refinement which might be desired would require more choices than the four presented here—perhaps all discrete integer values between 199 and 351. If, however, the profit distribution (payoffs) is known to be unimodal we could further restrict the range of strategies to those near the 300 unit level. If at 301 profits were greater than at the 300 level, we should proceed to investigate the payoffs in this direction until they begin to decrease. If the profits were a continuous function of the inventory level, the maximum value could be simply obtained by differential calculus.

The profits in this model are predicted. The use of this model for decision assumes these are predicted perfectly or with insignificant risk of significant error. If we can associate with certainty the profits that would result at some measurable time in the future for each inventory level or strategy, it is a model under certainty. Realistically, however, one cannot rely on these profit levels being obtained, given only information on inventory levels. Many other known and unknown factors influence the level of profits. In business decision, a state of certainty is the exception.

Risk

If the decision model does not assume certainty, but assumes risk, the various states of nature can be enumerated and the long-run relative frequency of their occurrence is assumed to be known. For example, it is known that a combination of seven appearing in a roll of a pair of two dice will occur in the long run with a relative frequency of 6/36. If eleven states of nature occur in the long run exactly as do the roll of two dice, probabilities can be assigned the eleven states. In other cases, the probability distribution may take on a continuous form such as a normal distribution. In this model, we assume we are certain about the relative frequency with which the given states of nature will occur in the long run. We do not assume any one state, but many; we do however assume that we know the probability of the occurrence of the various states.

There exists in this model more than one payoff for each of the strategies prior to the decision. After the decision has been made, obviously only one of the payoffs can occur as a result of the decision. A payoff exists for each combination of strategy and state of nature. In the table below there are three outcomes associated with each strategy.

STATES OF NATURE AND THEIR RESPECTIVE PROBABILITY OF OCCURRENCE

	States of Nature		
Strategies	A(.25)	B(.50)	C(.25)
1............................	P_{11}	P_{12}	P_{13}
2............................	P_{21}	P_{22}	P_{23}
3............................	P_{31}	P_{32}	P_{33}
4............................	P_{41}	P_{42}	P_{43}

If we were given a state of nature as having occurred and the selection of a particular strategy, the payoff would be assumed to be known with perfect precision, which in the actual case is seldom true. However, in any one decision, we do not know which of the states of nature will occur but only have expectations as to their relative occurrence.

A considerable amount of care needs to be exercised in assuming the risk model. The probability distribution of the states of nature is assumed to be known. Decision theory requires that the risk model should be used only when this is the case, although this assumption is frequently overlooked.

The number of states sufficient to use the risk model with confidence is a subject deserving further discussion and development. As with the certainty model, the prediction of the payoffs in the matrix is assumed to be perfect. In some circumstances, when certainty assumes one state of nature and the payoffs cannot be accurately predicted, a change to a risk model which permits specification of different conditions produces more accurate payoff predictions. The number of states of nature should be sufficient to provide accurate payoff predictions.

It should be emphasized that if the risk model is to be used properly and lead to the correct decisions, the time in which the outcome as a payoff is to be determined must be sufficient to encompass all of the results of the decision. In the interest of reasonableness of operation, it is desirable to establish some cutoff point for measurement purposes It is within this period that we seek perfect prediction of the payoffs. Part of the outcome beyond this point is ignored, but should not be of significant importance if the cutoff time is appropriately established.

Uncertainty

Uncertainty exists when one does not know the long-term relative frequency with which the states of nature will occur.

(1) Based upon past objective experience, one may be *relatively* confident of the nature of the probability distribution of states of nature;

(2) Based upon one's judgment, one may estimate the probability distribution;

(3) One may guess at the probability distribution of the states of nature based upon his subjective impressions; or,

(4) There exists no information whatsoever as to the relative frequency with which the states of nature will occur.

Uncertainty in decision theory describes all shades of knowledge of the probability distribution of the states of nature ranging from near accurate estimates based upon objective experience to an extreme case in which no knowledge exists. It is this type of model which most frequently applies to management decision. Uncertainty varies from the extreme of no information up to but excluding the condition of risk in which the probability distribution of the states of nature is known. Short of risk conditions, exists uncertainty.

DECISIONS UNDER RISK

In the certainty decision model the decision between alternative strategies is relatively obvious—namely *select the strategy whose payoff is largest or smallest depending upon whether the decision-maker is maximizing or minimizing.* In the case of risk the decision is not so obvious.

Expected Value

Under conditions of risk, the decision-maker must review the payoff matrix (his knowledge of the various payoffs), which represents combinations of states of nature with their probabilities of occurrence and strategies, in order to arrive at a decision. At first glance, one might be inclined simply to average the payoffs for each strategy, but this does not give proper weight to the relative frequency with which the payoffs are expected to occur. The payoff should be weighed by the probabilities involved. As the probabilities themselves add to one it is not necessary to divide the weighted sum by any factor. The "expected value" of a strategy is the sum of the payoffs each multiplied by its respective probability of occurrence. An expected value may be derived for each strategy.

The appropriate decision is to select the strategy with *optimizing expected value* (largest, for maximization of the payoff unit).

	States of Nature			
Strategies: Inventory levels	A(.25)	B(.50)	C(.25)	*Expected Values*
200.........................	100	100	50	87.5
250.........................	90	120	100	107.5
300.........................	70	120	140	112.5
350.........................	40	90	190	102.5
400.........................	0	50	160	65.0

In this example, the payoffs are profits which the decision-maker wishes to maximize. The optimal strategy is therefore the stocking of 300 units, for the expected value (the average profits from such a decision in the long run) is higher ($112.5) than for any other strategy.

However, if the probability distribution were uniform (the probabilities of the states of nature were known to be equal), the optimal choice is to stock 350 units.

	States of Nature			
Strategies: Inventory levels	A(⅓)	B(⅓)	C(⅓)	Expected Values
200..........................	100	100	50	83⅓
250..........................	90	120	100	103⅓
300..........................	70	105	140	105
350..........................	40	90	190	106⅔
400..........................	0	50	160	70

The expected values in the table are the weighted averages for each of the strategies. A solution to this decision problem was to select that strategy with the highest expected value. This is the most common decision-making criteria under the condition of risk. It will produce satisfactory results in many cases.

Consider, however, the decision between two alternative strategies one of which will give a payoff of 8 million dollars with a probability of one and the other strategy, a payoff of 10 million dollars with a probability of .9 and a loss payoff of minus 10 million dollars with a probability of .1. The expected value in each case is 8 million and thus, under the expected value criteria, each strategy would be equally desirable. Upon introspection, however, the preferred strategy is that leading to payoff of 8 million dollars with certainty rather than the one with a possible loss of 10 million dollars, even though the probability of occurrence is relatively small, particularly when the event is a one shot affair. It may appear that the expected value method in this particular example is less than satisfactory. The criticism levied against expected value (as implied) as a criteria is not a proper criticism of the technique of taking weighted averages of the payoffs; the fault lies in the manner of expressing payoffs in the traditional form such as profits or sales.

The issue is one of payoff measurement rather than one of expected value. Even though the payoffs may be quantifiable they may not have been measured in terms of the values we wish to optimize. If one is seeking to maximize utility (via some mix of goals), profit may, in many situations, be an inadequate measurement of utility. Frequently, one may indicate that he is not interested in profits, but survival of the firm, survival of the managers in their present positions, and so on. However, one usually proceeds to state the firm shall be assumed to be maximizing profits. Upon observing the results of decisions based upon profit maximization, some complain our techniques of decision-making are inadequate. The criteria used—profit maximization—simply ignores other aspects of utility, primarily variability of the returns. Doubling profits will not likely double utility. To arrive at the proper strategy necessitates converting the payoffs to relative utilities from which we may then compute the expected values. The best strategy is that with the maximum expected utility or minimum disutility.

In the example above, the payoff of minus 10 million, in utility terms, would be given a greater weight in the averaging process due to the disutility and consequently the expected value computed would be less than the expected value of the certainty alternative.

The reader may tend to back away from utility considerations because of the near-universally-accepted criticism of any type of utility measurement. At least theoretically, utility cannot be ignored for it is maximum satisfaction which is the real objective of the manager. If we assume we are dealing with only one manager, and we are interested only in one mental decision process, we are not forced into the argument of the lack of comparability of utilities between two individuals. For any one individual, one may state that a payoff to an individual may be less or greater than another payoff to him in terms of utility. That is, one ought to be able to rank the payoffs in terms of satisfaction to him as a manager.

Ranking, however, is not completely satisfactory for it tends to ignore degrees of preference which a manager may have for one payoff over another. The payoffs can be converted to relative utilities by a technique referred to as "standard gamble" method[2] which may be used to assign payoffs to positions on a utility scale from zero to one with reasonable reliability, if properly used.

Let us assume a particular strategy will result in the occurrence of three possible payoffs, *a, b,* and *c.* Although the technique does *not* require that the payoff be in dollars of profit, let us assign a gain of $0 to *a,* $100 to *b,* and $200 to *c.* Without knowing anything at this point about the relative frequency or probability of occurrence of *a, b,* or *c,* let us set down their utility to the decision maker. We can rank these on any relative scale such as 0 to 10, 0 to 1,000,000 or 0 to 1; let us choose the latter. We know *a* is the least desirable to the decision maker so we assign it a relative value of 0. We know that *c* is the most desirable so we assign it a value of 1; *b* should have some intermediate value. For each intermediate outcome, determine when a decision maker is indifferent to (1) receiving that outcome for certain and (2) a lottery between the extreme values with an assigned probability. For example, a decision-maker is offered the choice between (1) *b* for certain and (2) a result with probability *p* of getting *c* and a 1-*p* chance of getting *a.* If *p* is equal to 1 then he would choose alternative (2). If *p* were 0 he would choose alternative (1) and take the $100. At some *p* between 0 and 1 he would be indifferent to (1) and (2).

If we assume his particular utility pattern causes him to choose p equal to .8, we have thus assigned relative weights (0.8 and 1) to the outcomes a, b, and c—a scale of relative utilities of the payoffs.

INDIFFERENCE CURVES

Another method for solving the decision-making problem may be used. This one is similar to the expected value method when used with utility payoffs. As before, each strategy that may be chosen has a distribution of possible payoffs. The specific payoff that will occur depends upon the actual state of nature that does in fact occur. We have before the decision is made, information only on the expected relative occurrence of these states and therefore the expected relative frequency of the payoffs associated with each strategy.

The average payoff is nothing more than the expected value—computed as a weighted average of the payoffs for each strategy. As before, one is inclined to select the strategy with the largest return, in the case of, say, profits. This result may lead to unsatisfactory decisions as indicated in the discussion of expected value criteria using non-utility payoffs. One may, however, increase the dimensions of the evaluation of strategies and study each strategy, not only with respect to average payoff, but also with respect to the variability of expected returns and their expected variance.

The problem facing the decision-maker is to choose a strategy giving a combination for expected payoff and variance which is optimal, giving him the greatest satisfaction. He may enumerate all the strategies and observe the expected returns and the expected variability involved for each of them. Markowitz developed a technique for dealing with combinations of variance and returns in investment portfolio analysis.[3] He indicated that "efficient" strategies or portfolios (combinations of securities) are a subset of all strategies. Non-efficient strategies may be immediately eliminated as the managers choose portfolios or strategies such that: (1) among strategies of equal variability, he would select the one yielding the greatest expected payoff and (2) among strategies with the same expected payoff, the manager would prefer the one with the smallest variance. All the remaining strategies can be approximately represented by a curve (assuming continuity) of strategies constituting a set of efficient strategies. Without going into subtle explanations here, such a curve would have an appearance similar to the curve in Figure 1.

At high levels of expected return a decision-maker would be willing to accept greater variance. Consequently, the curve is upward sloping to the right. It reflects combinations of variance and average returns which must be superior to all other possible combinations. Each point along the curve represents a single strategy—a single combination of average payoff and the variability of payoffs. Given the set of strategies all of which are efficient, which strategy should the manager choose? Which combination

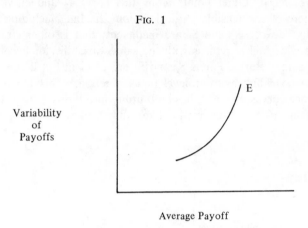

FIG. 1

Variability of Payoffs

Average Payoff

of return and variance is optimal in terms of his satisfaction? How much of the greater variance is the manager willing to bear in order to receive a greater return?

A device for summarizing the manager's attitude toward these combinations may be constructed and is commonly known as the indifference curve. As the curve reflects the manager's attitude to the average payoffs versus the variability of payoffs, it performs a function similar to the transference of standard payoffs into utility terms. It evaluates *two* dimensions of each strategy—the average and the variance payoffs, whereas the utility payoff measurement permits inclusion of any number of dimensions. This is an advantage only if more than two dimensions are felt necessary to evaluate the strategies.

The family of indifference curves can be drawn or constructed. At all points (strategies) along any indifference curve, the manager is indifferent to the choice of one strategy (combination of risk and payoff) over another. Figure 2 illustrates a family of indifference curves. One can construct an almost infinite number of indifference curves for the individual manager. They slope upward, reflecting the manager's liking for payoff and his dislike of risk; the curve is more likely to become flatter as it rises; to induce him to take on greater variability, he must be compensated with a greater return. Each indifference curve represents a set of strategies to which the manager is indifferent. A strategy is a point in two-dimensional space; not all of these are feasible or even available. Only those on the "E curve" are feasible strategies, from which the manager must choose one.

The manager's decision would be to select the strategy at the point of tangency of one of the indifference curves and the efficiency-strategy curve as shown in Figure 3. At the tangent point S_1, the optimal strategy is obtained—the combination of average payoff and variance which is optimal for this manager. Other points along this curve I_2 and curve I_3 do not include any of the feasible strategies along its line, including S_2 and S_3. All points between S_2 and S_3 are inefficient; that is other strategies exist which provide higher returns with the same variability or lower variability with the same returns. Points S_2 and S_3 are efficient but lie on an indifference curve yielding a lower level of satisfaction.[4] This technique of the indifference curves, in effect, has built utility into the system. The individual manager in this curve reflects his likes and dislikes for risk and return.

FIG. 2

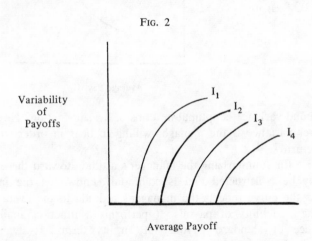

Average Payoff

The measure of dispersion or variability about the average payoff is customarily referred to as the *risk* associated with the selection of the particular strategy. Risk of the variability of the payoffs may be identified, in the use of this technique, as something less than the complete probability distribution itself. A convenient measure of risk may be used which measures only the dispersion of the distribution of payoffs. A satisfactory measure of dispersion for most cases is a form of the standard deviation. The standard deviation is usually expressed in absolute quantities. It is desirable, in order to make comparisons of levels of risk, to measure these standard deviations on a comparable basis relative to the mean of the distribution. Consequently we introduce the coefficient of variation which is defined as the standard deviation divided by the mean. This one value represents the relative dispersion of the distribution about the mean, representative of the risk involved in a particular strategy.

The problem of expressing risk in quantitative terms is one which has not been fully solved. The coefficient of variation is sometimes criticized as not satisfactorily expressing the risk involved. Some critics argue that the absolute standard deviation of two expected payoffs of say, five, and the same absolute standard of an expected payoff of say, ten, would involve the same risk even if the mean were higher in the second case. The probability distribution has the same absolute standard deviation but is based on a different mean.

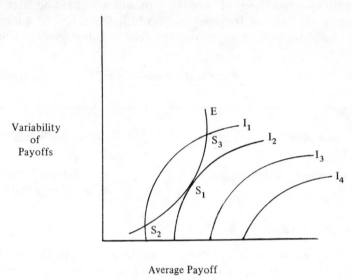

Average Payoff

On the other hand, for equal risks, one may inquire whether, due to the higher mean, we should require a proportionally higher standard deviation. If one does accept a proportionally higher standard deviation at a higher mean, he should prefer the coefficient of variation—a relative measure of risk.

Another concept for the measurement of risk is one used in information theory: that of "entropy," which has certain properties of advantage in measuring risk. In this case, the shape of the distribution need not be assumed to be the same as it is in standard deviation. Entropy measure uses all values of the probability distribution and will have a low value for a uniform distribution and will have a higher value for a more concentrated distribution. A possible difficulty with the use of entropy as a measure of risk is that it will give different values depending upon the number of possible outcomes enumerated (in the case of the discrete distribution). If the outcomes were ten in one case and five in another, different values of entropy would be obtained even though the range of dispersion might be the same. However, for most decision problems, the number of outcomes for each strategy could be stated as the same, even if it meant assigning zero probabilities to those outcomes.

DECISION UNDER UNCERTAINTY

Decision under *uncertainty involves a range of conditions* in which the probability distribution of states of nature varies from one in which we have considerable confidence, based upon objective experience, to the other extreme—conditions of uncertainty on which we have no information concerning the relative frequency with which the states of nature will occur. We shall look at uncertainty models at a few points along this continuum.

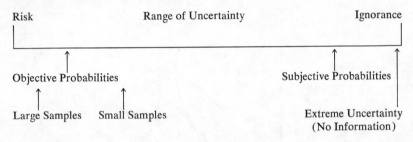

Objectively Obtained Probabilities

Under this class of decision problems, the selection of a particular strategy is based upon probabilities of the states of nature that are expected to occur; the probabilities in this case are estimated by use of objectively obtained experience. The relative frequency of the occurrence of the states of nature in the past has been accumulated; however the amount of experience recorded usually varies from a small amount of experience to considerable experience.

The information secured about the probability distribution may have been obtained through the accumulation of data on past experience or may be obtained, as it is in many cases, through a current investigation such as that based on sampling techniques. (There is a strong inclination to digress into the area of statistics at this point; however, in the interest of progress in our main topic, we shall avoid this diversion.)

In any case, the confidence that a decision-maker has in the probability distribution depends upon the number of observations which have been accumulated either from experience or by sampling. The acceptability of the accumulation of past experience, on which to base estimates of the relative frequencies of occurrence in the future, depends on the belief that the process under study is stable over time. This assumption, of course, is also necessary in the acceptance of the inference about future probability distributions based on a sample result. Statisticians tell us that uncertainty decreases as the size of the sample or experience increases; that is, the likelihood of error in the distribution will decrease as the number of observations increases. We may use as the distribution for the decision problem the relative frequencies as they were accumulated, or we may fit a distribution (binomial, normal, poisson, etc.) to the data, particularly if we have enough knowledge of the events and how they occur to know the shape of the actual population about which we are making inferences. Presumably, as the sample was taken by scientific (systematized and unbiased) procedures, we may measure the error involved in estimating the parameters of a particular probability distribution, a problem of statistical estimation.

The decision procedure for this type of model is similar to others. After the probability distribution has been decided, one may compute the expected value of utility payoff or the risk in the case of indifference curve analysis. The decision procedures are the same as they were under risk, when we knew the "population" probability distribution.

There is, however, a difference in this case. The probability distribution used may not be the same as the "population" distribution due to sampling error. The probable range of error and the impact upon the decision *may* be determined.[5]

Subjective Probabilities

The second class of decisions under uncertainty involves those where the decision-maker has no objective experience on which to rely, but on which he will desire to act on the basis of his best judgment. His judgment is based on past experience in the form of observations but the observations are not scientifically obtained. His statements are subjective. Schlaifer and others have suggested that the decision-maker, even though relying on judgment, ought to formalize his decision process by constructing a subjective probability distribution.[6] The subjective probabilities can be estimated by the decision-maker using his best judgment as to the relative frequency with which the states of nature would be expected to occur. The internal consistency of these probability estimates can be improved through the use of a lottery procedure similar to the standard gamble procedure.[7]

Given a subjective probability distribution of different states of nature, the selection of a particular strategy may be carried out as before, namely through the use of expected value of the utilities of outcomes or the indifference curve analysis.

The use of the subjective probability distribution in decision-making, however, cannot be assumed to have the same attributes as the objectively secured distribution. The objective distribution permitted us in many cases to estimate objectively the possible errors involved in relying on it. However the subjective distribution suffers from the lack of that attribute. Different individuals will likely express different distributions for the same problem and each will likely have varying degrees of confidence in the distribution.

It would be desirable to develop a technique to approximate our confidence or credibility in subjective distributions. It would also be useful to establish methods of combining judgments of distributions of different individuals so as to increase the confidence of reliability in the estimate of the distribution.

A recent exercise by a graduate student compared the results of combining subjective distributions of many individuals in order to observe the behavior in the estimate of population values. It was necessary to select something about which those sampled could give reasonable subjective impressions and for which actual population values were available. These were also compared to random samples from the population taken objectively via a random number table. The pooled percentages for each class of the student age distribution compared with the objective sample results, for a sample of size 50, is shown in the table below.[8]

SUBJECTIVE, OBJECTIVE AND POPULATION PROPORTIONS

Age Class	Subjective Pooled Values	Objective Sample Values	Population, True Values
15 through 17	4.4%	0.1%	0.6%
18 through 20	40.8	36.0	41.0
21 through 23	24.1	42.0	26.6
24 through 26	13.9	10.0	13.2
27 through 29	7.3	8.0	7.1
30 through 34	4.4	2.0	5.9
35 through 39	2.6	2.0	2.7
40 and over	2.4	0.0	3.0

The subjective distribution improved as an estimate of population values as the size of the sample increased from ten to fifty. A similar exercise was completed for the distribution of automobile manufacturers and bore out substantially the same results.

Other advances have been made toward methodology for combining subjective and objective data. When objective data are limited, how much weight should be assigned the subjective distribution(s)? Bayesian analysis has suggested the application of objective experience to subjective prior distributions in order to arrive at revised, posterior distributions.[9] If a sample of only one can be secured, the subjective distribution will have a strong influence on the posterior probabilities. As successive observations are added, the influence of the subjective distribution decreases. If only one observation can be secured, however, it would be desirable to differentiate between a subjective distribution in which we have considerable confidence and one in which we have little credence.

A solution to the problem of evaluating confidence in subjective distributions would help us both in combining subjective information and in combining objective and subjective information. It would also help in determining the point at which sufficient objective data permit us to ignore the subjective information. Sufficient sequential sampling will, in any case, eventually almost entirely eliminate the influence of the original subjective prior distribution.

At some point the lack of confidence in the subjective distribution, if no objective data can be obtained, warrants dropping the idea of using any of the above models. In such cases, the decision-maker assumes complete ignorance and must turn to models of decision-making under extreme uncertainty.

Decisions Under Extreme Uncertainty

In this class of decision problems the decision-maker is assumed to have no information available to him about the relative frequency of occurrence of the various states of nature; he does not have even subjective judgments concerning such probability distribution. In these cases, it would be hopeless to attempt to assign any such probabilities to the states of nature. An attempt to place the decision process in such a framework may result in a poorer decision than with other assumptions such as ignorance about the probability of the states of nature.

The criteria offered for use in arriving at a decision under extreme uncertainty are many and include such descriptive titles as rationality, pessimism, optimism, regret, and surprise. All of these have been suggested in the literature. Rationality, for instance, assumes that the decision-maker has no idea as to the relevant probability assignments and due to insufficient reason, it is assumed that all states are equally likely to occur. Equal probabilities to all states of nature are assigned and in this case the simple expected value (equivalent to an unweighted average of payoffs) is computed and the decision-maker simply selects the strategy with the highest expected payoff. This criteria of rationality has also been referred to in the literature as the criterion of Insufficient reason or the Laplace criterion.

Another criterion suggested by Abraham Wald and others is based upon a pessimistic outlook by the decision-maker who then chooses the strategy with the maximum of all minimum returns. An opposite rule, the optimistic criteria, selects the maximax criterion, in which case the decision-maker selects the strategy with the maximum of the maximums. Hurwicz has constructed and presented yet another criteria which takes into consideration the decision-maker's varying degree of optimism in their views on particular decisions.[10]

Another criteria, introduced by Savage, is called the criterion of regret; the decision-maker is assumed to minimize regret.[11] Regret is measured as the difference between an actual and the expected payoffs.

A potential surprise function was presented by G. L. S. Shackle for his criterion.[12] Those particular outcomes most likely to occur have least potential surprise whereas the outcomes with greater likelihood of occurrence in the decision-maker's mind have a low potential surprise. The potential surprise function is then combined with an individual indifference function in order to arrive at the best strategy selection. The best outcome is the one considered to be producing the largest gain for the decision-maker.

A thorough discussion of all the criteria is unwarranted in this paper.[13] The various criteria for strategy selection under conditions of ignorance or extreme uncertainty have received a good deal of attention. The intellectual game of "how many ways can you make a decision sound reasonable" has been well-played, but insufficient attention has been given to the more important problems of when ignorance should be assumed for decisions under less complete uncertainty.

SUMMARY

The decision-making model under certainty assumes one state of nature in which the payoffs of the various strategies may be predicted perfectly. When the payoffs are presented in optimizing quantities, such as utility, the rule states that the strategy with the largest payoff (under maximization) is selected.

Under conditions of risk, the model constraint of one state of nature can be relaxed and a finite or an infinite number of states may be assumed. Given the stated conditions, the prediction of payoffs is again assumed to be perfect. Under this model, given (1) the proper strategy alternatives, (2) the payoffs expressed in terms of the value to be optimized, (3) perfect payoff prediction, and (4) a known probability distribution of the states of nature, an optimal strategy may be selected as the best decision. This may be found by selecting the strategy with the largest expected value (to maximize) of payoffs or through an indifference analysis.

The decision-making model most common to the business and managerial field is that involving uncertainty, in various degrees, but usually not total ignorance. Uncertainty may exist when some objective experience is available but not enough to precisely determine the probability distribution of the various states of nature. The case tends to approach risk, but decision-making under risk assumes that a probability distribution is known. As the amount of objective experience decreases, the decision-maker must rely more upon the personal feelings or judgment concerning the selection of various strategies. Significant problems in this field are (1) to determine when the objective experience becomes so small that it should be replaced by a subjective probability analysis, or an assumption of ignorance, (2) what techniques can be used to combine effectively subjective probability information, and (3) in general, we need a confidence measure for subjective probability distributions.

Other problems consist of (1) the proper method of measuring risk, (2) the problems of the proper time within which to measure payoffs, (3) the problem of proper enumeration of a reasonable number of payoffs, (4) the problem of measurement of the payoff itself—how precise are the measurement requirements, (5) the use of the appropriate units in which to measure payoffs, and (6) the cost of securing information necessary to determine strategies; states of nature and payoffs.

REFERENCES

[1] Miller and Starr, *Executive Decisions and Operations Research* (Englewood Cliffs, New Jersey: Prentice-Hall, Inc., 1960), p. 68.

[2] John Von Neumann and Oskar Morgenstern, *Theory of Games and Economic Behavior* (Princeton: Princeton University Press, 1947). See also Miller and Starr, *op. cit.*, pp. 69–72.

[3] Harry M. Markowitz, *Portfolio Selection* (New York: John Wiley and Sons, Inc., 1959).

[4] William S. Sharpe of the University of Washington has supplied this type of analysis to capital allocation models for the firm, which appears in an unpublished text entitled *Business Finance; Theory and Management,* written by S. H. Archer and C. A. D'Ambrosio.

[5] See R. Schlaifer, *Introduction to Statistics for Business Decisions* (New York: McGraw-Hill Book Company, Inc., 1961), Chapters 10, 11, 17, 18.

[6] *Ibid.,* pp. 13–22.

[7] *Ibid.,* pp. 13–14.

[8] L. E. Richards, *A Study of Pooled Subjective Distributions Toward Approximation of the Objective Distributions* (unpublished research report, University of Washington, 1963), pg. 48. Fifty students (random sample) were asked what they believed was the age distribution of all students on campus. The proportions they estimated for each class were then averaged (pooled). In the objective case, 50 students' ages were randomly selected and placed in the age classes. Both of these estimates were then compared with the registrar's figures on ages of enrolled students.

[9] Schlaifer, *op cit.,* Chapters 12, 13.

[10] Leonid Hurwicz, *Optimality Criteria for Decision Making Under Ignorance* (Cowles Commission mimeographed discussion paper, Statistics No. 370, 1951).

[11] L. J. Savage, "The Theory of Statistical Decision," *Journal of the American Statistical Association*, Vol. 46 (1951), pp. 55–67.

[12] G. L. S. Shackle, *Uncertainty in Economics and Other Reflections* (Cambridge University Press, 1955).

[13] A more thorough discussion of most of these criteria can be found in Miller and Starr, *op. cit.*, pp. 85–94.

SELECTION 10

What Is a Decision?*

Samuel Eilon

DEFINITIONS

An examination of the literature reveals the somewhat perplexing fact that most books on management and decision theory do not contain a specific definition of what is meant by a *decision*. One can find detailed descriptions of decision trees, discussions of game theory and analyses of various statistical treatments of payoffs matrices under conditions of uncertainty, but the definition of the decision activity itself is often taken for granted and is associated with making a choice between alternative courses of action. As Fishburn puts it:

> Solving the decision model consists of finding a strategy for action the expected relative value of which is at least as great as the expected relative value of any other strategy in a specified set. The prescriptive criterion of a strategy will be maximization of the decision maker's total expected relative value. [3, p. 11]

A concise description of alternative definitions of a decision is given by Ofstad, who says:

> To say that a person has made a decision may mean (1) that he has started a series of behavioral reactions in favor of something, or it may mean (2) that he has made up his mind to *do* a certain action, which he has no doubts that he ought to do. But perhaps the most common use of the term is this: 'to make a decision' means (3) to make a judgment regarding what one *ought* to do in a certain situation after having deliberated on some alternative courses of action. [4, p. 15]

He then adds that (3) has the support of philosophical tradition. To quote Churchman, "The manager is the man who decides among alternative choices. He must decide which choice he believes will lead to a certain desired objective or set of objectives." [1, p. 17] The essential ingredients in this definition are that the decision-maker has *several alternatives* and that his choice involves a *comparison* between these alternatives and the *evaluation of their outcomes*.

---

* *Management Science*, vol. 16, no. 4, December, 1969.

THE DECISION PROCESS

But before we concentrate on the final selection of a course of action, it is necessary to consider the decision activity as a whole. What are the mental processes that the decision maker goes through before he arrives at his conclusion?

Figure 1 is an attempt to describe the decision process. in a schematic

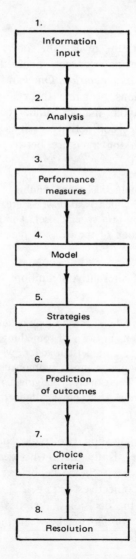

FIG. 1. The decision process

form: First, there is an information input, say from some data processing machinery. This is followed by an analysis of the information material with the purpose of ascertaining its validity and discriminating between its significant and insignificant parts. The analysis leads to the specification of performance measures, which provide the basis for determining how a particular course of action is to be judged, and then to the construction of a model in order to describe the behaviour of the system for which the manager is asked to make a decision.

In a production-marketing system, for example, the measures of performance may include profit, mean level and/or variance of plant utilization, level of meeting customer demand, and so on. Thus, any given courses of action, whether they represent existing policies or whether they are hypothetical propositions for new policies, can be described by arrays of the measures of performance that are thought to be most relevant.

A set of alternatives (or "strategies" in the language of the theory of games) is enumerated and predictions are then made regarding the possible outcomes of each alternative. In order to be able to select between them, a criterion for comparing outcomes in the light of their respective measures of performance is set up and finally the selection (called here *resolution*) is made.

There are several comments that should be made here. First, the term *decision* is identified in many people's minds with what is called here *resolution,* while some would argue that a decision includes the determination of selection criteria as well. Most students of statistical decision theory insist that the prediction of outcomes of events is an indispensable part of the decision activity, and some suggest that the enumeration of strategies is also an integral component of decision-making. It will become clear from the following discussion, I hope, that the various steps in the decision process are so interrelated and that each may have such significant implications for others, that it is essential to examine all these steps in order to identify the crucial links in the chain of events that leads to the final selection of a particular course of action.

Secondly, there is a need to distinguish between *rational* and *irrational* resolution. Dictionary definitions of the term *rational* ("endowed with reason, sensible, sane, moderate," etc.) are not entirely adequate for our purposes. Churchman discusses the concept of reason at some length and comments that

> perhaps the most predominant in the history of thought has been a definition of reason that has tied it closely to logic. The general idea here is that reason consists of logical and consistent steps that go from first principles to rigidly derived conclusions. The steps satisfy all the requirements that formal logic imposes on the so-called reasoning process. [1, p. 95]

Churchman is not satisfied with this concept and strongly suggests that "rationality has to do with goals as well as the means of the attainment of goals" [1, p. 102] and disagrees with those to whom "it will seem futile to ascribe rationality to goals, unless the goals are regarded as intermediate means to further goals," [1, p. 121]. The implication of Churchman's arguments is that questions of ethics and morality cannot be divorced from the concept of rationality, since they are often embedded in the determination of goals, otherwise we can never tell "what is absolutely right." The proposition that rationality should be judged in terms of what an individual wishes to attain, that if his intentions are good he is rational and if they are evil he is irrational, is of course contentious. For the sake of our discussion, however, I propose a more restricted definition of rational behaviour. What I mean by rational resolution is that the decision-maker conforms to the selection criterion, namely that if after applying the criterion a course of action A is shown to be superior to B, the decision-maker does in fact select A in preference to B. If he does not, then the resolution is *irrational*. Further aspects of rationality in decision-making are discussed later.

Thirdly, if the discussion of the decision-making process is confined to rational decisions, it follows that every step in the process described in Figure 1 is indispensable and that the steps must proceed in the order specified: Information is essential for analysis and for defining measures of performance; without these preliminaries, no model building related to the real world is possible, and without a model to describe the behaviour of the system that the decision maker is trying to control, no alternative courses of action (or strategies) can be considered; the prediction of outcomes is meaningless unless it corresponds to a set of alternative strategies, and the method for choosing between them may well have to be delayed until the expected outcomes have been listed. The final act, that of resolution, is specified by the criterion of choice.

Each step in this process has as its input the outcome of activities in preceding steps and in turn it provides an input to the next step. The use that is made of these inputs varies from step to step: All the relevant information, for example, is useful for analysis and for model building, but all the detailed data are rarely needed to define performance measures, and once the model has been constructed it embodies the previous steps to an extent that many information details may be ignored in subsequent steps.

Fourthly, it should be noted that while—for the sake of simplicity—the decision process is depicted in Figure 1 as a chain of sequential activities, it very often takes the form of recurrent chains with feedback. Figure 2 described in schematic form the model building process with feedback. Model building is very similar to proposing a hypothesis in the hypothetico-

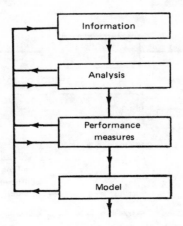

Fɪɢ. 2. Model building with feed-back

deductive scientific method. The model describes the interrelationships between variables in the system; it attempts to show cause and effect; in short, it is designed to provide a predictive tool, so that the controller of the system can proceed to manipulate the variables under his control in order to achieve some desired objectives. But in structuring a theory any given hypothesis needs to be tested and scrutinised, through the design of new experiments and the collection of fresh information, and a model constructed as a part of the decision process must be examined in very much the same way. At any stage in this process questions may arise as to the validity of the information, the adequacy of the analysis, the meaning of performance measures, the need for fresh evidence to test the model and some of its implications. This recurrent procedure permeates throughout the decision process.

HOW DATA PROCESSING IMPINGES ON ANALYSIS

The decision process starts with an information input and it is often asserted that information processing that precedes this input is quite distinct from the subsequent analysis that marks the beginning of the decision process proper.

If we examine, however, the activities that are involved in data or information processing on the one hand and in analysis on the other, we find that the line of demarcation is far from being distinct, if it can be drawn at all. Data processing consists of three major activities [2]; data and information storage, data handling and the presentation of information, and these activities may be further divided into several categories, as shown in Figure 3.

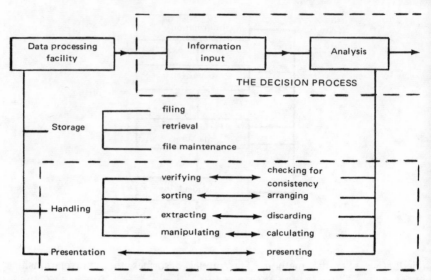

FIG. 3. Data processing and analysis

Let us now turn to analysis. What does the decision-maker do when he is engaged in analysis? First, he checks for consistency of the data that he is presented with, and if he detects inconsistencies, he demands an explanation. This activity of *checking for consistency* is not very different from *verifying,* which is part of data handling. Secondly, he arranges the information in a certain sequence and in a form that allows him and his colleagues to comprehend the full import of the information, and this activity of *arranging* is very similar to *sorting* in data handling.

The decision-maker then discards that information which he considers to be less significant for his analysis than the information that he chooses to retain for further examination, and this is precisely what *extracting* in data handling is designed to do. He then carried out *calculations,* which are akin to *data manipulating* in data handling, and finally he presents the results in a form that is most convenient and useful for the model building stage.

All these activities, that form a part of what I call "analysis" (namely, checking data to eliminate inconsistencies, arranging data, discriminating between more significant and less significant information, computing new sets of data and finally summarising and presenting the results), are precisely mirrored by those listed under the heading "data processing" (except for data storage). Data processing is, therefore, not distinct from analysis and the two greatly overlap.

In fact, if the decision-maker were clearly to specify in advance how the information should be handled prior to presentation, then the whole function of analysis could be transferred to the data processing facility, so that information input to the decision-maker is then already presented in a digested and convenient form for him to proceed immediately to the next stages in the decision process, namely to determining performance measures and to constructing a model.

In reality, of course, there are many circumstances in which the whole function of analysis cannot be transferred in this way. First, we find that many decision makers loathe delegating this function and thereby allowing the data processing facility to encroach on their domain of responsibility. Secondly, and this is perhaps fundamentally more important, the decision-maker is not always in a position to specify in advance what analysis should be undertaken. As already intimated in the diagram in Figure 2, analysis, setting performance measures and model building, are parts of an iterative process. Very often, it is only after an attempt has been made to construct a model and after its weaknesses have been exposed, that the need for further analysis can be realised and a re-evaluation of the specified performance measure can be undertaken.

There is, therefore, a limit to the degree of transfer of the analysis function from the decision-maker to the data processing facility, even when the decision-maker genuinely acquiesces in such a move. However, the point is worth making that when model building processes are comparatively routine with few novel features—and administration in industry and government abounds with such instances—a remarkable slice of the analysis function *can* be transferred from the decision process to data processing and there is a great deal of evidence to suggest that this transfer is accelerated when the data processing facility takes the form of a computer-based information centre.

What must be realised is that even when the computer centre assumes an increasingly important role in the analysis function, the decision-maker must retain the responsibility for drawing specifications for the output of the computer centre, not just to ensure that this output is relevant to the subsequent model building stage, but to underline the maxim that the output should be properly geared and in tune with the decision as a whole.

THE HALLMARKS OF RATIONALITY

It is sensible to analyse the decision process in all its ramifications only against the assumption of rational behavior on the part of the decision-maker. If he behaves irrationally, namely if he does not (when he makes a resolution) abide by an agreed criterion that specifies how a choice between alternatives is to be made, then much of what is accomplished in the preceding states of the decision process may be irrelevant or immaterial to his final resolution. Consequently, rationality in this context is best defined by reference to the decision itself: each time the final resolution deviates from what would be expected from following the process, then the resolution can not be said to be rational.

The decision-maker may argue that though his resolution does not conform to the official decision process, it should still be regarded as rational, because it would conform if an alternative decision process is agreed upon, namely a procedure that he approves of. But the question still remains: Does he or does he not adhere to this alternative decision process? If he does, namely if it is possible to discern such an alternative process (which we may conveniently term "the informal decision process," as opposed to the formal, or official, one) then the decision-maker acts rationally from his viewpoint, but alas irrationally from the organisation's viewpoint. If, on the other hand, this alternative decision process has not been clearly prespecified and is little more than a figment of the decision-maker's imagination, then his behaviour is irrational from every viewpoint.

Determination of Choice Criteria

A distinction must, therefore, be made between the situation where the decision-maker has been responsible for or a party to the determination of the choice criterion and the situation where he has not. In the latter, "rationality" and "irrationality" must be judged with reference either to the organisation or to the individual decision-maker. If he makes a resolution that conforms to the criterion imposed by the organisation, but one that he profoundly disagrees with, then from the organisation's viewpoint the resolution is perfectly rational, while from the individual's standpoint it is irrational. If he makes a resolution that conforms to his own criterion in opposition to the one specified by the organisation, then the position is reversed. In either case, there is a conflict between the decision-maker and the organisation.

If the decision-maker is responsible for the criterion of choice, the decision process is *personalistic* in character, namely the resolution at the end of the process becomes a function of the decision-maker's own personality, his beliefs, his attitudes and his value judgements. His resolution for given circumstances may well be different from that of another individual, though both may still behave rationally by our definition. If, on the other hand, the decision-maker does not participate in the determination of a choice criterion, the decision process is *impersonalistic* and the outcome must be the same for different decision-makers, if they all behave rationally.

Some Corollaries of Rational Choice

If the discussion is confined to rational choice, the following observations can be made about the final resolution by the decision-maker:

1. If the decision process produces only one alternative, there can obviously be no free choice exercised by the decision-maker, and therefore no decision. The essence of a *decision* is that the decision-maker has several alternatives open to him, so that he can exercise the prerogative of a conscious choice. In the case of a single alternative being presented, the decision-maker can clearly be dispensed with.

2. If there are several alternatives and if an agreed criterion allows complete ranking in terms of a composite measure of performance (which incorporates several measures or yardsticks), then the ranking process automatically causes one alternative to be superior to others. If the decision-maker behaves rationally, he must resolve to select this superior alternative. In that sense, therefore, he does not really exercise any free choice; the choice has already been made for him by the ranking criterion. Thus, once a choice criterion is agreed upon, the final resolution, or choice, is *automatic,* and again the decision-maker becomes redundant at that stage of the decision process.

3. If ranking of alternatives is possible and if several alternatives have equal ranking, then the selection criterion fails to discriminate between them. Unless the existing criterion for choice is modified, or a new one is employed, there is no way in which the decision-maker can be guided in giving preference to one alternative over another, and any choice he makes under such conditions may be regarded as a random choice. Once again, the decision-maker is made redundant, since random choices can be made equally well through the use of electro-mechanical devices.

4. If the available information is inadequate, or the analysis of the information is not penetrating enough, to allow the alternative strategies to be ranked at all, then any choice between them can only be made at random, irrespective of how refined and robust the criterion of choice is, and this random choice can be made mechanically.

The perhaps obvious conclusion to be drawn from this discussion is that if a free choice by the decision-maker exists at all, it does not lie at the stage called "resolution" in the decision process, but at the stage where the criterion of choice is determined. If alternatives can be ranked, then for any criterion of choice, resolution is automatic and trivial. The only excuse for including it in the decision process in Figure 1 is to provide a landmark to indicate that the process has come to a final conclusion.

Formal and Informal Procedures

The crux of the decision process lies in the model building stage and in the determination of the criterion of choice. It is mainly in the context of these two stages in the process that the degree of initiative allowed to the decision-maker should be viewed, since these are the significant components in the process that characterise the control mechanism as being formal or informal, personalistic or impersonalistic (see Figure 4).

The distinction between personalistic and impersonalistic control is somewhat more complicated than suggested in this diagram and a more detailed discussion of this problem is given later, but crude as it is the diagram suggests an interesting hierarchy of four control procedures. Random control is at one extreme end of the scale and impersonalistic-formal control at the other. Observations of the development of control procedures in industry suggest that they have a tendency to move in a direction shown by the arrows: Starting with a situation in which decisions and corrective actions are taken in a haphazard fashion (random control) in the absence of any directives, an individual emerges and tried to regularise these actions and mould them into a systematic and consistent pattern. As long as his procedure does not have the formal blessing of the organisation, it may be characterised as personalistic-informal. Subsequently the procedure is formalised and when eventually it tends to be independent of the individual it becomes impersonalistic-formal. The growth of enterprises from family concerns to large companies, the introduction of computer systems, the aftermath of developing a new product—all these are examples in which process of formalisation and impersonalisation can very often be detected.

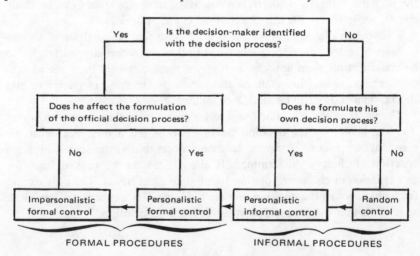

FIG. 4. Formal and informal procedures

Maximising Utility

So far the discussion of rationality has been confined to the final stages of the decision process. But what about the earlier stages? One way of considering a decision-maker who is engaged in constructing a model and weighing alternative strategies, is to regard him as a problem solver. When is his behaviour as a problem solver to be regarded as rational? Von Neumann and Morgenstern briefly discuss the concept of rationality in problem solving and say that an individual who attempts to obtain the maximum utility is said to act rationally and this definition is not at variance with the one suggested here. They go on to say:

> But it may safely be stated that there exists, at present, no satisfactory treatment of the question of rational behavior. There may, for example, exist several ways by which to reach the optimum position; they may depend on the knowledge and understanding which the individual has and upon the paths of action open to him. [6, p. 9]

There may be an implication in this statement that rationality is to be regarded as a function of the method used to arrive at the optimum solution, that if an optimum solution to a problem exists, an individual is said to behave rationally if he arrives at the solution through the use of the best (most efficient?) generally known method. This train of thought would suggest that rationality should be defined in absolute terms, which are determined by the problem and by the general consensus of opinion as to how to solve it, so that if an individual is seen to follow this path, his behaviour is considered to be rational.

This is certainly not the implication that I wish to convey in the definition of rationality suggested here. If an individual fails to follow the generally accepted path because of his ignorance of the existence of this path, and if he persists in following his own path, then from his point of view he behaves perfectly rationally, even if he does not attain the best solution and even if his actions appear to make no sense to a knowledgeable outsider. It seems to me that the first statement of von Neumann and Morgenstern is adequate to describe rationality in the context of this discussion, namely that *an individual is said to behave rationally if he attempts to obtain the maximum utility*. Rationality is, therefore, a relative concept. What is utility to one individual (let alone maximum utility) may not be utility to another. In a personalistic type of control, the goals, the utilities, the criterion of choice between alternatives and the final result of the decision process, may be very different for different individuals, even though all may behave rationally in the context of the definition given here.

The Method of Solution

What happens, one might ask, when an individual has followed his own method of solution and refuses to adopt what is generally acknowledged to be a superior method, in other words the individual can no longer argue that he is unaware of the existence of this other method? Does he behave rationally?

The answer, it seems to me, lies in whether the alleged superior method yields a better solution or not. The criterion as to what is "better" has already been determined and agreed by the individual prior to or in the course of his following his own path to arrive at a solution. If a new method is brought to his attention and is shown to produce a better result, better as judged by this criterion, and if the individual persists in ignoring this method, how can he claim to act rationally? In our definition, he no longer attempts to obtain the maximum utility, and therefore he ceases to behave rationally.

If, on the other hand, the new method produces the same or as good a solution as the one derived by the individual's method, then superiority of one method over another can be claimed only on grounds of efficiency (speed of calculations or economy in procedure), rigour, convenience or elegance. And here the answer to the question whether the individual continues to behave rationally depends on whether he accepts these arguments. If he does, yet refuses to change his method, he is irrational; if he does not, his behaviour from his viewpoint continues to be rational, though to others it may seem rather eccentric.

FREEDOM OF CHOICE

The many references to the ability of an individual to make a choice from among a number of available alternatives naturally raises the question: How and under what circumstances can an individual be said to have a freedom of choice?

This problem has exercised the minds of philosophers throughout the ages and has been the subject of numerous treatises. Of all the various approaches to this subject I have chosen to discuss here briefly the view of Ofstad, who provides a comprehensive review of the literature on this topic and suggests his own definition of freedom of choice.

Ofstad's View

Ofstad discusses freedom from determinism (or "freedom as indeterminancy," as he puts it) at some length [4, chapter III] and proceeds to consider four other possible definitions of free will: "freedom as self-expression," "freedom as rationality," "freedom as virtue" and "freedom as power." Some of the arguments under these various headings are very closely related to the discussion on determinism, others are covered in my previous discussion of the concepts of rationality and personalistic control and need not concern us any further here. What is, perhaps, more interesting is that after a detailed discourse of free will in relation to ethical criteria, Ofstad concludes with his own definition of a free person:

> P is a *free person* if, and only if, the following three conditions are fulfilled: (1) P's ethical system is oriented towards such values as love, tolerance and human dignity, (2) he has knowledge of his ethical system, his motivation and choice-situations so that he is able to find out which course of action will be best in accordance with this system, and (3) he is so strongly and whole-heartedly disposed to decide in favor of the course of action which he believes to be the right one, that he does not have to make any efforts in order to decide. [4, pp. 305–306]

This definition is not very satisfactory. The first condition requires definition of love, tolerance and human dignity, and above all it requires a definition of the degrees of orientation towards these values that would allow a person to be identified as free or otherwise. The second condition imposes similar difficulties of definition: what level of intimate knowledge does a person have to possess of his ethical system, motivation and alternative strategies to satisfy this condition? And do we ever get a situation where full knowledge of these issues does in fact exist? The first part of condition (3) is reminiscent of what I called personalistic control, but the second part is too ambiguous to be helpful: if the individual does not require to make any effort to make a decision, then the implication is that the outcomes of possible alternatives have already been arranged in a complete ranking order and in terms of Fig. 1 all that is left is to make the final selection, which then—as already pointed out—becomes a trivial component in the decision process.

One implication of Ofstad's definition is that freedom of choice is a matter of degree, and while we have as yet no way of ranking this degree of freedom (except, perhaps, in some trivial cases), the notion of partial freedom may be thought by some to be useful. As Ofstad says in his preface:

> Power to decide is not something which we have either in full or not at all. It is a matter of degrees and individual variations. What one man can do is not necessarily what another can do. What we can do in one situation may be different from what we can accomplish in another. [4, p. ix]

The other implication of Ofstad's definition, in the context of our discussion of the decision process, is that personalistic control does (or may) involve free choice whereas impersonalistic control does not (this is my own interpretation) and this is an implication that I fully endorse. It seems, however, that this result may be obtained by adopting the definition that freedom of choice exists when an individual has two or more alternative courses of action available to him and when there is no external compulsion to choose a particular alternative. This definition avoids many of the difficulties that are presented by a wider concept based on the absence of compulsion (some of these difficulties were discussed earlier) and it ignores the circumstances that have led to delimiting the range of available alternatives. Admittedly, if two individuals P_1 and P_2 are placed in identical situations and if P_1 is allowed three alternative courses of action and P_2 is allowed only two, then P_1's scope is wider than that of P_2. However, *both individuals are free to make a choice.* Some concept to indicate and even to measure this difference in scope would, therefore, be useful and while I am not proposing to define such a concept here, I suggest that it need not be part of the definition of freedom of choice.

ON UTILITY

The criterion of choice involves the determination of a measure of utility which incorporates the various entities defined as measures of performance and gives expression to the objective that the decision process is designed to attain. Take, for example, a production system in which capacity constraints lead to a conflict between several products. If the measures of performance are defined as the profit values for these products, and if the profit for one product can be increased at the expense of that derived from another product, then the purpose of the single utility scale is to take account of all the individual measures of performance, and in the example cited it may simply be the algebraic sum of all the profit values. If the total profit for all the products is defined as the utility function, and thereby implies that the objective of the decision process is to secure as high a value of this function as possible, then the decision-maker need no longer consider the effect of possible strategies on any one particular product; the conflict between the products is reconciled by the introduction of the utility scale.

Or take the case of controlling inventory to meet variable demand. If stock is depleted, demand cannot be met and if customers are not prepared to wait until the stock is replenished, then loss of revenue is incurred during the stock runout period, coupled with a loss in customer goodwill. The incidence of runouts (or alternatively, the percentage of the amount of stock not available on demand) can be reduced if the average stock holding is increased. The relationship between these two performance measures is shown in Figure 5, where strategy 1 associated with R_1 of runouts requires Q_1 average stock level and is compared with strategy 2, for which the corresponding values are R_2 and Q_2 respectively and $R_1 > R_2$ but $Q_2 > Q_1$. If both measures can be translated to cost figures, for example

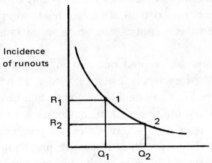

FIG. 5. Trading-off stock level against stock runout

by considering linear cost parameters a and b for the two measures respectively (namely a is the cost of increasing runout incidence by one unit and b is the cost of increasing the average stock level by one unit), then the utility function becomes $aR_1 + bQ_1$ for strategy 1 and $aR_2 + bQ_2$ for strategy 2 and the one that has the lower value (since the implied objective is to minimise the total cost) is preferable.

It may be useful to pause here and state some axioms and corrolaries associated with utility theory and which are due to Von Neumann and Morgenstern [6, Chapter 3]:

1. If there are two entities u and v and an individual is asked to state his preference, then only one of three relationships exists:

   $u > v$ which means that he prefers u to v

   $u < v$ which means that he prefers v to u

   $u = v$ which means that he has no preference, namely both are equally or undesirable.

2. If there are three entities u, v and w and if he states that $u > w$ and $w > v$, then $u > v$. This axiom implies transitivity of preference.

3. A weighting parameter α is defined in the interval $0 < \alpha < 1$. If there are three entities $u > w > v$ then a number α exists such that

   (1) $\alpha u + (1 - \alpha)v = w$

   i.e. u and v are given complimentary weights, such that the decision-maker becomes indifferent to the weighted sum or to w. Similarly, a value of α exists so that

   (2) $\alpha u + (1 - \alpha)v > w$

   and a value of α also exists so that

   (3) $\alpha u + (1 - \alpha)v < w.$

It follows that if there are three entities $u = w = v$, then equation (1) is true for any value of α.

4. If there are two entities $u > v$ then

$$(4) \qquad u > \alpha u + (1 - \alpha) v > v$$

for any value of α (in the prescribed interval 0 to 1).

5. If there are n entities or utilities $u_1, u_2, \cdots, u_n$ such that for any three entities a number α exists to produce a relationship as stated in equation (1), then the n entities can be arranged in a complete ranking order.

It should, perhaps, be pointed out that in discussing the parameter α Von Neumann and Morgenstern often refer to it as a measure of probability. Thus, if there are two possible outcomes to a given course of action and the corresponding utilities of these outcomes are u and v respectively then the expression $\alpha u + (1 - \alpha)v$ states the combination of these two events when α and $1 - \alpha$ are their respective probabilities. This combination describes the *expected utility* of the two possible events and, as we shall see later, allows for alternative strategies to be compared when each strategy may result in one of several outcomes and when each outcome has a single utility. By not specifically stating that α is a measure of probability, it is possible to extend these considerations to the case where each outcome or event has several utilities associated with it.

Let us now examine the way in which such a theory of utility can be applied for single and multiple objectives in deterministic and probabilistic systems.

1. *Deterministic outcomes with a single objective.* Suppose that a decision-maker has m strategies to choose from and a single measure of performance has been defined. If we consider for a moment a deterministic system, so that the utility (described by the measure of performance) or the outcome for each strategy is known, then the decision-maker's task is reduced to identifying the highest utility from an array of m values (each corresponding to one of the strategies), and as the theory of utility assumes that complete ranking is possible, there is no difficulty for the decision-maker in completing his task.

2. *Deterministic outcomes with multiple objective.* What we often encounter in reality is the existence of multiple objectives, as we have seen from the few examples cited earlier. Let us confine our discussion to the deterministic case and consider a set of N measures of performance that are assigned to each objective. For any given strategy there are N utilities $u_1, u_2, \cdots, u_N$ that describe the corresponding outcome.

The result of arranging N utilities $u_1, u_2, \cdots, u_N$ in a complete ranking order and the computation of weighting parameters, such as α in equation (1), is to produce a set of weighting constants $a_1, a_2, \cdots, a_N$ so that the composite utility U becomes the weighted sum of the N utilities

$$(5) \qquad U = a_1u_1 + a_2u_2 + \cdots + a_Nu_N.$$

If this utility function U is computed for all the available alternative strategies, the results for U can be arranged in a complete ranking order and the best strategy is then immediately identified. This is shown in Table 1 which consists of m rows for m alternative strategies; each row lists N utilities for any one strategy, so that u_{ij} is the utility j for performance measure j, and the composite utility U_i for strategy i is given in the last column. The values of U_i are all related to one composite numerical scale and the one with the highest value signifies the best strategy that should be selected.

3. *Probabilistic outcomes with a single objective.* The discussion so far has been confined to decision making under conditions of certainty, namely each strategy is assumed to be associated with a particular outcome. If only a single measure of performance applies, then ordering the strategies on a scale is automatic; if several measures of performance have to be considered, the reconciliation between them follows equation (5) and Table 1.

What happens under conditions of risk, when the outcome of any particular strategy is associated with a known probability? It is not difficult to see that composite utilities can be constructed in a similar way. Take first the case of a single measure of performance, so that u_j is the utility of

TABLE 1
A UTILITY TABLE

| Measures of Performance ..... | 1 | 2 | ... | j | N | Composite |
Weights	a_1	a_2	...	a_j	a_N	Utility
Strategies 1	u_{11}	u_{12}		u_{1j}	u_{1N}	U_1
$\vdots$						
i	...			u_{ij}		U_i
$\vdots$						
m	...				u_{mN}	U_m

TABLE 2
PROBABILITY MATRIX FOR A SINGLE MEASURE OF PERFORMANCE

| Outcomes .... | 1 | 2 | ... | j | ... | n | Total | Expected |
Utility	u_1	u_2	...	u_j	...	u_n	Prob.	Utility
Strategies 1	p_{11}	p_{12}		p_{1j}		p_{1n}	1	U_1
$\vdots$								
i	...		p_{ij}				1	U_i
$\vdots$								
m	...					p_{mn}	1	U_m

outcome j. In Table 2 there are m strategies and n outcomes and the probability matrix p_{ij} is the probability that strategy i will lead to outcome j.

The expected utility from strategy 1 is

(6) $$U_1 = p_{11}u_1 + p_{12}u_2 + \cdots + p_{1j}u_j + \cdots + p_{1n}u_n$$

where

$$p_{11} + p_{12} + \cdots + p_{ij} + \cdots + p_{1n} = 1$$

and similarly the expected utility for each of the m strategies can be found. There is a certain analogy between Table 1 and Table 2 and between equations (5) and (6). In view of the axioms enumerated earlier, the values of U_i can be ordered on a ranking scale and the optimal strategy can therefore be immediately identified.

4. *Probabilistic outcomes with multiple objectives.* The case of multi-performance measures is handled in the following way: A utility matrix is constructed similar to Table 1. Composite utilities are then calculated for the various outcomes and these are fed as the utility values in Table 2, from which the expected utilities for the available strategies are computed. The procedure is summarised in Table 3, in which, for convenience of presentation, the top part is an inverted version of Table 1 (i.e. now each column enumerates the utilities for the corresponding outcome) and the bottom part duplicates Table 2.

The Notion of Probability

Circumstances of risk are characterized by the fact that the matrix of decisions and outcomes has occurred many times in the past and that the general pattern of events suggests that steady state conditions prevail to allow an inference for future outcomes to be based on frequencies of past events. But such conditions rarely exist in a business environment, where decisions have to be made under conditions of uncertainty rather than risk, namely where probabilities of future outcomes cannot be equated to frequencies of past outcomes, either because such information is too meagre or nonexistent, or because present and future circumstances are believed to be significantly different from the past.

Diverse and often conflicting views are found among decision theorists on how to handle decision making under conditions of uncertainty. Some suggest methods for determining subjective probability measures, with which the problem of uncertainty can then be handled as if conditions of known risk prevail. Others argue that the conventional concept of probability be abandoned and that other procedures should be employed in order to compare the relative merit of outcomes and hence to identify the most desirable strategy. A fairly detailed account of the various schools of thought on this subject is given by Fishburn [3, Chapter 5] and this is not an appropriate place to elaborate on the subject, except to draw attention to the fact that fundamental differences in points of view are very much in existence.

TABLE 3
THE CASE OF MULTI-PERFORMANCE MEASURES UNDER CONDITIONS OF RISK

Outcomes		1	j	n		Weights
Measures of performance	1					a_1
	⋮					⋮
	k		u_{kj}			a_k
	⋮					⋮
	N					a_N
Outcomes Composite		u_1	u_j	u_n		

↓

Outcomes .... Composite Utility		1 u_1	j u_j	n u_n	Total	Expected Utility
Strategies	1				1	U_1
	⋮					⋮
	i		p_{ij}		1	U_i
	⋮					⋮
	m				1	U_m

It should perhaps also be pointed out that the very issue of whether a given situation may be described as one of risk or uncertainty is often also open to judgment and dispute. When it comes to making inferences about the future, historical records may well be interpreted in several ways, let alone the challenge that may be levelled at the assertion that such inference is at all valid. What seems to one individual a perfectly legitimate case of decision under risk may be argued by another as being a case of uncertainty, and the case of uncertainty is then amenable to interpretation in several ways, depending on the school of thought that the individual professes to be a disciple of.

THE RELATION BETWEEN UTILITY THEORY AND RATIONALITY

To summarize for the purpose of this discussion, the significant assumptions in the theory of utility suggested by Von Neumann and Morgenstern are:

(a) An individual is capable of ranking utilities. This assumption also implies consistency, or the need to avoid contradiction: If he prefers u to v then he cannot at the same time prefer v to u or be indifferent as to which utility he prefers.

(b) There is transitivity of preference.

(c) Weighting factors can be determined to compare utilities and hence to establish a composite utility scale.

It is worthwhile repeating these assumptions because of the significance that has been attributed to these axioms in relation to the concept of rationality. Von Neumann and Morgenstern lay great emphasis on the need for quantitative measurements in economics and after discussing their proposed axioms state that their purpose is "to find the mathematically complete principles which define 'rational behavior' for the participants in a social economy, and to derive from them the general characteristics of that behavior" [6, p. 31]. Many decision theorists go further and specifically identify the axioms of utility theory as axioms of rational behavior.

By this test most decisions in reality will probably have to be regarded as irrational. Take, for example, the assumption that by assigning appropriate weights a multi-objective array can be tranformed to a single measure on a composite utility scale. Individuals may have very strong views about the desirability of attaining each of the stated objectives, but may find it impossible to compare and reconcile them.

When, in "As You Like It," Corin asked Touchstone "and how like you this shepherd's life?," Touchstone replied:

> Truly shepherd, in respect of itself, it is a good life; but in respect that it is a shepherd's life, it is naught. In respect that it is solitary, I like it very well: but in respect that it is private, it is a very vile life. Now in respect it is in the fields, it pleaseth me well: but in respect it is not in the Court, it is tedious. As it is a sparse life (look you) it fits my humour well: but as there is no more plenty in it, it goes much against my stomach. Hast any philosophy in thee shepherd? [5]

In terms of any one objective an individual may find it possible to rank alternatives without much difficulty, but when it comes to declaring how much he is prepared to trade off one utility against another, he may be quite helpless.

Or suppose, for the sake of argument, that a man is faced with the prospect of enjoying the company of one of three ladies, A, B or C. He can enumerate many of the qualities of these splendid ladies—their physical dimensions, the complexion of their skins, the colour of their eyes, their I.Q.'s, the number of pimples per square inch, etc.—but he finds it impossible to come up with a composite measure of utility. The whole idea of a trade off between any two qualities he finds totally unacceptable. How is he to equate the level of intellect with the density of pimples, he asks? The utility of any one quality may well depend on the presence of other qualities. For example, he may regard a high density of pimples a positive asset when accompanied with certain skin and hair colouring, but a liability in other combinations. Nevertheless, he feels that he can compare two ladies at a time on the basis of an overall evaluation. If, having done this, he states that he prefers A to B and B to C and C to A, he does not abide by the axiom of transitivity of preference. The violation of this axiom undermines the elegant mathematical structure of utility theory and many decision theorists have no patience for such an individual and would simply regard him as irrational.

It should perhaps be pointed out that a "circular ranking," such as the one just described, does not necessarily violate the axiom of consistency. Our man may be perfectly consistent in always preferring (within a given space of time) A to B, etc., and avoiding any contradiction between any two of his statements. Admittedly, faced with a set of preferences as stated so far, he is unable to make a choice, since for any choice that he makes a better one (as judged by his own preferences) can be pointed out. Does the fact that he cannot act prove that he is irrational? In our discussion we have drawn a distinction between the determination of choice criteria and the act of selecting between alternatives; our man can argue that he truly *attempts to obtain the maximum utility* (which is our definition of rational behavior), but the choice criteria do not provide him with a means of making a final selection.

To base a concept of rationality on the axioms of utility theory that were listed earlier is therefore to take a rather narrow view and to exclude from the realm of rationality a significant proportion of decisions that do take place in daily life.

Let us now return to further considerations of personalistic control.

PERSONALISTIC AND IMPERSONALISTIC CONTROL

A distinction was made in Figure 4 between personalistic and impersonalistic control by examining whether an individual does or does not affect the formulation of the decision process. In the light of the foregoing discussion it would appear that personalistic and impersonalistic control are not two entirely mutually exclusive categories, but that several shades and degrees of personalistic involvement in the decision process can be identified. Consider the following two groups of questions about an individual:

Group (a): First order of personalistic involvement (conditions of certainty):

1. Does the individual set up the number and identity of the measures of performance?
2. In case of multi-objectives, does he specify the weighting coefficients that determine the composite utility function? If this is not possible, does he rank the outcomes and does he determine the criterion of choice?

3. Does he specify the array of available strategies?
4. Does he specify the array of possible outcomes?
5. Does he specify whether the decision making does or does not take place under conditions of certainty?

Group (b): *Second order of personalistic involvement* (when the decision is not under conditions of certainty):

6. Does he specify which decision theory to apply?
7. If probabilities of possible outcomes are required for the decision process, does he determine their values?
8. Does he determine the value of any subjective parameters (other than probabilities) that may be required in the application of a given decision theory (e.g. the coefficient of optimism if the Hurwicz criterion is adopted)?

Group (a) consists of questions that may be posed for every decision process. Group (b) is only relevant if the decision process is not subject to conditions of certainty.

There are four possible answers to each of these eight questions:

Yes— where the individual does carry out the activity described in the question, and even if his specification may subsequently be modified in the light of criticisms and suggestions by other people, those modifications are comparatively slight or the responsibility for the final specifications clearly lies with the individual.

No— when the specifications described by the question are laid down or are the responsibility of someone else, or when they are covered by standing orders and procedures.

Participates—when the individual is a member of a group of people responsible for the activity described in the question (e.g. when the group is a committee, or when specifications are based on averages of values suggested by several individuals).

Irrelevant— when the question does not apply (any one or several of questions 2, 6, 7 and 8 may become irrelevant in the light of answers to the other questions).

It should be emphasised that answers to the eight questions are to some extent a matter of subjective interpretation on the part of the questioner or investigator. It may be difficult in some circumstances to determine whether an individual should give the first or the third answer to a particular question. Nevertheless, the purpose of these questions is not to compute a crisp numerical value for the level of personalistic involvement of a particular individual, but to produce a profile of his involvement, as demonstrated by the answers in the example shown below (pertaining to a given task or decision process):

Question	Answer		
1	N		
2	P		
3	Y	Legend	Y—yes
4	Y		N—no
5	N		P—partipates
6	N		—question irrelevant
7	P		
8	—		

If answers to relevant questions are all "no," then control is strictly formal and impersonalistic, if all the answers are "yes" then control is purely personalistic, and between these two extremes there is a whole spectrum of alternative combinations.

It is in this context that the tendency of a decision process to become formal and impersonalistic in character may be traced: if answers to the eight questions are monitored over a period of time, then this tendency can be documented, as in the example below:

Question	Time⟶			
1	N	N	N	N
2	P	N	N	N
3	Y	Y	N	N
4	Y	Y	Y	P
5	N	N	N	N
6	N	N	N	N
7	P	P	N	N
8	—	—	—	—

Where Does the Decision Lie?

Having examined the various stages of the decision process, we may now return to Figure 1 and ask: Where are the crucial points in this process? Where can the decision maker be said to affect the turn of events?

The answer lies in the degree of personalistic control that he retains. We have already seen how a data processing facility can encroach on the decision-maker's domain by taking over parts or the whole function of analysis. Similarly, when the decision process as a whole becomes more and more impersonalistic, it simply follows the rules, and the rules are sufficiently detailed to cater for an ever increasing number of contingencies to obliterate the effect of the individual decision-maker. In the extreme case, when control is completely impersonalistic, the decision-maker ceases to have a meaningful role; he ceases to be a decision-maker.

REFERENCES

1. CHURCHMAN, C. W., *Challenge to reason,* McGraw Hill, 1968.
2. EILON, S., "Some notes on information processing," *Journal of Management Studies,* Vol. 5, No. 2 (1968), pp. 139–153.
3. FISHBURN, P. C., *Decision and value theory,* Wiley, 1964.
4. OFSTAD, H., *An inquiry into the freedom of decision,* Allen and Unwin, 1961.
5. SHAKESPEARE, W., *As you like it,* Act 3, Scene 3, 1623.
6. VON NEUMANN, J. AND MORGENSTERN, O., *Theory of games and economic behavior,* Princeton Univ. Press, 1953.

Chapter 5

Decision-Making, Objectives, and Conflict

5.1 INTRODUCTION

Regardless of the nature or type of decision, an important element in the process of decision-making is the choice and measurement of objectives and goals. This is because, in all types of decision-making (individual, organization or public), we must contend with the existence of multiple rather than single objectives. The fact of multiple objectives forces the manager to answer two questions. First, of the enumerated set of objectives, which ones are to be formally included in the decision problem? Secondly, what is the relative degree of importance of the chosen subset and the scale of measurement for each objective? These issues must be resolved before the manager proceeds to consider other elements of decision-making listed in Chapter 4 (section 4.5). Resolution of conflict* (conflict between objectives, individuals, groups, organizations, institutions, and so on) is the essence of the decision problem. In this chapter we will consider some aspects of objectives; discuss the problem of measurement of objectives; and mention different types and sources of conflict related to decision-making.

5.2 THE NATURE OF OBJECTIVES

A logical construction of the decision model would start with the obvious question: Why must a decision be made? The answer is that a need for decision exists, or that the decision-maker *perceives* a state of affairs which requires an act of choice. The result of the decision is a general or specific guide for action. The decision-maker has a set of objectives and

---

* The occurrence of conflict, its sources, and its resolution is an important area of study in behavioral sciences. See, for example, [Thompson, 1961, Chapter 5], [March and Simon, 1958, Chapter 5], [Hampton et al., 1968, Chapter 6].

goals and the *intended purpose* of his decisions is to so move the system (individuals, organizations, man-machine systems) that a maximum likelihood for the achievement of his objectives is created. We note here some of the characteristics associated with the question of objectives and goals.

Both individuals and organizations have multiple rather than single objectives (Miller and Starr, 1969, Chapter 3). Objectives serve both as targets to be achieved and tools for appraising performance, coordination and control. Objectives and goals are personal as well as role defined, and in most cases there is an inherent conflict between different types of individual as well as organizational objectives. It is the number of different goals (and hence measures of performance) involved in a decision problem that characterizes its dimension. If a decision problem involves a single measure of performance, we *optimize* (maximize or minimize) because the achievement of one goal is assumed *not* to adversely affect the achievement of other goals. On the other hand, if the decision is of a multidimensional nature, as is often the case, the conflict between goals forces the decision-maker to suboptimize.*

Another important aspect of objectives is the process through which individual, as well as organizational objectives are formed. Psychologists have tried to explain the formation of individual objectives through their research on "aspiration level." The aspiration level is some "satisfactory" value of goal attainment. It is a variable which depends upon previous levels of attainment; success tends to raise it while failure tends to lower it. The aspiration level has a negative correlation with satisfaction [March and Simon, 1958, p. 49]; is influenced by reference groups; and is usually greater than the most recent performance level [March, 1965, p. 633]. At the organizational level, the goal formation process can be examined in several ways. Cyert and March explain organizational goals as the result of a continuing bargaining-learning process [Cyert and March, 1963, pp. 26–28]. The goals of an organization are viewed as "a series of more or less independent constraints imposed on the organization through a process of bargaining among potential coalition members and elaborated over time in response to short-run pressures" [Cyert and March, 1963, p. 43].

Yet another aspect of objectives and goals is that they are hierarchical in nature. Top management goals are translated into division or department goals in such a way that they can be clearly communicated and used for performance appraisal. In the organizational setting, managerial effectiveness† is determined by the degree to which individual and organizational

---

* Suboptimization exists not only because of conflict between goals, it is also created because of imperfect knowledge, uncertain future, and because of changes in the value system of the decision-maker. In this sense, optimization is an ideal which can never be achieved (except in the theoretical models of a single dimensional problem under certainty—such as linear programming).

† [Reddin, 1970, p. 3]. Reddin defines managerial effectiveness in terms of output

goals are operationally integrated. If the nature of objectives is such that they cannot easily be made operational, the decision-maker must decide on some proxy variables* which are related, in a predictable way, to the original objectives.

5.3   THE MEASUREMENT OF OBJECTIVES

The question of measurement of objectives enters the decision model in two ways. First, is the objective single-dimensional and can it be operationally measured by a single measure of performance? Secondly, how can we handle those decision problems which operate in more than one dimension and which require more than one measure of performance? The decision problem with a single objective does not suffer from the complications that arise due to conflict between two or more objectives. However, the measurement problem remains to be resolved even in single-dimensional problems. The chosen objective may or may not have an objective scale of measurement. In such a case a "subjective" scale will have to be employed.† If an objective scale of measurement exists, then the decision-maker must specify its dimension and a target value.‡ The problem of measurement is more complicated in multi-dimensional decision problems, because of potential conflict between multiple objectives and also because of difficulties of measurement. The conflict between objectives is recognized and the decision-maker can resort to several means in order to resolve it.§ First, multi-dimensional objectives (with various measures of performance) can be assigned different weights so that the problem can be solved by dimensional analysis [Starr, 1971, pp. 278–284].

---

rather than input. What the manager achieves rather than what he does is managerial effectiveness. The authors of this book distinguish between "effectiveness" and "efficiency" in terms of the multiple dimensionality of the decision problem. In a single-dimension problem, efficiency implies effectiveness. In multiple-dimensional problems (where conflict can exist between different goals) efficiency along one dimension may well mean inefficiency along other dimensions. The net result in such a case could be a lack of effectiveness from the global point of view.

* See [Ansoff, 1965, p. 43–74]. Ansoff establishes a practical system of objectives for the business firm. Long-term and "flexibility" objectives are measured by employing a set of operational proxy variables. A similar approach may well be desirable in the health field (i.e., the long-term objective of "optimum" health must be operationalized through some measurable "proxy" variables).

† Subjective scales can be converted into objective scales by rank-order methods or by the application of utility theory. See [Von Neumann and Morgenstern, 1947], [Swalm, 1966], [Terry, 1963], [Hammond, 1967], [Starr, 1971, p. 50], [Torgerson, 1958] and [Green and Tull, 1970, Chapters 6 and 7]. A concise review of modern utility theory can be found in Chapter 2 of [Luce and Raiffa, 1958].

‡ Objective scales of measurement have been classified into four categories: (1) nominal scale, (2) ordinal scale, (3) interval scale, and (4) ratio scale. See [Starr, 1971, pp. 50–53]. Also see [Green and Tull, 1970, pp. 176–181].

§ See [Miller and Starr, 1959, Chapter 7].

The multi-dimensionality can also be handled by: (1) arriving at a single measure of performance (e.g., utility) by means of somehow transforming* multi-dimensional objectives to a single measure of performance; (2) optimizing with respect to one objective and "satisficing" with respect to the others (this is accomplished by structuring the problem into a programming format in which the most important objective is optimized subject to constraints which contain "acceptable" values of the other objectives).†

5.4 CONFLICT

Conflict arises whenever an individual or a group is involved in making decisions. In a sense, decision-making can be defined as the resolution of conflict. Conflict is a natural consequence of complex organizations characterized by interdependent relationships between individuals, and among groups of diverse skills, ambitions, values, and professional orientations. Conflict arises as two or more individuals or complex social units are deliberately interacting in order to "define or redefine the terms of their interdependence."‡ Thompson§ [1960] defines conflict "as that behavior by organization members which is expended in opposition to other members." March and Simon [1958, p. 112] comment on conflict:

> Conflict is a term of many uses. Most generally, the term is applied to a breakdown in the standard mechanisms of decision-making so that an individual or group experiences difficulty in selecting an action alternative . . . Thus, conflict occurs whenever an individual or group experiences a decision problem.

Conflict, bargaining, stress, and the resolution of conflict are common phenomena in individual experiences and organizational life. March and Simon [1958, p. 112] discuss three main classes of conflict phenomena: (1) individual conflict (conflict faced in individual decision-making), (2) organizational conflict (individual or group conflict within an organization), and (3) interorganizational conflict (conflict between organizations and groups).‖ A variety of mechanisms designed to cope with con-

---

* This can be done mathematically or by constructing trade-off functions. Trade-off functions may be either objective or subjective in nature. See [Ackoff and Sasieni, 1968, p. 35 and pp. 46–49]. The "indifference curve" of the economist is also an example of the trade-off function.
† For a discussion of the concept of "satisficing" (as opposed to maximizing) see [Simon, 1957, pp. 204–205].
‡ Walton and McKersie quoted in [Hampton et al., 1968, p. 356].
§ Thompson's paper reproduced in [Baker et al., 1969] explores: (1) the sources of conflict within organizations, (2) the vulnerabilities of different organizations to conflict, and (3) the devices employed by organizations to control conflict.
‖ Each class of conflict is explained and illustrated in [March and Simon, 1958, Chapter 6].

flict can be identified; specific reactions being a function of the source of conflict [March and Simon, 1958, p. 115].

A classification of the types of organizational conflict, their respective sources and defense devices is summarized in Figure 5.1.

FIG. 5.1
A CLASSIFICATION OF THE TYPES OF ORGANIZATIONAL CONFLICT

Type of Conflict	Source of Conflict	Defense Device
Administrative allocation.	Technology.	Organizational structure.
Latent roles.	Labor force.	Recruitment and selection.
Competing pressures.	Task environment.	Organizational posture.

Source: [Thompson in Baker et al., 1969, p. 144].

The role of objectives as the source of conflict has already been mentioned. Victor Thompson [1960] has used the relationship between specialist and hierarchical roles in the accomplishment of organizational and personal goals as a basis for the analysis of conflict in organizations. He describes and explains three sources of conflict: (1) conflict due to the violation of role expectation; (2) conflict concerning the reality of interdependence; and (3) conflict arising from blocks to spontaneous communications. Hampton et al. [1968, p. 358] identify as one source of conflict the stress caused by structurally determined interactions between the individual personality characteristics and organizational units. A considerable amount of empirical research is being directed towards exploring various aspects of conflict and their relationships to organizational effectiveness.* An account of the potential benefits which may be found in inter- and intra-professional conflict is given by Gross [1967].

Organizational conflict can be constructive or destructive, depending upon the way conflict is perceived, traced to its genuine source, and managed. Kelly [1970] has argued that "the way conflict is managed— rather than suppressed, ignored, or avoided—contributes significantly" to organizational effectiveness. Says Kelly [1970, p. 103]:

Contrary to conventional wisdom, the most important thing about conflict is that it is good for you. While this is not a scientific statement of fact, it reflects a basic and unprecedented shift of emphasis—a move away from the old human relations point of view where all conflict was basically seen as bad.

---

* See, for example, [Pondy, 1969], [Corwin, 1969], [Walton et al., 1969], [Lammers, 1969], [Assael, 1969], and references cited in the bibliography sections of these articles published in the December, 1969 issue of *Administrative Science Quarterly*.

In their survey of the literature on role conflict and role ambiguity in complex organizations, Rizzo et al. [1970] refer to Ben-David's [1958], Zawacki's [1963], and Perrow's [1965] treatment of sources of conflict in hospitals. Conflict in hospitals stems mainly from the fact that hospitals are characterized by multiple authority or multiple subordination systems.

5.5 CONCLUDING REMARKS

The purpose of this chapter was to mention some important aspects of objectives and goals (e.g., the question of multiple objectives, the process of individual and organizational goal formulation,* hierarchy of objectives, measurement of objectives) and consider the relationship between decision-making and conflict. Conflict between objectives, individuals, groups, and organizations is an important fact of organizational life; and the resolution of conflict is the essence of decision-making. An illustration of how a multi-dimensional problem in the health field was structured for utility measurement and choosing the most effective course of action is provided by Stimson (Selection 11).

Stimson's article describes an attempt to measure utilities that twelve key decision-makers in a large public health agency attached to a set of seven objectives. An effectiveness model was constructed in which the "best" alternative was identified by calculating and comparing the weighted sum of "efficiencies" for each alternative. This required that decision-makers place relative value (utility) on each objective, and assign efficiency ratings to various alternatives (i.e., respective probabilities that a given alternative will achieve a specific goal). The experimental method of measuring utilities consisted of three tasks. The first two measured the relative values (utilities) of the seven objectives, and the third obtained efficiencies of eight alternatives to achieve these objectives. The author, then, calculated the relative effectiveness of the various alternatives. The model was applied for the allocation of a federal grant to improve the outpatient care of the chronically ill and aged. The normal solution derived from the model compared favorably with the solution already decided upon by the agency. The article is important because it gives an illustration of one method (Churchman-Ackoff method) of measuring utility.

Schulz and Johnson (Selection 12) present a brief review of empirical research on conflict reported in the management, sociology, and hospital literature. Different types of conflict (e.g., hospital-client, interpersonal, administration-medical staff) were considered and some of the sources of conflict listed. Finally, some mitigators of conflict, for each type of conflict considered, were suggested. Conflict is positively related to inter-

---

* See, also [Selection 6 in Chapter 3].

dependence, specialization and heterogeneity of personnel and levels of authority. Hospitals are specially prone to conflict because "over 300 different professional societies and associations" exert diverse influence on the heterogeneous health team caring for the patient. The authors contend that "while conflict might foster institutional innovation and progress, the individual patient is best served by minimizing conflict and by creating institutional stability and harmony."

Managerial decision-making is an extremely complex task, as is evident from the topics mentioned in Chapters 4 and 5. Health administrators can draw on the concepts, tools and techniques, research, and approaches to decision-making provided by management science and behavioral models.

REFERENCES

Ackoff, R. L., and M. W. Sasieni, *Fundamentals of Operations Research,* New 1968   York: John Wiley & Sons.

Ansoff, H. I., *Corporate Strategy,* New York: McGraw-Hill. 1965

Assael, H., "Constructive Role of Interorganizational Conflict," *Administrative* 1969   *Science Quarterly,* vol. 14, no. 4, December, pp. 573–582.

Ben-David, J., "The Professional Role of the Physician in Bureaucratized 1958   Medicine: A Study in Role Conflict," *Human Relations,* vol. 2, pp. 255–257.

Corwin, R. C., "Patterns of Organizational Conflict," *Administrative Science* 1969   *Quarterly,* vol. 14, no. 4, December, pp. 507–520.

Cyert, A. M., and J. G. March, *A Behavioral Theory of the Firm,* Englewood Cliffs, N.J.: Prentice-Hall.

Green, P. E., and D. S. Tull, *Research for Marketing Decisions,* Englewood 1970   Cliffs, N.J., Prentice-Hall.

Gross, E., "When Occupations Meet: Professions in Trouble," *Hospital Ad-* 1967   *ministration,* vol. 12, no. 3, pp. 40–59.

Hammond, J. S., III, "Better Decisions with Preference Theory," *Harvard* 1967   *Business Review,* November–December, pp. 123–141.

Hampton, D. R., S. E. Summer, and R. A. Webber, *Organizational Behavior* 1968   *and the Practice of Management,* Glenview, Ill.: Scott, Foresman and Co.

Kelly, J., "Make Conflict Work for You," *Harvard Business Review,* July- 1970   August, pp. 103–113.

Lammers, C. J. "Strikes and Mutinies: A Comparative Study of Organizational 1969   Conflicts Between Rulers and Ruled," *Administrative Science Quarterly,* vol. 14, no. 4, December, pp. 558–572.

Luce, R. D., and H. Raiffa, *Games and Decisions,* New York: John Wiley & 1958   Sons.

March, J. G., *Handbook of Organizations,* Chicago: Rand McNally. 1965

March, J. G., and H. A. Simon, *Organizations,* New York: John Wiley & Sons. 1958

Miller, D. W., and M. K. Starr, *Executive Decisions and Operations,* 2nd edi-
1969   tion, Englewood Cliffs, N.J.: Prentice-Hall.
Perrow, C., "Hospitals: Technology, Structure, and Goals," in J. G. March
1965   [ed.), *Handbook of Organizations,* Chicago: Rand McNally, pp.
910–971.
Pondy, L. R., "Varieties of Organizational Conflict," *Administrative Science*
1969   *Quarterly,* vol. 14, no. 4, December, pp. 499–505.
Reddin, W. J. *Managerial Effectiveness,* New York: McGraw-Hill.
1970
Rizzo, J. R., R. J. House, S. I. Lirtzman, "Role of Conflict and Ambiguity in
1970   Complex Organizations," *Administrative Science Quarterly,* vol. 15,
no. 2, June, pp. 150–163.
Simon, H. A., *Models of Man,* New York: John Wiley & Sons.
1957
Starr, M. K., *Management: A Modern Approach,* New York: Harcourt, Brace,
1971   Jovanovich.
Swalm, R. O., "Utility Theory—Insights into Risk Taking," *Harvard Business*
1966   *Review,* November-December, pp. 123–136.
Terry, H., "Comparative Evaluation of Performance Using Multiple Criteria,"
1963   *Management Science,* vol. 9, pp. 431–442.
Thompson, J. D., "Organizational Management of Conflict," in *Industrial*
1960   *Organizations and Health,* F. Baker et al. (eds.], London: Tavistock
Publications Ltd., 1969.
Thompson, V. A., *Modern Organization, A General Theory,* New York:
1961   Alfred A. Knopf.
Torgerson, W. S., *Theory and Methods of Scaling,* New York: John Wiley &
1958   Sons.
Von Neumann, J., and O. Morgenstern, *Theory of Games and Economic,*
1947   *Behavior,* Princeton, N.J.: Princeton University Press.
Walton, R. E., J. M. Dutton, and T. P. Cafferty, "Organizational Context and
1969   Interdepartmental Conflict," *Administrative Science Quarterly,* vol.
14, no. 4, December, pp. 522–542.
Walton, R. E., and R. B. McKersie, *A Behavioral Theory of Labor Negotiations*
1963   *—An Analysis of a Social Interaction System,* New York: McGraw-
Hill.
Zawacki, J. S., "A System of Unofficial Rules of a Bureaucracy: A Study of
1963   Hospitals," Doctoral dissertation, University of Pittsburgh.

SELECTION 11

Utility Measurement in Public Health Decision Making*

David H. Stimson

The attempt to use utility as a criterion for choosing among actions goes back at least to an article written by Bernouilli in 1783 [7]. However, until recently economists have tended to talk about utility rather than to measure it experimentally. What little desire there was to measure utility slackened after it was demonstrated that indifference curve analysis based on ordinal utility was sufficient to sustain the theory of riskless choice [26]. Thus much of the economic theory of consumer behavior could be explained without a quantitative concept of utility.

The modern revival of interest in the measurement of utility stems from publication by von Neumann and Morgenstern in 1944 of *The Theory of Games and Economic Behavior* [43]. These authors demonstrated that under conditions on which indifference curve analysis is based very little extra effort is needed to obtain a numerical utility. The post-World War II popularity of research on decision making under conditions of risk and uncertainty and the use of utilities in decision theory models[1] have led to several experiments involving the measurement of utility. In general, the experiments have taken place in a laboratory setting, often with students as subjects. Usually the objects whose utilities were measured were sums of money or household items [11, 12, 13, 27, 31, 33, 40, 41]. There are only a few reports of experiments which took place in an organizational setting and used managers as subjects [22, 23].

THE EFFECTIVENESS MODEL

An operations research study made by the author of decision making and resource allocation in a large public health agency resulted in the construction of a model for the allocation of a federal grant to improve the out-of-hospital care of the chronically ill and aged.[2] The model, based on a method suggested by Churchman and Ackoff [9], requires the measurement of the relative values (utilities) of objectives sought by decision makers in the agency. This method has a wide range of applicability. For example, it may be used to assign relative values to outcomes, whether or not they are

* *Management Science*, vol. 16, October, 1969.

objectives, and to assign relative values to objects or properties of objects.

The model for the allocation of the federal grant attempts to measure the effectiveness of alternative courses of action under consideration by members of the public health agency. The procedure for measuring effectiveness requires two component measures: (1) the relative value (utility) of each objective, and (2) the efficiency of each alternative in achieving each objective, i.e., the probability that the selection of a particular alternative will achieve a particular objective.

Some of the critical assumptions underlying the effectiveness model are:

1. For every objective O_j, there corresponds a real nonnegative number V_j, to be interpreted as a measure of the true importance of O_j.
2. If O_j is more important than O_k, then $V_j > V_k$, and if O_j and O_k are equally important, then $V_j = V_k$.
3. If V_j and V_k correspond to O_j and O_k respectively, then $V_j + V_k$ corresponds to the combined objective O_j and O_k.

The third assumption permits values to be added. Because it implies that the objectives are independent and are valued individually rather than in clusters, the assumption is a strong one. An analogous situation in economics would be the assumption that the utility of a bundle of goods is the sum of the utilities of the different goods making up the bundle, with no allowance made for complementary or competitive goods.

A schematic representation of the effectiveness model is given in Figure 1.

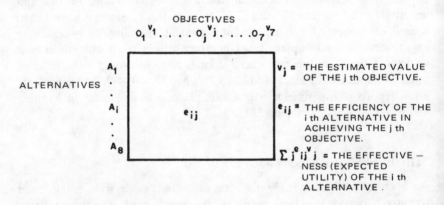

FIG. 1. The Effectiveness Model

The criterion used to select the "best" alternative calls for the calculation of the effectiveness, the weighted sum of the efficiencies $(\Sigma_j e_{ij} v_j)$ of each alternative, and calls for the selection of the alternative with the highest weighted sum. The effectiveness model can be rephrased in standard decision theory terms. When this is done, the weighted sum of the efficiencies in the effectiveness model turns out to be the same as the expected utility in the standard decision theory model.[3]

The difficulty of program evaluation caused the head of the public health agency and his key staff members to be uncertain about the effectiveness of their present method, let alone of alternative methods, of allocating the federal grant. Because of this and because the objectives were difficult to measure in terms of a common scale, the model had to be based on the information actually available. The effectiveness model is well adapted to such situations. In addition to the literature previously cited, there is other evidence that two of the basic assumptions of the model, additivity of values [2, 24, 39, 41] and the use of the maximization of expected utility as an indication of rational behavior [8, 30, 34] are useful in studies of decision making.

EXPERIMENTAL METHOD

Twelve key agency members closely involved with the federal grant program were interviewed individually. The interviews lasted between one hour and fifteen minutes and one hour and thirty minutes. During that time each participant was asked to complete three tasks. The first two tasks measured the utilities of the objectives and the third task obtained the efficiencies of the alternatives to achieve the objectives.

The general objectives of the health agency are "the prevention of disease and the provision of a healthful environment." These objectives are stated in such broad terms that it was necessary as part of this study to determine a set of objectives pertinent to the agency's allocation of the federal grant. It was important for the experiment that the meaning of each objective was the same for the agency members as for the author. Therefore, the language of the objectives was edited several times in order to insure agreement on meaning. Successive drafts of the set of objectives were read by the persons who would participate in the experiment and revisions were made based upon their comments.

Seven objectives were used in the model to encompass medical and scientific goals, the relationship of the health agency with its environment, and the psychological needs of agency members. The behavior of those connected with the federal grant program and the decisions reached were consistent with the pursuit of one or more of these seven goals:

1. To increase the availability, scope, and quality of out-of-hospital community health services for the chronically ill and aged. This is a personal health care objective.
2. To strengthen and support local health departments by providing funds for new or improved services in chronic disease programs. This

objective includes the maintenance of good relations with the local health departments.

3. To add to knowledge in the field of chronic illness and aging by doing and supporting significant demonstrations and specific investigations aimed at improving and extending outside-the-hospital services for the chronically ill and aged.

4. To show the Public Health Service that the states can do a good job with federal formula grant funds so that the trend to centralizing the funding of individual projects in Washington does not continue. This objective also includes the maintenance of good relations with the Public Health Service.

5. To conduct the federal grant program in such a manner that the state government acting through its appropriate departments is satisfied with the health agency's administration of the grant.

6. To get the support of various community and voluntary agencies in carrying out the federal grant program. This objective includes the maintenance of good relations with state and county medical societies and many other voluntary agencies.

7. To achieve self-fulfillment and enhance the prestige of those who administer the federal grant program in the health agency. This objective includes the natural desire to be identified with a good, well-respected program.

The procedure for obtaining a set of values consisted of several steps. In the first task the subject ranked the seven objectives in order of their importance to him and made choices among subsets of the objectives. From the ranking and the choices the author imputed values—not necessarily unique—to the objectives which were consistent with the subject's responses.

After the subject ranked the seven objectives, the author divided the objectives into two groups. The objective the subject had ranked as most important was placed in both groups. One group contained objectives the subject had ranked first, second, third and sixth (01, 02, 03, and 06). The other group contained objectives the subject had ranked first, fourth, fifth, and seventh (01, 04, 05, and 07). The subject was then asked to consider the group containing 01, 02, 03, and 06 and to state which he would prefer to achieve, the objective he had ranked as most important (01) or the combination of 02, 03, and 06. If the combination was preferred, the subject was asked to indicate his preference between 01 and the combination of 02 and 03. The final question about the subset of objectives was whether the subject would prefer to achieve 02 or the combination of 03 and 06. The same series of questions was repeated with the other subset of objectives (01, 04, 05, and 07).[4]

The choices involving the two subsets of objectives were checked to see if they were compatible. If they were not, the author pointed out the inconsistency to the subject and asked him to reconsider his choices and make adjustments to achieve consistency. An example of an inconsistency between the two subsets of objectives would be if the subject responded that he preferred 01 to the combination of 02, 03 and 06 and that he also preferred the combination of 04, 05 and 07 to 01.

Finally the choices involving the two subsets of objectives were checked with the original ranking of the seven objectives. Again any inconsistencies were pointed out, and the subject was asked to reconsider and to make adjustments to achieve consistency.

In the second task a unique set of values for the objectives was obtained by asking the subjects to rate the objectives on a ratio scale. The ratio scale in the second task was presented as an extension of the ranking the subjects had done in the first task.[5] The objective that the subject had ranked as most important was arbitrarily given a value of 100. A vertical scale marked off from 0 to 100 was placed in front of the subject and an arrow marked "1" was placed opposite 100. The subject then placed the remaining six arrows numbered "2" through "7" on the scale to indicate the ratio he believed each objective had to the value of 100 assigned to the first objective.

After the subjects had indicated a value on the ratio scale for each objective, their number assignments on this scale were compared with their verbal choices of the first task to arrive at a final numerical value for each objective. For example, if a subject had stated in the first (verbal) task that he would rather achieve the objective he had ranked as most important than achieve the combination of objectives he had ranked second and third in importance, the numerical value he had assigned on the ratio scale to the first objective would have to be greater than the sum of the values assigned to the second and third objectives. If not, the subject was asked to change his verbal choice or to change his number assignment to achieve consistency.

The third task was a complex one which asked the subjects to evaluate the efficiency of each alternative[6] to achieve each objective. The subject had to consider seven cards with the objectives on them, eight cards of a different color with the alternatives on them, and a scale with probabilities marked off from 0 to 100. The author went over the scale with the subject to familiarize him with the responses required for the task. Then the subject was given the card with the first alternative on it and the seven cards with the objectives on them. He was asked to give the probability that the selection of the first alternative would achieve each of the seven objectives. He responded with a number ranging from 0 to 100. A "0" meant that the selection of the alternative was practically certain not to achieve the objective; a "100" meant that the selection of the alternative was practically certain to achieve a particular objective.

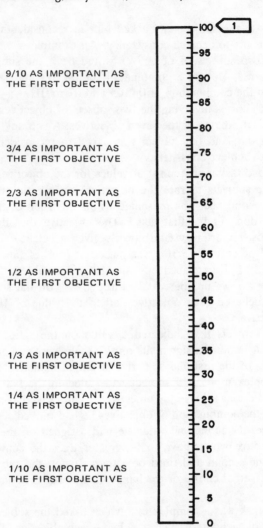

FIG. 2. Ratio Scale for the Second Task

The author recorded each probability on a score card which was kept where the subject could see it at all times. The procedure was repeated with the second alternative, and so on through all eight alternatives.

After the probabilities were recorded for all alternatives, the subject was asked to reread the cards with the alternatives on them and to indicate which alternative he thought would be the best way to allocate the federal grant and which would be the second best way.

Later the author calculated the effectiveness of each alternative. If the

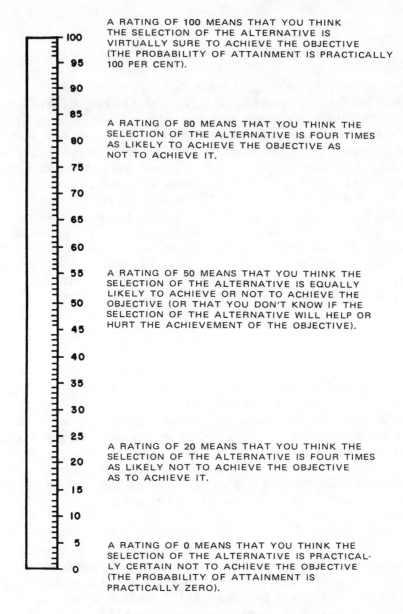

A RATING OF 100 MEANS THAT YOU THINK
THE SELECTION OF THE ALTERNATIVE IS
VIRTUALLY SURE TO ACHIEVE THE OBJECTIVE
(THE PROBABILITY OF ATTAINMENT IS PRACTICALLY
100 PER CENT).

A RATING OF 80 MEANS THAT YOU THINK THE
SELECTION OF THE ALTERNATIVE IS FOUR TIMES
AS LIKELY TO ACHIEVE THE OBJECTIVE AS
NOT TO ACHIEVE IT.

A RATING OF 50 MEANS THAT YOU THINK THE
SELECTION OF THE ALTERNATIVE IS EQUALLY
LIKELY TO ACHIEVE OR NOT TO ACHIEVE THE
OBJECTIVE (OR THAT YOU DON'T KNOW IF THE
SELECTION OF THE ALTERNATIVE WILL HELP OR
HURT THE ACHIEVEMENT OF THE OBJECTIVE).

A RATING OF 20 MEANS THAT YOU THINK THE
SELECTION OF THE ALTERNATIVE IS FOUR TIMES
AS LIKELY NOT TO ACHIEVE THE OBJECTIVE
AS TO ACHIEVE IT.

A RATING OF 0 MEANS THAT YOU THINK THE
SELECTION OF THE ALTERNATIVE IS PRACTICAL-
LY CERTAIN NOT TO ACHIEVE THE OBJECTIVE
(THE PROBABILITY OF ATTAINMENT IS
PRACTICALLY ZERO).

FIG. 3. Probability Scale for the Third Task

alternative with the highest effectiveness had not been rated by the subject
as his first or second choice, the subject was reinterviewed and asked to
comment on why he had not chosen that alternative.

RESULTS

First Task

The first task, the assigning of values to the seven objectives, was the easiest task for the subjects because the concept of ranking was familiar to them. Nevertheless, there were some problems.

The first choice among the subsets of objectives caused most of the subjects some difficulty and caused considerable difficulty in two cases. This was the choice between the objective the subjects had ranked as most important and the combination of the second, third, and sixth ranked objectives. It was hard for the subject to conceive of the value of an objective alone. The tendency was to think of these objectives as a cluster rather than individually. One subject commented that there was "some overlap" in the choice situation. Another said, "Choices are never this absolute, not all black or all white." The additivity assumption used in the experiment implies the objectives are independent, but the members of the agency are not used to valuing an objective by itself. It was the first choice that was hard to make; the rest of the choices caused no trouble.

Second Task

The purpose of the second task was to compare the assignment of numerical values to objectives implicit in the choices of the first task with the ratings of the objectives in the second task in order to get a unique set of values for the objectives. Of the eleven subjects who completed the experiment, only one had no inconsistencies between the first and second tasks. Of the remaining ten who had inconsistencies, six changed their numerical ratings only, three changed their verbal choices and numerical ratings, and one changed the rank order of his three lowest ranked objectives and also changed his numerical ratings.

The number of shifts in numerical ratings makes it doubtful whether the subjects' original ratings on the ratio scale expressed their actual values of the objectives. Nevertheless, the second task provided good check on the number assignment implicit in the first task. Faced with a numerical scale and their verbal choices, the subjects had to reconsider if they really preferred one subset of objectives to another. The use of the ratio scale also makes the additivity assumption explicit and permits the subjects to react to it. With two exceptions, the idea of additive values was readily grasped by the subjects and they were able to adjust their values and choices to achieve consistency.

Two subjects had trouble with the additivity assumption. In his verbal choice one subject preferred the first objective to the combination of the second, third, and sixth. But his ratings on the numerical scale for the combination of the three objectives added up to well over 100. When the inconsistency was pointed out, the subject argued that the average of the three objectives should be considered rather than their sum. The choices of the second subject showed the same inconsistency. Moreover, he had difficulty in recognizing the inconsistency.

Third Task

The third task was designed to obtain the efficiency of each alternative to achieve each objective. Although this task was a complex one, the subjects with one exception were able to do it successfully. One subject was unable to respond to this task. After he read the first alternative and was asked the probability that the selection of the first alternative would achieve the various objectives, he said, "I'm getting a headache trying to think out these possibilities. This is like a cross-word puzzle." He went on to say, "I don't think of these things in relation to each other [the probability that an alternative would achieve on objective] and I don't think of them in numerical terms." Referring to the scale of probabilities, he said, "When you start talking about 90 or 50 or 75, I just don't think that way."

The comments made by the subjects during this task showed that they thought seriously about the consequences of each alternative before arriving at their estimates of probabilities. Usually the subjects commented briefly before estimating the probability that an alternative would achieve an objective. They made such statements as these:

The Department of Finance would think that the State might have to pick up support of State level programs if federal funds were withdrawn, so they wouldn't like it.

The big local health departments would like it; the little local health departments wouldn't.

I think it is good for the local health department to do some thinking and planning. It pushes them a little.

The Public Health Service would accept it but they wouldn't be so happy so [the rating] would go down to 65.

Analysis Using the Model

The criterion for the selection of one alternative from the eight alternatives in the model is the maximization of effectiveness. This criterion is essentially the same as the criterion of the maximization of expected utility. "Rational" behavior in terms of this study is defined as selecting the alternative with the highest effectiveness.

The experimental procedure used to obtain the utilities and the probabilities was such that it would have been very difficult for a subject to see how the answers he gave in the three tasks would be put together to make a measure of effectiveness. Thus, it is doubtful that the subjects in this experiment deliberately tried to give answers which would make the measure of effectiveness of alternatives (when calculated later by the author) coincide with their choice of the two alternatives they really preferred. In addition, the subjects did not know in advance the tasks they would be asked to do during the interview.[7]

In the original study upon which this paper is based [37] the details of the actual decision making process for the allocation of the federal grant and the parts played by the head of the agency and others who participated in the experiment were set forth. In the review of what actually happened it was clear that the head of the agency was the one who made the basic decisions which controlled the agency's handling of the federal grant. Specifically, he chose the way the grant would be allocated. Therefore, a comparison of his choices of alternatives with the rankings by the model is given first. He selected the first alternative as his first choice. This is the choice he had actually made for the grant a few months earlier. In this experiment he picked the third alternative as his second choice. Calculations using the model showed that the first alternative had the highest effectiveness and the third alternative had the second highest effectiveness. Thus, in terms of the model for allocating the federal grant, he was a "rational" decision maker, i.e., his behavior was consistent with the hypothesis that he chose his alternatives as if he were maximizing expected utility.[8]

Of the eleven participants who completed the tasks in the experiment, seven selected as their first or second choice the alternative the model ranked first. Of these seven there were four whose first and second choices were also ranked first and second by the model. The complete results are:

The probability that four of the eleven subjects would have made "perfect choices" by chance is .0000545.[9] (A "perfect choice" is one in which the subject's first and second choices of alternatives are the same as the alternatives ranked first and second in effectiveness by the model.) Strictly speaking, this finding means that for four of the subjects the hypothesis, i.e., that they chose among alternatives as if they were maximizing expected utility, cannot be rejected. However, the overall agreement between the choices of the subjects and the rankings by the model is fairly good. Of the twenty-two first and second choices made by the eleven subjects, the model ranked nineteen of them as first, second, or third, in effectiveness.

TABLE 1
COMPARISON OF MODEL RANKINGS WITH SUBJECT'S STATED RANKINGS

Subjects	Model Ranking of Subject's 1st Choice	Model Ranking of Subject's 2nd Choice
A	2	3
B	1	2
C	1	2
D	1	6
E	3	1
F	N/A	N/A
G	6	1
H	2	3
I	5	2
J	1	2
K	1	2
L	2	3

Note: N/A means not available and refers to the one subject who was unable to complete the third task.

As stated earlier, if the subject had not rated the alternative with the highest effectiveness as his first or second choice, he was reinterviewed and asked to comment on why he had not chosen that alternative. The comments reveal some of the problems which arise in measuring utilities in complex decision processes and some of the difficulties in studying "rational" decision making in large organizations.

The first and second choices of four subjects (A, H, I, L) did not include the alternative the model ranked first in effectiveness. In addition, the first choice of subject G was ranked sixth by the model.

During the experiment subject A hesitated between alternative seven and alternative eight for his second choice. "If I were outside the Agency I'd pick number seven, but being in the Agency I'll pick number eight." Alternative seven was the alternative the model ranked first and alternative eight was the alternative the model ranked third.

Subject H was asked to comment on the sixth alternative, the alternative the model had ranked first. He said that this alternative would be all right after the out-of-hospital care programs were established in local health departments. However, he did not think this alternative was the way to get new programs started because the assurance of continuing support for local health departments was lacking.

The sixth alternative was the alternative the model ranked first for Subject I. When this subject was looking over the alternatives at the end of the final task prior to making his selections, he pulled out the sixth alternative as his first choice. Then he rejected it saying that the project grants called for in the sixth alternative were not feasible for the coming fiscal year. However, he added that the sixth alternative was something "we should work for as a goal for two or three years from now."

When subject L selected his first and second choices of alternatives at the end of the final task he eliminated the fifth alternative because it was "just a change in reporting requirements." The fifth alternative is the one the model ranked highest for him in effectiveness. When asked to comment on this alternative he said "I agree with it. We have asked for too many reports from local health departments."

Subject G was asked about his first choice which was ranked sixth by the model. The subject had had some difficulty with the scale of probabilities during the last task. During the experiment he said with reference to the final task, "It's too complex for me." Changing one probability to agree with a pattern he had followed on other alternatives would have raised the rank of the alternative he selected from sixth to second, but the change was not made.

These comments bear out the qualifications about rational decision making stated by Marschak in a study reporting experimental evidence that subjects chose the acts with the highest expected utility. He stressed the conditions conducive to rational behavior: ". . . when and only when stress is absent (e.g., memory is not overloaded, ample time is provided, etc.) and, above all, when and only when the structure of the problem is very simple and is laid bare, by the use of lucid syntax, tubular presentation, etc. [30, p. 105]."

DISCUSSION

Utility measuring techniques which rely on incremental changes in the object or objects being valued are not suitable for measuring the utility of indivisible objects such as the seven objectives in this study. In contrast, the divisibility of money allowed Davidson, Suppes, and Siegel [13] and other researchers to make very small changes in the amounts gambled in order to obtain the subject's utility scale for money. Small changes enabled the experimenters to be precise in their measurements.

The experiment using linear programming [13] and the experiments involving choices which result in an ordered metric scale [11, 12, 33] lead to non-unique solutions. For that matter, so does the first task of the Churchman-Ackoff method, but the non-uniqueness of the solution set obtained by this task warrants further discussion.[10] The set of questions asked the subjects about their preferences among subsets of the set of objectives orders some of the utility differences. It does not give a complete ordering and thus is not an ordered metric scale. The set of linear inequalities obtained from the questions used in the first task has a convex solution set. Which solution should be chosen for the values of the objectives? When faced with a similar situation, Davidson, Suppes, and Siegel [13] took the first solution they obtained and Suzuki [41] took the centroid of the solution set. There is no compelling reason to select any one of the infinite number of solutions.

There is one way, which, with luck, eliminates the need to answer the question about which solution to choose. In principle, linear programming could be used to obtain all the extremal points of the solution set. Then the expected utility of each of the eight alternatives in this study could be calculated using one extremal point for the values of the objectives. The alternative with the greatest expected utility would be noted. The procedure would be repeated with each extremal point. If every extremal point resulted in the same alternative having the greatest expected utility, so would every point within the solution set and there would be no need to proceed further. Under these circumstances an interval scale would not be needed. But rather than venture into what could have been a very time-consuming job with no assurance of success and rather than arbitrarily selecting one solution to use for the values of the objectives, the author adopted the procedure suggested by Churchman and Ackoff [9]. Their procedure includes a second task which has the subject assign values to the objectives on a scale marked off from 0 to 100.[11] Then the number assignments on the scale are compared to the subject's verbal choices in the first task. The subject is asked to resolve any inconsistencies between the number assignments and his verbal choices. After the resolution of any inconsistencies the number assignment of the second task is taken as the solution to be used in the effectiveness model.

It could be argued that if a technique had been used in the first task to rank the objectives on a higher ordered metric scale, checking the results of a subject's verbal choices in the first task against his placement of the objectives on a numerical scale in the second task would have achieved an even better final assignment of utilities to objectives. Apart from a desire on the author's part to test the Churchman-Ackoff approximate measure of value method, there is the practical consideration of the amount of time that can be spent in an experiment under field conditions. The subjects of experiments such as the one in this study are not students being paid by the hour for their participation; they are busy executives whose interest the researcher must hold during the experiment and whose assistance the researcher will need in subsequent interviews and informal discussions.

Seven objectives means the twenty-one possible combinations of contiguous intervals would have to be ranked to obtain a higher ordered metric scale. Because the procedure adopted in this experiment was to force consistency during the experiment, the checking of intervals could have been time-consuming. The Churchman-Ackoff method gave four to six preferences among subsets of the objectives that had to be checked against the numerical ratings on the ratio scale. Usually the inconsistencies were resolved without much trouble. A priori it would appear that consistency between the ranking of twenty-one intervals generated by verbal choices and the ranking of twenty-one intervals generated by numerical ratings would be difficult to achieve without confusing the subject or losing his interest.

One way to get the utilities of the seven objectives on an interval scale, after a subject has ranked the objectives in order of preference, would be to ask the subject to place the objectives on a numerical scale in such a way that the intervals between pairs of objectives would reflect his beliefs. For example, if the subject believed that the difference in utility between objectives 1 and 2 was twice as great as the difference in utility between objectives 4 and 5, he should place the objectives on the scale so that this interval ordering is preserved. Pretesting by the author showed that the concept of comparing differences in values of objectives was difficult to explain and the author's attempt to do so did not succeed. Because of the pretest, this approach was dropped.

All methods of measuring utility have their drawbacks. The Churchman-Ackoff method was selected because (1) it is well adapted to the situation of qualitative, indivisible objectives, (2) it can be administered in a reasonable length of time and thus is a practical way to proceed under field conditions, (3) it does not make use of a gamble to obtain a utility function and thus the possible confounding factor of an individual's like or dislike of gambling doesn't arise, (4) the questions asked in the Churchman-Ackoff method are probably easier for subjects to understand than the questions asked about the gamble in the Von Neumann-Morgenstern method [43] or in the Davidson, Suppes, and Siegel [13] method,[12] and (5) the accounts in the literature of the application of the Churchman-Ackoff method [9, 10, 36] are not given in nearly as much detail as the reports on the use of the von Neumann-Morgenstern method and the Davidson, Suppes, and Siegel method. In general, for this particular problem, the measuring utility which achieves an interval scale has advantages over those methods which fail to achieve an interval scale.

NOTES

[1] The literature of utility measurement and related fields is extremely large. Several surveys are available [1, 3, 5, 15, 16, 17, 18, 29, 44].

[2] The Chronically Ill and Aged Services federal formula grant was authorized by Public Law 87-395. A provision of this law permitted the federal government to make matching grants to states to assist in meeting the out-of-hospital health needs of the chronically ill and aged.

[3] The proof of this is given in [38].

4 Procedures to be used for handling different numbers of objectives are given in [9].

5 Stevens [35] suggested that it might be easier to measure utility on a ratio scale than on an interval scale. He proposed that methods of psychophysical scaling which ask subjects to make direct judgments of utility be tested experimentally rather than rejected on *a priori* grounds. His article contained the preliminary results of an experiment by Galanter [19] which were favorable to the attempt to measure utility on a ratio scale.

6 There was an extremely large number of alternative ways in which the federal grant might have been allocated by the agency. Merely shifting a few dollars from one category to another would have resulted in a different allocation. In this study eight alternatives were selected. These covered a wide range of feasible agency programs, yet the number was small enough for a decision maker to evaluate in terms of the seven objectives.

7 The use of members of an organization as experts to provide rankings and ratings in organizational studies is a well recognized research technique. It has been used to assign electronic equipment to naval ships [4] and to evaluate defects in product packaging [36]. A short discussion of this technique and other examples of its use are given in [32].

8 One major conclusion of the study was that the agency's information gathering and processing system did not generate all the data needed to judge whether more effective use could have been made of the federal grant by changes in its allocation. To increase the effectiveness of the administration of the federal grant different information was needed but not more information. The different information would permit the decision makers to prepare better estimates of the probabilities that alternatives would achieve objectives. There is no reason to believe that the cost of a new information gathering and processing system would exceed the cost of the existing system.

9 The probability of a subject selecting by chance as his first and second choices from the eight alternatives the two alternatives the model ranked first and second is 1/56. Because $\lambda = np$ is a small number in this study ($11 \times 1/56 = .196$) the Poisson approximation of the binomial distribution was used to calculate P (4 out of 11 "perfect choices," $p = 1/56$). For $\lambda = .20$, the probability of four or more perfect choices is .0000568 and the probability of five or more is .0000023. The difference, .0000545, is the probability of getting four perfect choices out of eleven by chance.

10 The problem created by the lack of uniqueness of utility function is that difficulties may arise when the utilities are used in a model to select alternatives. Examples can be constructed which show two sets of utilities, each consistent with the subject's choices, leading to the selection of different alternatives. One alternative has the maximum expected utility with one set of utilities and another alternative has the maximum expected utility with the other set of utilities [25]. In such a situation the criterion of "maximize expected utility" does not lead to a unique choice among the alternatives.

11 The assigning of weights to components of a variable to form a composite measure is a well known and frequently used technique in psychology [see, for example, 14, 20, 21, 42].

12 Two methods were used by Davidson, Suppes, and Siegel. The one referred to here is the one which uses an event whose subjective probability is empirically determined to be one-half. The event is a die whose sides have nonsense syllables on them.

REFERENCES

1. ADAMS, E. W., "Survey of Bernoullian Utility Theory," *Mathematical Thinking in the Measurement of Behavior,* H. Solomon (ed.), The Free Press, Glencoe, Illinois, 1960.

2. —— AND FAGOT, R., "A Model of Riskless Choice," *Behavioral Science,* 4 (1959), pp. 1–10.

3. ARROW, K., "Utilities, Attitudes, Choices: A Review Note," *Econometrica*, 26 (1958), pp. 1–23.

4. AUMANN, R. AND KRUSKAL, J., "Assigning Quantitative Values to Qualitative Factors in the Naval Electronics Problem," *Naval Research Logistics Quarterly*, 6 (1959), pp. 1–16.

5. BECKER, G. AND McCLINTOCK, C., "Value: Behavioral Decision Theory," *Annual Review of Psychology*, 18 (1967), pp. 239–286.

6. BENTHAM, J., "Of the Principle of Utility," *Source Readings in Economic Thought*, P. C. Newman, A. D. Gayer, and M. H. Spencer (eds.), W. W. Norton, New York, 1954.

7. BERNOULLI, D., "Specimen Theoriae Novae de Mensura Sortis," *Commentarii Academiae Scientiarum Imperialis Petropolitanae*, 5 (1738); translated by L. Sommers in *Econometrica*, 22 (1954), pp. 22–36.

8. BRIM, O., JR. ET AL., *Personality and Decision Processes*, Stanford University Press, Stanford, 1962.

9. CHURCHMAN, C. W., AND ACKOFF, R., "An Approximate Measure of Value," *Operations Research*, 2 (1954), pp. 172–181.

10. ——, ——, AND ARNOFF, E., *Introduction to Operations Research*, John Wiley & Sons, New York, 1957.

11. COOMBS, C. AND BEARDSLEE, D., "On Decision Making Under Uncertainty," *Decision Processes*, R. Thrall, C. Coombs, and R. Davis (eds.), John Wiley & Sons, New York, 1954, pp. 255–286.

12. ——AND KOMORITA, S., "Measuring Utility of Money Through Decisions," *American Journal of Psychology*, 71 (1958), pp. 383–389.

13. DAVIDSON, D., SUPPES, P., AND SIEGEL, S., *Decision Making: An Experimental Approach*, Stanford University Press, Stanford, 1957.

14. DUNNETTE, M. D., *Personal Selection and Placement*, Wadsworth Publishing Co., Belmont, California, 1966.

15. EDWARDS, W., "The Theory of Decision Making," *Psychological Bulletin*, 51 (1954), pp. 380–417.

16. ——, "Behavioral Decision Theory," *Annual Review of Psychology*, 12 (1961), pp. 473–498.

17. FISHBURN, P., "Methods of Estimating Additive Utilities," *Management Science*, 7 (1967), pp. 435–453.

18. ——, "Utility Theory," *Management Science*, 14 (1968), pp. 335–378.

19. GALANTER, E., "The Direct Measurement of Utility and Subjective Probability." *American Journal of Psychology*, 75 (1962), pp. 208–220.

20. GHISELLI, E. E., *Theory of Psychological Measurement*, McGraw-Hill, New York, 1964.

21. ——, AND BROWN, C. W., *Personal and Industrial Psychology*, second edition, McGraw-Hill, New York, 1955.

22. GRAYSON, C. JR., *Decisions Under Uncertainty: Drilling Decisions by Oil and Gas Operators*, Harvard Business School, Boston, 1960.

23. GREEN, P., "Risk Attitudes and Chemical Investment Decisions," *Chemical Engineering Progress*, 59 (1963), pp. 35–40.

24. GULLIKSEN, H., "Measurement of Subjective Values," *Psychometrika*, 21 (1956), pp. 229–244.

25. HALL, A., *A Methodology for Systems Engineering*, D. Van Nostrand Company, Princeton, 1962.

26. HICKS, J. R. AND ALLEN, R. G. D., "A Reconsideration of the Theory of Value," *Economica*, 1 (1934), pp. 52–76, 196–219.

27. HURST, P., AND SIEGEL, S., "Prediction of Decision from a Higher Ordered Metric Scale of Utility," *Journal of Experimental Psychology*, 52 (1956), 138–144.

28. LUCE, R., AND RAIFFA, H., *Games and Decisions*, John Wiley & Sons, New York, 1957.

29. —— AND SUPPES, P., "Preference, Utility, and Subjective Probability," *Handbook of Mathematical Psychology*, Vol. III, R. Luce, R. Bush, and E. Galanter (eds.), John Wiley & Sons, New York, 1965, pp. 252–410.

30. MARSCHAK, J., "Actual Versus Consistent Decision Behavior," *Behavioral Science,* 9 (1964), pp. 103–110.
31. MOSTELLER, F., AND NOGEE, P., "An Experimental Measurement of Utility," *Journal of Political Economy,* 59 (1961), pp. 371–404.
32. SCOTT, W. R., "Field Methods in the Study of Organizations," *Handbook of Organizations,* J. G. March (ed.), Rand McNally & Company, Chicago, 1965, pp. 293–294.
33. SIEGEL, S., "A Method for Obtaining an Ordered Metric Scale," *Psychometrika,* 21 (1956), pp. 207–216.
34. ———, SIEGEL, A., AND ANDREWS, J., *Choice, Strategy and Utility,* McGraw-Hill, New York, 1964.
35. STEVENS, S., "Measurement, Psychophysics, an Utility," *Measurement: Definitions and Theories,* C. W. Churchman and P. Ratoosh (eds.), John Wiley & Sons, New York, 1959, pp. 18–63.
36. STILLSON, P., "A Method for Defect Evaluation," *Industrial Quality Control,* 11 (1954), pp. 9–12.
37. STIMSON, D., "Decision Making and Resource Allocation in a Public Health Agency," Internal Working Paper, Social Sciences Project, Space Sciences Laboratory, University of California (Berkeley), February, 1967 (revised).
38. ———, "A Resource Allocation Problem in a Public Health Agency," *Management Action: Models of Administrative Decisions,* C. E. Weber and G. Peters (eds.), International Textbook Company, Scranton, Pa., 1969.
39. STOUFFER, S., "The Point System for Redeployment and Discharge," *The American Soldier,* S. Stouffer, et al. (eds.), Vol. 2, Princeton University Press, Princeton, 1949, pp. 520–548.
40. SUPPES, P. AND WINET, M., "An Axiomatization of Utility Based on the Notion of Utility Differences," *Management Science,* 1 (1955), pp. 259–270.
41. SUZUKI, G., "Procurement and Allocation of Naval Electronic Equipment," *Naval Research Logistics Quarterly,* 4 (1957), pp. 1–7.
42. TIFFEN, J. AND MCCORMICK, E. J., *Industrial Psychology,* 5th edition, Prentice-Hall, Englewood Cliffs, New Jersey, 1965.
43. VON NEUMANN, J., AND MORGENSTERN, O., *Theory of Games and Economic Behavior,* second edition, Princeton University Press, Princeton, 1947.
44. WASSERMAN, P., AND SILANDER, F., *Decision-making: An Annotated Bibliography, Supplement, 1958–1963,* Graduate School of Business and Public Administration, Cornell University, Ithaca, New York, 1964.

SELECTION 12

Conflict in Hospitals*

Rockwell Schulz and *Alton C. Johnson*

Evidence of conflict in hospitals is readily apparent. Nurse and nonprofessional hospital employee strikes receive wide publicity. Periodically, administrator-medical staff conflicts break into public view. Furthermore, hospital-client conflicts seem to be increasing as consumers of hospital service level charges of inefficiency and inattention to consumer expectations. Internally, the administrator is continually faced with eruptions of personal or departmental conflicts.

The first step in resolving conflict is to identify the underlying forces fostering it. This paper reviews empirical research reported in management, sociological and hospital literature for insight into some of these underlying forces. The scope of this review includes a brief consideration of hospital-client, interpersonal and individual conflicts. Conflicts related to administrators, medical staff and nursing groups are discussed in somewhat greater depth. Finally, some mitigators of conflict are suggested.

Modern management literature describes benefits that are derived from a reasonable amount of organizational and individual conflict.[1] Indeed, confrontation is sometimes necessary in order to achieve overdue reforms. Just how serious, then, is conflict in hospitals?

One might expect conflict to affect quality of patient care adversely. This tends to be confirmed by studies of Georgopoulos and Mann, who found higher quality care in hospitals where physicians and nurses had a greater understanding of each other's work, problems and needs.[2] Studies in mental hospitals report patients are affected adversely by staff conflict.[3] While conflict might foster institutional innovation and progress, the welfare of the individual patient is served more effectively with institutional stability and harmony. Moreover, conflict can be debilitating for participants, rigidify the social system in which it occurs, and lead to gross distortions of reality.[4] Thus, this paper assumes that minimizing conflict is an important goal and it suggests sources and mitigators of conflict.

Institutional Conflict

Evidence of client-hospital conflict is increasing; however, few empirical studies have been conducted to examine this problem. Patients have very

* *Hospital Administration*, Summer, 1971.

little voice in hospital matters, nor, until quite recently, have they seemed
to desire one; largely we suspect, because they've assumed that professionals know what's best for them. Etzioni notes that only in public monopolies
(e.g., the post office) do clients have less influence than in hospitals.[5]
Apparently, he does not see current constituencies of hospital governing
boards as an effective voice for the client. The recent report by the Urban
Coalition tends to support the view that patients, especially the poor, do
not have a proper voice in decision-making.[6]

A lack of clearly defined community service goals could be an underlying factor in hospital-client hospital conflict. Etzioni suggests that "sometimes an organizational goal becomes the servant of the organization rather
than its master. . . . Goals can be distorted by frequent measuring of organizational efforts, because as a rule, some aspects of its output are more
measurable than others."[7] Certainly, hospitals are susceptible to this in-
version of ends and means. The hospital financial statement, for example,
is one of the few easily understood measurements available to trustees and
administrators and it usually stresses institutional goals as opposed to patient goals.

Conflict or competition between hospitals is evident from the major
programs, such as comprehensive health planning, designed to reduce it.
*However, there appears to be little empirical research on the seriousness,
underlying sources, or measurable effects of such conflict.* It can be assumed that displacement of community service goals by institutional goals
would be an important factor in such conflicts. What is best for an individual hospital is not always best for the society it serves.

Conflict Within Institutions

Certain internal characteristics inherent in the hospital organization foster
conflict. For example, interdependence, specialization and heterogeneity of
personnel and levels of authority, all appear to be related positively to
conflict.[8] In fact, few organizations are composed of as many diverse skills
as the hospital, which generally has nearly three employees for each patient
and a heterogeneous health team influenced by over 300 different professional societies and associations.

Individual Conflict

An individual's role in the hospital can have a major effect on conflict to
which he is subjected. His personal characteristics and past environment
will determine the impact and his coping mechanisms to role conflict. Role
theory, including role conflict, has received considerable study, although

not in a hospital setting. It is easy to imagine role conflict faced by physicians, nurses and administrators. The physician, for example, functions as an agent for an individual patient, his specialty, his profession, his staff, his institution, his community and his own welfare as an individual practitioner. The welfare of these individuals and groups and obligations of the physician to them and to himself are periodically in conflict. *The nurse is frequently caught between multiple lines of authority.* The administrator usually functions in a boundary role; that is, he is frequently in a position between the nurse and physician, two physicians, patient and employee, etc.

Role ambiguity is related to role conflict. Role ambiguity can be defined as uncertainty about the way one's work is evaluated by superiors, uncertainty about scope of responsibility, opportunities for advancement, and expectations of others for job performance. A variety of studies have demonstrated that there is frequently a wide disparity between what a superior expects of his subordinate and what the subordinate thinks the superior expects of him. In an industrial setting Kahn found the individual consequences of role ambiguity generally comparable to individual effects of role conflict. They include, "low job satisfaction, low self-confidence, a high sense of futility, and a high score on the tension index."[9]

A Coping Mechanism: Retreat

Surveys in industrial enterprises found that tension and strain increase directly with occupational status. Individuals in professional and technical occupations experienced the most tension followed by managerial, then clerical and sales.[10] However, Kahn found the medical administrator in the industrial plant who works under conditions of high role conflict scored low on tension.[11] In a case study he found the administrator kept potential conflicts in a delicate balance by retreating into his own section of expertise, i.e., statistical and financial management. The obvious implication is that the administrator can minimize conflict and tension by restricting his role. While this represents one case study in a non-hospital setting, one can logically assume a relationship between the scope of an administrator's role and his effort to effect changes and administrative conflict. Such a coping mechanism may aid the equanimity of the administrator but will not help him fulfill his broader obligations and responsibilities. Kahn's studies also relate personality variables to experiences of strain from conflict.[12] He found tension more pronounced for introverts, for emotionally sensitive people, and individuals who are strongly achievement-oriented. Personality characteristics also affected exposure to role conflict and tension. Individuals who are relatively flexible and those who are achievement-oriented are more subjected to conflict pressures.

Interpersonal Conflict

Interpersonal conflict is defined broadly to include both (*a*) interpersonal disagreements over substantive issues, such as policies and practices, and (*b*) interpersonal antagonisms, that is, the more personal and emotional differences which arise between interdependent human beings.[13] Both forms are broadly evident in the hospital setting. Interpersonal antagonisms would seem to be more prevalent in hospital operations because by nature they deal with emotions. However, no studies were found related to relative frequency, severity or source of interpersonal conflict in hospitals.

Administration-Medical Staff Conflict

Whereas in industry top executives usually enjoy both formal and informal power and status, power and status do not appear to be centered in the same individuals in the hospital organization. This characteristic, rather unique to hospital organization, is a basic source of administration-medical staff conflict.

Power has been defined as the maximum ability of a person or group to influence individuals or groups. Influence is understood as the degree of change that may be effected in individuals or groups. Authority has been defined as legitimate power.[14] In reviewing a variety of authors, Filley and House have summarized the basis of power being derived from (1) legitimacy, (2) control of rewards and sanctions, including money, (3) expertise, (4) personal liking, and (5) coercion.[15] Observation tells us that the hospital administrator usually has (1) legitimacy from delegated authority for hospital affairs from the governing board, (2) effective control of funds, beds, and other resources, (3) increasing expertise, particularly as management information systems improve, (4) personal liking, and (5) ability to coerce through demands of such sources as the Joint Commission on the Accreditation of Hospitals. Studies by Perrow and Georgopoulos and Mann tend to confirm the increasing dominance of the administrator.[16] Recent demands by the American Medical Association and medical staffs in many hospitals for medical staff representation on hospital boards tend to confirm their protestations of declining influence.

The Factors of Status

Other studies are somewhat conflicting; however, they appear to relate more to factors of status. For example, Georgopoulos and Mann, after describing the administrator as most influential, describe his source of influence as delegated authority from trustees, while sources of physicians' influence include their expertise, prestige, status and power among patients and the community.[17] A recent survey reported that "trustees and medical staffs do not view the administrator as a leader, but as a generally passive influence caught between the board and doctors."[18]

Goss suggests that physicians tend to view administration as a less prestigious kind of work.[19]

The hospital administrator's drive for professionalism and his desire for more prestigious titles such as president or executive vice-president, tend to suggest that he believes he needs to improve his status. As physicians attempt to maintain or increase their power, and administrators improve their status, presumably, both tend to feel threatened. Under such circumstances conflict increases.

Physicians and nurses, like professionals in other fields, have primary allegiance to professional status rather than to organizational status.[20] Hence, the potential for professional-institutional goal conflict is present.

The hospital organization is sometimes referred to as a duopoly with essentially autonomous administrative and medical staff organizations. Croog suggests that each system is oriented to a different set of values, one emphasizing provision of service, one emphasizing maintenance of operation of organization.[21] The Barr report related hospital inefficiences to this dual management authority.[22] Other studies tend to confirm the presence of a conflict between bureaucratic routine and individualized patient care.[23] Perhaps a more flexible organizational structure with emphasis upon project teams would reduce this type of conflict.

Nursing Conflict

Considerable basic conflict in nursing is evident from many studies. Most of these inquiries indicate that nurses are satisfied with their vocation, but dissatisfied with specific conditions of salary, work load, working hours, etc.[24] However, Argyris suggests more basic problems, such as frustration of the dominant predispositions of nurses.[25] He reports nurses in the hospital he studied were not able to fulfill effectively important predispositions, such as being self-controlled, indispensable, compatible, and expert. Findings of Corwin, Taves and Scott, reported later in this paper, seem to support these conclusions.

Status may be a source of basic conflict among nurses. In years past, nursing was one of the few careers a woman could enter and attain some degree of professional prestige. Today, more vocational opportunities are opening to women as sex discrimination continues to decline. Women can, or at least sometimes believe they can, gain greater recognition in such fields as business, government, medicine and teaching.[26] Whereas nurses had been virtually the only professionals in the hospital outside of the physicians, they are now receiving increasing competition for status from a proliferation of allied health professionals, many of whom have higher standards of education, pay, and autonomy. In his survey of student nurses and personnel in three major hospitals, Taves found that "compared to student nurses who have a relatively high image of nursing on the average, the image that the general duty nurse holds seems to be especially low. . . . Head nurses have a somewhat better image of nursing than general duty nurses." He also found that other hospital personnel had an even lower image of nursing.[27]

Struggle for Professionalism

Frustrations are evident in nursing's struggle for professionalism. Corwin and Taves suggest that "the drive to gain professional status and achieve a unique place of importance within the hospital's division of labor, inevitably brings the group into conflict with the lay administration and physicians who are jealous of their prima donna status within the hospital scheme."[28] Scott states that the nurses' drive for professionalism may be based on carving out a special niche for themselves in which they can operate relatively independently from control by other groups and which allows them some claim to superior status.[29]

Organizational factors present conflicts for nurses. Nurses' career advancement has shifted from an individual to an organizational context wherein a nurse must move through the bureaucratic hierarchy to gain recognition. Rewards in this hierachy, however, do not reflect professional patient care, but administrative duties. Argyris suggests that nurses believe that an administrator is a second-class citizen. He also suggests that the only area where a nurse is free to "blow her top" is in the administrative area and this adds another factor which keeps administration in a low status function.[30] On the other hand, Taves found that nursing personnel who have higher ranking official positions in the organization are more satisfied with their jobs than lower ranking personnel.[31]

The Need to Mitigate and Control Conflict

Others suggest sources of nursing conflict can be a lack of role and job concensus,[32] type of care,[33] and dislike of working with non-professionals.[34]

Regardless of the source, it is evident that a considerable degree of conflict exists in hospitals. The problem then, is one of developing ways and means of mitigating or at least controlling conflict. The next section suggests some approaches to the resolution of this problem.

ACTION PROGRAM

Figure I presents a decision model related to diagnosing and mitigating conflict. It lists conflict participants and some of the underlying sources of conflicts presented in this paper. A brief description of the mitigators listed in the exhibit follows below:

Comprehensive Institutional Goal Setting

Comprehensive institutional goal setting is a formalized program to define goals and objectives *explicitly*. Too often goals are defined implicitly, such as "high quality care at low cost." Explicit goals state measures affecting quality and costs. Often goals can be stated in terms of specially attainable objectives.

Goal definition should begin with a study of the needs of the society the institution intends to serve in order to obviate displacement of goals. Medical staff members and employees, in addition to administrators and trustees, should participate in setting goals. Sociologists, political scientists and economists, as well as planners and citizens of the public served, can provide appropriate resource personnel to deliberations. Explicit institutional goals aid community understanding, assist internal and external evaluation of outputs reducing overemphasis on inputs such as costs and facilities, help to sublimate personal differences by focusing efforts on end results, and help to marshall required resources for attaining goals.

Organizational Changes, Public Relations Programs

Communications can be improved by broadening official lines of communication with citizens served by the institution. Policies for governing board membership might be revised to represent more appropriately the constituencies served. Or, an advisory board might be established to review expressed needs of constituencies and hospital programs to meet needs. A public relations program based on appropriate client attitude surveys can be beneficial.

Community Goal Setting

While many communities are preparing plans for community health services, few have effectively articulated explicit goals and objectives that

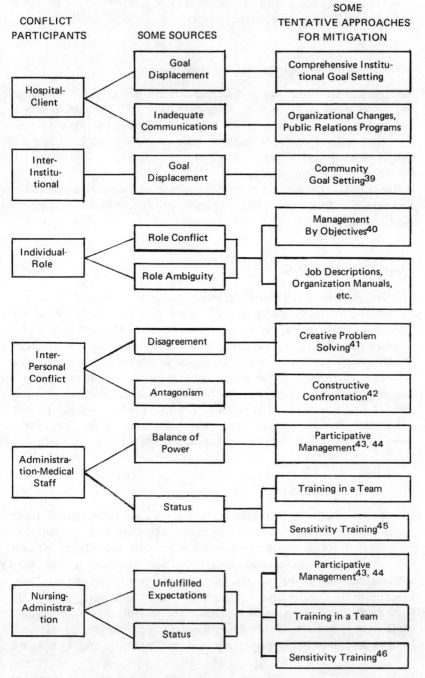

Figure 1*
DECISION MODEL
FOR DIAGNOSING AND MITIGATING HOSPITAL CONFLICT

*See text footnotes 39-46 for numbered references in figure.

plans should serve. The City of Dallas is a notable exception.[35] There, community goals for health services provide a framework for institutions to coordinate individual goals and plans.

Management by Objectives and Role Definition

Management by objectives is the participation between the subordinate and his superior in setting the subordinate's goal.[36] Through interaction and discussion, a subordinate can determine precisely what is expected of him, thus reducing anxiety resulting from ambiguity, while at the same time improving worker independence in task performance and at the same time increasing accountability.

Role definition through job descriptions and administrative manuals can also help to reduce role conflict and ambiguity. These tools are familiar to most administrators.

Creative Problem Solving

Creative problem-solving utilizes techniques that sublimate antagonistic conflict and fosters creativity in participative problem-solving. Maier notes the distinction between "choice behavior" which is an examination and a selection from the alternatives, and "problem-solving," which is a searching or idea getting process.[37] By turning choice situations into problem-solving situations, participants are more apt to focus on end results rather than on who is presenting or standing for what. It maximizes creativity and sublimates hostility, self-pity and rigidity. Creative problem-solving promotes end results wherein everyone wins, rather than a choice situation in which there is a winner and loser or a compromise wherein everyone loses.

Constructive Confrontation

Issues of conflict tend to proliferate when there are interpersonal antagonisms between individuals. A manager can take steps to avoid issues that may result in open interpersonal conflict between individuals. However, indirect effects of interpersonal antagonism will frequently persist and in the long run may be more damaging than an open confrontation. Walton suggests using constructive confrontation with third party intervention, particularly by consultants from outside the institution.[38] Components of confrontation include, 1) clarifying the issues with parties, 2) expressing feelings descriptively, 3) expressing facts and fantasies, and 4) resolution and agreement. It would appear, however, that third party intervention should be utilized sparingly.

Participative Management

Participative management is a philosophy of management in which hospital employees and physicians participate in a meaningful way in the administration of the hospital. It is a philosophy espoused by Rensis Likert and by the late Douglas McGregor, who wrote of "theory X and theory Y."[39] Studies by Coleman, Gamson and Corwin support the view that broad participation in authority systems minimizes major incidents of conflict, although minor incidents may be more frequent.[40]

Management by objectives and comprehensive institutional goal setting are examples of participative management. The administrator does not abdicate his responsibility, he shares it. By sharing planning, coordination, control and management information, the administrator can actually gain more control over his responsibilities.[41]

Sensitivity Training

Sensitivity training, with emphasis on institutional social system development, can help to overcome "hang-ups" related to concerns over status.[42] Laboratory training based on the more traditional group dynamics training is suggested rather than the recent individual self-awareness training which at times borders on therapy. It is the latter, personal development training, that has been maligned recently.

Training in a Team

Health workers are expected to function as a team, yet they are seldom trained for this role. Hospital administrators spend more time with physicians and nurses than any other group. It would be beneficial if they had meaningful dialogue in the formative educational period. This could be easily arranged through seminars or research projects on such subjects as ethics, legal problems, group dynamics, contemporary problems in health, to name just a few. Opportunities for informal as well as formal associations should be arranged. Interdisciplinary study or informal association can also be arranged through the work environment.

Combined degree programs between medicine and hospital administration and/or nursing and hospital administration should be considered seriously. In addition to improving team associations at the educational level, it would help to improve administrative skills of those who actually administer a large part of health service and health team.

In Summary

Conflict in hospitals is an incredibly complex issue. While it deserves considerably more research, much can be done to apply current knowledge of sources and mitigating activities. In general, increased demand for services and attempts to diagnose and lessen conflicts will result in new policies and procedures. Among these will be research studies to identify the impact of various conflict situations. In addition, one can expect to see changes in goal setting, planning, organizational relationships and training programs.

FURTHER READINGS SUGGESTED BY THE AUTHORS

CORWIN, RONALD. "Patterns of Organizational Conflict," *Administrative Science Quarterly,* Dec. 1969, pp. 507–521.

DODDS, RICHARD W., M.D. "A Framework for Political Mapping of Conflict in Organized Medicine—Especially Pediatrics," *Medical Care Review,* Vol. 27, 10, Nov. 1970, pp. 1035+.

KAHN, ROBERT L. *Organizational Stress* (New York: John Wiley & Sons, 1964).

KELLY, JOE. "Make Conflict Work for You," *Harvard Business Review,* July–Aug. 1970, pp. 103–113.

LEWIN, KURT. *Resolving Social Conflicts: Selected Papers on Group Dynamics* (New York: Harper & Bros., 1948).

PERROW, CHARLES. "Goals and Power Structure," *The Hospitals and Modern Society,* Eliot Friedson, editor (New York: The Free Press, 1963), pp. 112–146.

PONDY, LOUIS R. "Varieties of Organizational Conflict," *Administrative Science Quarterly,* 14:4, Dec. 1969, pp. 499–505.

REFERENCES

[1] Among them are: Amitai Etzioni, *Complex Organizations,* Holt, Rinehart & Winston, 1961, pp. 124–126; Mason Haire, *Modern Organization Theory,* Wiley, 1965; and Robert L. Kahn, *Organizational Stress,* Wiley, 1964.

[2] Georgopoulos, Basil S. and Floyd C. Mann, *The Community General Hospital.* Macmillan Company, 1962, p. 400.

[3] Stanton, Alfred H., and Morris S. Schwartz, *The Mental Hospital.* Basic Books, 1954, pp. 342–365; and William A. Caudill, *The Psychiatric Hospital as a Small Society.* Howard University Press, 1958, pp. 87–127, as reported by Peter M. Blau and Richard W. Scott, *Formal Organizations.* Chandler, 1962, pp. 53–54.

[4] Walton, Richard, *Interpersonal Peacemaking.* Addison Wesley, 1969, p. 5.

[5] Etzioni, Amitai, *Modern Organizations.* New York: Prentice-Hall, 1964, p. 95.

[6] *Rx for Action,* Report of the Health Task Force of the Urban Coalition. John Gardner, Chairman. Washington, 1969.

[7] Etzioni, *op. cit.,* pp. 4–11.

[8] Thompson, Victor, "Hierarchy, Specialization & Organizational Conflict," in *Administrative Science Quarterly,* p. 519, and Corwin, Ronald, "Patterns of Organizational Conflict," *Administrative Science Quarterly,* Dec. 1969, pp. 507–521.

[9] Kahn, Robert L., *Organizational Stress.* Wiley, 1964, p. 380.

[10] *Ibid.,* p. 144.

[11] *Ibid.,* pp. 362–371.

[12] *Ibid.,* pp. 225–335.

[13] Walton, *op. cit.,* p. 3.

[14] Filley, Alan C., and Robert J. House, *Managerial Process and Organization Behavior.* New York: Scott, Foresman & Co., 1969, p. 55.

[15] *Ibid.,* p. 61.

[16] Perrow, Charles, "Goals and Power Structure," *The Hospitals and Modern Society.* Eliot Friedson, editor. Free Press, 1963, pp. 112–146, and article in *Handbook of Organizations;* and Georgopoulos, *op. cit.,* p. 567.

[17] Georgopoulos, *op. cit.,* p. 567.

[18] "Trustee's View of Administrators Told," *Modern Hospital,* October 1968, p. 29.

[19] Goss, Mary E. W., "Patterns of Bureaucracy Among Staff Physicians," *The Hospital,* p. 180.

[20] Argyris, Chris, *Diagnosing Human Relations in Organizations: A Case Study of a Hospital.* New Haven: Yale University, Labor and Management Center, 1965, p. 62; and W. G. Bennis et al., "Reference Groups and Loyalties in the Outpatient Department," *Administrative Science Quarterly,* March 1958.

[21] Croog, S. H., "Interpersonal Relations in Medical Settings," *Handbook of Medical Sociology,* H. E. Freeman, S. Levine, and L. G. Reeder, editors. Prentice-Hall, 1963, p. 256.

[22] Secretary's Advisory Committee on Hospital Effectiveness, Department of Health, Education, and Welfare, 1967.

[23] *Abstracts of Hospital Management Studies,* Vol. IV, June 1968. University of Michigan, pp. 137–140 and 196.

[24] Corwin, R. G., and Marvin J. Taves. "Nursing and Other Health Professions," *Handbook of Medical Sociology,* pp. 187–212, and Argyris, *op. cit.*

[25] Argyris, *op. cit.,* p. 189.

[26] Corwin, and Taves, *op. cit.,* note that studies in two states indicated teaching outranked nursing in prestige (p. 193).

[27] Corwin and Taves, *op. cit.,* p. 189.

[28] *Ibid.,* p. 206.

[29] Scott, W. Richard, "Some Implications of Organization Theory for Research on Health Services," *Milbank Memorial Fund Quarterly,* Vol. XLIV, No. 4, Part 2, October 1966, p. 52.

[30] Argyris, *op. cit.,* pp. 67–69.

[31] Taves, *op. cit.,* p. 51.

[32] *Ibid.,* p. 74 and p. 965. Georgopolis, *op. cit.,* p. 398, and Argyris, *op. cit.,* p. 10.

[33] Perrow reported a study by Coser which found nurses giving only custodial care were alienated because they were "unable to implement a single goal."

[34] Argyris, *op. cit.,* p. 70.

[35] *Goals for Dallas,* Dallas, Texas, 1966.

[36] Odiorne, George, *Management by Objectives,* Pitman, 1965.

[37] Maier, Norman F., "Maximizing Personal Creativity Through Better Problem Solving," *Personal Administration.* Vol. 27, 1964 and Filley, Alan C. and Andre Delbecq, "On the Possibility of a Better World," University of Wisconsin (unpublished).

[38] Walton, Richard E., *Third Party Consultation,* Addison-Wesley, 1969.

[39] Likert, R., *New Patterns in Management,* McGraw-Hill, 1961; and McGregor, D., *The Human Side of Enterprise,* McGraw-Hill, 1960.

[40] Coleman, James S., *Community Conflict,* Glencoe, Ill., Free Press, 1957; William Gamson, "Rancorous Conflict in Community Politics," *American Sociological Re-*

view, Vol. 31, pp. 71–81; and Ronald G. Corwin, "Patterns in Organizational Conflict," *Administrative Science Quarterly,* December 1969, pp. 507–520.

41 Tannenbaum, A. S., "Control in Organizations: Individual Adjustment and Organizational Performance," *Administrative Science Quarterly,* September 1962, p. 236.

42 Buchanan, Paul C., "Laboratory Training and Organization Development," *Administrative Science Quarterly,* September 1969, pp. 466–477; Lewin, Kurt, *Resolving Social Conflicts: Selected Papers on Group Dynamics,* Harper, 1948.

Part III

Planning

PART III
Planning

Chapter 6.
Aspects of Planning

6.1   Introduction

6.2   On Planning
     6.2.1 Planning and
         Decision-Making

6.3   Planning Defined

6.4   Some Characteristics of
     Planning

6.5   Planning Philosophies

6.6   Types of Planning
     6.6.1 Strategic Planning
         Cycle
     6.6.2 Planning Structure

6.7   The Role of Planning in
     Health Care Systems

6.8   Concluding Remarks

Two selected articles

Chapter 7.
Planning, Programming
and Budgeting

7.1   Introduction

7.2   Techniques of PPB
     7.2.1 Programming
     7.2.2 Cost-effectiveness
         Analysis

7.3   Methodology of PPB

7.4   Concluding Remarks

Two selected articles

Chapter 8.
Health Information Systems

8.1   Introduction

8.2   What Is Information?

8.3   Management and Health
     Information Systems

8.4   Information System
     Design

8.5   Applied Health
     Information Systems

8.6   Concluding Remarks

Two selected articles

Chapter 6

Aspects of Planning

6.1 INTRODUCTION

Health care entities are complex and dynamic systems; always subject to a mixture of strong political, economic, social, and technological forces. Such systems do not run by themselves; they must be understood, designed, improved, administered, and controlled. This requires planning—either formal or informal, but always *conscious* and deliberate. Planning is a very broad and interdisciplinary subject, and we found it difficult to draw boundaries for the purpose of writing this chapter. There was, on the one hand, the temptation to strictly limit our discussion to health care organizations. We decided against this approach because we considered its scope to be rather narrow. The other approach, which we also rejected, would have concentrated exclusively on the mechanistic aspects of planning. The mechanics of planning can differ from organization to organization, but the *process* of planning is based on the same principles of management. Our discussion of planning is therefore oriented to the *process* of planning, particularly business planning, because we feel that the health care administrator can and should transfer the accumulated knowledge in the business planning literature to health planning.

We recognize that the nature of services generated by health care systems imposes special considerations in health planning which may not always be present in the business context. For example, the role of competition is severely limited, and payment for institutional services is usually through third parties. We feel, however, that not enough "hard" planning has occurred in the health area, and our premise is that attempts to break this impasse will succeed only when techniques from the business arena are deliberately transferred to the health sector.

In this chapter we present a general discussion of planning followed by several definitions of planning; provide a brief discussion of planning philosophies; describe its salient characteristics; give a classification of different types of planning; and examine the role of planning in health care systems.

269

6.2 ON PLANNING

To plan is to prepare for tomorrow. Planning is the process of making decisions in the present to affect future outcomes. Planning has been considered as one of the basic managerial functions.* Through planning the manager determines in advance, the *what, when, who* and *how* of possible courses of action to cope with the future. Planning, in other words, sets the framework to guide the future behavior of an organization, health related or otherwise, and its constituents. The central purpose of planning is to develop processes (creative aspects), mechanisms (implementation aspects), and managerial attitudes (motivation aspects) in order to make today's decisions with a better understanding of the future, and to make future decisions "more rapidly, more economically and without disruption to the ongoing business" [Warren, 1966, p. 29]. The result of planning is a plan (usually a structure of plans) which describes contemplated actions and their outcomes; and thus serves as a formal means of coordination and integration.

Viewed broadly, planning is the device or process through which a planner, or a group of planners, strives to move a system from one state of affairs to another and more valued state of affairs. Since we are always concerned with systems, in one form or the other, at one level or the other, our involvement in planning is both necessary and continuous. Planning is indeed the central task in any organized activity. We cannot, for example, think of any major managerial function (e.g., organizing, staffing, directing, controlling, etc.) that does not require either formal or informal planning. In fact all managerial functions are inextricably related to planning; their need emerges either as a result of planning or they are undertaken for the purpose of planning. Planning is ubiquitous. It is as essential for individuals as it is for corporations,† hospitals,‡ government agencies, colleges, political parties, churches, nations and international bodies. As expressed by Ackoff [1970, p. 1], "Planning is one of the most complex and difficult intellectual activities in which man can engage. Not to do it well is not a sin, but to settle for doing it less than well is."

Planning is neither a new discipline nor a novel concept.§ What is new is the acceptance by business, health care, and government organizations

---

* See, for example [Koontz and O'Donnell, 1968], [Newman et al., 1967] and [Fayol, 1949].

† See, for example [Argenti, 1968], [Aguilar, 1967], [Payne, 1963], [Steiner, 1963], [Steiner and Cannon, 1966], and [Ewing, 1958].

‡ See, for example [Allemand, 1964], [Arnold, 1968], [Barry and Sheps, 1969], [Feldstein, 1967], [Frieden and Peters, 1970], [Hamburg, 1967], [Kaufman, 1969], [Lentz, 1970], [Peters, 1964], [Somers, 1968], [Strauss, 1969], and [Sigmond, 1967].

§ See, for example [Scott, 1965, Chapter 3] for a review of the historical evolution of long-range planning.

of formal planning as a means to more effectively meet their objectives. Several professional planning societies in a variety of disciplines, including health care, have been organized during the last two decades.* The role and rise of the planner in the corporate hierarchy has been documented in the literature [Steiner, 1970]. Attempts have also been made to evolve a general theory of planning which relates various steps in planning to more established theories.† Somers [1968] lists a set of general principles of community health planning and defines the special role of the teaching hospital in the community planning process.

Management has accepted the necessity and virtue of planning for reasons other than developing formal plans. There is logic behind the claim that the process of formal planning is perhaps just as useful as the results of planning.‡ Indeed, one of the major benefits of a formal planning system is the fact that managers are required to put down on paper, in concrete terms, the informal plans which would otherwise guide their actions. In this fashion, they are forced to examine the present, learn from the past and focus on the future. Glaring inconsistencies between stated goals and actual actions, or between different parts of the organization are immediately brought to the surface, and corrective measures are adopted. Many such opportunities for improving current operations, if not discovered because of a formal planning effort, would be lost forever.

6.2.1 *Planning and Decision-Making*

Planning and decision-making processes are very similar—but with one important difference. In certain cases, one can decide without planning, but every aspect of formal planning by definition requires decision-making.§ Planning is, in effect, *anticipatory decision-making* [Ackoff, 1970, p. 2]. Planning is required whenever the desired future state involves a set of interdependent decisions, decisions that are too large and hence must be subdivided into phases and stages, and decisions requiring inputs from various parts of the organization. [Ackoff, 1970, pp. 2–3].

Planning and doing are intimately related. It is perhaps easier to accept the separation of deciding and doing as compared to a separation between

---

* In addition, professional management groups such as TIMS and Academy of Management have organized special planning groups.
† See, for example [Le Breton and Henning, 1961]. The authors outline 13 steps and relate them to the following theories and roles: (1) Theory of Need Determination, (2) Theory of Choice, (3) Theory of Data Collection and Processing, (4) Theory of Testing, (5) Theory of Organizing for Planning, (6) The Role of Communication Theory in Planning, and (7) the Role of Persuasion Theory in Planning.
‡ See Eric Trust quoted in [Ackoff, 1970, p. 15].
§ See Mockler [1972, p. 11] for a comparison of decision-making and planning processes.

planning and doing.* In practice, organizational tasks will exhibit different mixtures of planning and doing, depending upon the level of organizational hierarchy. The higher the organizational level, the more is the planning content of the manager's job. Considerations of human motivation require that, as far as possible, a planning system permit maximum participation in the *process* of planning of those individuals who are to implement the plans.

Ansoff and Brandenburg present an analysis of planning with reference to a schematic model of a Management Decision Cycle which we produce in Figure 6.1.

FIG. 6.1. MANAGEMENT DECISION CYCLE

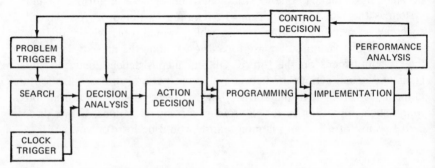

Source: [Ansoff and Brandenburg, 1967, p. B-224].

They maintain that planners have traditionally concerned themselves only with programming; but future opportunities lie in developing integrated planning models which encompass not one but all phases of the decision cycle. They view the planner as a specialist within management science and summarize his role thus:

1. His interest is directed to models which are of direct relevance and usefulness to the firm. In a compromise between "formalism" and "realism," which each management scientist has to make, the planner inclines toward the latter.

2. The planner's job is "on line." As a part of management he is a daily "real time" participant in the ongoing management process. By contrast, many other management scientists within the firms operate "off line" [in OR or management science groups) on special problems and assignments.

3. A consequence of the on line responsibility is the planner's concern with

---

* There are two schools of thought on this issue. The *separationists* claim that the pressures of routine work tend to undermine systematic planning and hence a separate planning staff should be organized for making formal plans. The *nonseparationists* believe that "planning and doing are separate parts of the same job; they are not separate jobs." The arguments are summarized in Scott [1965, pp. 170–171].

programming, again in contrast to many other management scientists who consider the problem "solved" when the preferred alternative is chosen.

4. Similarly, the planner is concerned with organizational acceptance of planning, with implementation, with measurement, and feedback into the planning process.

Planning requires a blend of scientific analysis, human judgment, and experience. To quote Branch [1966, p. 245] "Many of the requisites of the successful staff planner—flexibility, inclusiveness of thinking, deductive ability, intuitive perception, sensitivity to human considerations, and capacity to learn—depend as much on his emotional maturity as specific business experience or professional training."

6.3 PLANNING DEFINED

Several formal definitions of planning can be found in the literature.* As defined by Drucker, planning is "a continuous process of making present entrepreneurial† decisions systematically and with the best possible knowledge of their futurity, organizing systematically the effort needed to carry out these decisions, and measuring the results of those decisions against expectations through organized systematic feedback." [Drucker, 1959, p. 240] Ansoff and Brandenburg [1967, p. 230] define planning as "a process of setting formal guidelines and constraints for the behavior of the firm." This process of planning "includes search for threats and opportunities, analysis of these, selecting preferred ones, scheduling their implementation and using performance feedback to improve the performance." The essence of planning is contained in the following descriptive definition which the authors have evolved from their experience.

Planning is the process of analyzing and understanding a system, formulating its goals and objectives, assessing its capabilities, designing alternative courses of action or plans for the purpose of achieving these goals and objectives, evaluating the effectiveness of these plans, choosing the preferred plan, initiating necessary actions for its implementation, and engaging in continuous surveillance of the system in order to arrive at an optimal relationship between the plan and the system.

This definition implies that planning includes the tasks of measuring the outputs of the plan in order to compare them with the goals of the

---

* See, for example [Steiner, 1969, pp. 6–7], [Warren, 1966, p. 21], [Scott, 1965, p. 20–21] and other references given at the end of Chapter 6. The reader will find 18 different definitions of planning reviewed by Y. Dror, "The Planning Process: A Facet Design," in Lyden and Miller [1967, pp. 96–99].

† Although commonly used with reference to a profit-oriented organization, the term "entrepreneurial" has relevance to all types of managerial situations. It refers to an ability to devise imaginative alternatives and configurations of resources, adapt to changing environment, and act with foresight.

system and, if necessary, making necessary changes either in the plan itself or in the goals of the system or both. This constant and mutual "rematching" of the system's goals and objectives with the components of the plan is necessary because most real-life systems operate in dynamic rather than static environments.

6.4 SOME CHARACTERISTICS OF PLANNING

From our definition of planning, we can distill several characteristics or requirements of planning and identify several types of plans.

1. Planning must be purposeful; hence, planning always starts with a statement of goals and objectives.

2. Planning is not an act; it is a *process* consisting of a series of interrelated steps or phases. Furthermore, the planning process is continuous and iterative (it converges to a desired state through several repetitions of the planning cycle).

3. Planning is required whenever we are dealing with large, complex, and interdependent decisions. That is, planning is an integral part of the process of managing a system.

4. Planning is hierarchical in nature. In general, the manager designs a *system* of plans, rather than an individual plan.

5. Planning must have an organizational identification. In other words, plans are caused by and made for certain parts of organizations.

6. Allowing for the socio-political environment of the organization, planning should be deliberate, rational, and objective. An important point of reference for planning is the current capability profile* of the system.

7. Planning deals with the future, and as such, requires an input of forecasts of economic variables, patient needs and demands, utilization of health services, social environment, and direction of political forces. Internal assessment of the system's capabilities plus input from external appraisal provide the basis for alternative plans.

8. Planning can have as many dimensions as the dimensions of the system for which the plans are being made. In planning, these key dimensions† can be identified: (A) Time (short range, medium range, long range); (B) Organizational Level (regional, hospital-wide, departmental); (C) Functional Area (patient services, financial, maintenance); (D) Orientation (internal or external) and (E) Scope of the Plan (comprehensive plan, master plan, strategic plan, tactical plan, implementation plan, etc.).

9. Planning implies standards which become the basis of the corresponding control system.

---

* See, for example [Ansoff, 1965, Chapter 5].
† For further elaboration, see [Steiner, 1969, p. 12].

10. Since planning premises, internal requirements, and external influences can change over time, the elements of flexibility must be built into the very design of a plan.

If we examine the operational implications of these characteristics or requirements of planning, we come to the conclusion that planning must take place at all levels and in each part of the organization. Furthermore, planning involves an infinity of considerations because of the constantly changing nature of the organization as well as its environment. There is, logically, no end to the planning process. In order to have a successful planning system, certain supporting elements must be provided* (e.g., an effective management information system, a formally organized planning group, clearly defined planning methodology and planning cycle).

6.5 PLANNING PHILOSOPHIES

The philosophical base of planning lies in the conception that any organization (family, business firm, hospital, military, government, or society) can more effectively attain its objectives if it engages in systematic planning. As expressed by Branch [1966, p. 309] "Planning philosophy presupposes that man must influence his future to some degree by present actions to survive. It considers this effort ethically desirable. It implies that human knowledge and rationality are cumulative, and presumes the existence of goals sufficiently definite for planning." Planning philosophies can be discussed both at the macro and micro level. At the macro level, we are concerned with such issues as centralized versus decentralized economic planning, form and structure of national, regional, and area-wide planning of health care facilities, and the relationship between the central government and major sectors of industry. At the micro level, health care planning has been directed at such "operational" problems as patient scheduling, bed utilization, inventory control, purchasing, diet planning and so on. The "macro" and "micro" aspects are interrelated; "macro" sets the framework for, and guides the direction of, "micro" efforts. The two "pure" forms of planning philosophies (in the macro context) are completely centralized and completely decentralized planning. In varying degrees, the socialist countries, and many developing countries, engage in centralized planning. Economic, social and industrial plans in these countries are developed and implemented through the direct authority of the central government.† On the other end of the spectrum, decentralized planning philosophy assumes that the needs of the society are best served

---

* See Clee in [Steiner and Cannon, 1966].
† The highly publicized 5-year or 4-year plans of these countries are examples of such planning.

when the production of goods and services is guided by freely operating market forces—rather than by a centralized planning authority. The United States and most of the European countries rely on the principle of a free market economy. However, in practice, most nations practice a *changing* mixture of these two pure philosophies in order to meet specific demands of the times. Realities of circumstances, rather than doctrinaire considerations, decide the policy issues.* For example, an overwhelming majority of the countries in the "free-market economy" category, have introduced national health plans. Even in the United States, the last bastion of individualistic health care philosophy, the question is no longer *if* a national health care plan should be instituted. It is, rather, *when* to institute it and *how* to organize and finance it. At the micro level, the philosophical considerations relate essentially to the behavioral attributes of top management. This is true in all organizations, although the statement has more relevance to corporate planning than to health care planning.

An operationally useful classification of planning philosophies has recently been advanced by Ackoff [1970, p. 6], who suggests three categories of planning philosophies: (1) *satisficing*,† (2) *optimizing,* and (3) *adaptivizing.* The philosophy of "satisficing" rejects the idea that the objective of the businessman is to maximize profits. On the other hand, the *satisficer* planner sets goals and objectives which he considers to be "good enough." They may not be the best possible goals, but they are desirable, feasible, and in the judgment of the decision-maker, they are above the organization's aspiration level.

In comparison to the satisficer, the *optimizer* seeks to either maximize or minimize some measure of performance. His orientation is quantitative in nature, and he is prone to model building. This philosophy has achieved its success in solving "operational" problems of organizations. While the quantitative models have great potential, most seem to optimize only a part of the system—without clearly establishing the relationship of the part with the overall organizational purpose or strategy. This tendency of looking only at part of the system, rather than the overall system and its behavior, threatens the potential of optimization techniques for solving more important policy decisions of the organization. The failure on the part of management to take full advantage of optimization techniques is unwittingly being perpetuated by its preoccupation with the mechanics, while ignoring the true implications of the philosophy underlying these techniques. The fault of course does not lie with the techniques; they are only as good as the adeptness of the user. Until and unless management men can overcome this type of "myopia" [Leavitt, 1960], they will always

---

* For example, it was not the Democratic but the Republican administration which imposed the first peace time wage and price controls in 1971.
† The concept of "satisficing" was originated by Herbert Simon [1957, pp. 204–205].

be open to the following well-known criticism, narrated by Simon [1960, pp. 17–18].

> Some relatively simple management problems—for example, many problems of factory scheduling—turn out to be far too large for even such a powerful tool as linear programming. It is easy for the operations research enthusiast to underestimate the stringency of these conditions. This leads to an ailment that might be called mathematicians' aphasia. The victim abstracts the original problem until the mathematical intractabilities have been removed (and all semblance to reality lost), solves the new simplified problem, and then pretends that this was the problem he wanted to solve all along. He expects the manager to be so dazzled by the beauty of the mathematical results that he will not remember that his practical operating problem has not been handled.

It is for the reasons just mentioned that techniques of optimization have in general been more successful in tactical rather than strategic planning, and their domain is recognized to be well-structured rather than ill-structured problems.

The third type of planner, the *adaptivizer,* believes in creating "a response to a change (stimulus) that actually or potentially reduces the efficiency of a system's behavior, a response which prevents that reduction from occurring" [Ackoff, 1970, p. 17]. The optimizing planner generally takes the system structure for granted and seeks a course of action that best solves the problem. The adaptive planner on the other hand, tries to change the system in such a way that more efficient behavior follows "naturally" [Ackoff, 1970, p. 20].

The three philosophies of planning, which we have discussed very briefly, have their own adherents in all phases and levels of management. Health care administrators should understand the significance of these approaches in solving the myriad problems that arise in the health setting. Our current social priorities demand a more formal and forceful participation of administrators in shaping the strategic decisions of health care organizations. While there appears to be a gap in terms of the administrator's contribution to the resolution of strategic planning problems, it is precisely the capacity to attack such problems that will result in the creation of an effective and efficient delivery system for health care.

6.6 TYPES OF PLANNING

Planning and its output, the plans, can be classified according to a variety of criteria such as scope, level, time, subject, degree of detail, purpose, degree of control, etc.* These criteria are not necessarily mutually ex-

---

* See, for example [Steiner, 1969, p. 12], [Branch, 1962, p. 26–27], [LeBreton and Henning, 1961, Chapter 2]. LeBreton and Henning list 13 dimensions of a plan each of which can be used as a criterion of classification.

clusive; nor are they absolute. For example, the scope of a national health plan is subject to extensive bargaining and political consensus; it may include or exclude a number of specialized benefits. The level at which planning is done can be national, regional, or local—but the terms "regional" and "local" are subject to changing boundaries. Plans can be long-range, medium-range, or short-range; but "long" and "short" are also relative terms. The criterion of subject matter can yield such classifications as hospital planning, physical planning, functional planning (finance, production, inventory, scheduling, etc.), business planning, military planning, economic planning, government planning, and so on. We can similarly cite classifications of plans according to several other criteria. One classification deserves special emphasis, however. This is the classification of *strategic* planning as opposed to *tactical* planning. Strategic planning refers to the process of setting the *basic* purpose and direction of the organization. Strategic planning is long-run, broad, and is concerned with both ends and means. Tactical planning is usually short-range, narrow, gives more details, and is concerned with means of implementation. Once set in motion, strategic plans cannot easily be reversed. In addition, they usually require commitments of large investments. Tactical plans contain a greater degree of flexibility. Tactical plans are developed in support of strategic plans, and the two are, of course, intimately related. Strategic and tactical planning are "like the head and tail of a coin: we can look at them separately, but we cannot separate them in fact" [Ackoff, 1970, p. 4]. Examples of strategic planning in the health field are: construction and location of a new hospital, degree of inter-institutional affiliation, scope of health services of an institution. Tactical planning includes such considerations as: patient scheduling, purchasing, inventory control, and maintenance.

The subject of strategic and tactical planning has received considerable attention in the management literature.* The stages in the strategic planning cycle are discussed below; some models of tactical planning are covered in Chapters 12 and 13.

6.6.1 *Strategic Planning Cycle*

As mentioned earlier, planning is not a single act. It is a process consisting of interrelated and inter-dependent stages. Regardless of the type or scope of planning, these stages of the process must be completed: (1) analysis and understanding of the system, (2) formulation of objectives and goals, (3) assessment of current organizational capabilities, (4) designing alternative courses of action, (5) evaluating the effectiveness of alternative

---

* See, for example [Ansoff, 1965], [Steiner, 1969], [Ewing, 1958], [Aguilar, 1967], [Mason, 1971], [Ansoff, 1958], [Simon and Newell, 1958], [Tilles, 1963] and other references given at the end of Chapter 6.

plans and choice, (6) implementation, and (7) surveillance and control. Since planning is a continuous process, there is no natural beginning or ending of strategic planning. It is logical, however, (at least for purposes of analysis) to view strategic planning as a cycle—starting with an analysis of the system, the formulation of organizational objectives* and goals, and culminating with the implementation and control of the strategic plans.†

We can now proceed to discuss seven phases that constitute the planning cycle.

PHASE *1. Analysis and Understanding of the System*

The analysis and understanding of the system is the first step in formulating strategic plans. This involves five basic considerations as outlined by Churchman [1968, pp. 29–30].

A) The total system objectives and, more specifically, the performance measures of the whole system;

B) the system's environment: the fixed constraint;

C) the resources of the system;

D) the components of the system, their activities, goals and measures of performance;

E) management of the system.

The implications of this phase are twofold. First, by forcing the administrator to define what the "system" is and what particular measure or measures of performance must be assigned to the system, his sights are raised from just tactical planning to that of the overall mission of the system. Secondly, a detailed analysis of the system's resources and constraints yields the information and data needed to develop organizational strategy. This step, in the language of the practitioner, answers the question of: "Where are we at the present time?"—a question which must be faced if concrete answers to two other important questions "Where do we want to go?", and "How do we get there?" are to be satisfactorily derived.

PHASE *2. Formulation of Objectives and Goals*

This phase answers the question of "Where do we want to go?" In other words, it specifies the *ends* towards which management would *like* the

---

* Ansoff [1965, p. 40] views an objective as made up of three elements; *attribute, scale* and *goal*. An attribute specifies the dimensions along which the achievement of objective is to be measured; the scale provides the yardstick for measurement; and goal is a specific value on the scale to be obtained within a specified time.

† Subsidiary, divisional, departmental, and all other plans are derived from strategic plans. Several models representing the relationship of the "system" of plans can be found in the literature. [Steiner, 1969], [Gilmore and Brandenburg, 1962], [Anthony, 1965], [SRI Report No. 183].

system to move during a specified period of time. This requires that a *schedule* of achieving these goals be established. The process of goal (and objective) formulation has received a great deal of attention from social scientists and behavioral scientists [Simon, 1964]. The fact that organizational objectives are hierarchical in nature establishes the operational necessity and framework for interdependence of strategic planning with tactical and project planning. It has been suggested by Cyert and March [1963] that organizational goals are the "result of a continuous bargaining-learning process." This aspect of organizational life implies that health administrators should assume the central role in formulating strategic plans. For the effectiveness of health care organizations is in large part dependent on them, and they must contribute their share of effort in designing organizational goals and strategy.

How do we go about developing a system of objectives and assigning target values which become goals to be achieved over a specified period of time? Although the practice in terms of the types, coverage, and degree of detail will differ from organization to organization, a very useful and practical system of objectives is presented by Ansoff [1965, pp. 43–74].

It should be noted that most organizational objectives are interacting rather than independent categories and, hence, objective setting is a complex and dynamic process. Yet this is a task which must be performed—each organization must reach a consensus on specific target levels—both for short-run and long-run plans. One practical procedure for establishing target levels consists of forecasting the future, assuming no change in the present posture of the organization (*reference projection*); comparing it with the aspirations of top management (*aspiration projection*); and deciding to choose a realistic value in view of the organization's capability profile (*planned target*). A comparison between the reference projection and the planned target establishes what is known as the *planning gap* [Ansoff, 1965, Chapter 8]. The purpose of planning is to close this gap.

PHASE 3.* *Assessment of Current Organizational Capabilities*

It is obvious that realistic goals and objectives cannot be established without knowing the current capabilities of the organization. This task requires an internal audit or self-appraisal in order to determine the current "state" of the system—from which a list of the *strengths* and *weaknesses* of the organization can be extracted. The self-appraisal reaches every level

---

* It is here that health care institutions suffer from serious difficulties including the fact that their product or output is difficult to assess. While the principal goal of the health facility is patient care, the establishment of suitable parameters for its measurement has long been regarded as virtually impossible. We strongly suggest, however, that suitable proxy measures be uncovered on an interdisciplinary basis.

and every part of the organization. Data must be obtained on operations, delivery systems, finance, research, personnel, purchasing, maintenance, and all other identifiable functions of the organization. Although individual forms to suit the particular needs of an organization can be designed, it is useful to evolve a generalized form for each area of activity to be used in the initial stages of the program. Later, as the planning cycle is repeated and as the momentum of experience gathers, the contents of the self-appraisal forms can be changed to suit the individual needs of specific units of the institution.

Assessment of current organizational capabilities yields information on: (1) available resources, (2) strengths and weaknesses, and (3) estimates of external opportunities and constraints.

PHASE 4. *Designing Alternative Courses of Action*

This phase deals with the specification of *means* by which organizational goals and objectives are to be achieved. In particular, alternatives (e.g., different methods for meeting patient and community demands and needs) must be considered in terms of: (a) their feasibility, and (b) their potential impact on health status. Various alternatives such as expansion of current facilities, development of satellite clinics, sharing services, and mergers can be considered.*

Once particular proposals have been designed, plans must be formulated specifying the types and amounts of various resources that must be employed, their method of acquisition, and the necessary programs and procedures to support the implementation of these courses of action.

PHASE 5. *Evaluating the Effectiveness of Alternative Plans and Choice*

This phase calls for projecting the consequences of the various plans enumerated in Phase 4. The projections must be made along the dimensions of the goals agreed upon in Phase 2; and they must then be compared with the established target levels for the duration of the plan. Those courses of action which either do not meet the target levels or are politically not viable must be discarded; and the remaining should be evaluated not only in terms of their goal-achieving properties, but also in terms of a set of priorities.

PHASE 6. *Implementation*

The result of Phase 5 brings us to the stage where a definite resource allocation commitment must be made. The task of implementation requires

---

* In the business context, see [Ansoff, 1965, p. 109].

that decision-making procedures be spelled out for all parts of the organization. This is the "action" stage in which the detailed questions of *what, who, how* and *when* must be answered.

PHASE 7. *Surveillance and Control*

A *system* of control is an integral part of the overall *system* of management. Plans, strategic or tactical, will have no impact on the organization if they are not kept under proper surveillance and control. The familiar elements of a control system are: (1) standard or target stated in the dimension of the goal to be achieved, (2) means of gathering information and measuring performance, (3) comparing actual performance with the stated target, (4) analyzing the deviations between actual and target performance, and instituting measures (which could involve either changing the plan target or plan implementation procedure or both) to restore a balance between the plan and the system.

6.6.2 *Planning Structure*

Planning structure refers to two things. The first is organization for planning which involves the assignment of responsibility for developing different types of plans to various units of the organization. Planning details are specified; planning schedule is fixed; and inter-relationships between different units are established.* The second refers to the hierarchy of plans themselves, that is, how different plans dovetail with each other. For example, if we accept Ansoff's classification of business decisions [1965, p. 8], planning activities will be roughly divided into a) strategic planning, b) administrative planning, and c) operational planning. At the top of planning structure is strategic planning which provides the framework for making strategic decisions aimed at producing an overall strategy for the organization. Administrative planning deals with the acquisition and organization of resources in order to facilitate the implementation of strategic plans; whereas operational planning concerns itself with the actual scheduling of operations (and all other attendant activities) in as efficient and effective a manner as is possible within the organizational constraints.

The planning structure must be built to suit organizational and environmental realities. For example, planning for relationships between patient care, research, and teaching functions will vary according to category of

---

* For a discussion on "organizing for planning," see [Scott, 1965, Chapter 10], [Ewing, 1958, pp. 145–212], and [Payne, 1963, Chapter 9].

hospital, degree of community involvement, and type of medical staff organization.

6.7 THE ROLE OF PLANNING IN HEALTH CARE SYSTEMS

The ideas of business planning are as relevant to health care organizations as they are to corporations. The concepts of strategy, expansion, diversification, mergers, acquisitions—the whole range of terms, techniques, and tools—can and should be brought to bear in a *conscious* manner in the management of health care facilities. One could speculate that an important factor in rising health costs during the last decade has been a lack of management orientation. We are now witnessing the beginnings of a planning movement in the health field—both in the macro and micro sense.

At the macro level, the Hill-Burton Act of 1946 provided a great incentive for coordinated planning in the health care field. For example, in order to obtain Hill-Burton funds for hospital construction, each state was required to prepare a comprehensive plan, on an area basis, designed to produce a coordinated network of hospitals and public health centers. The major objective of health planning has been frequently stated as the organization and delivery of "optimum health"* services to the population of a defined region. Comprehensive planning in the health field is necessary because "except in very unusual circumstances, a single hospital—by itself—cannot be expected to provide optimum health services." [Sigmond, 1967, p. 32]. Planning programs are increasingly being organized in the health care field. For example, formal planning groups in the health field have expanded by more than tenfold during the past decade. Most cities with a population of over 250,000 have a health planning group, although their planning activities may not extend beyond collecting demographic and utilization data [Battistella and Weil, 1969, p. 2352]. The Comprehensive Health Planning Act (public law 89–749) has given further impetus to health planning by making provisions for: "(1) categorical grants for special circumstance projects, that is, services to meet health needs of limited geographic scope or of special regional or national significance; (2) extension of assistance for personnel among federal, state and local levels [Battistella and Weil, 1969, p. 2364].

---

* See [Sigmond, 1967, p. 31] for a listing of six "optimum health" characteristics. Developed by the American Hospital Association, they are: (1) a team approach to care of the individual under the leadership of the physician; (2) a spectrum of services, including diagnosis, treatment, rehabilitation, education, and prevention; (3) a coordinated community and regional system; (4) continuity between hospital and nonhospital aspects of patient care; (5) continuity between hospital inpatient and out-patient services; and (6) continuing programs of evaluation and adequacy in meeting the needs of the community.

Klarman [1967] describes the role and impact of economic* factors in hospital planning with reference to urban areas. He considers planning as a vehicle of social control, an economic intervention by the government, and notes the unique nature of hospital planning. A special feature of health planning is its emphasis on *collective* planning (Selection 14). That is, consumers, physicians, administrators, community-representatives, and planners from non-health areas are all encouraged by the government to pool their opinions and resources. At this time, we can say that health planning is in a transition stage. The present dependent facilities will have to be woven into a coordinate system of health through well-designed comprehensive planning programs.

At the micro level, there is increasing awareness of the potentials of planning. Newer tools and techniques of planning are being applied to better manage the internal workings of health care facilities.† Young [1968] describes a series of models for the allocation of nursing and logistic resources, utilization of facilities, and medical information analysis. Allemand and Turney [1964] give a statistical approach to project patient load for hospital planning. Arnold [1968] has discussed the application of management concepts and tools to health planning. Barry and Sheps [1969] describe the process by which the Cleveland Metropolitan community developed a community health planning model. Feldstein [1967] suggests the possibility of building an econometric model of a health care center.

Tools and techniques of planning range all the way from rules of thumb to modern techniques of management science. A classification of major tools and techniques is given by Steiner [1969, p. 336]. It is beyond the scope of this book to discuss the entire range of these topics each of which is an important subject by itself. However, we have chosen to discuss two topics: "Planning-Programming-Budgeting" (Chapter 7) and "Health Information Systems" (Chapter 8). In our judgment, these two topics are of special significance in the implementation of policy as well as operational decisions in the health field.

6.8 CONCLUDING REMARKS

In this chapter we have given a brief discussion of planning, planning philosophies, types of planning, and the role of planning in health care

---

* The following economic factors are examined in terms of their importance as links between community planning and area-wide hospital care: (1) the waste of a low rate of occupancy, (2) adapting to random variation in admissions, (3) the trend toward larger hospitals, (4) the indivisibility of equipment and teams, (5) the Hill-Burton program, rising unit costs, and Roemer's law, (6) the long life of the physical plant, (7) changes in the population of the cities and the growth of suburbs, and (8) federal grants-in-aid.

† A representative bibliography of the field will be found in Part V.

systems. Planning for health is a very complex and demanding task because of the need for comprehensiveness and the diversity of factors involved in health. The "thesis" of Blum and Sully's article (Selection 13) is that "planning for health *cannot* be described as comprehensive if it is directed solely to health services or even to traditional health concerns." It must, instead, consider and coordinate all the determinants of health. The authors identify four major categories of determinants of health. The first category is *environment,* consisting of the physical (housing, transport, air, and water quality), the educational, the economic, and the social components. The second set includes *personal habits and health behavior* which determine the degree of good health and longevity; while *genetic heritage* is the third category. The fourth set determining health is the system of *health services*—their range, quality and availability. The implications of these diverse sources of influence on health is that planners must consider all four categories, rather than focus exclusively on the system of delivering services. The needs and tasks of health planners are identified. An illustration of the planning process is provided by considering the problem of automobile accidents. The authors maintain that comprehensive planning is undertaken to create a systems model of the interlocking relationships for the health problem and to identify the specific points where it is possible to intervene. The following steps in planning are elaborated: (1) statement of the problem and of the goal; (2) analysis of the problem or system; (3) analysis of the client subsystem involved; (4) determination of the possible alternative interventions; and (5) comparative evaluation of the utility of the alternative solutions of courses of action.

Frieden and Peters (Selection 14) suggest that urban planning information and methods can contribute significantly to the development of future health systems. New directions, scope, and goals for the health service system are reviewed. A major goal is the "more deliberate integration of hospitals into a network of health facilities and services." The authors emphasize the need for special planning mechanisms—both to create new systems of health care and to keep them responsive to the changing health needs of society. Health planning is moving from voluntary associations for studying problems and exchanging information to agencies authorized by law to plan delivery of services. The authors list several characteristics of health planning and present a classification of most common types of health plans. Also discussed are the issues of defining goals and objectives, health information data, resources, and ecological information. The authors give examples to illustrate how information about the community's general characteristics is integrated with health data. This is done by considering three components of health plans: (1) projections of future bed needs; (2) definitions of health facility services areas; and (3) studies of housing conditions. Finally, the authors outline several possible ways in which health and city planning agencies might benefit from closer coordination.

REFERENCES

Ackoff, R. L., *A Concept of Corporate Planning*, New York: John Wiley & 1970 Sons.

Aguilar, F. J., *Scanning the Business Environment*, New York: Macmillan. 1967

Allemand, D. M., and W. G. Turney, "Simplified Statistical Approach to Hos- 1964 pital Planning," *Hospital Progress*, December, pp. 85–91.

Ansoff, H. I., "A Model for Diversification," *Management Science*, vol. 4, no. 1958 4, July, pp. 392–414.

Ansoff, H. I., *Corporate Strategy*, New York: McGraw-Hill. 1965

Ansoff, H. I., and R. C. Brandenburg, "A Program of Research in Business 1967 Planning," *Management Science*, vol. 13, no. 6, February, pp. B-219 —B-239.

Anthony, R., *Planning and Control Systems: A Framework for Analysis* Bos- 1965 ton: Graduate School of Business, Harvard University.

Argenti, J., *Corporate Planning: A Practical Guide*, London: George Allen and 1968 Unwin Ltd.

Arnold, M. F., "Use of Management Tools in Health Planning," *Public Health* 1968 *Reports*, vol. 83, no. 10, October, pp. 820–825.

Barnard, C. I., *The Functions of the Executive*, Cambridge, Mass.: Harvard 1966 University Press.

Barry, M. C., and C. G. Sheps, "A New Model for Community Health Plan- 1969 ning," *American Journal of Public Health*, vol. 59, no. 2 February, pp. 226–236.

Battistella, R. M., and T. P. Weil, "Comprehensive Health Care Planning." 1969 *New York Journal of Medicine*, September, vol. 69, no. 17, pp. 2350–2370.

Branch, M. C., *The Corporate Planning Process*, American Management 1962 Association.

Branch, M. C., *Planning—Aspects and Applications*, New York: John Wiley & 1966 Sons.

Churchman, C. W., *The Systems Approach*, Delacorte Press, New York. 1968

Clee, G. H., "Organizing for Multinational Planning," in George A. Steiner 1966 and Warren M. Cannon *Multinational Corporate Planning*, New York: Macmillan.

Cyert, R. M., and J. G. March, *A Behavioral Theory of the Firm*, Englewood 1963 Cliffs, N.J.: Prentice-Hall.

Dror, Y., "The Planning Process: A Facet Design," in F. J. Lyden and E. G. 1967 Miller (eds.), *Planning, Programming, Budgeting: A Systems Ap- proach to Management*, Chicago, Ill.: Markham Publishing Co.

Drucker, Peter F., "Long-Range Planning: Challenge to Management Science," 1959 *Management Science*, vol. 5, no. 3, pp. 238–249.

Emery, James C., *Organizational Planning and Control Systems*, New York: 1969 Macmillan.

Ewing, David W. (ed.), *Long-Range Planning for Management,* New York:
1958   Harper & Row.
Fayol, Henri, *General and Industrial Management,* New York: Pitman Pub-
1949   lishing Corp.
Feldstein, M. S., "An Aggregate Planning Model of the Health Care Sector,"
1967   *Medical Care,* vol. V, no. 6, November–December, pp. 369–381.
Frieden, B. J. and J. Peters, "Urban Planning and Health Services: Op-
1970   portunities for Cooperation," *Journal of the American Institute of
Planners,* vol. XXXVI, no. 2, March, pp. 82–95.
Gehrig, Leo J., "Comprehensive Planning for Health," *Journal of Medical Edu-
1968   cation,* vol. 43, April, pp. 464–470.
Gilmore, Frank F., and Richard G. Brandenburg, "Anatomy of Corporate
1962   Planning," *Harvard Business Review,* November–December, pp. 61–
69.
Graning, H. M., "The Institution Needs of the Health Industry," *Public Health
1969   Reports,* vol. 84, no. 4, April, pp. 305–310.
Hamburg, A. Z., "Using Census Data in Local Planning," *Hospitals,* vol. 4,
1967   September, pp. 60–63.
Kaufman, H., "The Politics of Health Planning," *American Journal of Public
1969   Health,* vol. 59, no. 5, May, pp. 795–797.
Klarman, H. E., "Economic Factors in Hospital Planning in Urban Areas,"
1967   *Public Health Reports,* vol. 82, no. 8, August, pp. 721–728.
Koontz, H., and C. O'Donnell, *Management: A Book of Readings,* New York:
1968   McGraw-Hill.
Leavitt, T., "Marketing Myopia," *Harvard Business Review,* July–August, pp.
1960   45–56.
LeBreton, P. P., and D. A. Henning, *Planning Theory,* Englewood Cliffs, N.J.:
1961   Prentice-Hall.
Lentz, E. A., "Health Care Planning," *Hospitals,* vol. 44, April 1, pp. 93–95.
1970
Lyden, F. J., and E. G. Miller (eds.), *Planning, Programming, Budgeting: A
1967   Systems Approach to Management,* Chicago, Ill.: Markham Publishing Co.
Mason, R. H., et al., "Corporate Strategy: A Point of View," *California Man-
1971   agement Review,* Spring, vol. XIII, no. 3, pp. 5–12.
Mockler, R. J., *Business Planning and Policy Formulation,* New York: Ap-
1972   pleton-Century-Crofts.
Newman, W., et al., *The Process of Management,* Second Edition, Englewood
1967   Cliffs, N.J.: Prentice-Hall.
Payne, B., *Planning for Company Growth,* New York: McGraw-Hill.
1963
Peters, J. P., "The Problem of Community Planning," *Hospital Progress,*
1964   May, pp. 142–144.
Scott, B., *Long Range Planning in American Industry,* American Management
1965   Association.
Sigmond, R. M., "Health Planning," *Medical Care,* vol. V, no. 3, May–June,
1967   pp. 117–128.
Simon, H. A., *Models of Man: Social and Rational,* New York: John Wiley &
1957   Sons.
Simon, H. A., *The New Science of Management Decision,* New York:
1960   Harper & Row.

Simon, H. A., "On the Concept of Organizational Goal," *Administrative*
1964   *Science Quarterly,* vol. 9, no. 1, June, pp. 1–22.

Simon, H. A., and A. Newell, "Heuristic Problem Solving: The Next Advance
1958   in Operations Research," *Operations Research,* vol. 6, no. 1, January–February.

Somers, A. R., "Some Suggested Principles for Community Health Planning
1968   and for the Role of the Teaching Hospital," *Journal of Medical Education,* vol. 43, April, pp. 479–494.

Stanford Research Institute, *Report No. 183,* September, Stanford Research
1963   Institute, Menlo Park, Cal.

Steiner, G. A., *Managerial Long-range Planning,* New York: McGraw-Hill.
1963

Steiner, G. A., *Top Management Planning,* Toronto: Collier-Macmillan Can-
1969   ada, Ltd.

Steiner, G. A., "Rise of the Corporate Planner," *Harvard Business Review,*
1970   vol. 48, no. 5, September–October, pp. 133–139.

Steiner, G. A., and W. M. Cannon, *Multinational Corporate Planning,* New
1966   York: Macmillan.

Tilles, S., "How to Evaluate Corporate Strategy," *Harvard Business Review,*
1963   vol. 41, no. 4, July–August, pp. 111–121.

Viguers, R. T., "Tomorrow's Voluntary Health Care System: The Challenge
1969   for the Hospital," *Hospital Progress,* June, pp. 68–71.

Warren, E. K., *Long-Range Planning: The Executive Viewpoint,* Englewood
1966   Cliffs, N.J.: Prentice-Hall.

Young, J. P., "A Conceptual Framework for Hospital Administrative Decision
1968   Systems," *Health Services Research,* Summer, pp. 79–95.

SELECTION 13

What Is Comprehensive Planning for Health?*

Henrik L. Blum, M.D. and Eleanor Kunitz Sully

By grace of Public Law 89–749 and Federal funding, the phrase *comprehensive health planning* is becoming broadly familiar to those concerned with problems of health and well-being. If we choose to turn the words around and talk about *comprehensive planning for health,* this is no quibble but a question of where we focus our attention. The authors will not be dealing here with the nature of nor the necessities for comprehensive health services. Planning to deliver the full range of health care to all our citizens is a major challenge and carries its own load of problems— how best to provide coordinated preventive, therapeutic and rehabilitative services; how to organize a comprehensive health care center for a neighborhood, or set up a service plan which covers financing, health education and quality medical care. But these concerns are only one part of a much broader subject.

Health may be seen as determined by four major influences. The first of these is *environment,* in which we include the physical (housing, transport, air and water quality), the educational, the economic, and the social. All of these are important and closely related determinants of how healthy people are.

Even the way individuals respond to the signals of illness or dysfunction, the way in which they avail themselves of health services, are in large part functions of environmental influences. Do they take preventive health precautions? Do they seek medical care in other than acute situations? Do they smoke, drink, use drugs unwisely, drive safely, undereat, overeat? These patterns of response make up the sum of personal *habits and health behavior* which constitute a second major influence on how long one survives and with what degree of good health. Research dollars and health education programs have pursued solutions in this area but the problems still outrun the answers.

*Inquiry, vol. 6, no. 2, 1969.

Genetic heritage is a third basic factor influencing health and well-being, a "given" which had commonly been considered impervious to intervention until the development of recent preventive programs such as early diagnostic evaluation and genetic counseling.

The fourth factor determining health is the system of *health services*—their range, quality and availability. This, of course, is the traditional practice field for health professionals. To our way of thinking, however, health services *per se* come too little and too late in trying to overcome the effects of critical deficiencies manifested as excessive or premature morbidity, disability and death. We present as our thesis, therefore, that planning for health cannot be described as comprehensive if it is directed solely to health services or even to traditional health concerns.

THE STATISTICAL PICTURE

Let us take a quick look to see if this notion that health status is related to factors other than the availability of health care services is borne out by national statistics. For six conditions causing serious limitation of activity (heart conditions, mental and nervous conditions, arthritis and rheumatism, high blood pressure, orthopedic impairments, visual impairments), there is, according to the National Center for Health Statistics, an average six-fold increase in prevalence for family income under $2,000 over those with an income of $7,000 or more. For heart conditions, this ratio is 11.9 per 1,000 population for incomes over $7,000 to 53.8 per 1,000 for incomes under $2,000. For mental and nervous conditions, the ratio is 4.2 to 26.4. In arthritis and rheumatic conditions, the ratio is 8.7 to 59.3; high blood pressure, 3.9 to 23.8. For orthopedic impairments (other than paralysis), the ratio is 14.9 to 54.4; for visual impairments, 2.7 to 23.4. Variations according to race, probably largely an expression of poverty and educational lacks, show nonwhite infant mortality for the United States to be 43.2 (infant deaths per 1,000 live births) as against 22.9 for the white population. In 10 major cities, the infant mortality ratio ranges from a low of 21.6 for whites to 46.5 for nonwhites.[1]

Figures such as these are commonly interpreted as a reflection of the unavailability or under-utilization of health services by the poverty population. There is no question but that the utilization of health care services, as expressed by the number of bed-disability days per year and of physician-visits per year, shows a continuing rise with a rise in income; those with the greatest frequency and extent of disability, the poor, actually get the least health care. However, the causal relationships involved here may not be so simple as they seem.

Questions Planners Must Ask

In spite of greatly increased national expenditures and expanded programs in the health sector, the relative infant mortality rate in the United States continues to deteriorate year by year in comparison with other countries, many of which are spending far less on health care. At the same time, longevity or life expectancy for adults in the older age brackets are also not improving in comparison with other countries, nor have they improved to any significant degree for those over 65 since the year 1900. This suggests that not only poverty, but affluence as well, may be shortening the average life span through the maintenance of a life style few other countries can afford. If mounting expenditures in the health field have not produced any significant proportional improvements over the years, is it because things would have been much worse without this high cost of care? Or might the money have been spent to more effect elsewhere? Will increased or even reorganized health care services, without a concomitant attack on poverty, ignorance and discrimination really improve this record? Will massive infusions of health services bring about any marked improvement without radical changes in patterns of living? These are questions planners must ask.

Physicians and other health professionals are not unaware of these problems. To date, however, the solutions have been almost exclusively concerned with the system of delivering services. It would be most unfortunate if the medical community were to be trapped, in volunteering to correct the significant health deficiencies in this country, by recommending increased national expenditures in a sector where dollar for dollar they will very probably do the least good. If, instead, physicians would contribute the analytic skills which are the heart of their training and practice to a diagnosis of the ills of the total community, we could begin to look for interventions which are the earlier, or the less expensive, or the more easily attained means of solving our major health problems. Before inventing solutions we need to undertake problem definition and analysis. The scope of comprehensive planning for health suggests that what may be needed most is a look around us to see what can be done outside, as well as inside, the traditional medical care field.

THE NATURE OF PLANNING

If planning for health is to be comprehensive, all aspects of health problems, all health aspects of social problems, and all services directed to the prevention or amelioration of these problems must be at least considered. Since in the first round planners will not be able to tackle all of the problems involved, we suggest earmarking for initial study those conditions whose consequences we all agree we *do not like,* whether they involve criminality, addiction, heart disease, automobile accidents, lung cancer or measles. Such an approach will lead to an examination of those conditions which are taking an inordinate proportion of the services of the community through its health, welfare, police and other major social service agencies, and those where there is a marked deficit in services.

Complex Interrelationships Considered

The interrelationships between the various physical, emotional and social dysfunctions labeled as illness or deviancy and the community agencies set up to deal with them are extraordinarily complex. More than one "label" per person is common, and persons or populations having significant problems in one area of disability may be expected to have them in others.[2] As a consequence, assignments of responsibility for any one category of disability are typically shared by several agencies, most persons seriously in need of help requiring services from more than one sector. Preventive services customarily come from one source, treatment from others, rehabilitation services from still others. Furthermore, since the social definition of needs and the traditions of service may vary widely from one situation to another, no two communities will necessarily make the same assignments. In one instance, a category of disability or deviancy may be perceived in terms of its etiology, in another in terms of its danger to others, or of the resources most readily at hand.[3]

In considering departures from well-being, the approach which planners use will have a tremendous impact on the way in which they look at a problem. If we define disability or deviancy as a limitation on the individual's ability to function in his normal roles, whether socially assigned or self-assumed, we come up with a totally different set of casualty figures than that derived from the traditional morbidity and mortality approach. At least during the initial planning stages, the "role disability" concept is useful in setting up priorities for study and determining which social agencies will need to be included along with health agencies in the planning process.

THE TECHNIQUES OF ASSESSMENT

One of the early tasks to be undertaken by a comprehensive health planning group is the rapid evaluation of its particular community, the unique panorama of social and health problems and the services available. A population breakdown needs to be carried out on the basis of age groupings and educational, racial, social and cultural backgrounds; then, the various educational, cultural, political, economic and religious institutions that serve the community need to be identified. Once the basic data have been collected, the evaluation can be carried a step further in terms of whether or not the community provides services for all those who want them, what limitations are imposed, what groups do not or cannot receive services.[4] The capability of these same institutions for the training of the various kinds of people necessary to the provision of services must also be considered.

If changes are to be made in the patterns of disability through improved services, the community landscape will determine both what is needed and whether proposed changes can be achieved. Planners need to know such things as the proportion of educated persons and those with adequate incomes, the nature of the tax structure, the sources of economic and political power, the opportunities offered for work and for achievement at all levels. Assessment of a community includes an accounting of its total resources above and beyond health services *per se*. Job opportunities, transportation, recreational facilities, social and political outlets, the flow of communication, the degree of citizen involvement, the effectiveness of political action—all of these are critical factors.

Community Trend Lines Analyzed

Yet even the panoramic view we have described is not enough. In collecting and analyzing data, planners must look backward along the line of each of the major indicators in order to see whether there has been any significant change over time. It is important to know whether the community is static, or whether it has improved or worsened in one or more of these measurable phenomena. If data are assembled for points in time separated by 10 or 20 year intervals, it is possible for any particular phenomenon to have reversed its field more than once since the last sounding was taken. Shorter intervals are necessary in order to judge whether the trend line is currently rising, falling, or holding steady. Planning hinges upon an assessment of where we are and how we got where we are—both the circumstances and the rate. From this moving set of bases, the planner attempts to predict where we are going to be at some appropriate point in the future.

The choice of a reasonable period of time over which to project and plan is built around the scope of the particular problem. For example, the supply and utilization of physicians cannot be looked at in terms of one, two, or five years because physicians aren't produced in less than a decade of college and post-college training and are in no position to make great changes in the practice of medicine for perhaps another decade after they enter practice. Other changes may be achieved in a much shorter period. Timetables need to be cross-related if the goals for one projected plan are dependent on the achievement of others.

As we project the trend line for a health problem into the future, at the same time establishing trend lines for the resources and services required, often we will find we do not like what we see today and even less what the trend lines indicate will be the situation in five or ten years. It is therefore desirable to intervene in such fashion that we will *not* come out where our present rate and way of doing things are taking us. This is the heart of planning: the intent to intervene, the knowledge of where and how interventions can be made most effectively, and the rate at which changes are to be introduced.[5]

THE TECHNIQUES OF CREATING INTERVENTIONS

Many of us are experienced in program planning, making minimal projections into the future, outlining a vision of what we would like to have in some one situation at a point in time and calling that the objective. We then proceed to create a scheme which will presumably deliver us to that point. This version of planning (which might better be called scheming) is devoid of most of the elements of modern planning technology.

After settling on the problem to be tackled and making a statement of the probable goal, e.g., reducing the incidence of automobile accidents, there are four necessary steps to be taken. These are: 1) analysis of the problem or condition-system; 2) analysis of the client subsystems involved; 3) determination of the possible alternative interventions; and 4) comparative evaluation of the utility of the alternative solutions or courses of action.[6]

Analysis of the Problem or System

To continue with our concern for automobile accidents, by way of example, the analysis of the motor-accident *system* is the first task. A model of the system can be constructed by drawing up a series of statements which describe the relationships involved. It is known that even many new automobiles are far from safe—so unsafe, in fact, the suggestion has been made that it would be cheaper for the government to pay the manufacturers x dollars per car for a safety package than for the country as a whole to bear the expense of the loss of life, property and productivity represented by accidents due to unsafe automobiles. Rough figures are available by which we can determine which automobile safety hazards account for what numbers of accidents, injuries and deaths. These in turn can be translated into such costs as damaged property, lost earnings, medical care and dependency. A second important relationship in the occurrence of automobile accidents is the inadequate construction of even the most modern freeways. Built-in death traps such as narrow lanes, unexpected merging of lanes, confusion in entrances, exits, signs and markings are by no means rare. The consequences and costs of these factors can also be estimated. A third relationship is indicated by the high proportion of fatalities which occur as a result of accidents in rural areas. Recent investigations suggest that deaths due to rural highway accidents are less attributable to excessively high speeds than to the dearth of quickly available emergency medical care outside of urban centers.

Another aspect of the "auto accident model" is concerned with the *driver's* contribution to lack of safety in auto travel. Calculable excessive contributions are made by age, or by the use of various medications which diminish the drivers' ability to perceive and react. Still another relationship is between drinking and driving upon which tremendous emphasis has been placed. Recent studies have shown, however, that alcohol-related accidents are more often the problem of the chronic alcoholic than of the social drinker.[7]

Analysis of the Client Subsystems

It becomes apparent that a fuller understanding of the condition-system under scrutiny includes not only an analysis of who or what is exposed to which forces, but also of the individuals exposed. Both current victims and potential susceptibles or future victims are considered as "clients" for our purposes. In analyzing the client-system, we need to look at such factors as susceptibility, receptivity, "protectability." For example, when we consider the relationships between alcoholism and unsafe driving, we must ask ourselves what do we know about alcoholics. It is easy enough to collect evidence as to what makes the alcoholic an accident-susceptible driver. But beyond that we have great difficulty in finding out what underlying forces make people susceptible to alcoholism. If more were known about this client-system in relation to the susceptibility to alcohol, susceptibility to auto accidents might be dealt with more intelligently.

In addition to determining factors of susceptibility in the clients, we must find out something about their receptivity to existing and potential controls. The effects of education about alcohol, in the schools or through mass media, the exposure to social drinking, detection of early problems in drinking, treatment, detention, more stringent licensing of drivers with a history of alcoholism might be considerations. In each community which is studying this particular client-subsystem we have the opportunity to evaluate the contributions that are presently made to prevent alcoholism by formal education, to treat by case-finding and appropriate therapy, to control by police enforcement and the use of punitive measures.

Other client subsystems requiring analysis would include the aged driver suffering from chronic illness, or, at the other end of the scale, the accident-susceptible teenage driver. The so-called "normal" driver subsystem also needs study, and evidence is mounting that even the good driver may no longer be able to cope with the rigors of modern freeway travel without electronic assistance.

Determination of Possible Alternative Interventions

Once a model is accurately constructed in relation to the health problem under consideration, we can identify the points where it may be possible to intervene. For each relationship described, there are potentially a number of alternative methods for intervention. The issue of the unsafe automobile, for example, can be attacked from any one of several approaches. The government could pay car manufacturers what is necessary to make a safe car. Legislation could be sought to require safety features with the cost falling upon the *person* who buys the car. Individual car owners could be required to install and use various safety devices such as safety harnesses. Whether legislation or education is the best method in dealing with individual car owners remains an open option.

The issue of freeway construction and safety introduces the question of whether the vast urban use of freeways is an efficient method of moving people, not only because of accidents but for additional considerations of cost, deterioration of property values, aid pollution, etc. If freeways are not to be eliminated altogether, the appropriate intervention might be safer design, or the introduction of electronic guidance devices. Better patrol is another possible approach to freeway safety (albeit another area where there is little evidence). Rapid mass transit is a major alternative. Options still remain as to whether the costs will be borne by the entire community, by those using the transportation system, or by those using the freeways.

Comparative Evaluation of Alternative Solutions or Actions

The benefits anticipated from each intervention can in most cases be documented by people competent in the field. To help determine the costs or inputs required for each benefit obtained, several factors need to be considered. The total direct cost of the proposed intervention can usually be estimated. However, if a particular measure can be put into effect at a presumed cost of so many dollars per capita, it must be decided what proportion of the population will be involved and what proportion will be effectively aided. The true cost figure for the results achieved may be quite different from the initial cost figures estimated for the procedure. For example, in a tuberculosis control program if skin testing is to be done, it must be remembered that for a given population at best only 90 percent will be reached by the promotion campaign; that the remaining 10 percent may have as much disease as the 90 percent tested; that the test is only 95 percent accurate; that only 90 percent of those tested will return for a reading; that only 50 percent of the identified positives will agree to go on drug therapy; that perhaps only half of those beginning treatment will finish it; and that the treatment is only 90 percent effective for those completing therapy. A simple calculation will give us the probable first year cost, and the continuing cost for a program serving a population containing a certain number of susceptibles and a certain number of potential cases. Under the assumptions noted, the number of cases actually prevented may be estimated as being 10 or 15 percent of the target population defined in the original program.

Benefits are the tangible expression of whatever it was that we intended to achieve. It is not enough to say that we are going to eradicate tuberculosis or that we are going to skin test everybody. Nor is it an accurate measure of the benefits to count the number of people found positive and placed under treatment. What must be determined is what proportion of the people tested and placed under treatment as a result of the expenditures involved are cured or rendered noninfective. Moreover, the new benefits are limited to those who would not have been brought to treatment under existing schemes. The final estimate of benefits can only be based on the whole picture of the number of potential cases prevented, of lives and years of productivity saved as a result of dollars spent on the particular intervention.

Determining Value of Benefits

There are devices to give these benefits a dollar value so that the sum of the benefits achieved can be compared directly with the total cost of the new program in dollars. According to prevailing economic theory, the dollar value of a life may be equated with its potential in terms of production.[8] Loss of productivity due to premature death or disability is a dollar loss. However, putting benefits into dollar terms is not always a happy maneuver in health programming. For example, programs directed toward saving or prolonging the lives of the elderly would show low dollar-benefits, since the aged have little potential for significant production. The total or per capita years of life saved for this group might also be small in comparison to other age groups. Moreover, the years of life saved might be spent in a hospital bed or in a nursing home at a high social cost.

If every life is to be given a value depending upon age, sex, race, education and earning capacity, can we ever justify programs other than those showing the best benefits-to-cost ratio? Favorable ratios would force us to tilt the scales in the direction of programs which serve the young adult, white college male because he has the highest expected earnings running for the longest period of time. In the same vein, how does one measure the dollar value of a birth control program which prevents potentially valuable lives from coming into existence? Even if birth control programs are to be directed primarily to the poorly-educated nonwhite with a low earning record and a high incidence of so-called damaged or retarded offspring, the benefits would probably always be less than the cost plus losses of predictable earnings.

From these examples it becomes apparent that the cost-benefit formula may easily be carried to a *reductio ad absurdum* in the field of public health where humane values are still important. The worth of a mother, of a child to his parents, of a wage earner to his family may be weighed on a different value scale from that of social productivity. It is possible, however, to talk in terms of years of life saved and indicate the probable degree of utility such lives will have without getting embroiled in the issue of whether or not dollar value can be assigned to human life. Certainly in health planning, we can let values other than dollar values help us decide in which areas we wish to spend what proportion of the money available to us. Having done so, it is perfectly valid to choose from among equally acceptable interventions directed toward the same goal the one that costs the least or makes the least use of resources in short supply. We might, for instance, face the growing physician shortage by creating in the next decade 80 new medical schools costing at least $75 million apiece. Alternatively, we might take cognizance of the studies which indicate that 50 percent or more of the physician's working hours do not require his level of skill, and work out a system for substituting bookkeeping, clerical and lesser health skills for scarce physician time. In this case no new medical schools need be created.

Spillover Effects of Interventions

Comprehensiveness in planning calls not only for looking at the costs and benefits of various alternative courses of action but for looking ahead to see what spillover effects each intervention might lead to, either desirable or undesirable. Current analysis reported from the health field tells us that we need 100 percent more radiologists, 100 percent more general practitioners, 50 percent more nurses, and so on. Interventions proposed on the basis of such projections fail to consider the future implications of solving health manpower shortages simply by training more people in the traditional modes. If, for example, the elite of the student population is pulled into the health industry by the tremendous economic incentives that would result from opening 80 new medical schools in the next decade, there is going to be a dearth of the same caliber persons in engineering, science, education and other professions. Obviously, faculty resources would be strained beyond sensible limits to support this number of schools and would abstract a disproportionate number of the better practitioners from practice. The scramble to produce new doctors might well divert us from considering the evidence that physician skills are at present poorly utilized. On the other hand, if the intelligent use of aides, preventive approaches and automated procedures were to be developed along with the doubling of physician outputs, in 20 years we would probably find ourselves with a surplus of physicians.

Secondary benefits accruing from the substitutive use of health personnel at lower levels of skill are not insignificant either. The approximate million-man vacancies in health manpower cited at every manpower conference could probably be filled from the bottom of the ladder by the unskilled who need jobs, resulting in a real secondary economic and social good for the country. Obviously, costs and benefits to society at large will not always be synonymous with the distribution of costs and/or benefits to various groups of individuals. In certain instances, some pay and also gain; in others, those who pay may not be those who gain. Questions of equity and concern for future generations must necessarily enter into the choice between alternative courses of action.

FIRMING UP THE GOALS

No final decision can be made in choosing the most appropriate method for intervention without careful review of both short-term and long-term goals. In a complex society such as ours, there exist hierarchies of goals moving from the immediate and specific to the abstract or ideal and closely related to prevailing value systems. Health planning is naturally concerned with specific program goals, often the control or eradication of a socially undesirable condition: V.D. control, control over water pollution, family planning, etc. At the next level on a ladder from the concrete to the more general, we have institutional goals, in part a cluster of program goals, in part an expression of broader social needs. A higher level still brings us to the widely accepted goals of human well-being: healthy families, healthy communities, affluence, creative leisure, peace. At the top are the goals of our democratic society: freedom, personal liberty, security, diversity of choice; and finally the highest level, that of self-fulfillment. As health planners, we work toward tangible program goals, but the high level societal goals must be kept in view lest gunbarrel vision threaten some of our most treasured values.

We do not know how to make logic chains from the highest level goals to workaday objectives. We can do the reverse, however, keeping the higher goals in mind as we set program goals. Tight planning at the program level by technologists who insist on holding the authority to enforce their plans might force us into abandoning democratic ways of making public policy. At the same time, singleminded concentration on one higher level goal, such as security, could wipe out diversity of choice or, if it calls for police state approaches and regimentation, could adversely affect goals at all levels.

The Developmental Approach

Comprehensive planning takes the developmental approach. We determine trends and choose the direction that is seen as most desirable, create the relevant plans, earmark the resources, undertake the increment proposed for a particular program year, and watch for both expected and unexpected results. Final decisions in setting significant health goals can rarely be made by a health planning body acting alone because of the extensive interrelationships involved. Setting priorities and determining appropriate mixes will require the involvement of other community policy groups. Elements judged to be of consequence to the system under consideration, but determined in practice by another sector of the economy, must be called to the attention of that other sector. Even if assigned to another sector of the community, it cannot then be forgotten. If it is, some essential ingredient may be lost and the health plan go forward only in a limited sphere or at the expense of other benefits. This suggests that trade-offs must be used, and that marginally increasing or decreasing costs need to be kept in mind so that no one critical area gets 90 percent while another gets little or no attention, becoming the weak link by which an important set of interventions is lost.

There can be no assumption that high goal levels imply the need for planning at higher government levels; that is, that Federal planning is concerned with higher goals than local. This has often been the case, but in terms of comprehensive planning the different levels of government cannot be equated with a comparable position in the hierarchy of goals. In fact, the scrutiny of individuals in their home neighborhoods is probably the most relevant way of determining how well we are approaching our high level goals. Planning on the neighborhood level, with individual men and their values in sight and mind, is probably more likely to result in high level goal achievement than exercises in planning carried out at a great distance and guided primarily by statistics. For a keen discussion on values, see Williams, "Individual and Group Values."[10]

Perhaps the "marble cake" image of the way in which all levels of government mix as they undertake specific programs in a community is not complex enough to convey an accurate picture of how levels and spheres of planning interrelate with goal levels.[11] The concept of goal levels and the ubiquitous evidence that there are a multiplicity of goals equally salient for the majority of people create a twofold demand: 1) for acceptable trade-offs, 2) for a center of policy decision-making at appropriate levels where priorities can be set, plans designed, and resources allocated accordingly.

ASSIGNMENT OF PROPOSED INTERVENTIONS FOR IMPLEMENTATION

We come now to a final stage in the planning process: assembly of the packages of skills, facilities and community approaches representing the interventions with the highest payoff, each intervention directed to a vulnerable point in the system we wish to control. A central planning unit then has the job of assigning these packages for determination of feasibility by those most competent to decide. Some proposals emanating from the health planners, such as those for making the automobile safer, will go to the industrial planning sector. Plans to make highways safer will go to the public works sector. Education of drivers will go to the educational sector. Emergency care, problems of aging, senility and drug usage will remain in the health sector for more definitive planning and programming. Obviously, some issues (for example, the training of physicians) will be referred to state or national levels of health and education planning.

Within the health sector, planners must reexamine the kinds of skills and facilities needed for each assignment. For example, the control of tuberculosis may call for a massive skin testing program. If the present laws and licensure demands are to be followed, a physician (occasionally a nurse) must do the test. This will be a waste of highly skilled persons doing work that an adept individual with no training could learn to do in two weeks. If this consideration is of enough economic significance, plans will call for changes in state laws and prevailing practices, even in educational procedures and employment opportunities. Similarly, it may be that the demand for certain types of X-ray films will be doubled or tripled under new screening programs for chest diseases, breast cancer, etc. These films could probably be read by technicians who have had three months training.

Perhaps 5 to 10 percent of the pictures read then need to be seen by a radiologist for definitive diagnosis.

There is equal need for a review of when hospitalization is necessary and when it is not in relation to any number of programs. The use of hospitalization for diagnostic purposes in order to get insurance coverage for expensive laboratory procedures has squandered high cost hospital services. Restrictions on outpatient services irrationally designed to hold down costs in the insurance sector of the health economy can, in this way, add as much as $75 to the cost of a $25 procedure for the health care sector overall. The deployment of skills, old and new, may have a decisive bearing on the concentration or the distribution of facilities. The multipurpose "well-being worker," for example, would probably be based in the neighborhood, as would the independently operating "assistant physician" in order to provide maximum accessibility; moreover, these persons would need only a minimum of equipment.

Reconsideration of Professional Standards

Planning approaches such as these also demand a complete reconsideration of the present "merit badge" approach to professional standards, which really says very little about the quality of service. If a health worker has a certain kind of badge, we assume that he can and will do a certain level or quality of job and that all the duties he performs require the skills he is presumably capable of applying. These assumptions are hard to verify, and we must face the possibility that a technician, for example, can be trained to read most X-ray films or fill most tooth cavities. An analysis of job responsibilities and the skills required in terms of the quality and quantity of work needed would seem much more to the point than blanket qualification by an M.D., a D.D.S. or a specialty board rating. In fact, degrees often allow unlimited license to perform tasks that are either too simple or too complicated for the skill level of the practitioner. Social waste is high when costly skills are not used to maximum advantage. Both individual patient and social losses are also high when incompetent operators having the required merit badges do work beyond their capacity.

So-called high professional standards adopted statewide or nationwide may in fact mean that many areas will have no one at all to provide service. On the other hand, if persons with lesser skills are utilized under appropriate supervision in procedures for which their skills are adequate, a better distribution of services will be possible. At the same time, there will be a saving of the higher level skills for jobs where there can be no substitutions and which usually call for parallel high overhead backup facilities. Both high level skills and expensive facilities need to be used to capacity if they are to be maintained.

Are there examples where this kind of thinking has been carried out in our health system? The intensive care or coronary units created by many hospitals may be one such example. Obviously, some patients were in need of levels of skill and intensity of services that could not be maintained routinely on each ward. Special skills and facilities were therefore concentrated in a given unit and the chances of survival for critically ill patients were tremendously increased. In the rest of the wards there was concurrently a decreased need for special skills. Although this might be interpreted by some as a lowering of general ward standards, the net result was an overall improvement in hospital care as shown by patient survival.

Overall Community Need Examined

In similar fashion, a community must be examined in terms of its overall need. Can each of its hospitals have a coronary care unit, equipment for open heart surgery, a cobalt therapy unit? Or should just some have such facilities? Might only certain hospitals in strategic communities have this kind of equipment so that each unit will get maximum usage and maintain adequate skills at a reasonable cost? At the community level this kind of approach has been used but rarely. For example, we hear a great deal about promoting periodic health examinations although their value has not yet been accurately determined. There are no convincing studies to show what the dollar of preventive care will provide in the way of benefits if spent on annual examinations. Multiphasic health checkups, even those which do not use physician time directly, may, in terms of the numbers of referrals for unimportant or borderline conditions, very easily take up the time of one-fifth of all the physicians in the United States and place a premium on getting medical care when it is critically needed. Cost-benefit analysis of the alternatives in this situation has not been carried out.

Similarly, incentives around group practice are being set into motion before a substantial analysis has been undertaken of what group practice contributes to effective delivery of health care. It can be observed that some group practices change the style of service to patients and that more ancillary services are probably utilized.[12] But there is only dubious evidence that the group practitioner sees more patients, provides his patients a less expensive service, or that in the long run group practice is more efficient or effective in protecting health.

Traditional delivery systems in the health field are not only well established (hospitals, private medical practice, health departments), but also render many billions of dollars' worth of service annually. At the same time the needs and opportunities for modifying the machinery whereby they render care are increasing. In many cases, the advantages of creating new internal operating relationships or of utilizing new techniques is irresistibly advantageous in spite of often significant capital outlays or continuing operating costs. The specific promises of more effective diagnosis and therapy and the saving of lives or amelioration of disability provide ample justification for introducing changes.

What happens then to our thesis that health problems should be subjected to an analysis first so that the "best" interventions are selected before any changes are introduced into the machinery of health services? Obviously, we cannot stop the machine and wait for the completely "logical" analytical approach to be carried out for each health problem before any changes in the delivery system are to be made. But neither can we continue to move only in a narrow-gauge service planning approach which is often wasteful of limited resources and ineffective in improving the health status of the community.

After the first round of comprehensive planning, health planners will begin to extend their knowledge and look at newly established services to evaluate their effectiveness. Certainly it is not possible to review all the related programs established during the year, but there is reason for the rhythm of periodic evaluation. The results of some programs cannot be measured for several years. In these cases evaluations are scheduled at appropriate intervals, perhaps not in final terms but to see whether the intervening steps are moving according to plan. One can then make a good guess as to whether future steps will proceed as originally set up or whether modifications of the initial interventions are called for. In other situations, the first year's results may clearly indicate there was a failure to estimate correctly the effects of various forces, or that countervailing forces have arisen in response to the program initiated. Evaluation leads us to a continued awareness of the anticipated results, and thus to opportunities for learning about relationships that were either unperceived or misread when plans were formulated. On this basis we are able to utilize new knowledge and redeploy technologies and resources for the next round of planning.

WHO IS TO DO THE PLANNING?

Modern planning is rapidly developing its own technology—PPBS, cost-benefit analysis, etc.—which will not infrequently be totally unfamiliar to members of comprehensive health planning councils. On the other hand, the technical experts may want to plan the whole game themselves, listening only reluctantly to suggestions from outside their circle. The same is too often true of health professionals. We suggest that only through the broadest possible representation from a variety of interest groups can the issues at stake be brought into the forum of public discussion. For example, it would seem impossible to go into any depth on the problem of providing medical insurance without representation from the insurance industry. We suspect that it is equally impossible to design a plan to fund health care services for those unable to pay for them without representatives of the taxpaying public and the lawmakers at the planning table. Programs for teenage drug, V.D. and illegitimate pregnancy victims probably will not be very relevant until the "consumers" take part in the planning and help the professionals understand the nature of the problems as well as the possibilities for intervention. Similarly, if we hope to develop new ways of rendering health care services through the utilization of new skills, both those with presently used skills and those who will be called on to create new skills must be included as partners in the planning. Since planners must ultimately ask for implementation of the interventions they design and for the changes in behavior needed to insure utilization of new services, both those who will be asked to carry out the plans and those who will be the consumers must be represented from the beginning.

This does not mean that everybody has to be on a planning body. Central planning bodies having as many as 50 to 75 members can make judicious use of committees which involve representatives of each sector of the community and the client groups at risk. With this kind of community outreach, planning proposals can be assured of support when it is needed to move plans into action.

There is another critical aspect to the question of who will do the planning. Participants are needed who can provide perspective. We grant that the only kind of comprehensive health planning meaningful to most of us is that concerned with our own communities—neighborhood, city or county. Since, however, this familiar community may not be large enough or have adequate resources to support significant skills or facilities, it will often be necessary to merge a number of communities for planning. Some programs can only materialize through regional compacts or contracts with neighbors. Planning, therefore, will have to go on at this higher level even though there may be no official governmental machinery or traditional ways of negotiating at the metro or multi-state regional level.

Problems Involve Differing Areas

It is also important to realize that many problems coexist which involve vast but differing areas. Air pollution, transport, waste removal and water pollution interrelate closely, but may each have a different problem shed.

The possibility of doing something about any one of these (which may involve all the others) will force us to work at higher and broader levels of community. The technical skills, resources and enablement necessary could ultimately involve a whole state or, in fact, the nation. The ability to collect taxes (the basis of many of our health and well-being services), is more and more centered in Federal government because while the big combines of taxable resources typically have offices in one state, their plants, workers, services and resources, as well as their stockholders, are dispersed throughout the country or the world. At the same time, the mobility of the American population means that people need to have some guarantee not only of equal employment opportunities, but of environmental safeguards and adequate health services anywhere in the United States.

Planning, therefore, has to be carried on not only with the full range of local interests, but with representation from each of the levels of community or government related to the problem under consideration, up to the Federal level. On any given problem, the view may be quite different from each community level. The so-called "rape" of Boston's West End was designed by the city of Boston to improve its tax position by removing an old slum and improving the outlook of the whole city for the future. Agencies at the national level authorized to fund urban redevelopment acquiesced in this particular view. If, however, there had been study of the situation at the West End neighborhood level, it soon would have been apparent that thousands of self-reliant people, with a level of delinquency and dependency lower than that for most such communities, were to be socially dislocated and separated from the homes and small businesses by which they had been able to raise and provide for their families through a number of generations. The uprooted West Enders very likely became an increased burden for Boston social agencies. The welfare of the surrounding neighborhoods that had to pick up the homeless was certainly affected. In all probability the outlying communities of Greater Boston and the state of Massachusetts ultimately experienced costly secondary effects that may have more than negated any benefits to Boston in this piece of redevelopment.[13]

Determining Spillover Effects in Advance

One way of looking for secondary or spillover effects in advance is by looking at the possible solutions to problems through the eyes of individuals or agencies that represent several levels of community. The neighborhood, of course, is the most critical because that is where one can come closest to seeing what the individuals involved are likely to gain or lose. It is equally important to look at what effects a plan will have for neighboring communities and the rest of the region, and in some cases for the state or even the whole country.

Obviously, planning structures are not going to be set up simply under PL 89-749, nor can health planning bodies all conform to a given pattern since the communities whose problems they are designed to solve are not necessarily similar. But they must be organized to be responsive to the public which pays the bills and receives the services. Theirs is the continuing responsibility to receive and to disseminate information on health problems, the possible alternative solutions, objectives, costs and benefits. Everyone then will have a chance to see whose interests are at issue, why certain alternatives are more suitable than others, and what kind of price tag is attached. We do not see comprehensive planning bodies as those that make final policy. Planning groups analyze, prepare, publicize, give the public and their elected representatives the data by which they can make better decisions—even decisions which may on occasion overrule the planners.

It cannot be said too often that with the limitation on resources in any one year, the decision to spend money in one direction in order to save lives determines that lives will be lost in some other direction. Planning decisions must be clear and firm on where and why we give preference. As all of us begin to face up to our judgments in terms of the values that underly them, we may learn how to respect the values held by others, how to resolve value difference, and thereby how to improve the quality of public policy-making in trying to improve the health status of this country.

Health may be an ideal vehicle for thrashing out old and new values through the processes of comprehensive planning. Many concerns related to health problems are shared by individuals of all shades of political belief and economic background. Perhaps the extension of thinking about cause and effect, and the development of acceptable interventions formulated around health issues, will make it possible to reestablish meaningful sharing of actions. Planning is only now coming into use as a tool by which we can create futures.

SUMMARY

Comprehensive planning to improve health status must consider factors outside as well as inside the medical care field. Modern planning techniques allow us to construct a system-model of the interlocking relationships for any major health problem. On this basis we can identify the points where it is possible to intervene. Alternative interventions can be compared in terms of costs, benefits and long-term effects to determine the most effective course of action. Successful implementation will depend on the capacity of comprehensive planning councils to represent all the interest groups in the community and to transmit relevant information to policy-making bodies.[14]

REFERENCES

1. U.S. National Center for Health Statistics. *Medical Care, Health Status and Family Income,* Series 10, No. 9 (Washington, D.C.: GPO, 1967), p. 7.
2. THURLOW, H. J. "General Susceptibility To Illness: A Selective Review," *Canad. Med. Assoc. J.,* Vol. 97 (December 2, 1963), pp. 1–8.
3. BLUM, H. L. AND ASSOCIATES. *Notes On Comprehensive Planning For Health* (San Francisco: American Public Health Association, Western Regional Office, 1968), p. 3.11.
4. *Ibid.,* ch. 7.
5. FRIEDMAN, J. "A Conceptual Model For The Analysis of Planning Behavior," *Administrative Science Quart.,* Vol. 12, No. 2 (September, 1967), pp. 225–252.
6. NOVICK, DAVID. *Program Budgeting* (Cambridge: Harvard University Press, 1968).
7. WALLER, J. "Use and Misuse of Alcoholic Beverages As A Factor In Motor Vehicle Accidents," *Pub. Health Rep.,* Vol: 81 (July, 1966), pp. 591–597.
8. U.S. Public Health Service. *Estimating the Cost Of Illness,* Health Economics Series No. 6 (Washington, D.C.: GPO, 1966).
9. PREST, A. R., AND TURVEY, R. "Cost-Benefit Analysis: A Survey," *Econ. J.* (December, 1965), pp. 683–735.
10. WILLIAMS, R. M., JR. "Individual and Group Values," *Ann. Amer. Acad. Pol. & Soc. Sci.,* Vol. 1 (May, 1967), pp. 20–30.
11. GRODZINS, M. "The Federal System," *Goals For Americans: The Report of the President's Commission on National Goals* (Englewood Cliffs, N.J.: Prentice Hall, 1960).
12. BAILEY, R. M. "Economies of Scale In Outpatient Medical Practice," *Group Pract.* (July, 1968); and Bailey, R. M. "Appraisals of Experience In Fee-For-Service Group Practice in the San Francisco Bay Area: A Comparison of Internists In Solo and Group Practice," *Bull. N.Y. Acad. Med.* (November, 1968).
13. GANS, H. J. *The Urban Villagers* (New York: Free Press, 1962).
14. Much of the content of this article has been condensed from the senior author's "Notes On Comprehensive Planning For Health," *op. cit.*

SELECTION 14

Urban Planning and Health Services: Opportunities for Cooperation*

Bernard J. Frieden and *James Peters*

The crisis in medical care has led to many proposals for change in the health service system and to a variety of health planning structures. The work of health planners parallels that of urban planners in a number of ways; yet there has been little contact between these two fields. A survey of published health plans indicates that few have moved very far toward proposing future health system alternatives and that urban planning information and methods can contribute directly to the development of such proposals.

Health care, a matter of deep public concern for many years, is now emerging as one of the central social policy issues on the national agenda. Dissatisfaction with the state of health care in the United States has centered on its soaring cost, uneven quality, and limited availability—particularly to the poor. Criticisms of the health service system have attracted widespread attention. Less well known, perhaps, is the ferment of ideas and proposals that are being advanced by a number of hospital administrators, medical economists, public health officials, and specialists in preventive medicine. The general outlines of new and alternative health service patterns are becoming apparent in recent literature on medical care and in experimental programs in many parts of the country.

New Directions in Health Services

Out of the many separate proposals that are being advanced and tested today, it is possible to give a composite picture of the new directions in this field.[1] First, current interpretations advance several new goals for the health service system: to make care readily accessible and regularly available to everyone; to provide continuing care; to offer flexibility and choices to the public; and to make extensive use of prepayment and insurance mechanisms so that ability to pay will not be an obstacle. Other goals

* *Journal of the American Institute of Planners*, vol. XXXVI, no. 2, March, 1970.

sought through more limited proposals are extension of services, holding down costs, and improvement in quality of health care.

Many proposals aim at minimizing costly hospital stays by providing a wide variety of services for patients who can remain at home or do not need full hospital care. These services include preventive programs, diagnostic and treatment services for out-patients, home care, after care, rehabilitation, and social services. Some proposals would extend hospitals into the community by expanding out-patient departments and establishing local clinics, half-way houses, and home care programs outside the hospital. Other proposals would build service systems around neighborhood health centers rather than around major hospitals. These centers would provide basic medical services and would take responsibility for continuing patient care but would draw on hospitals for specialized testing, major surgery, and other services that cannot be efficiently provided at the neighborhood level.

In addition to emphasizing out-of-hospital services, most conceptions of the future health system call for more deliberate integration of hospitals into a network of health facilities and services. In an integrated system, the expansion of individual hospitals would be limited by the area's needs and by availability of services and equipment elsewhere. The current tendency of each hospital to add specialized, expensive services—such as open-heart surgery and cobalt bombs—has been subject to much criticism as a contributor to high hospital costs and under-utilization of scarce resources. Thus, the President's Commission on Heart Disease, Cancer, and Stroke found that 30 percent of the 777 hospitals equipped for closed-heart surgery had no such cases during the year of its study, and 41 percent of the hospitals equipped to do open-heart surgery averaged less than one operation per month. This under-utilization not only adds to hospital costs, but fails to maintain the skills needed for highly specialized procedures. The Commission found far higher mortality rates in hospitals that performed few of these operations than in those with a full work load.[2]

A regionalized approach would work against unnecessary duplication of facilities. It would also promote closer relationships between hospitals and other types of facilities, such as nursing homes, in order to assure greater continuity of care and more consistent standards of quality. Closer linkages within the system would also make medical care more accessible by providing many points of entry for patients. Regional health information systems have also been proposed to facilitate data exchange on individual medical histories as well as on the state of community health.

Other new directions in the health field concern development and use of medical personnel. More efficient utilization of medical and nursing staffs, laboratory technicians, and other hospital personnel is needed not only to deal with chronic manpower shortages and to limit cost increases, but also to provide an acceptable quality of care. The poor coordination and inflexibility of present personnel arrangements have led one recent study to characterize hospital staffs as "a collection of guilds."[3] Proposed solutions range from managerial reforms within hospitals to reallocation of staff functions to relieve highly trained professionals of work that can be performed by para-medical personnel, such as health aides. In some experimental programs, patients maintain relationships with a health team rather than a single physician.

Finally, no vision of a future health system would be very persuasive without a vision of how to pay for it. Various forms of insurance are proposed; almost all depart from present private health insurance by doing more than supplying payment for existing services. Most proposals conceive of prepayment arrangements as planning tools that provide certain incentives for development and use of a medical system. Typically, they call for providing comprehensive coverage for preventive, diagnostic, treatment, and after-care services both in and out of hospitals. Some proposals link prepayment to special health delivery systems, such as group practice. Recognizing health care as a social responsibility, proposals for future service would expand programs such as Medicare and Medicaid and would build in mechanisms to assure a higher quality of care.

Planning Structures

These conceptions of future health systems imply that individual decision-making units will somehow work together to a far greater extent than they do now. *Moving from the present collection of independent, often unrelated, services and facilities toward a future system of health care will require new social interventions and new limits on the decision-making of individual institutions.* In many ways, the problems are similar to those of urban development, where attempts are also made to shape many individual decisions so that the resulting pattern promotes social objectives. As in urban development, special planning mechanisms are needed both to create new systems of health care and to keep them responsive to the changing health needs of the American people.

Recent studies of the health system reach fairly consistent conclusions about who should do the planning. The principle that consumers as well as providers of health care should be involved in decision-making is widely accepted. Active participation of the poor, who are most in need of medical care, is increasingly seen as essential. The mixed public-private nature of health care argues strongly for a governmental-private partnership in health planning. The distribution of medical services along with the patterning of service areas warrant health planning at the state, regional, and local levels. The complexity of the health system means that planning at any one level must draw on resources from other levels. A recently established neighborhood center in West Oakland, California, involves resources and activities of three federal agencies, the city health department, local medical, dental, and other health professional groups, and a neighborhood citizens organization that is sponsoring the project.

Many kinds of health planning structures have already been formed. Their number has increased dramatically in the past few years, and their character has been shifting from that of voluntary associations for studying problems and exchanging information to agencies authorized by law to plan delivery of services. Examples of health planning organizations include individual hospitals planning their own expansion, areawide hospital or health facility planning councils, health and welfare councils, public health departments, medical societies, and specialized health organizations such as those dealing with mental health or tuberculosis.

Areawide health facility agencies are important planning bodies. Prompted by federal encouragement and financing, their number grew from four in 1946 to sixty-five in 1966. They are concerned with coordinating individual hospitals' facility and service plans, measuring future needs, and promoting services to meet these needs. Some councils have claimed success in preventing unnecessary construction and raising funds for needed expansion, but others have had relatively little influence on hospital decisions. These agencies depend on voluntary membership and voluntary compliance, except in a few states where Blue Cross threatens its member hospitals with financial penalties if they expand without planning council endorsement.

Federal health programs have led to other forms of planning with a statutory base and governmental authority. Since 1946, Hill-Burton funds for hospital construction and modernization have required annual state plans for setting priorities. In 1963, federal grants were made available for comprehensive state mental health planning, and each state is now required to have a mental health plan as well as plans for services to the mentally retarded. Legislation in 1965 provided federal funds for planning major medical centers to treat heart disease, cancer, and stroke. The Partnership for Health program, established in 1966, offers flexible block grants to states for health services in place of previous categorical grants for specific services. Under the new program, a comprehensive health planning process is required as a basis for allocating federal funds. Federal grants are authorized to pay the full cost of comprehensive state health planning, and 75 percent planning grants are made available for metropolitan and areawide planning. All fifty states have now established the required health planning agencies and by June 1969, ninety-four grants for areawide health planning had been made under this act.

Growing federal commitments to health services are likely to lead to other innovations in planning. Grants for health services in poverty areas, for example, stress involvement of local residents in policy-making and development of new training and employment opportunities. Medicare and Medicaid started without creating special planning structures, but there is growing concern over the results of these massive programs. Both help low-income people pay for medical services provided through the existing system. The federal government, which is now a major purchaser of health services, will not be able to ignore the problem of holding down costs and maintaining the high quality of these services.

CONTRIBUTIONS OF URBAN PLANNING

Health planning agencies have had relatively little contact with their city planning counterparts or with city planning as a profession.[4] Most of their staff members have backgrounds in social welfare and health services, particularly public health and hospital administration. Yet as health planning has shifted its focus from individual hospitals to large service systems and their interaction with the community, its concerns have come to overlap those of urban planning. Understanding and projecting the urban context is basic to anticipating future health needs. Changes in urban development patterns, population distribution, and transportation systems will influence local health needs and should affect choices of health programs and sites for facilities. City planners are in a position to help health planning by supplying information on community development.

When health planning moves beyond adjusting the present service system and advances alternative health care arrangements, other planning skills will also be relevant. City planning's experience with goal formulation, invention and testing of alternatives, implementation methods, and monitoring of results has potential applicability to health planning. Two reservations are important: (1) formal methods for managing these elements of city planning are not yet very advanced; and (2) city planners who want to apply what they know to health planning will have to acquire a good understanding of the health service system.

We have found it useful to undertake a state-of-the-art survey of area-wide health planning to explore possible interactions with urban planning. To establish a basis for cooperation, we have attempted to provide an understanding of *several characteristics of present health planning:*

Its institutional setting—who prepares health plans.
The nature and purpose of health plans.
Information needed for health planning and how it is used.
Health planning recommendations and how they are to be implemented.

The only common element of the thirty-three plans we surveyed was their areawide orientation. We did not consider plans for the expansion of an individual hospital or for a single neighborhood clinic. Some of the plans included were recommended by professionals in the health planning field; some were brought to our attention by published bibliographies; others, by chance. Therefore, there is no statistical validity to this survey, but certain elements of planning philosophy and method are repeated often enough to suggest that the impressionistic generalizations are reasonably valid.

A glance at the bibliography will give an idea of the range of issues that may be covered in areawide health plans. Topics include physical and mental health services—prevention, treatment, and rehabilitation. Many plans also consider environmental health issues and the regulatory activities of public health departments (inspection and licensing). The Prince George's County "self-study" (27), one of the most complete, covered medical treatment programs and facilities, as well as water supply, air and water pollution, sewage and refuse disposal, noise control, swimming facilities, vector (vermin) and nuisance control, housing (including transient housing), food and milk sanitation, and radiological and occupational health. None of the studies considered traffic safety or other types of accident control.

Since our examples are drawn from published plans, they do not include some of the newer varieties of health planning, such as projects in urban poverty areas or plans undertaken as part of the Partnership for Health program. Subject to this qualification, our survey shows health planning moving toward development and presentation of health system alternatives, but still far from that goal. In the present state of the art, there are already many opportunities for cooperation. As health planning becomes more comprehensive and more concerned with health in a community setting and as urban planning continues in a state of rapid change —from land use to broader community development—we see many advantages in cultivating closer ties between these two fields.

Health Plans and Planners

When the health planner uses the term "plan," he is referring to a variety of surveys and special studies quite different from the traditional comprehensive city plan. Typically, the reports do not include a description of the health service framework desired at the end of the planning period. The most common types of plans are:

1. *Plans for planning:* These studies discuss the need for health planning and propose an organizational framework for that purpose.

2. *Special studies:* These are studies that are not meant to be comprehensive, but instead attempt to answer a narrow question of areawide significance; for example, how many hospital beds will be needed in the community in five, ten, or twenty-five years? Questions of this type are often answered with only a minimum of attention to other related aspects of the health service system.

3. *Surveys of health services:* These are inventories and analyses of existing health problems and services. Many have specific recommendations for incremental improvements within the present health service system.

4. *Health service system plans:* These plans bear a closer resemblance to the *ideal* city plan. They take a hard look at the overall service system, evaluate possible alternatives, and propose basic reorganization where necessary.

In this country, city and regional planning had its beginnings in the private efforts of community-minded citizen organizations. Increasingly it has become a public function until, with a few exceptions, planning agencies are units of state and local governments or groups of governments. But American medicine has a long tradition of stubborn autonomy. Health planning—even "comprehensive" health planning—is still done by a bewildering array of organizations. They may be temporary or permanent bodies; they may operate under public or private auspices; they may be staffed by volunteers or full-time professionals; they may be independent of the institutions that actually provide health services, or they may be directly related to these institutions. Clearly, these health planning organizations do not fall into neat categories, but the following seven types can be identified:

1. *State hospital and medical facilities agencies* are responsible for allocating federal funds under the state's Hill-Burton health facilities construction programs.

2. *Statewide health planning organizations* are usually non-profit corporations that have been established with Hill-Burton funds and funds from a variety of other public and private sources. They provide information and technical assistance to local planning bodies, prepare regional and statewide planning studies, and act as advisor to state Hill-Burton agencies.

3. *State health departments* perform area planning (usually statewide) both with staff and through consultants.

4. *Areawide hospital or health facilities planning councils* are non-profit corporations whose members may be independent citizens, representatives of other health organizations (Blue Cross, United Fund, Hospital Association), or representatives of community health planning bodies. In general, their task is to coordinate health facilities planning in

a metropolitan area. They may advise the state Hill-Burton agency by evaluating local projects that will involve Hill-Burton funds.

5. *Local health and welfare councils* have generally been established to coordinate the work of public and nonprofit social service organizations. They may have jurisdiction over the distribution of United Fund support. Health services will usually be only a part of their total concern.

6. *National Commission on Community Health Services* has sponsored community self-studies in twenty-one communities across the country. The studies were generally conducted by ad hoc planning organizations made up chiefly of volunteers from the medical professions, staff members of local government and private welfare agencies, and representatives of the community at large. The studies received endorsement, funds, advice, and staff from a variety of local public and private health and welfare organizations. They were the only studies in our survey that considered both environmental and personal health.

7. *City and county health departments may plan* for the delivery of traditional public health services, environmental health programs, total health care for the poor (7), or, in cooperation with other agencies, they may be involved in comprehensive health planning covering both public and private services (11).

Health planning studies are generally directed by physicians and/or holders of MPH degrees, although some of the community self-studies were coordinated by social workers. City and regional planners are conspicuous by their absence from the ranks of study directors or consultants. Exceptions include the work of John Dyckman for the California Department of Mental Hygiene (17)—this was considered a highly experimental undertaking, and the work of Reginald Isaacs (as a member of Associated Consultants) for the Department of Health in Puerto Rico (3).

The participation of laymen is the rule in areawide health planning activities, but it seems to be generally limited to middle class community leaders—the same people who have traditionally served on city planning commissions. They not only overrepresent higher income groups, but they also overrepresent those citizens who have a particularly thorough knowledge of the community and who can most easily make use of existing health services. While the published reports do not necessarily identify every member of planning boards or working committees, almost none indicates that any effort was made to involve representatives of low-income groups in planning. The Chicago plan is a partial exception; the staff included a sociologist who surveyed community organizations and individuals in poverty areas in order to give the planners a better understanding of local health problems and patterns of obtaining medical care. (Low-income citizen participation has been used more extensively in planning for health services within individual neighborhoods, such as Columbia Point in Boston and Cooper Square in New York City.)

Goals and Objectives

The health plans in our survey devote scant attention to formulation and selection of alternative long-range goals and short-range objectives. This may be intentional. Areawide health plans involve many independent health services, each with its own jurisdiction and interests. An effort to formulate detailed goals might create more problems among the autonomous health services than it would solve. Most plans in the survey contain no statement of goals whatsoever. When goals are stated, they are seldom specific: ". . . more efficient health services in Bucks County through better coordination of efforts in the health field . . ." (4); "coordination of human and physical resources within the present major hospital organizations" (31).

The Santa Clara Hospital Commission was slightly more specific:

> Planning and administration of health facilities must foster good medical care. Such care depends on:
> a. The comprehensiveness of services, personnel and programs;
> b. The continuity provided through established patient flow channels between facilities and system of cooperation between agencies as directed by the physician (15).

These last two goals, *comprehensiveness* and *continuity* of services, would be subscribed to by any health planning agency, but at least such statements begin to establish helpful criteria for measuring the adequacy of existing services. Still more specific goals might be added, such as *accessibility* of care.

Broad goals need to be further defined. Accessibility, for example, is affected by cost of care, travel time, and waiting time. Health planning agencies have seldom adopted specific policies in regard to these issues, although a few make use of rule-of-thumb standards similar to those once so prevalent in city planning. Associated Consultants' regionalization plan for Puerto Rico proposes a measurable objective:

> Presently, access to district hospital services for everyone is not possible within the desired thirty minutes. This cannot be attained even when the full highway program is completed. The more immediate goal will be one hour travel time (3).

HEALTH INFORMATION

Many different kinds of health information are collected by health planning agencies to describe general community characteristics, to identify health problems and health services, to delineate hospital service areas, and to estimate present and future needs. Generally, the information falls into three categories: (1) *prevalence* (the number of people with a certain condition); (2) *utilization* (the number and characteristics of people currently using a facility); (3) *resources* (an inventory of the components of the health system). A potential fourth category, which could examine patient attitudes toward medical services, personal use of facilities, and opinions of health care, was overlooked by all but two of the plans (7, 8). Unfortunately, many of the so-called plans publish health information but virtually neglect to examine its implications or to relate it to specific policy issues bearing on future health service systems.

Prevalence

Information on prevalence—that is, how many people have a specific condition—can be useful in assessing unmet needs, projecting changes in patterns of use, and establishing service priorities. Often, available prevalence data are inadequate to assess unmet needs since cases are seldom counted until they are brought to the attention of the physician. Not all persons with VD will see a doctor and not all cases diagnosed by doctors will be reported to public health agencies.

Many health plans state their need for more accurate information regarding the prevalence of chronic illness. The Rourke plan for Lincoln, Nebraska (31), for example, uses scattered data from studies in other communities in an attempt to estimate the *need* for long-term care beds. The consultant finally falls back to the suggestion that the hospitals take a "cautious" approach to the provision of long-term care beds until *demand* is documented. But the only way to get an accurate estimate of local prevalence of chronic disease would be to conduct a sample survey of the local community. The only way to be sure that all persons were receiving the care they needed—that is, to convert potential need into actual demand—would be to make a broad range of services available and accessible and then to persuade people to use them.

A second use of prevalence data is to project changes in patterns of use. Information reflecting trends in the incidence of various diseases can be of assistance in decisions concerning the use of special facilities. For example, a steady decrease in the rate of tuberculosis may indicate that existing TB facilities could be abandoned or used for the treatment of other diseases. The figures may suggest that additional TB beds should be provided in general hospitals where they can be easily converted to other uses.

A third use of prevalence data is to establish service priorities. In theory, resource allocation decisions might be based, in part, on the relative incidence of various diseases. (The Federal Heart, Cancer, and Stroke program was certainly established as a result of the high incidence of these diseases as causes of death.) Only one of the plans, however, makes explicit use of comparative rates to establish priorities or adopt one program rather than another. These choices are usually based on more informal—and often inscrutable—grounds.

The Chicago Board of Health plan uses comparative incidence data as a means of establishing priorities for location of services. The plan first establishes that residents of Chicago poverty areas have a greater need for additional health services than do residents of nonpoverty areas. This was established by comparing data obtained from local and state health departments on infant mortality, total mortality, mortality from selected major causes, and incidence of diseases (TB, VD). Most of the indicators demonstrated the greater health problems of the poor in spite of the fact that the poverty area population was younger than that of non-poverty areas. These data were then used to rank the relative "health level" of each of twenty-four poverty areas on the basis of absolute number of cases as well as on a per capita basis.

Utilization

Health plans are full of information concerning the current use of existing health facilities. Such data may be gathered for any type of service—the number of children seen in a well-baby clinic, visits by public health nurses, and so on. It may be analyzed on the basis of a number of user characteristics—age, income, residence, mode of payment. It can be used to help answer many questions: Is the service being used? Is there a need for additional personnel? For more beds? Where do the people who are using the service live?

Typical hospital utilization data include: (1) number of admissions; (2) average length of stay; (3) patient census; (4) occupancy rate; (5) patient origin. Trends in length of stay, by type of service, can help to achieve greater accuracy in estimating future bed needs. The patient census may be a one-day count or an average daily census derived from annual records. Optimum occupancy rates vary with the size of the hospital and the type of service. The ideal rate will be high enough for economical operation and low enough for flexibility.

Patient origin is used to determine the future bed needs of a particular hospital and the pattern of hospital choice. The Santa Clara Hospital Commission collected this data by census tracts, "in order to coordinate health planning with other types of long-range community planning carried out by the county Planning Department" (15).

Information on the use of physicians' services is particularly difficult to obtain. The Chicago planners had hoped to compare poverty and non-poverty areas on this basis, but discovered that "such data are not available on a small area basis for any city in the United States, and Chicago is no exception in this regard." The only data came from the Department of Public Aid and it concerned the use of doctors by public assistance recipients. Columbia University's Puerto Rico study asked the patients themselves about their use of doctors. The Chicago and Puerto Rico planners were the only ones to go to the patients themselves for information concerning their use of medical services. The Chicago plan was based in part on discussions with community organizations on local health problems and interviews with about 300 people on welfare whose medical expenses were paid from public funds. The Puerto Rico study included a survey of almost 3,000 families, covering utilization of private and public services, medical costs, and attitudes toward specific services.

Resources

An inventory of health resources is, naturally enough, a vital part of any plan. It may cover facilities, personnel, and services and may include hundreds of items, depending upon the goals of the plan and the nature of the service. In general, inventories describe the type of service, restrictions on clientele, facilities, cost, capacity, staff, and organization. From the city planner's point of view, health planners seem relatively unconcerned with the exact location of resources; areawide plans are somewhat map shy. (One plan used a paragraph—rather than a map—to describe the area's highway system.)

Columbia's study of medical care in Puerto Rico was the only plan that attempted a detailed areawide survey of the *quality* of care in individual hospitals. Most studies are chiefly concerned with questions of organization, administration, and program. They ask, "Are there enough nurses?" not, "Are patients receiving good nursing care?" But the Puerto Rico planners sent an internist, pediatrician, obstetrician, and surgeon to visit hospitals of different sizes under private, state, and municipal ownership. The team examined sample case records from the previous year and studied the physical plant, equipment, organization, and personnel of each hospital.

Ecological Information

Most of the health plans in our survey included ecological information to describe the area. To varying degrees the plans discuss: (1) total population—present and projected; (2) population characteristics; (3) the economy; (4) housing; (5) water supply and waste disposal; (6) government; (7) transportation. Very often this information is reported without analysis, since areawide health studies rarely develop detailed system proposals requiring integration and interpretation of such data. For example, a discussion of the locational issues involved in a projected facility would require an understanding of the *interaction* between diverse aspects of the community, such as transportation, the economy, population, political structure, and the labor force. Since city planning agencies typically collect ecological information and, more to the point, use it when making decisions, this area might be a good place to begin collaboration.

1. *Total population—present and projected:* This information is obtained from a variety of sources, frequently from the local city planning department. This seems to be the type of ecological information most used by health planners.

2. *Population characteristics—present and projected:* Overall trends in age distribution are often used to suggest future service needs. Lehman and Dyckman's *A Pattern of Community Mental Health Services* and Associated Consultants' studies for Puerto Rico examine geographical distribution of population characteristics as clues to the particular service needs of each area. Lehman and Dyckman, for example, examine income group distribution as a clue to the ability to pay for services, ethnic group distribution as an indication of areas where there may be cultural barriers between doctor and patient, and differential age distribution to indicate where special mental health services will be required for children or the elderly. Otherwise, consideration of the different charactristics of subarea populations seems to be rare in health planning.

3. *Economic base:* Most major health planning reports include some discussion of the local economic situation as part of a general description of the area; overall income distribution, unemployment rate, principal industries, and public health and welfare expenditures are typical data. However, only a few plans make substantial use of economic data as an aid in decision-making. Lehman and Dyckman point out that unemployment and mental disability are likely to be positively related, suggesting a greater need for mental health services in areas with high unemployment rates. The Massachusetts mental health plan uses census data on income, unemployment, and housing value as part of a socioeconomic index used to rank the state's mental health areas on the basis of need.

4. *Housing:* Discussions of local housing problems include census data on housing conditions and reports of renewal and other programs affecting the area's housing supply. Since health planning agencies often are responsible for developing adequate housing codes and establishing inspection programs, some studies contain brief discussions of adequate sanitary standards, codes, and inspection programs.

5. *Water supply and waste disposal:* The studies reviewed make use of a wide variety of readily available information describing the existing systems; for example, construction of sewage lines, adequacy of treatment process, number of homes served, and expansion plans. Typically these studies do not discuss plans for future development of utility systems, possibly because the necessary data or techniques to make such projections are unfamiliar.

6. *Government:* Most health plans contain a description of local government for background purposes only. Lehman and Dyckman found a need for more "information on present political decision processes which influence the allocation of mental health resources."

7. *Transportation:* Since only a few plans were seriously concerned with locational issues, it is not surprising that transportation factors are treated briefly in most reports. A few plans, primarily those in which city planners played major roles, use data on automobile ownership and travel time as indicators of accessibility of health services. Lehman and Dyckman examined variations in automobile ownership rates throughout the San Gabriel Valley. They concluded that "the great majority of the population are able to move by automobile quite freely. Only in the lower income areas will there be a major significance for service location to be accessible to non-drivers."

Data on travel time were used in a few plans to measure accessibility of health services. A maximum travel time may be set as one of the criteria for determining the future need for an existing or proposed facility. This may have to be balanced against conflicting criteria: the Hawaii planners had to decide whether to maintain a hospital that served a population below economical size or to force people to travel more than one hour to a general hospital. The planners in California and Puerto Rico used comparative travel times—present and projected—as a test of alternative schemes for the regionalization and location of major health facilities.

Uses of Health Information: Three Examples

Three components of health plans illustrate how information about the community's general characteristics is integrated with health data: (1)

projections of future bed needs; (2) definitions of health facility service areas; and (3) studies of housing conditions.

I. PROJECTIONS OF FUTURE BED NEEDS

The future utilization of health services might logically be projected by synthesizing information about the general characteristics of the community, changes in its population, predicted transportation and housing development, medical advances, and future benefit and payment plans. Into the calculation could be added the group of people, often the elderly and the poor, who do not make full use of medical facilities when they need care. Extended government payment programs that will reduce economic barriers and revised hospital procedures, such as the establishment of neighborhood clinics to make medical care less forbidding, should encourage a larger number of people to use health services.

Presently, however, the most common way to project utilization trends is simply to apply a population growth factor to extend current utilization rates. For example, some estimates of bed needs are made on the basis of a formula for the ratio of beds to population, such as 4.5 beds/1,000. (The formula may be derived from the guidelines of the state's Hill-Burton agency.) Health planners first define the service area, then estimate its bed requirements. But this rule-of-thumb formula can lead to some absurdities. The first Lincoln, Nebraska, plan (24) indicated that the area suffered a deficiency of beds, when, in fact, occupancy rates were already too low for economical operation. APHA's St. Louis plan (1) casts some doubt on the value of projecting long-range bed needs because of uncertainties about future patterns of care. But it is easy to defend the time spent getting accurate short-range projections of five years or so, since they are required to determine immediate construction needs.

2. SERVICE AREA

Every areawide report assumes that a health service area exists—that is, an area for which coordinated facilities and service should be planned. But only a few reports discuss the criteria for defining a service area, indicate the importance of defined standards, or state the basic assumptions.

Service areas can be viewed in terms of the *area actually served* by a particular hospital or group of hospitals. A service area, in this sense, must be determined—or assumed—as a basis for estimating future bed needs. Then, planners can project population trends, health conditions, and other characteristics that may affect future demand for beds. The patients of particular hospitals do not all come from a single area, however, and there is much overlapping of areas served by different hospitals in the same region. A study of locational factors in the utilization of Massachusetts General Hospital, conducted as part of this research project, indicated a complex pattern with different areas of patient origin for different socioeconomic groups.[5] Although a few plans in our survey acknowledged that lower income people have special problems of access, none dealt directly with this issue in delineating service areas.

Anthony Rourke's hospital plan for Lincoln, Nebraska, recognizes the overlapping of service areas for individual hospitals. Rourke uses patient residence data to delineate a three-part service area: (1) a base service area in which the three major hospitals serve most medical needs; (2) a peripheral service area from which patients come for special services or because of particular preference for a Lincoln hospital; (3) a regional service area from which patients come only for special services. Each service area sends patients at a different rate. Rourke also divided the entire region into four quadrants and determined the rate at which each hospital received patients from each of the quadrants. Thus, the location of population growth can be related with some precision to the demand for beds in the three hospitals. This approach to serve area analysis illustrates the need for detailed patient origin data.

A second concept sees the service area as a logical or *ideal area* for which to plan a health program. This concept demands consideration of transportation systems, location of existing resources, political boundaries, and desirable standards of access (for example, that no person should be more than ten miles—or one hour's travel time—from a general hospital). Associated Consultants' plan for Puerto Rico illustrates the application of this second concept in its thorough review and revision of the government's general hospital service areas. Under this scheme each region is to be served by a system of municipal health centers linked to a central hospital. The study reviews the factors relevant to the delineation of regions, recommends changes, and recommends one of the two alternative locations for a medical center in the proposed Mayaguez region. The factors considered included "size of area and topography; population; present and planned means of transportation; social, economic, and political factors; availability of personnel; and the experiences of the Board of Health." Regionalization schemes designed for other special purposes (economic planning, police administration) were reviewed. Certainly the issues involved in this phase of health planning call for the collaboration of health and city planners. Both were represented on the Puerto Rico project.

For most areawide planning groups a central problem is delineation of the service area within which needs are to be analyzed and resources allocated. Frequently, planning areas are established on the basis of the political realities of resources allocation, rather than on the basis of actual or desired patterns of utilization. At present, the priorities for allocation of federal grants for hospital construction and modernization are established on the basis of the extent to which present supply of hospital beds within a service area meets the estimated "need" for such facilities. In practice, service areas usually coincide with political boundaries (boundaries of cities and towns, individual municipalities, or counties) and are assumed to be mutually exclusive. Standard procedure is to make a patient flow study (that is, determine what portion of each hospital's patients come from what city or town), and then assign hospitals to those areas from which they draw the majority of their patients.

Since the population in need of hospital services is not distributed uniformly across the state or even within a metropolitan area, the manner in which service areas are defined becomes a crucial determinant of estimated need and priorities. Accessibility, reputation of the hospital, its economic accessibility, formal and informal referral patterns, ethnic, religious, and personal ties produce a maze of overlapping service areas that make contiguous, mutually exclusive service areas difficult to justify. Regardless of whether "demand" or "need" becomes the basis for determining the adequacy of present hospital services and proposing new service systems for the future, neither standard can be meaningfully applied until the concept of service area is more adequately defined.

3. HOUSING

Housing is a subject of direct significance both for urban development and environmental health. Correlations between poor housing and poor health have been demonstrated, and the causal connections are fairly clear. A number of respiratory and other infectious diseases are linked to multiple use of toilet and water facilities, inadequate heating or ventilation, and inadequate and crowded sleeping arrangements. Certain digestive ailments are related to poor washing and toilet and food storage facilities. In addition, many injuries result from home accidents related to inadequate kitchens, poor electrical connections, and badly lighted and unstable stairs.[6]

The NCCHS "Study Guide" included a section on housing, raising questions on structure, heating, electrical supply, overcrowding, and ventilation. Most of the plans, however, contain little more than a superficial discussion of local housing problems and limit themselves to descriptions of existing conditions, reviews of licensing, zoning, and inspection programs, lists of code enforcement difficulties, and discussions of present and future activities. The typical description of housing conditions includes only the percentage of sound, deteriorated, and dilapidated housing. Some reports note the general problem of finding standard housing for low-income families. The Prince George's County report (27) mentions that the present inspection staff is too small to provide adequate housing code enforcement but states that the code itself is a good one. All the reports call for more detailed planning to solve housing problems; however, none of the plans gives an indication of what should be included in "more detailed planning."

Many health plans describe current urban renewal activity and its effect on housing supply, but they do not discuss relationships between renewal and the administration or distribution of health services. Urban renewal could, for example, provide funds for a diagnostic survey of neighborhood health needs; renewal plans could include health facilities and services.

On the other hand, Lehman and Dyckman make use of housing data as a guide to locational decisions in mental health planning. Subarea trends in housing costs were used to update census data on income. They also examine present and projected residential densities, relating high density areas, with their larger populations of single persons, including the widowed, the divorced, and the separated, to the need for mental health services.

Implementation

Only a few plans considered specific issues related to implementation of their recommendations. Relatively speaking, attention to implementation is a strong point of the Chicago Board of Health Medical Care Report (7). It raises questions of budget, administrative techniques, and sources of funds for neighborhood health centers; yet it does not discuss site or space requirements. Perhaps one reason more plans do not raise specific issues of implementation is that the health planning agency operates within the limits of multiple jurisdictions and historic autonomy of health services. Since the agency depends on consensus, it may try to avoid public discussion of issues that could expose conflict.

Few of the health plans covered in this survey give explicit attention to the political, legal, and financial context of health planning. This context may suggest ways in which health planning agencies can bring about changes in health services. An independent health planning agency, for example, may be able to influence health services if it controls important funds, such as Hill-Burton allocations or proceeds from United Fund campaigns. Public health departments can influence the operation of the private services from which they purchase care. Health planners may also be able to implement change through legislation (nursing home standards, for example).

The published health plan can, in any case, publicize facts, present a reasoned point of view, and influence public opinion. The exchange of information and opinion and the backstage bargaining that go into the creation of a health plan may be of even greater value, but the extent of such bargaining is difficult to establish solely by reading the published plan.[7]

RECOMMENDATIONS OF AREAWIDE HEALTH PLANS

There is obviously great variety in the recomendations found in areawide health plans. In varying proportions the plans: (1) make vague exhortations; (2) recommend specific policy; (3) recommend specific action; (4) recommend further research and planning.

1. *Vague exhortation*
   Better communication should be developed between the Department of Health, municipal hospitals, and others, and between personnel of different institutions concerned with the care of the patient.
2. *Specific policy*
   . . . objectives of hospital planning in this community should envisage general hospitals of a minimum 250–300 bed capacity.
3. *Specific action*
   In order to improve the health of the poor we must take steps to change (the existing) pattern. The proposal being made will accomplish this by developing a series of local health centers . . . wherein each family can identify with a specific person such as a health counselor. It should be our goal to set up centers in each of the poverty areas. (Program, staff, and budget are then discussed in detail.)
4. *Further research and planning*
   Many families who need existing community services fail to use them for a variety of reasons . . . further study of services offered in the community is needed to discover why they do or do not appeal to the people they are intended to serve.

How are the recommendations influenced by the nature of the planning organization? We cannot draw any firm conclusions, but several impressions may be worth noting. First, recommendations by agencies planning for themselves are usually more narrowly focused, more concerned with short-range program planning, and, therefore, far more detailed in regard to costs and other issues of implementation than are recommendations by broadly based groups trying to evaluate all community health services.

Another impression is that only organizations with control over distribution of funds (Hill-Burton money or private contributions) feel free to make specific policy recommendations to voluntary hospitals. Thus the New York State Department of Health, Division of Hospital Review and Planning will recommend—however politely—that a hospital close its doors. On the other hand, the Reno County (28) planners did a highly professional job of estimating future bed needs but did not presume to tell the county's two general hospitals how many of the beds should be provided by each institution, even though they were advising the Hill-Burton agency.

By contrast, and rightly, no health planning organization is hesitant to suggest changes in public health programs. For example, the final report of the Bucks County Community Health Study (4) contains fairly specific recommendations regarding public health services: "A medical clinic for family planning should be set up in each of the three locations of the Bucks County Department of Health." However, the report contains only a few general recommendations in regard to hospitals: "At least one of the hospitals in the county should consider the development of a chronic care unit."

Only a few of the plans emphasize long-range improvements or specify a target date for the implementation of recommendations, unless they are discussing hospital bed needs in relation to estimated population growth, in which case rough estimates are often made for the next twenty-five or thirty years. This reluctance to be specific about the timing of recommended action may be due, in part, to the fact that planning bodies are frequently independent of the institutions for which they are planning. There are exceptions. The Halifax County self-study (11), for example, includes recommended actions to be completed "now" (employ a full-time physical therapist in the county); in five years (establish a county building code ordinance); or in twenty years (combine municipal water supplies of three adjoining communities). However, forty-nine of the sixty-seven recommendations are to be carried out "now," and all but six of the recommendations are to be acted upon in less than five years. Like most of the plans surveyed, the Halifax plan recommends only incremental improvements to the existing health service system.

PLANNING FOR SYSTEM ALTERNATIVES

In view of the possibilities noted earlier for dramatic improvements in the health care system of the United States, it is pertinent to ask whether health planning is moving toward development of alternative health service systems. Although virtually all the plans we surveyed propose useful *incremental* changes in the present pattern of services, most stop far short of presenting *new* models of health care. In general, they do not describe or evaluate alternative approaches or consider the interrelationships of various elements of health service systems. Too often the plans give the impression that there are no hard choices or major decisions to be made, either openly or by default, and limit their goals to patching weak spots in existing services.

An exception, as usual, is Lehman and Dyckman's plan for mental health services in the San Gabriel Valley. This plan examines five alternative service patterns, based on combinations of six variables:

Controllable variables:

    1. Emphasis on direct provision of services (traditional medical pattern) *vs.* emphasis on indirect services by training community caretakers and agents.

    2. Concentration of services *vs.* dispersion of services.

Non-controllable variables:

    3. Pattern of services if large-scale mental health prepaid coverage becomes available *vs.* pattern of services with present small-scale mental health prepaid coverage.

    4. Limited funds *vs.* abundant funds.

    5. Scarcity of specialists *vs.* abundance of specialists.

    6. Patterns of urban development and transportation systems to follow present trends *vs.* major variations in area development.

Four illustrative alternatives are outlined and a fifth "most likely" alternative is developed in slightly greater detail. The outlines consider the sources of public funds and their allocation for administration, research, indirect services, and direct patient care, as well as the types and cost of facilities under each alternative.

The Chicago study describes two radically different approaches to health care:

> An approach in which comprehensive care is developed sequentially for sub-cohorts in the population. For the sake of identification, this is the vertical or cohort plan (neighborhood health centers).

> An approach which proposes to refine and supplement existing (programs) with an attempt to meet the needs in the most important areas of deficiency. For the sake of identification, this is the horizontal approach (community-wide services) (7).

While the Chicago planners recommend the first alternative for the major components of health care, they point out that some types of services are best provided on an areawide basis. These include services that deal specifically with relatively rare health problems and services requiring specialized, high-cost equipment.

Most plans in the survey fail to take proper account of interrelationships within the health service system. For example, a few plans briefly acknowledge that payment plans affect the demand for health services, but only the San Gabriel Valley plan considers thoroughly the effect that new private and federal payment plans may have on the use of mental health services. This plan also considers the effects of changes of public attitude toward mental health services, changes in manpower training, and changes in therapeutic approaches.

Many areawide health plans tend to avoid locational issues. They seldom indicate, with any degree of specificity, the physical distribution of proposed facilities. Even more rarely do they get around to the actual selection of sites. For example, the Chicago plan (7) includes specific program proposals and detailed budgets, but contains no discussion of site or space requirements for the proposed neighborhood health centers. The Hospital Commission of Santa Clara County had an ambitious goal:

> By integrating the hospital planning program into a county-wide land use study of the County Planning Department, the (Santa Clara Hospital Commission) hoped to establish fixed locations for future hospitals as was the case for schools and other public and semipublic facilities. It was believed important not to separate hospital planning from other planning (15).

The Commission's final report (1965), however, gives no indication that this work has been accomplished.

One is more surprised that many areawide health plans tend to plan for the health needs of the area as a whole, with little consideration of the special characteristics and special needs of subarea populations. Health plans often seem to view their respective areas as if the population were homogeneous, or at least thoroughly mixed. However, this approach is a natural result of a view of the health service system that emphasizes health care based in large general hospitals and specialized facilities designed to serve the entire area. There are only a few plans that devote attention to the needs of subareas (7, 17, 20).

The relative underdevelopment of alternative health system proposals in the plans we reviewed is probably indicative of the current state of areawide health planning. It may have another meaning as well. Conceivably, the most effective pathway to major changes in the health system may consist of a series of individual innovative programs rather than the systematic approach of comprehensive planning. Recent innovations have occurred in the planning of specific projects—such as neighborhood health centers or new hospital-based community programs—but they are hard to find in the plans covered in our survey. If individual projects do turn out to be the leading edge of systemwide improvement, the most relevant setting for interaction between urban development and health services may be in project planning rather than comprehensive health planning. The nature of the interaction between these fields need not differ greatly from what it might be in the setting of comprehensive planning. Project planning, too, involves clarifying goals, understanding the community setting, delineating service areas, projecting needs, and devising methods of implementation. In either case, the problems cross conventional professional boundaries and ought to stimulate cooperative work.

THE ROLE OF THE CITY AND REGIONAL PLANNER
IN HEALTH PLANNING

A recent survey of over 200 city planning agencies by the American Society of Planning Officials[8] suggests that there are very weak relationships between health planners and the city planners. Only 17 percent of the agencies have spent more than 2 percent of their time on health planning. Twenty-eight percent have staff members who are "particularly interested" in the health field; only 4 percent have staff members with some training or experience. Nineteen percent of the agencies claim that their involvement has been or would be resisted by health organizations. Perhaps this is due to medicine's historic dedication to autonomy and wariness of "outsiders."

But the lack of strong precedents for collaboration does not preclude the possibility of joint ventures. It does suggest, however, that although cooperation may be practical, economical, and mutually advantageous, it will not occur spontaneously. It will require forethought: contact between agencies will have to be carefully established and projects will have to be carefully articulated and well planned.

Our survey suggests nine ways in which health and city planning agencies might benefit from closer coordination:

1. Health planning organizations could contribute their knowledge of environmental health issues to agencies concerned with physical planning.

2. With the aid of health planners, city planners could add health indices to other indices (such as housing conditions, income, juvenile court cases, welfare recipients) used in neighborhood analyses.[9] The availability of adequate health services should be considered along with other services in the evaluation of subareas. This would help city planners to understand the problems of a community and set priorities more sensitively.

3. Although health planners are already finding city planning agencies to be a good source of information on population projections, housing, land, and development trends, they do not avail themselves of other relevant data that the city planner is likely to have.

4. It would be to the advantage of both fields if the locational aspects of health planning were better understood. Health planners seem to ignore the effects of site selection and transportation factors on the use of health services. Probably they do not feel sufficiently competent in this area. City planners need to know more about the locational requirements

of health facilities so that they may take these factors into consideration in land use planning, zoning, and urban renewal.

5. Since they are supposedly trained in planning method as much as in any particular subject matter, city planners should be able to contribute their methodological skills to health planning projects. Specifically, planners might help health organizations collect and analyze data, formulate goals, and identify and evaluate alternatives.

6. City planning agencies have a variety of implementation techniques that might be put at the service of health planning organizations, including capital budgeting, urban renewal, and, in the area of environmental health, various types of development control. Moreover, urban planning agencies usually operate within the context of local government and necessarily become familiar with the political factors involved in funding, acceptance, and implementation of their programs. Their familiarity with local political realities might be useful to the health agencies.

7. The city planning agency, because of its involvement in the rehabilitation and construction of housing, could work with the health agency to establish housing and sanitation codes and inspection programs. It could also help the health agency evaluate health service facilities in terms of physical standards. For example, health resource inventories should make a separate tally of beds in fire resistant and non-fire resistant buildings.

8. Since city planning agencies are already concerned with the projected use of land and demands for future facilities, they may be able to help health agencies anticipate changes in their service areas resulting from population shifts and new travel patterns.

9. Increasingly, city planning agencies are helping to prepare plans that combine environmental with social service components. These include community renewal programs, anti-poverty programs, Model Cities plans, and plans for new communities. New expertise is being developed in understanding the special needs of minority groups and in working directly with citizens to ensure that planned programs are sensitive to public needs and values. These methods should be shared with health planners.

Although this survey of health plans has prompted many critical observations on the methods and scope of health planning, no professional imperialism is intended or warranted. A similar survey of published city plans would no doubt reveal comparable weaknesses and omissions; but the problems of urban development and health care are related, and greater cooperation can yield benefits in both fields. The approach we propose is not an expansion of professional domain, but rather cooperation based on common concerns, mutual respect, and a pooling of knowledge.

NOTES

1 This discussion is drawn particularly from the following books, which give an excellent overview of health services: John H. Knowles (ed.), *Hospitals, Doctors, and the Public Interest* (Cambridge, Mass.: Harvard University Press, 1965); National Advisory Commission on Health Facilities, *A Report to the President, December 1968* (Washington, D.C.: Government Printing Office, 1968); National Commission on Community Health Services, *Health Is a Community Affair* (Cambridge: Harvard University Press, 1966); David D. Rutstein, *The Coming Revolution in Medicine* (Cambridge, Mass.: MIT Press, 1967); Herman M. Somers and Anne R. Somers, *Medicare and the Hospitals: Issues and Prospects* (Washington, D.C.: The Brookings Institution, 1967).

2 Somers and Somers, *Medicare and the Hospitals*, p. 198.

3 *Ibid.*, p. 121.

4 See, American Society of Planning Officials, *The Urban Planner in Health Planning* (Washington, D.C.: U.S. Department of Health, Education, and Welfare, Public Health Service, 1968). Possible contributions of urban planning to health planning are discussed in Bernard J. Frieden, "The Changing Prospects for Social Planning," *Journal of the American Institute of Planners*, XXXIII (September 1967), 311–23; Bernard J. Frieden, "New Roles in Social Policy Planning," A Paper presented to the American Institute of Planners 1968 Annual Conference, Pittsburgh, October 1968; Harold Herman, "Converging Interests in Health and Comprehensive Planning," *Planning 1967* (Chicago: American Society of Planning Officials, 1967), pp. 211–5; Michael L. Joroff, "A Significant But Limited Role," *ibid.*, pp. 206–10. The recent report of the American Institute of Planners committee on comprehensive health planning contains a series of proposals for increasing the sensitivity of urban planning to health factors and improving communications between city planners and health planners. See, *AIP Newsletter*, IV (September 1969), 5–8. Two current surveys provide good background on the state of comprehensive health planning: Donna Anderson and Nancy N. Anderson, "Comprehensive Health Planning in the States: A Current Status Report" (Minneapolis: Health Services Research Center, American Rehabilitation Foundation, 1969); and Lana B. Stone, "From Organization to Operation: The Evolving Areawide Comprehensive Health Planning Scene" (Minneapolis: Health Services Center, American Rehabilitation Foundation, 1969).

5 Laura G. Bruton, "Locational Factors in Hospital Utilization: A Case Study of Massachusetts General Hospital" (unpublished Master's thesis, Department of City and Regional Planning, MIT, 1967).

6 Alvin L. Schorr, *Slums and Social Insecurity* (Washington, D.C.: Government Printing Office, 1963), pp. 13–4.

7 See, Ralph Conant. *The Politics of Community Health* (Washington, D.C.: Public Affairs Press, 1968).

8 American Society of Planning Officials, *The Urban Planner in Health Planning* (Washington, D.C.: Government Printing Office, 1968), p. 81.

9 See, Helen M. Wallace *et al.*, *"Availability and Usefulness of Selected Health and Socioeconomic Data for Community Planning,"* *American Journal of Public Health*, LVII (May 1967), 762–71.

REFERENCES

1. American Public Health Association. *Public Health and Hospitals in the St. Louis Area: A Mid-Century Appraisal.* New York: APHA, 1957.

2. American Public Health Association. *Survey of the City of New Haven Department of Health, 1961–1962.*

3. Associated Consultants (Reginald R. Isaacs *et al.*). *Planning Studies for the Department of Health, Commonwealth of Puerto Rico.* Vol. 1: *Analysis and Evaluation of the General Hospital Service Area,* November 1959; Vol. 2: *Policies for the Planning of the Medical Center for Mayaquez,* March 1960; Vol. 3: *Program for the Planning of the Medical Center of Mayaquez,* April 1961.

4. Bucks County Community Health Study (Doylestown, Pa.). *Profile of Bucks County,* November 1964; "Section Reports," September 1965 (Mimeographed.); *Recommendations for Better Health in Bucks County,* January 1966.

5. Burlington (Vt.) Area Community Health Study. *Profile of the Community,* January 1964; *Environmental and Personal Health of the Community,* May 1964; *Goals and Recommendations,* September 1964.

6. California Department of Mental Hygiene. *Services for the Retarded in the Mid-Valley Region.* Sacramento: January 1966.

7. *Chicago Board of Health Medical Care Report,* November 1965.

8. Columbia University, School of Public Health and Administrative Medicine, and Department of Health of Puerto Rico. *Medical and Hospital Care in Puerto Rico.* February 1962.

9. Community Council of San Mateo County (California). Action Study on Community Health Services: *Community Profile,* May 1964; "Work Committee Reports" (mimeographed, various dates); *San Mateo County Plans for Health Action,* 1965.

10. Connecticut Mental Retardation Planning Project. *Miles to Go.* Hartford: 1966.

11. Halifax County (N.C.) Commission on Health Services. *Profile,* May 1964; *Action,* June 1965.

12. Hastings, John E. G. *Labour's Plan for a Medical Care Program for Toronto.* Toronto: Toronto Labour Health Center Organizing Committee, September 1962.

13. Health Facilities Planning Council of Hawaii. *Areawide Health Facilities Plan for County of Honolulu: 1965–1985.* Honolulu: February 1966.

14. Hood, Thomas R. *Survey of Health Departments in Jacksonville and Duval County, Florida.* Local Government Study Commission of Duval County, 1966.

15. Hospital Commission of Santa Clara County (California). *Health Facilities and Service Planning for the People of Santa Clara County.* 1963 edition: 1965 supplement.

16. Lake County, Illinois, Board of Health and Regional Planning Commission. *Planning the Environment: A Method of Achieving Public Health.* (Undated, c. 1960.)

17. Lehman, F. Guillermo and John W. Dyckman. *A Pattern of Community Health Services.* Sacramento: California Department of Mental Hygiene, October 1965.

18. Lucas County (Ohio) Community Health Study. *Steering Committee Report.* Toledo Council of Social Agencies, March 1967.

19. Maryland State Planning Commission, Committee on Medical Care. *An Integrated State-Wide Program for Mentally Retarded Children,* March 1960; *Report of the Subcommittee on Organization for Health,* June 1960; *Comprehensive Medical Rehabilitation Programs for Maryland,* August 1961; *Report on Convalescent Care Needs for Children in Maryland,* 1963; *Report on Community Health Services,* March 1963.

20. Massachusetts Mental Health Planning Project. *Mental Health for Massachusetts.* Boston: June 1965.

21. Metropolitan Council for Community Services, Inc. *Chattanooga Area Health Study.* (Undated, 1966?).

22. Metropolitan Washington Health Facilities Planning Council, Inc. *A Review of Short-Term General and Other Special Non-Federal Hospitals in the Metropolitan Area of Washington, D.C.* April 1963.

23. New York State Department of Health, Division of Hospital Review and Planning. *A Blueprint for the Hospitals of Rochester.* Albany: July 1961.

24. Norby, Joseph G. and John N. Hatfield. *A Comprehensive Survey of the Health Facilities of Lincoln, Nebraska.* Lincoln Community Hospital Fund, 1955.

25. Pennsylvania Economy League, Inc. (Western-Division). *Coordinated Planning for Hospitals.* Pittsburgh: February 1959.
26. Planning Services Group. *Hospitals and Public Welfare.* Springfield, Mass.: Lower Pioneer Valley Planning Commission, May 1965.
27. Prince George's County Community Health Study Council. *Report of the Prince George's Community Health Study Council.* Bladensburg, Md.: 1966.
28. Reno County Health Facilities Planning Council. *Reno County Health Facilities: Survey and Recommendations.* Topeka: Kansas Health Facilities Information Service, Inc., August 1964.
29. Rhode Island Advisory Council on Mental Retardation. *Rhode Island Plan for Mental Retardation: A Report to the Governor.* Providence: September 1965.
30. Richmond County Department of Health *et al. An Environmental Health Report of Augusta, Georgia,* August 1964.
31. Rourke, Anthony J. S. *A Study Report to the Lincoln Hospital Council: A Master Plan for Development of Facilities for Bryan Memorial Hospital, Lincoln General Hospitals, St. Elizabeth Hospital, Nebraska Orthopedic Hospital,* January 1964.
32. Springfield (Mass.) Area Community Health Study. *Community Profile Report,* March 1964; *Recommendations,* December 1965.
33. Springfield-Sangamon County (Ill.) Health Services Action Study Committee. *A Community Profile,* January 1964 (revised September 1964); *Assessment of Health Services,* June 1964; *A Plan for Health,* November 1964.

Chapter 7

Planning— Programming— Budgeting

7.1 INTRODUCTION

In this chapter we introduce the reader to the important concept of "Planning-Programming-Budgeting." We will present a very brief discussion of the two techniques of PPB (programming and cost-effectiveness analysis) and the steps involved in implementing this relatively new tool of management.

Planning-programming-budgeting (commonly known as PPB or just "program budgeting") is a technique of making allocation decisions. Although the terms planning (the process of making present decisions to cope with the future), programming (to schedule activities in support of planning decision), and budgeting (to allocate financial resources in support of programs) are not new, an operationally useful synthesis of these processes (planning-programming-budgeting system or PPBS) is of rather recent origin.* First introduced in the Department of Defense in 1961, PPB was extended by Presidential Order to all the executive offices and agencies of the United States Government in 1965.† Programming was the new element in PPB; it provided an objective-oriented link between planning and the old format of budgeting. In applying PPB, the format of the annual operating budget was not changed. Instead, a torque converter was developed for translating the five-year program into the budget format and

---

* For a history of PPB, see Hitch [1967], Novick [1967].
† The important government documents which explain the purpose, format, structure, and relation of the system to the budget processes are three bulletins issued by the United States Bureau of the Budget: Bulletin No. 66-3 (Oct. 12, 1965); a Supplement to Bulletin No. 66-3 (Feb. 21, 1966), Bulletin No. 68-2 (July 18, 1967). The last mentioned bulletin was to replace the first two. All three are reproduced as appendices in Lyden and Miller [1967].

vice-versa [Hitch 1967, p. 3]. Since that time, PPB has been applied in areas including health, education, natural resources, transportation, poverty, and crime.* There is evidence that PPB systems will soon become an integral part of the budget preparation process in state and local governments.† As opposed to traditional budgeting which is control oriented, PPB has a planning orientation. When objectives cannot be quantified (e.g., control of foreign relations, certain health programs) it is more meaningful to develop budgets with a planning orientation.

The planning orientation of PPB (as opposed to a control or management orientation)‡ has been emphasized by Schick in [Lyden and Miller, 1967, pp. 26–52].

> PPB is predicated on the primacy of the planning function; yet it strives for a multi-purpose budget system that gives adequate and necessary attention to the control and management areas. Even in embryonic stage, PPB envisions the development of crosswalk grids for the conversion of data from a planning to a management and control framework, and back again. PPB treats the three basic functions as compatible and complementary elements of a budget system, though not as co-equal aspects of central budgeting. In ideal form, PPB would centralize the planning function and delegate *primary* managerial and control responsibilities to the supervisory and operating levels respectively.

7.2 TECHNIQUES OF PPB

7.2.1 *Programming*

PPB essentially consists of two "management techniques (programming and cost-effectiveness analysis) which are related and mutually supporting, but distinct; in fact, they are so distinct that it is possible to use either without the other" [Hitch, 1967, p. 3]. The two techniques can be used in varying degrees, depending upon the nature of the problem. The first technique, programming, develops a *program structure* and long-range (5 to 8 years) resource and financial requirements to support the contemplated programs. The program structure starts from the general objectives of a department; then lists specific objectives and sub-objectives to attain the general objectives; and finally enumerates various program categories

---

* See Novick [1967, Chapters 4–9].
† For a discussion of limitations, problems and risks of PPB, see McKean and Anshen [in Novick 1965, pp. 85–307].
‡ The basis of Shick's arguments is Robert Anthony's classification of administrative processes into strategic planning, management control, and operational control [Anthony, 1965]. This classification corresponds to Ansoff's classification of business decisions which we discussed in Part II.

and programs that can help achieve specific objectives and sub-objectives. If desirable or possible, the programs are then broken down into *program elements* and activities. Program structure therefore represents a hierarchy of programs—each level containing a different aggregation and detail. Two things characterize the program structure. First of all, programs are classified by outputs* (which are objective-oriented) rather than inputs. Similarly, financial budgets are classified according to outputs—as opposed to the traditional budget classification by objective of expenditure (e.g., agency, or department or origin). Secondly, once the program structure is developed, its resource and financial requirements are projected from 5 to 8 years in the future. In this sense, PPB is long-range planning for public bodies.

7.2.2 *Cost-effectiveness Analysis*

Cost-effectiveness† analysis is the second part of the PPB system. The purpose of cost-effectiveness analysis is to choose that set of programs which achieves maximum value of the objectives for a given level of costs; or conversely, which minimizes costs for a given level of outputs. The program outputs can be measured either in physical units, monetary terms, or some other unit of measurement (e.g., length of stay in a hospital). Cost-effectiveness analysis permits comparison of program outputs per unit of cost input; in terms of quantity as well as quality. It thus ranks alternative programs according to a measure of effectiveness. A schematic representation of cost-effectiveness analysis is shown in Figure 7.1.

Hitch explains cost-effectiveness in these words [1967, p. 7]:

> Systems analysis in the sense of cost-effectiveness analysis is nothing more or less than economic analysis applied to the public sector of the economy or, indeed, to the private sector. Economic analysis is concerned with the allocation of resources. Its basic tenet is to maximize the value of the objectives achieved minus the value of the resources used. In business, this reduces itself to maximizing profits, because both income and outgo are measured in dollars. In defense and generally in the public sector, we lack a common valuation for objectives and resources. Therefore, we have to use one of two weaker maxims: maximize objectives for given resources, or minimize resources for given objectives.

---

* For example, in the case of some health programs, the output may be patient-days.
† Other terms used to denote the same concept are "cost-benefit analysis," "systems analysis," "cost-utility analysis," "operations analysis," "operations research." We prefer "cost-effectiveness" because in managerial decisions, the term of effectiveness has a pragmatic ring. For a statement aimed at distinguishing cost-effectiveness analysis from operations research, the reader is referred to a quote from David Novick given in Lyden and Miller [1967, p. 16].

FIG. 7.1
THE STRUCTURE OF ANALYSIS

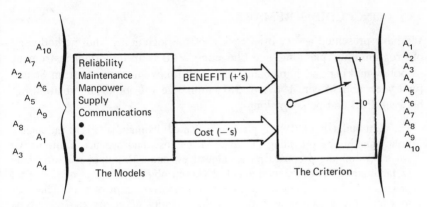

Source: [Quade, 1966, p. 9].

7.3 METHODOLOGY OF PPB

The methodology of PPB is reflected in the steps which each federal department was asked to follow in 1968 in order to implement the PPB system [Lyden and Miller, 1967, p. 5]:

1) Develop its objectives and goals, precisely and carefully;
2) Evaluate each of its programs to meet these objectives, weighing the benefits against the costs;
3) Examine, in every case, alternative means of achieving these objectives;
4) Shape its budget request on the basis of this analysis, and justify that request in the context of a long-range program and financial plan.

An operational PPB system must consist of three components, each contributing in varying degrees to the attainment of objectives in different parts of the organization. The first two, which we have already discussed, relate to the *structural* (program structure) and the *analytical* (cost-effectiveness analysis) process. The third is the required *information system* to support the first two. A sound information system is necessary for purposes of planning, feedback, and control. Its primary function, in a PPB system, is for "(1) progress reporting and control and (2) providing data and information to serve as a basis for the analytical process—especially to facilitate the development of estimating relationships that will permit making estimates of benefits and costs of alternative future courses of action."* The output of a PPB system is a comprehensive multi-year plan consisting of programs, resource requirements, and financial data. The plans are systematically reviewed and updated annually.

7.4 CONCLUDING REMARKS

We have presented a very brief review of the techniques and methodology of programming, planning, and budgeting. PPB is an important instrument of policy-making and implementation. The following excerpts from Schick [in Lyden and Miller, 1967, p. 38] emphasize the important relationship between PPB and policy-making.

> Program budgeting (PPB) is planning oriented; its main goal is to rationalize policy-making by providing (1) data on the costs and benefits of alternative ways of attaining proposed public objectives, and (2) output measurements to facilitate the effective attainment of chosen objectives. As a policy device, program budgeting departs from simple engineering models of efficiency in which the objectives is fixed and the quantity of inputs and outputs is adjusted to an optimal relationship. In PPB, the objective itself is variable; analysis may lead to a new statement of objectives.

It can be said that of the two related aspects of PPB (i.e., programming and cost-effectiveness analysis), programming is more general and should precede cost-effectiveness analysis. Our two selections for this chapter (Selections 15 and 16) focus on cost-effectiveness analysis—as this aspect of PPB is the key to choosing preferred health programs. The reader is referred to Frankel [in Novick, 1967, pp. 208–247] for a description of the development of a *program structure* for health.

A "program-budget" framework can be developed for budgeting health expenditures at the state as well as the federal level. Kissick [1967, p. 209] has listed five elements† of the PPB system as applied to the Public Health Service. He provides a schematic illustration [Figure 1, p. 211] of how a PPB system works in the health field. A summary of the applications of PPB (and cost-effectiveness analysis) is given by Klarman [1967].

A cost-effectiveness analysis of New York's emergency ambulance service was conducted by Savas [1969]. The cost-effectiveness of several alternatives for providing ambulance services was analyzed by using computer simulation. Bond et al. [1968] have provided an account of the

---

* Fisher [in Novick, 1967, p. 61].

† (1) Clearly defined statement of Public Health Service objectives and goals; (2) automated information systems; (3) continuing program analyses; (4) program plans including five-year financial plans and annual reviews; and (5) evaluation.

efforts for evaluating costs versus benefits of an occupational health program during its early development in a company with 27,000 employees.

Kirby [1971] describes the introduction of cost-benefit analysis in a large health care system.

Packer (Selection 15) investigates ways in which "the basic concepts of model building and cost-effectiveness can be applied to the health planning process." The scope* of the health problem is reviewed and the desirability of applying cost-effectiveness at all decision-making levels within the health system is indicated. A set of problems in health planning is enumerated and an approach to model building for cost-effectiveness analysis is described. The author discusses some of the methodological implications of the problem of planning the community health service system and recommends the use of digital computer simulation. Various measures of effectiveness for a health system are considered. One measure, stated in a negative manner as the absence of health, is a measure of ineffectiveness of the system (the measure of effectiveness is complementary to that of ineffectiveness). The proposed measure of ineffectiveness is defined as the expectation of the weighted sum of the population's expected duration of stay in specified disability states. Packer describes various types of costs alternatives: fixed and variable; sunk and future; actual (direct) and implied (indirect). Distinctions are also made among the various bearers of the costs: the government, the community, and the individual.

Smith's article (Selection 16) differentiates between cost-benefit and cost-effectiveness analyses. A simple example is employed to illustrate the two concepts; followed by a discussion of common errors made in using the analyses. An example of a cost-benefit study in public health programs is provided by citing a study in which several ways of preventing motor vehicle accidents were compared. Finally the author presents relevant aspects of a report (prepared for the Bureau of the Budget) in which the cost-effectiveness approach was utilized for comparing alternative ways in the treatment of kidney disease.

REFERENCES

Anthony, R. N., *Planning and Control Systems,* Boston: Graduate School of
1965   Business Administration.
Bond, M. B., et al., "An Occupational Health Program: Costs vs. Benefits,"
1968   *Archives of Environmental Health,* vol. 17, September, pp. 408–415.
Fisher, G. H., "The Role of Cost-Utility Analysis in Program Budgeting," in
1967   D. Novick (ed.], *Program Budgeting,* Cambridge, Mass.: Harvard
University Press, pp. 61–80.
Frankel, M., "Federal Health Expenditures in a Program Budget," in D.

---

* The statistics given are for Fiscal 1965. For more recent data, see Chapter 1.

1967   Novick (ed.), *Program Budgeting,* Cambridge, Mass.: Harvard University Press, pp. 208–247.

Hitch, C. J., *Decision-Making for Defense,* Los Angeles, Calif.: University of
1967   California Press.

Kirby, W. H., "Cost-Benefit Analysis in a Large Health Care System," in M. G.
1971   Kendall (ed.), *Cost Benefit Analysis,* New York: American Elsevier Publishing Co.

Kissick, W. L., "Planning, Programming, and Budgeting in Health," *Medical*
1967   *Care,* vol. V, no. 4, July–August, pp. 201–220.

Klarman, H. E., "Present Status of Cost-Benefit Analysis in the Health Field,"
1967   *American Journal of Public Health,* vol. 57, no. 11, November, pp. 1948–1953.

Lyden, F. J., and E. G. Miller, *Planning, Programming, Budgeting: A Systems*
1967   *Approach to Management,* Chicago, Ill.: Markham Publishing Co.

McKean, R. N., and M. Anshen, "Limitations, Risks, and Problems," in David
1967   Novick (ed.), *Program Budgeting,* Cambridge, Mass.: Harvard University Press, pp. 285–307.

Novick, D. (ed.), *Program Budgeting,* Cambridge, Mass.: Harvard University
1967   Press.

Novick, D. in F. J. Lyden, and E. G. Miller, *Planning, Programming, Budget-*
1967   *ing: A Systems Approach to Management,* Chicago, Ill.: Markham Publishing Co., p. 16.

Quade, E. S., "Systems Analysis Technique for Planning-Programming-Budget-
1966   ing," *P. 3322,* Santa Monica, Calif.: The RAND Corp., March.

Savas, E. S., "Simulation and Cost-Effectiveness Analysis of New York's
1969   Emergency Ambulance Service," *Management Science,* vol. 15, no. 12, August, pp. B608–B627.

Schick, A., "The Road to PPB: The Stages of Budget Reform," in F. J. Lyden
1967   and E. G. Miller (eds.], *Planning, Programming, Budgeting: A systems approach to management,* Chicago, Ill.: Markham Publishing Co., pp. 26–52.

SELECTION 15

Applying Cost-Effectiveness Concepts to the Community Health System[*]

A. H. Packer

The objective of this paper is to investigate some ways in which the basic concepts of model building and cost-effectiveness can be applied to the health planning process.

The first two sections describe the problem and the approach taken, and define the concepts involved.

The third section outlines the methodological implications that can be drawn and recommends large-scale digital computer simulation techniques as a potentially effective means of applying cost-effectiveness concepts to community health system planning.

The next section, a study of effectiveness measures, suggests that the system's basic purpose is to reduce the likelihood that individuals will be in a state of ill health. The proposed measure of ineffectiveness is defined as the expectation of the weighted sum of the population's expected duration of stay in each of m disability states. The applicability of this and other measures to specific health programs is also discussed.

The fifth section deals with the problem of estimating costs. Distinctions are made among the various kinds of costs, such as: fixed and variable; sunk (historic) and future; actual (direct) and implied (indirect). Distinctions are also made among the various bearers of the costs: the government, the community, and the individual.

The final section is a summary.

Scope of the Problem

Expenditures for health and medical care services in Fiscal 1965 totaled $38.4 billion, or 5.9 per cent of the Gross National Product (GNP); governmental expenditure amounted to almost $10 billion, or 26 per cent of this amount. Since 1955 the annual expenditure has increased 112 per cent; this represents a 25-per cent increase in the percentage of GNP expended for health and medical care.

[*] *Operations Research,* vol. 16, March–April, 1968.

The increased expenditure has not been uniformly borne. Insurance benefits accounted for 19 per cent of private personal health care expenditures in Fiscal 1955; in Fiscal 1965 the proportion had risen to 31.6 per cent. The government's expenditures have risen more rapidly than the total; its share has increased from 24.4 to 25.9 per cent for all types over the stated period. Also, the federal share of public expenditure has increased, from 45.2 to 51.2 per cent in ten years.[1]

An examination of these trends and public statements by national political leaders suggests that health and medical care expenditures will be subjected to greater influences, both directly and indirectly, from various government sources.

It is imperative under these circumstances that health services be rationalized, that the limited available resources be allocated to maximize benefits to society, and that the principles of cost-effectiveness be applied at all decision-making levels within the system.

Some educational institutions and research centers, certain specialized hospitals, and some portions of the pharmaceutical and medical insurance industries serve the entire nation or large regions; however, the great mass of health resources such as hospitals, nursing homes, public health organizations, clinics, treatment and diagnostic centers, private physicians and dentists, nurses, etc., serve individual communities. Since resources developed in national institutions are finally implemented at the community level, it is most appropriate to apply cost-effectiveness considerations at the individual community level.

The need for coordinated planning of community health resources has been recognized.[2, 3] This concept of planning is written as law under the Hill-Burton Act. The Bureau of State Services (Community Health) accepted as its mission "the advancement of a concept of community health in which public and private resources together deliver to all segments of the population a comprehensive range of preventive, curative, and restorative health services in the most efficient and effective manner feasible, with full utilization of relevant scientific advances.[4]

Difficulties in Planning

Recognition of the need for comprehensive planning is a necessary, but not sufficient, condition to its satisfaction. The nature of health services makes effective planning difficult. First, there is the problem to which this paper is addressed—adequate, operational measures of effectiveness are elusive and appropriate data are frequently unavailable. Second, some of the most important resources—doctors, hospitals, nursing homes, etc.—typically operate in an independent fashion. Third, many aspects of these resources (e.g., the hospital's location and basic physical layout, or the location, pattern, etc., of the private physician's practice) are fixed for long periods during which the various resources are continually subject to rapidly changing patterns of demand and utilization owing to factors such as advances of medical science, rapid growth of health insurance coverage, improvements in the standards of living, changes in population characteristics, and a greater degree of urbanization.[5] A fourth system characteristic that contributes to the difficulty of planning is the system's stochastic nature.[6] Fifth, because interaction between the health resources and the population occurs at the community level, effective planning must be adapted to the needs and resources of specific communities. Recognition of this fact is implicit in recent legislation (Public Law 89–749). One objective of this Act is the substitution of statewide planning and funding of health services for the current practice of categorical grants (i.e., TB, venereal disease, maternal and child care, etc.).

A General Approach

The five problems listed above are only a brief introduction to the conceptual difficulties involved in applying analytical techniques to interdisciplinary problems of socioeconomic planning; other difficulties will be described later in the paper. Viewed pessimistically the problem may appear to be impossible to solve. However, in spite of difficulties, planning decisions have been and will continue to be made. The realistic goal is progress towards improving these decisions and not an 'ultimate' solution.

This goal will *not* be achieved if the analytical technique is so simplified and rigid that it provides conclusions contrary to good judgment. For example, a measure that weights the effectiveness of health programs so heavily in terms of current earnings that programs directed towards the control of children's diseases are neglected is worse than useless.

The recommended approach is to begin the analysis with the problem defined in all its complexity and to proceed by abstracting from this complexity to a model of the problem that is simple enough to be conducive to analysis. During the abstracting process, simplifying assumptions should be made explicit so that it will be apparent whether the conclusions of the analysis should be supplemented or replaced by judgment. As progress is made in developing and using the model, it should be possible to add back those important aspects of reality that were initially 'assumed away.' Thus the analytical process and the degree to which complexity is recognized, is divided into two stages as illustrated in Fig. 1. The first is the conceptual stage in which the problem is taken in its full complexity and explicitly simplified until a manageable model is obtained. The second is the opera-

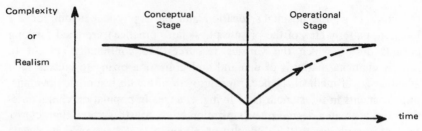

Fig. 1. The analytic process.

tional stage in which the simplified model is developed, validated, and made more realistic.

MODEL BUILDING FOR COST-EFFECTIVENESS ANALYSIS

Some Definitions

It may be helpful to define some of the terms used to describe the systems being modeled. The community, together with human and physical resources which serve its health needs, comprises a complex and dynamic system. The system's state is defined by the value of certain variables which describe the state of the individual system elements, e.g., the prevalence of particular diseases, the available hospital beds, etc.

The set of variables and the set of parameters can each be divided into two subsets. One subset contains variables and parameters which are generally controllable by the policymakers, while the complementary subset contains those that are relatively uncontrollable. Examples of each type are presented in Table I. It should be noted that "controllable" and "uncontrollable" are defined only in relative terms and depend on the time, the authority, and the resources available to the policymaker.

The policymakers are vitally interested in the values, or outcome, of one particular subset of the variables. This is the subset by which the cost and effectiveness of the system is measured. Any planning process requires a prediction of the changes to be anticipated in these crucial variables as a result of alternative actions.

Past model-building efforts have had, among others, the following three objectives:

1. To train people in the performance of complex tasks, including management activities.

2. To provide a research tool to aid in the study of complex systems.

3. To act as an aid in the decision-making process.[7]

This study is principally concerned with the third objective and, thus, the model must explicitly recognize the policy variables and provide for their convenient manipulation. Since the three objectives are not mutually exclusive, the suggested model should also be useful in meeting the remaining two objectives.

TABLE I
EXAMPLES OF SYSTEM ELEMENTS AND RELATIONS

	Less Controllable	*More Controllable*
Variables	Demographic characteristics including socioeconomic factors Current resources and economic capacity to support additional health activities	Insurance coverage Distribution of diagnostic clinics Extent of home nursing care services
Parameters or relations between the variables	Education and utilization of public health services Insurance coverage and medical care utilization Nutrition, air and water pollution, housing and health levels	Available resources and various health problem goals (e.g., priorities and timing) Responsibilities of health service organizations, or providers

The decision-making objective can be subclassified for those models that support planning:

1. To study complex systems for the purpose of system design, where the interactions are too complex to be understood and simulation can provide insight.

2. To test proposed solutions or hypotheses.

3. To quantify the improvement anticipated from the use of a proposed analytically derived solution.[8]

4. To prove the value of proposed changes and to present them in a manner that enhances acceptance of changes and facilitates implementation.[7]

For a model to be useful as an aid in decision-making, it should be of the following form:

$$V = f(a_i, X_i, b_j, Y_j), \quad (i = 1, 2, \cdots, n; j = 1, 2, \cdots, m) \quad (1)$$

where

V is a measure of the system's value,

X_i are the controllable elements or decision variables,

a_i are the controllable relations or parameters,

Y_j are the uncontrollable variables or elements, and

b_j are the uncontrollable relations or parameters.

If the relations can be defined and values assigned to the parameters and variables for two alternative system configurations, the model can be used to compare the proposed configurations.

Cost-Effectiveness

The planner's objective is to identify for the policymaker the state of the controllable variables and parameters that will maximize the value of the system subject to an assumed set of conditions. The assumed set of conditions is defined by the state of the uncontrollable variables and parameters. Budget constraints may or may not belong to this uncontrollable set. If the budget is in fact fixed, it is an uncontrollable variable and the objective is to maximize effectiveness under the budget (and other) constraints.

Some of the controllable variables and parameters can be varied, within limits, without incurring any appreciable cost; this subset of controllable variables generally includes allocation of a specified resource, establishment of the sequence or the priority of treatment, etc. On the other hand, there is a complementary subset of controllable variables and parameters that require significant expenditures to effect a change; increasing the total facility or personnel resources generally falls into this category.

For a specified expenditure level, or budget, and a specified set of values for uncontrollable variables, there are one or more optimum settings (i.e., optimum system configurations) for controllable variables that maximize the system's effectiveness. At a different expenditure level, a new configuration may maximize effectiveness. The decision as to whether the additional effectiveness is worth the additional cost is properly left to the policymaker. The analysis can provide cost-effectiveness ratios, indicate the marginal cost-effectiveness of additional investment, and eliminate from consideration any inferior alternatives—i.e., system configurations dominated by alternatives that are either more effective and no more costly, or less expensive and no less effective.

Uncertainty

The planning problem is complicated by the uncertainty associated with estimates of costs and effectiveness levels. Uncertainty results from the inability accurately to predict the variable and parameter values for the time period relevant to the alternative plans being considered. Prediction difficulties arise from two sources: first, many relations are only imperfectly known, and second, it is impossible to know whether the relations that currently prevail are stable and will persist. The imperfectly known relations between air pollution and lung cancer or between 'quality' of medical care and patient prognosis are examples of the first source of uncertainty. An example of the second type is a significant breakthrough in cancer prevention or treatment that makes existing or planned treatment facilities obsolete and thus invalidates conclusions drawn from models reflecting the current state of medical science.

Another planning difficulty is evaluating future expenditures or benefits. Most economic analyses discount future expenditures and income by applying an interest rate or cost to capital; a variant of this technique may prove useful in evaluating future benefits. Discounting future benefits raises all the conceptual difficulties of interpersonal welfare comparisons if the benefits are to be foregone by one generation so they may accrue to another. An example is the allocation of limited financial resources to a research effort for finding a cure rather than for extending current treatment facilties.

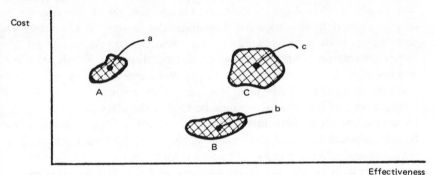

Fig. 2. Cost-effectiveness alternatives with uncertainty.

Figure 2 illustrates the above concepts. The cross-hatched areas (*A, B, C*) indicate the cost-effectiveness regions for three alternative configurations. The points (*a, b, c*) within the areas represent the expected value of cost and effectiveness. System *A* need not be considered further since it is dominated, under all circumstances, by system *B*. (The entire region *A* is less effective and more costly than *B*.) The choice between systems *B* and *C* is left to the policymaker.

The planning objective, illustrated in Fig. 2, is to provide the optimum system configuration (setting of the controllable elements and relations) for a number of budget levels.[9] Better information will reduce uncertainty and diminish the areas (*A, B, C*) surrounding the expected values.

METHODOLOGICAL REQUIREMENTS AND AN APPROACH

Requirements

This section discusses some of the methodological implications of the problem of planning the community health service system and attempts to show why a simulation approach may be appropriate. This should not be taken to mean that analytical models should not be used.* These latter models are generally to be preferred and should be used where possible and efficient. Frequently analytical submodels can be incorporated into a computer simulation program of larger scope.

Determining costs and effectiveness for existing programs, though a difficult task, is relatively simple compared to projecting accurately the future state of a rapidly changing environment. However, the prediction difficulty is alleviated somewhat because comparing alternative programs requires estimates of *relative* outcomes of alternative actions rather than accurate predictions. As the number of alternative programs to be considered increases, it is no longer appropriate to compare two or three programs at a time. What is necessary is a constant set of assumptions— or an unbiased framework—for measuring alternatives; if a new set of assumptions is to be considered, a means is needed to reevaluate all affected alternatives under the new conditions. In other words, the requirement is for a function that maps alternative decisions into their resulting costs and effectiveness. The only consequence of a prediction error, as long as it is unbiased, would be to shift the areas shown in Fig. 2. Of course the uncertainty that underlies the error will also generally increase the areas (A, B, C) surrounding the expected values and will, if large enough, make it impossible to discriminate among alternatives.

The elements comprising the community health system are synergistic. That is, the joint effect of changes in individual elements of the system will, in general, not be equal to the sum of the individual effects of the changes in each element. Thus, alternative combinations of programs will have to be evaluated jointly. Obviously, double counting on the cost and effectiveness side of the ledger must be avoided; this is an especially important consideration in situations where multiple health problems are prevalent.

A methodological consideration discussed in the section dealing with measures of effectiveness is that no single utility function that is appropriate for all programs is known. Even if a single measure of effectiveness is adopted for all programs, the present inability to quantify the relation between, for example, pollution levels or doctors' visits and this single measure, suggests the use of a multidimensional scale for measuring results. This typically precludes the use of an optimizing algorithm.

Intercommunity difference in population composition, climate, topography, economic conditions, existing health resources, political organizations,

---

* The dividing line between analytical and simulation models is rather vague. For the remainder of the paper, if a mathematical technique or algorithm (such as linear programming) can be used to find an optimum solution, the model is of the analytical type. If heuristic techniques are required to search for "good" (in place of optimum) solutions, the model is of the simulation type.

and other health-influencing factors demand that the methodology developed should be of a general nature applicable to this diversity. When applied to the relevant data of individual communities, however, the methodology must produce specific results for the individual situation.

Recommended Approach

There are alternative approaches that can produce the function required to relate decisions to estimates of their resulting costs and effectiveness. Obviously, the choice of approach should be dictated by the nature of the problem and decisions to be evaluated. One choice is between analytical and simulation models. (As noted previously, the line dividing these two classes of models is quite vague.) An analytical model is generally more efficient if the problem can be stated in terms such that available mathematical techniques can be used to 'solve' for an optimum solution. If heuristic methods of 'searching' for the optimum are required, or if Monte Carlo techniques are necessary, then simulation is usually more efficient. Another methodological question concerns the use of a computer; this must be answered in terms of the complexity of the model, the number of alternatives to be considered, the number of sets of assumptions under which the alternatives will be evaluated, etc.

For many of the more significant problems, the methodological requirements noted above can frequently be met best by a large-scale digital computer simulation model. This model or program should attempt to accomplish the following, insofar as is practical:

1. Tie together the analytical solutions or subprograms that describe parts of the system not only to provide a common data base and a set of assumptions but also to ensure the logical consistency of these various parts.

2. Provide a means to investigate, through heuristic procedures, those parts of the system that are too complex to be solved by explicit mathematical formulas.

3. Permit flexibility of output in terms of the various measures of effectiveness to be employed.

4. Be able to accept data describing the significant variables of a specific community; that is, become a model of the community specified by the input data.

5. Provide an analysis of the time path of the impact of the particular system configuration being evaluated. For example, if a new organization of hospital facilities is being considered, what will the transition period between the current organization and that proposed look like?

6. Provide a convenient device for testing the sensitivity of the projected results to errors in the data, relations, or assumptions.

If the final requirement for sensitivity testing is met, it should estimate (1) the expected error of the conclusions drawn from the simulation and (2) the relative significance to the error term of current gaps in knowledge of the system.

Because what will happen to a community and the health of its population is so much a function of uncertain internal as well as external factors, it is unlikely that any simulation model will accurately predict it. As noted previously, scientific breakthroughs, changes in national or community economic situations, changes in social and educational structure, etc., while generally excluded from the model, play important roles. The model should, however, be able to forecast what would happen, given a set of assumptions, in the absence of the exogenous occurrences noted above. Of more value, the model should provide estimates of the impact of changes in the controllable parameters or decision variables under various sets of assumptions.

The research strategy should be based upon a building-block approach. As research is performed, for example, which relates intensive preventive medical care to general health[10] or sociodemographic characteristics to the hospital experience of mental patients,[11] it should be possible to include these relations in the model. Also, the larger model should be capable of utilizing analytical [12, 13] or simulation models[14] of subsystems as they are developed. These smaller subsystem models are the building blocks with which the total system model will be constructed. The advantages of developing and testing each building block before its inclusion in a larger model include the following:

1. Testing and verifying the larger model is simpler.

2. The experience gained in developing the earlier models is increased to the benefit of subsequent efforts.

3. Perhaps most important, the completed subsystems can provide intermediate and worthwhile payoffs during the long, expensive modeling of a complex total system.

MEASURES OF SYSTEM EFFECTIVENESS

Basic Objective

Implicit throughout the previous discussion is the need for an operationally useful measure of effectiveness of the alternative systems (or subsystems) to be modeled.

A necessary precondition to the development of measures of effectiveness is an acceptable, perhaps qualitative, statement of the system's basic goals. Alternative programs, with specific aims, which are often strikingly diverse, must be evaluated against these basic goals. For example, certain programs such as those dealing with the control of communicable disease, vector control, and accident prevention, intend to reduce the incidence of specific health problems. Other resources such as hospitals, diagnostic and treatment centers, ambulances and other emergency equipment, and chronic disease and rehabilitation programs attempt to ameliorate the effects of specific diseases. Health education activities, environmental control efforts (e.g., sanitation; noise abatement; and air, water, and land pollution control), and certain preventive health programs are often related to a broad spectrum of health problems. The inclusion of mental and emotional health activities often requires a complete restatement of basic objectives. Objectives of other social welfare programs in economic development, education, health insurance, housing, poverty alleviation, etc., must also be evaluated. The yardstick (whether it is a general statement of goals or a precise measure of effectiveness), if it is to be universally applied, must be able to cope with this diversity.

One approach has been directed towards the development of a health index. This suggests that an index of community health could measure the effectiveness of alternative programs. An acceptable index that (1) is sensitive to the effectiveness of health programs and (2) is composed of measurable components has proved elusive. Indices of crude and age-adjusted death rates have previously been used. Since 1956, however, the death rates in the United States have been relatively constant; thus greater attention has been paid to morbidity. Since increased morbidity is often the result of reduced mortality (e.g., the longevity of diabetics has increased morbidity while decreasing mortality), the evaluation of mortality and morbidity rates is subject to much interpretation.

SULLIVAN suggests classifying morbidity by four categories of disability: confined, limited mobility, limited activity, and restricted activity.[15] CHIANG proposes an index composed of age-specific components derived from the death rate and the incidence and duration of illness.[16] SAUNDERS suggests measuring health rather than illness and uses a concept of the individual's functional adequacy to fulfill a social role.[17] In no case has the development progressed to the point of producing an operationally useful index.

Requirements of the Measures of Effectiveness and Alternative Approaches

Measures of effectiveness are functions of observable variables by which the degree of attainment of the basic goal (e.g., community health) can be measured. For instance, the basic goal of defense expenditures is the maintenance of peace; a secondary goal derived from the primary objective is to maintain an effective deterrent. To obtain a measurable variable, however, defense expenditure decisions attempt to maximize the number of kills of one sort or another.[18] The measure of effectiveness suggested in the next section will, for many health programs, be measurable in a primary sense. In certain instances, however, it will be necessary to use variables related in a secondary or tertiary manner to the basic goal.

Assume that a finite list of variables related to effectiveness can be agreed on; these might include such things as age-specific death rates, incidence and prevalence of disease, indications of mental health, etc. If the variables in the list are numbered 1, 2, ..., n, the list can be represented by an n-dimensional effectiveness vector, $(X_1, X_2, \ldots, X_n)$, where the X's take on different values for alternative system configurations. If each element in one vector takes a value preferable to that of the corresponding element in the alternative vector, there is no difficulty in selecting the superior or more effective system. The real problem arises because this unidirectional relation does not generally exist. According to the utility concept of value, or effectiveness, there exists a way to obtain a utility function to evaluate the alternative vectors: $\phi = \phi(X_1, X_2, \ldots, X_n)$.

At least three alternative approaches for measuring effectiveness can be identified. The first evaluation alternative, in accord with cardinal utility theory, is to derive a VON NEUMANN-MORGENSTERN utility function by which a numerical value can be assigned to ϕ for alternative effectiveness vectors. [19-21] This approach is implicit in placing a numerical scale on the abscissa of a cost-effectiveness graph such as that shown in Fig. 2. The second alternative is to rely on ordinal utility theory. Ordinal utility theorists would not assume that a numerical value can be assigned to each effectiveness vector, but would state that such vectors can be ordered—i.e., one vector is better, worse, or equal to another. The scale of the abscissa of Fig. 2 would then become indeterminate and a statement could be made about relative, but not absolute, effectiveness. For example, the system configuration represented by point c is more effective than point b, and point b is more effective than point a; however, there is no way to measure or even compare these differences. The decision as to whether the additional effectiveness is worth the additional cost must be left to the policymaker's value judgment. Accepting the premises of ordinal utility theory, the concepts of marginal effectiveness or cost-effectiveness ratios lose their meaning. The third alternative is to present the policymaker with the complete effectiveness vectors corresponding to the alternative system configurations and allow him to make his own choice. This has been the approach for most, if not all, evaluations that have been made of complex systems.

The three approaches are not necessarily mutually exclusive. A numerical-valued (cardinal) utility function can be both a useful conceptual device and a goal to be sought even if it cannot be achieved in an operational sense. Using this approach, an attempt can be made to combine as many elements as possible in an effectiveness vector. That is, if a number (say, m) of utility functions can be defined by combining sets of the n variables, then the policymaker can be presented with a shorter and more meaningful effectiveness vector of the form $\phi = \phi_1, \phi_2, \ldots, \phi_m$ where m is less than n. He must then reconcile these ultimate effectiveness measures.* Analogies can be observed in industrial situations: Ideally, the basic objective may be to maximize the vaguely defined 'long-run profit'; in fact, the policymaker must reconcile an effectiveness vector written in terms of current profit, market share, liquidity, public image, etc.

The Objective Function: A Case-Month Approach

The basic goal, or objective, of the system may be stated in a negative manner as the absence of ill health. The measure discussed below, then, is a measure of the ineffectiveness of the system; the measure of effectiveness is complementary to that of ineffectiveness.

First, consider the system as viewed by an individual. The system's ineffectiveness is some weighted sum of his chances of being in any state of ill health for some finite time period.† If m states of impairment are defined to represent various disability levels (and ultimately death), then from the individual's point of view the system's ineffectiveness is given by:

$$I^p = \sum_{i=1}^{i=m} c_i t_i, \qquad (3)$$

where c_i is the weighting factor for disability state i, and t_i is the duration of stay in state i. The m states are states of disability or restricted activity.

A reasonable starting point might be to use states corresponding to the four morbidity levels suggested by Sullivan and to add an initial state (controlled disease—minor disability) and a terminal state (premature death). The duration of stay in this terminal state is defined as the actuarially estimated reduction in life span that is due to bad health. Note that this

---

* By placing each of the n components of the original effectiveness vector into one or more (*not* mutually exclusive) sets $A, B, \ldots, m$, we can define m utility functions of the form

$$\phi_1 = \phi_A (X_i); i \text{ an element of } A,$$
$$\phi_2 = \phi_B (X_i); i \text{ an element of } B.$$

In this way the basic effectiveness vector $(X_1, X_2, \ldots, X_n)$ can be transformed into $(\phi_1, \phi_2, \ldots, \phi_m)$. If, in general, ϕ_j has more intuitive meaning in a policy sense than does x_i, and m is less than n, then the transformation is useful.

† It is not logically necessary that conclusions obtained using this definition will be contradictory to those arrived at using the definition of the World Health Organization: "Health is a state of complete physical, mental, and social well-being, not merely the absence of disease or infirmity." All that is required is that any perceived deviation from the ideal state be described as one of the disability states.

measure aggregates all diseases and accidents to which the individual is vulnerable. Thus the value of I^p must be built from an analysis of each potential hazard. One of the m impairment states must be assigned to each definable stage of the disease or accident and then the time in each state estimated. The appropriate aggregation can then be performed. To avoid double counting it is necessary to assign a single disability state when multiple diseases and/or accidents are involved.

I^p is an individual's measure of the system ineffectiveness. By focusing on the future and examining the probability of being in each state, one can avoid in a reasonable way the problem of the 'infinite' value of life. That is, we are all willing to incur a finite probability of a premature death to avoid a (larger) finite probability of ill health—e.g., to undergo an operation to avoid a serious disability.

Given I^p, the individual's measure of the system's ineffectiveness, a function is needed to relate the community's measure of ineffectiveness to the number of people in each state of ill health. That is, how can the individual measures be aggregated to obtain a measure for the community? Any attempt to aggregate over an individual utility function, such as that given in equation (3), encounters the difficulties of interpersonal welfare comparisons. Certainly the values imputed to each c_i may not only vary among individuals at any point in time but also vary for a single individual among different points in time. This is the essence of the 'index number problem' familiar to economic analysis.

The problem is not generally soluble because the solution requires a social indifference curve or a preference function for making interpersonal comparisons of welfare. [22] The general insolubility should not be taken to mean that important particular solutions are not available or that reasonable approximations cannot be made. In fact, for many of the real decisions that have to be made, this measure will provide an unambiguous choice. This results if the situation is analogous to Pareto optimality. In this instance, any possible alternative to the 'optimal' decision will create additional case-months in some disability state without any offsetting reductions in some other state. If it can be assumed that the disability states can be strictly ordered (e.g., limited mobility is strictly preferred to confinement), the area of unambiguous choice can be further extended. In this instance any possible alternative to the 'optimal' decision will create additional case-months in some less preferred state at least equal to the offsetting number of cases in the more preferred state.

These concepts may be illustrated by a simple example. Assume that five alternative disease control programs (A, B, C, D, E) are available and that the estimated case-months in each disability state associated with each are as given in Table II.

As a first guess, assume that Program C is the optimum program.

TABLE II

ESTIMATED CASE-MONTHS RESULTING FROM FIVE ALTERNATIVE PROGRAMS

Disability State	Disease Control Programs				
	A	B	C	D	E
1—Minor disability	1000	1000	1000	900	1000
2—Restricted activity	1100	1000	1000	1100	0
3—Limited activity	1200	1000	1000	900	1000
4—Limited mobility	1000	900	1000	900	1000
5—Confined	1000	1100	1000	900	1000
6—Death	1000	1000	1000	1300	1001

Program C is unambiguously superior to A on the basis of the analog with Pareto optimality; for each disability state the number of case-months associated with Program A equals or exceeds that for C. Program C is unambiguously superior to B by the second criterion. The relative reduction in the number of case-months in (the more preferred) state 4 associated with program B is at least offset by the increase in case-months in (the less preferred) state 5. A comparision between programs C and D is only a more complicated case of that between programs C and B. Again C is unambiguously superior, since reductions in case-months in more preferred states are at least offset by increases in case-months in less preferred states. A comparison between programs C and E illustrates the point previously made that no general solution can be found. The relative evaluation of 1,000 case-months of restricted activity against one additional month of premature death is ultimately a subjective judgment.

The remainder of this section is an attempt to derive possible utility (objective) functions that can map the number of case-months in each disability state into a single numerical measure of effectiveness and thus reduce the area of ambiguity. The particular functional forms presented below only illustrate the kind of development necessary to obtain a single-valued function.

The objective function should deal explicitly with the future and thus must be a function of the probabilities of future occurrences. The function should also distinguish between the individual's and the community's point of view and thus must aggregate the individual disutilities as given in equation (3).

Admittedly, choosing appropriate values for c_i (the disutility weights assigned to each disability state) is a task of subjective value judgments. It seems impossible to avoid this problem. Initial insights may, however, be obtained by determining the weights implicitly assigned by some current health programs. (It would be interesting to examine the consistency of these weights among various programs. For example: Is the implicit value of an extra year's life implied by current kidney disease or cancer programs equivalent to that implied by current accident prevention or preventive health programs?) Also, individuals reveal preferences by their expenditure decisions. Demand (income-expenditure) studies might indicate the relative value or disutility of certain health problems implicitly assigned by individuals in the marketplace.

Certainly the selected function should be monotonic and should increase with the number of ill persons. For each disability state, every additional individual in that state (1) will create an additional burden upon the community by demanding certain health resources and (2) will, because of his own reduced productivity, diminish the community's capacity to cope with the burden. Thus, in general the 'disutility' function will have an increasing derivative; that is, the disutility to the community of each additional person's ill health will be greater than that of those preceding him.

One possible aggregation scheme that satisfies this requirement would be to multiply the individual measures of ineffectiveness by a ratio of the form:

$$\frac{\text{number of people in disability state } i}{\text{total population–number in disability state } i}$$

In this scheme, each individual entering the state by both adding to the numerator and decreasing the denominator, would make more than a proportionate increase in the measure.

A second, more complex scheme is to concentrate on rate of change in health and to use a dynamic measure that concentrates on the time path of an individual's health state rather than on static values.

Another aggregation scheme with the above-mentioned characteristics is the exponential form. In this case, the cost to the community of having x individuals in disease state i is expressed as

$$k_i = c_i t_i e^{\alpha x_i}, \tag{4}$$

where k_i is the measure of the system's ineffectiveness from the community's point of view, x_i is the number of individuals in state i for time t_i, α is some appropriate constant (perhaps α should be replaced by α_i permitting the assignment of a second constant to each disability state), and t_i and c_i are as previously defined.

The expected value of the measure of ineffectiveness is then the sum of these weighted by the probability of their occurrence. That is,

$$E[k_i] = \bar{k}_i = \int_0^\infty k_i f(k_i) \, dk_i, \tag{5}$$

where $f(k_i)$, the probability distribution of k_i, is a function of the joint probability distribution x_i and t_i. If it can be assumed that these two variables—i.e., the number of individuals in the disability state i and the duration of stay in that state—are independent, then the expected measure of ineffectiveness is given by:

$$k_i = c_i E[t_i] E[e^{\alpha x_i}]$$

$$= \left[c_i \int_0^\infty t_i f(t_i) \, dt_i \right] \cdot \left[\int_0^N e^{\alpha x_i} p(x_i) \, dx_i \right], \qquad (6)$$

where $f(t_i)$ and $p(x_i)$ are the probability distributions associated with t_i and x_i respectively, and N is the total number in the population.

The assumption of the independence of x and t is not always valid. For example, if the disabilities in question are the result of communicable diseases, then the number of carriers—and thus the number of secondary infections—is a function of the time each individual spends in the infective state. Even in this case, the independence assumption may provide a good first approximation if the disease prevalence is small relative to the total population.*

The variance of the effectiveness measure is significant in choosing between alternatives; that is, a planner might prefer a program with an estimated value of 10 ± 1 to an alternative with an estimate of 11 ± 10. Under the same assumption of the independence of x and t, the variance of k_i is given by:

$$V[k_i] = E[t_i^2] \cdot E[e^{\alpha x 2i}] - E^2[k_i]$$

$$= \left[\int_0^\infty t_i^2 f(t_i) \, dt_i \right] \cdot \left[\int_0^N e^{2\alpha x_i} p(x_i) \, dx_i \right] - (\bar{k}_i)^2. \qquad (7)$$

Equations (6) and (7) evaluate the expected value and variance of the system ineffectiveness for a single disability state. If independence is assumed among the states,† then the total system's mean effectiveness is given by

$$\bar{K} = \sum_{i=1}^{i=m} \bar{k}_i, \qquad (8)$$

and the variance by $\qquad V[K] = \sum_{i=1}^{i=m} V[k_i]. \qquad (9)$

---

* It is possible to test this assumption for certain diseases or groups of diseases. Also note that the final integral implies that sufficient numbers of persons are in each state so that this discrete variable can be treated as a continuous one. Integrating the first bracketed term to infinity is a mathematical convenience since the maximum duration of stay in any disability state is limited to a lifetime.

† This assumption is obviously not perfectly valid. If the number of persons suffering from an illness is fixed, the size of the group in any disability category is a function of the number of persons in the remaining categories. Thus the off-diagonal elements in the variance-covariance matrix are, in general, different from zero, and equations (8) through (11) become more complex. The assumption may more reasonably be stated thus: Assume that the total number of disabled persons is small relative to the total population and that most entries into any disability category come from the well population, and that the off-diagonal elements in he variance-covariance matrix are small.

If the constants c_i and α are chosen so that $\bar{K}$ is restricted to values between 0 and 1, then the expected value of the effectiveness of the community health system is given by

$$\bar{E} = 1 - \bar{K} = 1 - \sum_{i=1}^{i=m} c_i E[t_i] E[e^{\alpha x_i}], \qquad (10)$$

and the variance by $\quad V[E] = V[K]$. $\qquad\qquad\qquad (11)$

If the probability distributions of the duration of disability states and the number of individuals in each state (t_i and x_i) are known, then $\bar{E}$ and $V[E]$ may be determined by performing the mathematical operations shown in equations (6) through (11). For some health problems, sufficient data are available to establish these functions and their parameters.

The measure of effectiveness of a program is the net increase in $\bar{E}$ anticipated over the program's life, i.e., the weighted sum of the probable net decrease in case-months in each disability state. Future benefits may be discounted. Once the admittedly difficult task of establishing the c_i's has been accomplished, a means will have been found to compare accident prevention programs with programs designed to facilitate emergency treatment, or to compare additional diagnostic centers with additional hospital beds. These comparisons can be made if the appropriate probabilities can be projected for each alternative plan considered.

Program-Specific Measures

In order to apply any of the case-month approaches suggested above, it is necessary to be able to relate the effects of alternative actions (e.g., prevention, treatment) to changes in the number of case-months. In some instances, the relations are well known from laboratory experiments or from many case histories, and the case-month method may be applied directly. For example, the effectiveness of immunization programs designed to control communicable diseases such as smallpox, diphtheria, influenza, etc., may be measured by the distribution of secondary cases following one or more initial cases. The effectiveness of detection and treatment programs intended to control communicable diseases such as venereal disease, tuberculosis, etc., could also be directly measured in terms of the probability distribution of the case-months in each disease (i.e., disability) state.

There are some programs for which the functional relations between disability state changes and controllable variables or parameters are not known with a high degree of certainty. Then it is often necessary to rely on expert judgment to obtain the required relations between prevention or treatment and illness. For programs in which these relations are not well known, it may be advisable to use more easily obtainable measures of effectiveness to make intraprogram decisions. This may be the case for some programs concerned with the utilization of health resources, namely: certain aspects of physician care and nursing services, and certain aspects of hospitals or other facility services. For example, while the beneficial emotional and physical effects of comfort care are recognized, it is difficult to quantify the relations or to establish the point at which further comfort no longer serves a useful purpose.

Comfort care is a good example of the 'consumption' characteristics of many aspects of health care. It has been observed that: ". . . medical services are probably more often demanded because of a desire to reduce the everyday aches and pains of life, which affect earning power little if at all, than for the treatment of the fatal diseases. . . ."[23] Despite conceptual measurement problems associated with consumption benefits, they must be considered to obtain a meaningful analysis.

In cases where definitive relations between treatment and result are not known, effectiveness will necessarily be measured in terms of availability and quality of care. Availability of care can be measured by the degree to which financial, administrative, spatial, or social considerations impede the necessary treatment for perceived problems. Forecast needs can be compared with available or proposed facilities to determine the probability distribution of expected service delays. Quality of care is more difficult to measure but may be estimated by comparing actual treatment with professionally accepted norms for diagnostic tests performed, specialists and other special services utilized, number of examinations, etc. Meaningful conclusions can also be drawn by observing whether variations in utilization are correlated with medical needs or with less relevant factors such as income, race, place of residence, etc.

In other instances the inability to quantify relations between suspected causative factors and incidence of disease precludes the direct application of the case-month approach. Environmental health programs (e.g., pollution control) are important examples of a health subsystem to which the case-month measure of effectiveness is currently inapplicable. For these programs, meaningful measures can be derived in terms of average and maximum concentrations of various pollutants. Also some weighting scheme could be used to assign values to the probabilities of encountering various pollutant levels; e.g., a high weight would be assigned to a finite probability of a 'dangerous' condition and a low weight for an 'uncomfortable' situation. Another possibility is to approximate the case-month approach if disability states are defined for corresponding levels of discomfort as well as for resulting illnesses.

Finally, mental health is an important subsystem lacking the relation between health status and both the causes and the treatment of the disease. Many criteria noted previously are applicable: e.g., available, appropriate treatment and probable detection at various disease stages. Also, some objective measures are available, such as the discharge rate from mental hospitals, recidivism rate, etc. For the foreseeable future, however, the absence of quantified relations implies that effectiveness will have to be measured in terms of professionally accepted notions of treatment.

Development of program-specific measures of effectiveness is important because: (1) except at the highest policy level, planners of health services are, and will continue to be, concerned primarily with the allocation of resources within (not among) specific programs and (2) even at the highest policy level, program-specific cost-effectiveness schedules are necessary if interprogram allocation decisions are to be made rationally. That is, decisions allocating funds between, for example, dental health and a communicable disease program should be made on the basis of the 'best' (or at least good) programs in each category.

The measures suggested in this section cannot generally and consistently be related to the over-all (case-month) measure suggested previously. However, it may prove valuable to attempt to calculate such a measure, using rough estimates if necessary, as a supplement to more specific program measures. This procedure will force a consideration of the over-all point of view, identify major gaps in information, and encourage development of an operationally useful over-all measure of effectiveness that can be universally applied to all programs.

MEASURING THE COSTS

General

Costs of alternatives, as well as effectiveness, must be estimated in order to rationally allocate scarce resources. Costs are considered easier to handle than effectiveness because dollars are homogeneous and measurable. However, accurately estimating future costs is not simple. Consideration must be given to uncertainty of the estimates, to inflation, to the time-value of money (i.e., the discount rate to be used), to the opportunity costs of alternative uses, etc.

Recent research in health economics has distinguished between actual (direct) and implied (indirect) costs of medical care. Actual costs are true expenditures; implied costs are usually foregone earnings.

Actual Costs

Actual costs include expenditures for hospital and nursing home care, physician and nursing services, drugs, medical research, construction, medical education, training of personnel, and miscellaneous expenditures for administrative costs of programs, information and referral services, public education, etc. The most common conceptual error made with cost data is the failure to distinguish between costs that are fixed and costs that are variable relative to the considered alternatives. Planning decisions should be concerned with the *differences* in future costs. Thus, in measuring hospital costs, the part of the daily rate for room and board that is applied to pay off the building bonds is irrelevant to most planning decisions; yet reduction of hospital utilization that will postpone or eliminate the need for construction of a new facility is pertinent. Thus, the 'cost' of utilization of any facility may vary depending on the community's rate of population growth. For purposes of control as well as planning, distinction must be made between fixed and variable costs.

What is the relation between resource utilization and the costs of the definable elements? The costs of things bought in very small (inexpensive) quantities vary with utilization in a continuous fashion. These are the variable cost elements of the system. The term *semivariable* is frequently applied to costs whose relation to utilization is best depicted by a step function. If the 'steps' become sufficiently large so that only one level is associated with the range of utilization under consideration, the costs are referred to as fixed.

Interest and obsolescence charges associated with sunk costs, such as past construction expenditures, are the most obvious examples of fixed costs. Other expenditures, such as those for administration, heat and light, etc., are generally fixed for most decision making. Because of their discrete nature, personnel and equipment costs are generally semivariable, i.e., 1.5 public health nurses or 2.4 X-ray machines are unobtainable. These costs become more nearly continuously variable as the number of personnel or equipment considered grows. For example, expenditures for new facilities can also be viewed as semivariable if the community is large enough. Materials and supplies and externally contracted services are common examples of variable costs.

Figure 3 illustrates these ideas. As an example let the figure represent the relation between costs and utilization of a hospital facility. Let the fixed-cost line represent the unavoidable costs associated with the current facility; let the semivariable line represent equipment, and let the variable cost line represent labor and material costs (this latter straight line is, in fact, a step function with small steps). Assume initially that alternatives *A* and *B* are the only ones available. For this analysis both facility and equipment costs are fixed, i.e., uncontrollable. If alternative C is made available, then equipment costs become a control variable that must be considered. If a fourth alternative with a utilization rate high enough to

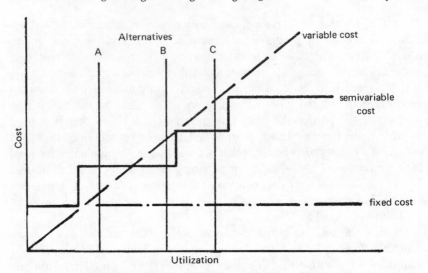

Fig. 3. Ways in which costs vary with utilization.

require additional investment in facilities is feasible, then the 'fixed' facility cost becomes a variable.

Planning (or budgeting) and control can be facilitated if costs are accumulated by cost centers or areas of responsibility. That is, the budget procedure should be such that expenditure estimates are initiated by the individual ultimately responsible for those funds and those areas of activity; the budgetary and management information systems should be designed to report the costs in the same manner. Thus, areas of authority and responsibility are made coincident and readily identifiable. Attempts to achieve these administrative goals may lead to more effective, functional organizations.

For example, if the state's chief public health officer is responsible for all state expenditures, budgets should be prepared and costs reported on that basis; but fixed costs for which he cannot be held responsible (e.g., for previously built facilities) should be excluded. On the other hand, if the officer in a specific clinic is responsible for only a few classes of personnel and inventory expenditures, these costs must be separately identified and reported. Only in this way can cost-effectiveness be applied at all levels of the organization and the budgeting, planning, and control functions be integrated.

Cost reporting considerations should be taken into account when building simulation models of the system; that is, the output should identify the relevant cost variables, where relevance of a variable is defined by its relation to the appropriate decision-maker. These remarks also apply to selecting the 'measure of effectiveness' variables included in the simulation output.

Implied Costs

Estimating the potential earnings lost because of the incidence of disease is more difficult than estimating actual expenditures made in its prevention and treatment (though the latter is difficult enough, especially for preventive programs not directed to a specific disease—e.g., community health education). Most calculations of implied costs are made in terms of the present value of future losses of output. Reduced efficiency, absenteeism, psychic, and other intangible costs are generally excluded. Values for productive time are calculated for each sex and age class within the labor force using average earnings and adjusting for unemployment rates. Wages for housewives' services are imputed as the mean earnings of domestic servants.[3] In other studies, attempts are made to estimate the earnings lost as a result of underemployment, and in one case a value is imputed to reduced earnings that are due to the social embarrassment of having had syphilis.[24]

Cost-Benefit Analysis

Cost-benefit analysis is an alternative to the cost-effectiveness approach to health planning. Cost-benefit analysis excludes consideration of those factors that cannot be ultimately measured in economic terms. In essence, it proposes that the sum of actual and implied costs be used as a single measure of effectiveness.[25, 26] As KLARMAN states:

> The total costs of a disease per case serve as the measure of benefits derived from preventing that case. In a cost-benefit calculation the comparison is between contemplated additional expenditures for health and medical services, on the one hand, and the anticipated reduction in costs (direct plus indirect), on the other hand. This is the essential conceptual framework.[27]

In this analysis, economic benefits that accrue to the individual (the implied costs) are lumped with cost-savings that accrue to the government. More useful results would be obtained if the bearer of the costs were identified: the individual, the community, or the government. If this is done, a straightforward cost-revenue evaluation could be made to determine the government's *net* cost of proposed programs: i.e., the cost of the program less the anticipated resultant reduction in other programs plus the tax yield from the anticipated additional earnings. Then the decision could be made on the basis of the net economic gain to society (the benefit) that can be obtained from a net public expenditure (the cost). The results of the cost-revenue analysis may also provide a boundary condition for initial program evaluation. (SILBERSTEIN has performed an interesting study along these lines in Israel.[28])

Cost-revenue and cost-benefit studies deal solely with elements that can be measured in economic terms; a cost-effectiveness study considers other 'benefits' in addition to those that are purely economic. However, it is still the net cost to the government of obtaining the economic and noneconomic benefits that is relevant. For instance, changes in productivity and changes in employment in the medical services industry that may result from alternative health programs are important economic factors that must be considered in determining the 'costs' of suggested programs.

The appropriate method of handling cost-benefit analyses or the economic aspects of cost-effectiveness analyses may be summarized as follows: For each examined alternative, first determine the resulting changes in income and expenditure streams of each party (public, private, community, etc.); then bring the streams to a single point in time (i.e., the present) by applying discount factors to determine the present value of each stream. The discount factors selected should reflect the opportunity costs, the time-value of money, and perhaps the costs of uncertainty. Concentrating on differences in net financial streams implies that fixed costs will be ignored in the decision-making and that semivariable costs will be considered only if they vary within the range contemplated by the analysis.

Though cost-benefit analysis is simple to handle mathematically, economic considerations cannot be the sole criterion for choosing among alternatives for an abundant society. (It may be more appropriate in a scarce manpower economy.) The cost-benefit approach distorts the conclusions by overemphasizing morbidity among males in their maximum earning years; by underestimating prevalent problems such as neurotic conditions, common colds, and certain allergenic conditions; and by ignoring intangible costs, etc. Actual and implied costs are important dimensions of any resource allocation decision; however, the cost-effectiveness framework permits (and demands) explicit consideration of variables that are measured not in dollars and cents but in terms of basic human values.

SUMMARY

The objective of this paper has been to investigate the applicability of current system design and evaluation concepts to planning community health service systems. The concepts include: systems analysis, model building and digital computer simulation, evaluation of system effectiveness, and cost estimating. Each of these topics requires considerably more attention than has been provided in this report. The more salient points and some tentative conclusions are summarized in the following paragraphs.

The costs and effectiveness of alternative system configurations are functions of many variables. System design requires identification of cost and effectiveness variables, specification of the relating functions or parameters, and estimation of their relative controllability.

Models of the total community health service system or significant subsystems within it can provide estimates of costs and effectiveness of alternative system configurations. Large-scale computer simulation models meet the methodological requirements for modeling such complex systems.

The measure of effectiveness of the community health system is essentially multidimensional. One approach has been suggested to reduce the many criteria to a single numerical value. Because of the incomparability of interpersonal utilities, a general solution cannot be achieved;* however, it is possible to restrict the area of ambiguity and to reduce the number of indistinguishable alternatives. For a large number of situations, it would appear that a single-valued measure is too restrictive and that the best results can be achieved by reducing the many criteria to a few significant measures to be ultimately reconciled by the policy-maker. The multidimensionality of the effectiveness measure is one of the significant considerations leading to the recommendation of the simulation approach.

Planning is ultimately concerned with future situations. Thus, the relevant costs, like the relevant measures of effectiveness, are those yet to be incurred. This requires that distinctions be made between fixed costs and those that vary owing to the decisions being made, that the degree of uncertainty be estimated, and that the opportunity value of money be considered.

REFERENCES

1. IDA C. MERRIAM, "Social Welfare Expenditures, 1964–1965," U.S. Department of Health, Education, and Welfare, Washington, D.C., U.S. Government Printing Office, 1965 (reprinted from *Social Security Bulletin,* October, 1965).
2. U.S. PUBLIC HEALTH SERVICE, *Principles for Planning the Future Hospital System,* Department of Health, Education, and Welfare, Washington, D.C., U.S. Government Printing Office, 1959.
3. SUBCOMMITTEE ON HEART DISEASE (The President's Commission on Heart Disease, Cancer, and Stroke), *A National Program to Conquer Heart Disease, Cancer, and Stroke,* U.S. Government Printing Office, Washington, D.C., 1965.
4. U.S. PUBLIC HEALTH SERVICE, *Research in Community Health,* Bureau of State Services, Department of Health, Education, and Welfare, U.S. Government Printing Office, Washington, D.C., 1962. (The Bureau of State Services' responsibilities have been reassigned under the most recent reorganization of the Public Health Service.)
5. AMERICAN MEDICAL ASSOCIATION, *Report to the Commission on the Cost of Medical Care,* Vol. I, pp. 8, 18, 26, 144, 145, (1964).

* A related, but somewhat different, approach to this problem is to view the decision-making process as an attempt to maximize a committee preference function subject to certain constraints.[29, 30]

6. CHARLES D. FLAGLE, "Operations Research in the Health Services," *Opns. Res.* **10**, 591–603 (1962).
7. D. G. MALCOLM, "The Use of Simulation Management Analysis," *Report of the Second System Simulation Symposium,* pp. 11–26, American Institute of Industrial Engineers, New York, 1959.
8. D. B. HERTZ, "Simulation for Problem Solving," *Report of the Second System Simulation Symposium,* pp. 27–29, New York: American Institute of Industrial Engineers, 1959.
9. PETER D. FOX, "A Theory of Cost-Effectiveness for Military Systems Analysis," *Opns. Res.* **13**, 191–202 (1965).
10. G. A. SILVER, *Family Medical Care,* Harvard University Press, Cambridge, Mass., 1963.
11. P. H. PERSON, JR., *The Relationship Between Selected Social and Demographic Characteristics of Hospitalized Mental Patients and the Outcome of Hospitalization,* American University, Washington, D.C., 1964.
12. DAVID G. KENDALL, "Mathematical Models of the Spread of Infection," *Mathematics and Computer Science in Biology and Medicine,* pp. 213–225, Mathematics Research Council, London, 1965.
13. M. ZELIN AND G. H. WEISS, *A Semi-Markov Model for Clinical Trials,* U.S. Army Mathematics Research Center, Madison, Wisc., 1963.
14. R. B. FETTER AND J. D. THOMPSON, "The Simulation of Hospital Systems," *Opns. Res.* **13**, 689–711 (1965).
15. NATIONAL CENTER FOR HEALTH STATISTICS, *Conceptual Problems in Developing an Index of Health,* U.S. Public Health Service Publication No. 1000-Series 2-No. 17, U.S. Government Printing Office, Washington, D.C., 1966.
16. ———, *An Index of Health—Mathematical Models,* U.S. Public Health Service Publication No. 1000-Series 2-No. 5, U.S. Government Printing Office, Washington, D.C., 1965.
17. B. S. SAUNDERS, "Measuring Community Health Levels," *American J. Public Health* **54**, 1063–1070 (1964).
18. A. BLUMSTEIN, "Operations Research Approach to the Problems of Law Enforcement and Criminal Juctice," presented at MIT seminar devoted to Operations Research in Public Affairs, September 10, 1966.
19. JOHN VON NEUMANN AND O. MORGENSTERN, *Theory of Games and Economic Behavior,* Princeton University Press, Princeton, N.J., 1944.
20. PETER C. FISHBURN, *Decision and Value Theory,* Wiley, New York, 1964.
21. H. CHERNOFF AND L. E. MOSES, *Elementary Decision Theory,* Wiley, New York, 1957.
22. GARDNER ACKLEY, *Macroeconomic Theory,* Macmillan, New York, 1961.
23. A. W. MARSHALL, *Cost/Benefit Analysis in Health,* p. 3, The Rand Corporation, Santa Monica, Calif., December, 1965.
24. HERBERT E. KLARMAN, "Syphilis Control Programs," *Measuring Benefits of Government Investment,* The Brookings Institution, Washington, D.C., 1965.
25. DOROTHY P. RICE, *Economic Cost of Cardiovascular Diseases and Cancer, 1962* ("Health Economics Series No. 5"), U.S. Public Health Service, May, 1965.
26. ———, *Estimating the Cost of Illness* ("Health Economics Series No. 6"), U.S. Public Health Service, May, 1966.
27. HERBERT E. KLARMAN, *The Economics of Health,* p. 163, Columbia University Press, New York, 1965.
28. J. SILBERSTEIN, "Cost of Non-Rehabilitation in Israel: A Pilot Study," *J. Chronic Disease* **17**, 991–1018 (1964).
29. K. J. ARROW, *Social Choice and Individual Value,* Cowles Commission Monograph No. 12, Wiley, New York, 1951.
30. H. THIEL, *Optimal Decision Rules for Government and Industry,* pp. 322–356, North-Holland Publishing Company, Amsterdam, 1964.

SELECTION 16

Cost-Effectiveness and Cost-Benefit Analyses for Public Health Programs*

Warren F. Smith

Cost effectiveness and cost benefit are subjects which, to those who are not professional economists, evoke a somewhat less than overwhelming response. They are, however, ingredients frequently mentioned in the recipes for planning-programing-budgeting systems and, if only for this reason, it becomes desirable to have a speaking acquaintance with these subjects.

Most persons who undertake a survey of the literature in this field quickly find the terms "cost effectiveness" and "cost benefit" used more or less interchangeably. Some writers, however, appear to make a firm distinction between the two terms, often without defining the difference.

I will attempt to differentiate between those expressions in this paper, although there is some lack of uniformity in the definition of terms even among economists.

In cost-benefit analysis, the monetary cost of a program is normally compared with its expected benefits, and normally these benefits are expressed in dollars. I use the word "normally" to indicate that there are exceptions. Costs, benefits, or both might be expressed in nondollar terms. An example of this is a comparison of different types of training programs for health service personnel. In such an example, "benefits" could be shown in number of persons trained, and "costs" could be shown in number of trainers needed, perhaps under different approaches. If training manpower is limited, the number of trainers could be more important than their salaries.

In a cost-benefit analysis of alternate programs, we compare the expected benefits to determine which is the best investment. Because of the frequent emphasis on the most effective use of money when given a choice of possible programs, both costs and benefits are usually expressed in dollars to permit ready comparison. For the same reason benefit divided by cost, the benefit-cost ratio, is often useful in making comparisons.

Cost-effectiveness analysis differs from cost-benefit analysis in that costs

* *Public Health Reports*, vol. 83, November, 1968.

are calculated and alternate ways are compared for achieving a specific set of results. Our objective is not just how to use funds most wisely; it also includes the constraint that a specified output must be achieved. Very often, this output is not expressed in dollars.

If we were told to determine the best program for training 1,000 nurses in a given time (to use the previous example of training) we could obtain costs of various training programs and make comparisons, and the study could be classified as one of cost effectiveness.

Cost-benefit studies expedite comparisons among several programs with differing objectives, whereas cost effectiveness generally refers to a comparison of different ways of reaching the same objective. In both cost-effectiveness and cost-benefit studies, we are frequently troubled because we have no satisfactory unit of measurement common to the benefits from various health programs.

Such indices as "years of gain in life expectancy" have been proposed as a useful yardstick to measure benefits. Some studies attempt to translate time into monetary terms by computing expected income loss because of premature death or disability.

Until we discover a universal unit for quantifying the value of health, ways to measure benefits will continue to hamper comparisons among alternate health programs. Perhaps of more importance, this lack complicates comparing benefits among health and nonhealth activities competing for limited funds.

Examples of Both Analyses

I will give some examples of these analyses, starting with a hypothetical benefit-cost ratio computation on a trivial scale. Assume that a pill X, which is on the market, will assure the user a day of good health and $20 for working that day. To make matters even more simple, also assume that without taking pill X the user will not be able to work and therefore will not earn the $20. If pill X costs $5, the benefit-cost ratio in dollars is 20 divided by 5 or 4.

Now before rushing out to buy pill X, we might also examine all other alternatives and discover that there are other similar pills with different probabilities of success or a different period of effectiveness. We might compute the ratios of all the alternatives, compare them, and from this information select what appears to be the best choice in terms of benefit-cost ratio.

As cost-benefit studies are used in health program planning, they often concern comparisons among different programs, each vying for financial support. It may be necessary to decide if an admittedly desirable program must be completely scrapped simply because other programs are more deserving of limited funds.

Unfortunately, we must often make these decisions with incomplete information. Still worse, there may be well-recognized factors affecting the analysis which are deliberately ignored, either because we do not know how to deal with them in a quantitative sense or because we believe their effect is too small to justify laborious computation, or a little of each.

Returning to the pill example, suppose that in our search of alternatives we find a pill Y for $4 which will give the same return (a day of good health) as pill X. We will consider the relative virtues of pills X and Y in determining a ratio of effectiveness to cost, and we might further assume that the user does not necessarily want to work. He values a day of good health just because it gives him some time free from disease or discomfort. To him it is only a day to be used as he chooses—working, playing, or just sleeping.

On a cost-effectiveness scale, the ratio with pill X is 1 to 5 or 0.2 and with pill Y, 1 to 4 or 0.25. The units are now days of good health per dollar and again pill Y is the winner, but now it is no longer clear if either pill is a good choice. The decision rests on someone's judgment as to whether or not the return is worth the cost.

According to my earlier distinction, the output now is specified as days of good health, and we seek a pill which will achieve this result most economically. In using this changed approach, a decision maker has the responsibility of imposing his judgment, whereas before he could claim his decision had some economic justification.

A benefit-cost dollar ratio gave him a magic number to work with because presumably any project with a ratio of 1 or larger could at least pay its own way, and anything with a ratio of less than 1 was a loser. This somewhat flippant description of cost-benefit analysis should not, however, be construed to minimize its real value. Much serious and valuable work is going on right now, using cost-benefit studies to assist authorities to reach decisions.

In 1966, Mr. Gardner, former Secretary of the Department of Health, Education, and Welfare, appointed study groups to make a series of health program analyses and to investigate the costs and benefits of certain health programs. In making their studies, the analysts (1) used purely economic costs and benefits, although they pointed out that "For the purposes of estimating benefits among diseases, it is recognized that economic loss or even death do not completely state the damage and harm caused by disease. Pain and the impact on family relationships are among the more obvious additional items. We do not know how to bring such items into this kind of analysis as yet. . . ."

Despite some shortcomings, these analyses can be highly useful. But before examining some actual analyses, I want to discuss briefly some pitfalls to avoid in making these studies.

Avoiding Errors in Using the Analyses

Comparing total rather than only marginal costs is an error that is difficult to avoid. What should be analyzed is the effect of change from the present situation, both in new benefits and new costs. For example, suppose we have an investment of $10 in a device which produces 50 units an hour and we learn of the invention of two improvements which will increase this machine's efficiency. Item A, an adapter costing $5, allows the device to produce 60 instead of 50 units per hour. Item B, costing $7, can increase the output to 65 units per hour. Assuming that we are going to buy one of the new adapters and that we will not consider operating costs, market conditions, or final equipment disposition, which adapter would be the best choice from a cost-effectiveness standpoint?

Wrong. The total cost, if we buy item A, will be the original $10 plus the added $5, or $15, and the total resultant output is 60 units per hour. Dividing output by cost gives us a ratio of 60 to 15 or 4. The total cost, using item B, will be the original $10 plus $7, or $17 with a resultant output of 65, or a ratio of 65 to 17 or 3.8. The conclusion using this misleading analysis is that item A is preferred because it seems to give the largest ratio of effectiveness to cost.

Right. The marginal or added cost for item A is $5, and the added output is 10 units per hour for a ratio of 10 to 5 or 2.0. The marginal cost using item B is $7 and the added output is 15, giving a ratio of 15 to 7 or 2.1. Our conclusion using this correct procedure is that item B is preferred because of its greater marginal ratio.

The point is that the level of expenditure made in the past, whether good, bad, or indifferent, won't affect the decision on items A and B, so the analysis should be limited to the effect of change only.

Another frequent problem is caused by trying to find a policy which simultaneously gives the greatest benefit and the least cost. Cost analysis studies may seek a policy which will realize the greatest benefit at a given cost, or a given benefit at the least cost, but not both at the same time. This fact can be seen very easily by comparing some hypothetical alternatives. Suppose we could spend $1 and gain $3 for the ratio of $3 to $1 or 3. Compare that with the expenditure of $100 for a benefit of $500 for a ratio of 5. The second choice certainly seems best and maybe it is—if we have the $100. If we don't, it is immaterial what the ratios are. The larger benefit is obtainable only with a larger cost.

Now assume that for $100 we could get a $300 benefit, again with a benefit-cost ratio of 3. We see that there is no preferred choice between this ratio and the previous one of $3 to $1, yet anyone can see by simple inspection that, despite what the ratios say, a profit of $200 is better than one of $2. To avoid this difficulty, some economists prefer not to use a ratio, but instead to compute marginal benefit minus marginal cost.

The fact that investments in the public sector tend to come in large chunks causes another type of problem in cost-benefit analysis. Only on paper is it possible to build half a water purification plant, and in reality most projects require large discrete expenditures. Sometimes particular combinations of projects, if they are possible under the total budget, are especially efficient but may get overlooked. To illustrate, suppose we have $100 to invest, with the following alternatives:

A brings a return of $600 for a cost of $60—the benefit-cost ratio is 600 to 60 or 10.

B brings a return of $500 for a cost of $40—the benefit-cost ratio is 500 to 40 or 12.5.

C brings a return of $1,000 for a cost of $70—the benefit-cost ratio is 1,000 to 70 or 14.3.

Using these ratios, C looks to be the preferred choice, because it has the highest ratio. But closer inspection shows that a combination of A and B with a combined ratio of 600 plus 500 over 60 plus 40, equaling 11 is pretty good too.

Combining A and B brings a return of $1,100 whereas C only returned $1,000. True, with C there was some money left over, but even if we count this in, we end up with only $1,000 plus $30 or $1,030 as compared with $1,100.

The difficulty, of course, is that in so readily taking the best individual bargain we reduced our budget to a point where we could no longer take advantage of any other opportunities. Cost-benefit analysis didn't really fall down on the job, because C is the best way to spend $70.

Are we to use our money (really the public's money) to find the best bargain? Or are we supposed to use it to get the greatest return? Unfortunately, we have seen that these two aren't necessarily the same. There is a need for a clear-cut statement of objectives as a prerequisite of any meaningful cost-benefit or cost-effectiveness analysis.

Another part of these analyses that cannot be overlooked is that of discounting, a procedure that is used extensively in dealing with future costs or benefits. The purpose of discounting is to convert the economic implications of actions taking place later to their equivalent value now. To do this, we use interest tables and a discount rate that supposedly represents the value of money over time. Just as by using interest tables we can find how much $1 invested today will be worth at some time in the future, so we can do the reverse and find out how much a dollar needed some years from now is worth today. For example, the present value of a dollar to be used 1 year from now is about 91 cents, if money is worth 10 percent interest.

It is important to know what interest rate to use. At first thought, this seems apparent, but further thought indicates that it is not so simple. The rate should represent what the money is worth if it were available for other uses. Now the difficulty is one of worth to whom and for what other uses. If we are limiting our thinking to government, you might say that money is worth what the government pays to borrow it, say interest that is paid on E bonds. Others think it should measure the cost of using private capital in the form of taxes to the government, private capital that might have been used elsewhere; therefore, the rate ought to be the going market rate of interest or more.

Another interesting fact about the time preference for money is that it tends to vary inversely with the life expectancy. In other words, younger persons seem willing to wait for a future payoff but, as you might expect, the older we get, the more interested we are in quick results if we are to use them.

Fairly small variations in the discount rate can often lead to big differences in the cost-benefit ratio. To illustrate this, consider an activity costing $100 a year. Assume that by the end of the year the $100 has been spent, and the resultant benefit is equivalent to $105. Without doing any discounting (zero percent), the net benefit in dollars is 105–100 or 5.

If a discount rate of 5 percent were used, the net program benefit in dollars would be zero, because at this rate of return, the $100 could have given a $105 benefit even without the activity. If a 10 percent discount rate were used, however, there would be an apparent $5 loss for this activity because the money it cost might have been used otherwise to obtain $110 in benefit instead of only $105.

Why all this fuss over a technical detail? Because discounting is particularly important when a long timespan is covered, as often happens with health programs in which some benefits accrue only many years after the outlay (2).

With so many difficulties to consider, are the results worth all the effort? Wildavsky, a nationally recognized cost-benefit analyst, says cost-benefit studies are shot through with political and social value choices and surrounded by uncertainties and difficulties of calculation (3).

But he also says that the method has great utility by telling decision makers what they will be giving up if they follow alternative plans. He admits that the cost-benefit formula does not always jibe with political realities—it omits political costs and benefits—and we can expect it to be twisted out of shape from time to time. Yet, he sees the method as being of great importance in getting rid of the worst projects and asserts that avoiding the worst when one can't get the best is no small accomplishment.

Example of a Cost-Benefit Study

Now that we have discussed some pros and cons of these methods, let's examine some actual studies made by professionals.

I will summarize briefly part of a cost-benefit analysis done in late 1966 (4). In this study, several ways of preventing motor vehicle accidents

TABLE 1

PRESENT PROGRAM COSTS AND ESTIMATED LOSSES IN THOUSANDS OF DOLLARS, BEFORE DISCOUNTING

| Year | Present Program Costs | Total Losses | Losses from Injury | | | Mortality Losses |
			Total	Direct Costs	Indirect Costs	
Total-----	$16,600	$32,700,000	$7,800,000	$4,300,000	$3,400,000	$24,900,000
1968 -----	3,200	6,200,000				
1969 -----	3,300	6,300,000				

were compared. Of all the alternatives, the list was narrowed down to nine that were considered both feasible and realistic. Of these nine possibilities, I have picked one for discussion. The goal of this program was to prevent motor vehicle injuries by improving driver training. This is how the analysts proceeded.

Step 1. A baseline was established from which to measure change. Remember that the increment of change is the essential ingredient in cost-benefit analysis. The baseline used was the present level of program activities, costs, fatalities, and injuries, which are listed in tabular form. Since some activities and some level of accidents will necessarily take place in the future even with no program change, it was also necessary to project what the future would hold even if nothing different were done.

It was assumed that the present level of effort would remain relatively constant through 1972. The number of fatalities and injuries was also projected through 1972, based on existing trends. Population projections were obtained from the census, mortality and injury data were obtained from the national health survey and other sources, and trend lines were plotted on graph paper.

Step 2. A common denominator was determined by converting fatalities

TABLE 2
ADDED PROGRAM COSTS IN THOUSANDS OF DOLLARS AND
REDUCTION IN INJURIES AND FATALITIES

Added Program Costs		Reductions	
Actual	Discounted	Number of Injuries	Number of Fatalities
$825,000	$750,550	665,300	8,515

and injuries into dollar costs. To do this, lost earnings as a result of premature death were determined. The cost of days lost from work as a result of injury and a number of other costs, such as those from days of hospitalization and physician visits, were also computed. Almost all these data were nonexistent and had to be developed from other records. Table 1, although incomplete, shows the general procedure used to calculate program costs and losses, assuming present levels.

I have presented the table primarily because the derivation of the information is important for analysts. Direct costs include hospital care, physician's services, nursing home care, drugs, and medical supplies. Indirect costs include loss of earnings by those whose injuries kept them from working. Mortality costs include the expected lifetime earnings (before conversion to present value by discounting) for the projected fatalities in each year, based on life expectancy tables. It was assumed that unemployment would average 4 percent and that earnings would be the same as in 1964.

It may be of interest to know how the study group handled housewives' services. Losses for housewives who were expected to be incapacitated because of motor vehicle accidents were based on the wages earned by domestic servants. After adjustment for wage supplements, a housewife's salary was estimated to be $2,767 annually, using 1964 data.

Step 3. The alternative, a program to improve driver education and training, was fully described.

Step 4. The change in status if this alternative were in effect was calculated (table 2).

Step 5. The costs and benefits were computed and the final ratio obtained (table 3).

Some of the major assumptions in this example were as follows: First, calculations were based on an assumption that improved methods of basic driver training, education, and retraining could reduce the number of deaths and injuries from motor vehicle accidents by 20 percent annually after the program has been in operation for 5 years.

Second, during the first 5 years an average reduction of 10 percent was expected. If this estimate is in error, and the actual death and injury reduction proves to be only 5 to 6 percent during these first years, the benefit-cost ratio becomes less than one. How sure was the study group of their estimate? They stated, "There is little doubt that some improvements are possible with better training and education, but how much remains a big question. Furthermore, methods to evaluate this program are crude and consist mainly in instituting the program and then either observing changes in accident rates with time or in comparing other comparable populations who don't have the program."

Our conclusion might be that this program appears to be worthwhile, but certainly we should not be overconfident that it will effectively reduce deaths and injuries. If a budget cut became necessary, this program might be one of the first to go because of its relatively low rank.

Example of a Cost-Effectiveness Study

My next example is a September 1967 report for the Bureau of the Budget, utilizing the cost-effectiveness approach (5). This study on the treatment of kidney disease was undertaken by a group of physicians, statisticians, and economists who specifically noted that they felt that a cost-benefit analysis was inappropriate partly because of the difficulty of putting a value on human life.

The study compares the effectiveness and cost of two alternate ways of prolonging the life of persons otherwise doomed to an early death because of end-stage kidney disease. New technological capabilities and the obvious consequences of no action (death) make this investigation unusual.

Two possible means of prolonging the life of persons suffering from end-stage uremia are a kidney transplant or the use of dialysis equipment, generally known as the artificial kidney. Both techniques can be used in various combinations, such as repeated transplants followed by dialysis.

Effectiveness is measured in a straightforward comparison of the number of years of life expected to be added, on the average, through transplantation or dialysis. This comparison originally assumed that a gain in years of life by one mode of treatment is the same in quality as that from another treatment method. The study group, however, could not accept this because the volume of evidence suggested a difference in the value of the added time.

A patient dependent on mechanical dialysis equipment must limit his actions to some extent—a geographic limitation, for example—because he must be able to get to the equipment when it is needed. Also, certain restrictions in diet must be followed by persons using the artificial kidney, restrictions that do not affect those with a transplant.

Although the committee did not go so far as to suggest that their weighting factor was the result of rigorous analysis, they did accept a factor of 1.25 to weight the value of a year of life gained after transplantation more heavily than that gained by hemodialysis. They stated that this factor was for illustrative purposes but even so it seems extremely significant that a committee of this status publicly went on record as accepting the difficult premise that life under some conditions could be 25 percent more valuable than under other conditions.

The philosophical point to be emphasized is that this in no way implies that some people's lives are more important than others. This fact is not the issue here, and it would be unfair to imply this. However, the concept of different values of time, because of the various uses to which time can be put, is an important and controversial one to many researchers.

On the cost side of the ledger, the computations were made more complex because the cost of failures as well as successes must be included on the presumption that all medically suitable patients will be treated.

A further complication of the dialysis alternative is the large difference in cost, depending on whether treatment is done at a center or in the home.

TABLE 3. ADDED PROGRAM COSTS AND SAVINGS, IN THOUSANDS OF DOLLARS, AND BENEFIT-COST RATIO

| Costs of added program | Total savings | Morbidity savings | | | Mortality savings | Benefit-cost ratio |
		Total	Direct	Indirect		
$750,550	$1,287,000	$213,000	$117,000	$96,000	$1,074,000	1.7

In making the calculations, life tables were constructed to show the life expectancies under each treatment mode. A further example of the committee's need for innovation was that not enough time has elapsed to permit reliable estimates of long-range life expectancies in this new field; estimates must therefore be based on speculation and the best testimony now available.

The results from computing effectiveness showed than an average marginal life expectancy of 9.0 years could be expected for a person on dialysis treatment compared with 17.2 years for one in the transplantation group (actually 13.3 added years from a successfully transplanted kidney followed by 3.9 more years on dialysis after eventual failure of the transplant). After adjustment at $13.3 \times 1.25 + 3.9$, an estimate of 20.5 quality-adjusted years of life is obtained—more than twice as much as that for persons under dialysis treatment (Table 4).

Adding another column (not in the report) to show the ratio of effectiveness to cost, using years of life gained as the effectiveness measure and costs in $10,000(s), yields the following figures:

	Years of life gained
Treatment	Costs in $10,000
Dialysis:	
Center	0.9
Home	2.4
Transplantation:	
Unadjusted	3.8
Adjusted for quality	4.6

These cost-effectiveness computations indicate that, in increasing the average life expectancy of end-stage uremia patients, the transplantation method provides the lowest cost per year of added life expectancy. Fortunately, it also appears to offer the greatest prospect for added length of life.

One early conclusion of the study group was reached, not as a direct result of this cost-effectiveness analysis, but because of the incidental gain in program understanding due to the study process. This conclusion was that there were not enough available kidneys for transplant and that many were lost after transplantation. The group recognized that research directed at organ storage and preservation and at tissue typing ought to be high on the priority list of kidney disease research.

They also saw that even sizable reductions in the cost of equipment were not likely to exert a radical effect on the overall cost of dialysis because costs were largely for personnel at dialysis centers. Therefore, efforts should be concentrated on possible means of minimizing staffing at dialysis centers rather than devoting significant funds to equipment refinements.

The committee concluded that "In terms of cost effectiveness there are advantages in an approach oriented toward transplantation . . . research activities directed at making transplantation more widely applicable and efficacious are likely to yield considerable economic benefits."

Conclusions

We have looked at some examples of cost-benefit and cost-effectiveness analysis, moving from trivial hypothetical instances to some reasonably complex examples of real analyses. Despite difficulties with these methods of analysis, they can be useful decision aids, although even their most ardent proponents would probably not suggest that they be decision determinants.

Prest and Turvey (6) stated recently that " . . . one can view cost-benefit analysis as anything from an infallible means of reaching the new Utopia to a waste of resources in attempting to measure the unmeasurable."

I think you will be seeing and hearing more about these techniques in

TABLE 4. Cost Per Year, Discounted, and Years of Life
Gained by Two Treatments for Kidney Disease

Treatment	Cost	Years of life gained	Cost per year
Dialysis:			
Center	$104,000	9	$11,600
Home	38,000	9	4,200
Transplantation:			
Unadjusted	44,500	17	2,600
Adjusted for quality ...	44,500	20.5	2,200

Source: Reference 5.

the future because they are a crucial element in the planning, programming, and budgeting systems. William Gorham, former Assistant Secretary of HEW (7) said, "A major task under PPB will be cost-effectiveness analyses of alternative solutions to particular social problems. The analyses will, at first, be crude. New measurements of effectiveness will have to be devised, experimented with, and refined. New data will have to be collected, both on cost and on effectiveness. 'Educated guesses' will have to be employed, tested, and revised."

Like most methodologies in a state of test and revision, there are bound to be successes and failures as refinements are made in these analyses.

REFERENCES

1. U.S. Department of Health, Education, and Welfare: Program analysis series. U.S. Government Printing Office, Washington, D.C., 1966.
2. Klarman, H. E.: Syphilis control program. *In* Measuring benefits of government investments, edited by R. Dorfman. The Brookings Institution, Washington, D.C., 1965.
3. Wildavsky, A.: The political economy of efficiency; cost-benefit analysis, systems analysis, and program budgeting. Public Admin Rev 26: 292–310, December 1966.
4. U.S. Department of Health, Education, and Welfare: Motor vehicle injury prevention program (analysis). U.S. Government Printing Office, Washington, D.C., 1966.
5. Report of the Committee on Chronic Kidney Disease. U.S. Government Printing Office, Washington, D.C., 1967.
6. Prest, A. R., and Turvey, R.: Cost-benefit analysis: A survey. Econ J 75:683–735, December 1965.
7. Gorham, W.: Allocating Federal resources among competing social needs. HEW Indicators, U.S. Government Printing Office, Washington, D.C., August 1966, pp. 1–11.

Chapter 8

Health Information Systems

8.1 INTRODUCTION

Communication and information are the lifeblood of an organization. Neither planning nor decision-making, or for that matter any other managerial process, is possible without communication and information. Communication can be viewed as the process of exchange of information; it provides the means of contact between organizational members and organizational decision centers. Included in the various ways in which an organization can be analyzed is the view of an organization as a communication network. According to this view, an organization consists of decision centers or "nodes" between which flow of information takes place. The design of an efficient and effective communication network is a fundamental requirement for managerial decision-making. The purpose of the network is to facilitate the flow of information between different decision centers of the organization. In this chapter we will define the term information; briefly describe its uses in managerial decision-making; discuss relationships between management or health information systems and the computer; and provide a methodology for designing an information system. Lastly, we cite some of the applied aspects of health information systems.

8.2 WHAT IS INFORMATION?

Information can be defined as *potential* knowledge. Information is valued for its capacity to increase knowledge, although in actuality it may or may not do so. [Wilson & Wilson, 1965, p. 22] No organization can function without an adequate exchange of information between its decision centers. Decision-making is based on the availability of the right type of information at the right time. Information must be gathered, processed, and transmitted to designated points in the organization. Information sources that

381

generate data* must be connected, directly, or indirectly, to information users. The important considerations in providing information relate to the *type, amount, form,* and *frequency* of information required in decision-making processes. In addition, in order to be effective, information must be timely relevant, valid, and properly processed.†

Information is transmitted in the form of symbols, images, descriptive statements, or "hard" data. Since information is relevant input for decision-making, data must be separated according to the needs of the various decision classes. For example, data can be grouped according to information requirements for strategic decisions, administrative decisions, and operational decisions. In the hospital setting, data can be separated to meet the needs of the medical or nursing staff, the administrator, the financial group, and various reimbursement agencies. Within each decision class, data can be further classified into: currently useful data, potentially useful data, and extraneous data.‡ The identification, collection, classification, processing, communication, interpretation, storage, and retrieval of relevant data are important aspects of an information system.

Information has always been the fundamental ingredient in managerial decision-making. Recently, however, we have witnessed an information explosion.§ The amount and variety of information have been growing at an exponential rate. Administrators must learn to cope with this phenomenon; they must *manage* information, not be buried by the avalanche of irrelevant data. Each organization must develop a system for the purpose of making more effective decisions. They must take advantage of modern information technology‖ to develop a structure or system out of inter-related data. The awareness of this need has resulted in the emergence of a new area called *Management Information Systems.*

---

* McDonough [1963, p. 71] describes "data" to be messages that have not been evaluated for their worth in a specific situation. "Information" is seen as *evaluated data,* and all communications in an organization is seen as some form of data processing.

† Information is a resource with its attendant *costs* and *benefits.* It is possible to conduct a cost-benefit analysis in designing an information system. Such an analysis is the purpose of economic feasibility studies before installing a formal information system. For a framework of information economics, see [McDonough, 1963, Chapters 5 and 6].

‡ Another way to classify data is by five dichotomies suggested by Dearden and McFarlan [1966, p. 6]: (1) Action and nonaction, (2) Recurring and nonrecurring, (3) Documentary and nondocumentary, (4) Internal and external, and (5) Historical and future.

§ See Toffler [1970].

‖ Myers [1967, p. 18] describes information technology as having three components: (1) The Computer, (2) Telecommunications, and (3) Management Science Techniques. The computer is viewed as an "engine" which is an "information converter, processer, transformer, and receptacle."

8.3 MANAGEMENT AND HEALTH INFORMATION SYSTEMS

Management information systems (referred to in the literature as MIS) derive their name and meaning from the fact that their focus is on the flow of information and that they represent a network rather than an isolated exchange of information required for management decisions. An information system is the set of "procedures, methodologies, organization, software, and hardware elements needed to insert and retrieve selected data as required for operating and managing a company" [Moravec, 1965, p. 38]. Health Information Systems or Hospital Information Systems (frequently labeled HIS) are management information systems for health-related organizations. The principles, methods, tools, and techniques for developing and installing MIS and HIS are essentially the same except that health care organizations have some unique problems. They encompass human life—the delivery of health care to prevent sickness, restore health, and for rehabilitation. As such they are all the more important and the experience with MIS accumulated in the business world can and should be utilized in developing computer based health information systems. This fact is increasingly being recognized by health care administrators [Jackson, 1970].

The boundaries of an information system can be drawn according to area of activity, level of sophistication and by scope. For example, we can study financial, personnel, logistics, or patient information systems.* Information systems can be simple (consists of elementary computer programs) or advanced (have on-line, real time capabilities†). Their scope can be "fundamental" as opposed to "total".‡ Information systems have been related to computer programs by Prince [1970, p. 39] on a continuum

---

* Prince [1970, p. 85] lists 6 dimensions of information that are relevant in each major or minor information system: (1) sources of information, (2) types of information, (3) measurement methods applied to the information, (4) the time dimensions of the requirements for information, (5) the location of the decision-maker requiring such information, and (6) the use of the information by the decision-maker.

† Donald Carroll [in Myers 1967, p. 143] gives this definition of an on-line, real-time system: Remotely located transaction-origination stations are connected directly ("on-line") to the central processor; and transactions are processed immediately upon origination (in "real time"), subject only to delays resulting from the processing of the transaction itself and from queuing behind transactions of earlier origination or otherwise higher priority. To fulfill the requirement of "real time," these delays must be negligible in the context of the particular application.

‡ For a concept comparison between "fundamental" and "total" information, see Moravec [1965, p. 38]. Briefly, a "fundamental" system is limited to data considered absolutely essential for the firms mission; whereas a "total" information system includes all data for "all the needs of all levels of management and operations."

running from 1 to 10, where a computer program has a rating of 1 and an advanced information system a rating of 10. (See Figure 8.1.)

FIG. 8.1
A CONTINUUM SHOWING RELATIVE POSITIONS OF PROGRAMS AND SYSTEMS

Computer Program	Activity Program	Functional Program	Operating System	Information System	Advanced Information System

←——→

1   5   10

Source: [Prince, 1970, p. 39].

The following definitions* will help clarify the terms shown in Figure 8.1.

Computer Program: A set of instructions to be followed by the computer.

Activity Program: A network of integrated computer programs directed at a specified activity (e.g., patient scheduling).

Functional Program: A much larger network of computer programs directed at a functional area (e.g., patient accounting).

Operating System: A self-contained unit of a computer-based integrated network that can monitor and control a significant grouping of activities. Human decision-makers are not an integral part of the system.

Information System: Consists of one or more operating systems with the additional provision that human decision-makers (management) are able to introduce desired changes in the system through appropriate mechanisms contained in the network.

Advanced Information System: The advanced (on-line, real time) form of the information system directed at the total organization.

Information systems and computers are intimately related. Any meaningful information system, especially in complex health care organizations, will be operationally unfeasible without the computer. Thus, Prince [1970, p. 40] defines a management information system as a *"computer-based* network containing one or more operating systems, which provides relevant data to management for decision-making purposes and also contains the necessary mechanism for implementing changes or responses made by management in this decision-making activity." However, the study, analysis, and design of an information system proceeds in stages in which the deci-

---

* These definitions are simplified versions of the descriptions in Prince [1970, pp. 35–46].

sion whether to acquire a computer can come last. This point is emphasized by several authorities in the field. "The important consideration for management," write Dearden and McFarlan [1966, p. 18], "is the effectiveness of the information system and not whether to acquire computer capability." The effectiveness of information systems and of the computer system "are not necessarily the same." Withington [1966, p. 3] states that the study of information systems is not the study of computers. "It is the study of how the organization communicates and processes information to maximize the effectiveness of management and further the objectives of the organization." Our view on the matter is that computers are necessary but not a sufficient condition for building an effective health care system. The health care administrator need not be a computer expert, but he must be familiar with the issues involved (from a management point of view) and should be able to communicate with the computer specialists. We subscribe to the view expressed by Prince [1970, p. 59]:

. . . the majority of the (information system) team members should intentionally not be too deeply aware of the "state of art" in regard to computer systems, transmission equipment, and other supporting facilities. Instead the team members should be predominantly management-types with a strong orientation to the organization and to its environment.

8.4 INFORMATION SYSTEM DESIGN

Although there does not seem to be any unique management science method to select an optimum configuration for an information system, our own experience suggests the following steps for designing a formal system:*

Step 1. *Determine the organizational need for information.*
This involves a study of decision-making activities in the organization. What types of decisions are made? At what levels and where in the organization are these decisions made? What type of information is needed for making these decisions? This step identifies the requirements for information.

Step 2. *Identify the sources of information.*
Identification of original and intermediate sources of information can be made by drawing an input-output type schematic for each center. The decision center is treated as a "black box"; only its inputs and outputs are identified and shown on the schematic for each decision center.

---

* Prince [1970, pp. 47–60] discusses five phases in planning and implementing an information system: (1) planning, including commitment and orientation by executive management, (2) organization review and administrative study, (3) conceptual systems design, (4) equipment selection and program design, and (5) implementation. The reader is also referred to a schematic plan for designing an information system [Moravec, 1965, Fig. 6].

Step 3. *Synthesize the results of steps 1 and 2.*
The product of this is a network connecting all decision centers in the organization.

Step 4. *Decide on the amount, form, and frequency of information.*
This step involves eliminating unwanted information, streamlining required information. In this step we evolve the essential elements of the information system.

Step 5. *Choose the means of information communication and information processing.*
It is in this step that we select computer software, hardware, and other supporting equipment.

Step 6. *Implement the system.*
The step involves installing the system, improving it, and securing cooperation from organizational members.

8.5 APPLIED HEALTH INFORMATION SYSTEMS

The operational consequences of some major elements of an information system for hospital management, as outlined by Griffith,* are reproduced below:

—Basic measures of resource utilization and output will be generated essentially as a by-product of computerized accounting processes.

—Data on the quality and utilization of medical care will be obtained from an abstracting process very similar to the present PAS system. This will be manual until the record itself is computerized. It may remain a manual process, at least in part, some time after that.

—Additional information on the state of the demand upon the system, and the quality of performance will be input to the computer at frequent intervals (daily or more often). This information will be used in staffing, scheduling, inventory reorder and quality control models, to advise middle management of hospitals in a variety of areas.

—There will be provisions to include specialized data of various kinds pertinent to specific planning or control problems. This will include special sampling studies and opinion surveys. Computer routines will facilitate analysis, while data collection will be largely manual.

—Data banks of historical information in output, resource consumption, quality and other statistics of interest will be available on either magnetic tape or disk storage. These data will be organized to facilitate either routine or special computer analysis. They will include comparative information among hospitals and regional compilations.

—Computer programs will be available for most analytic tasks. These will include general programs for multiple regression and analysis of variance,

* See Chapter XIV of John R. Griffith's manuscript *Quantitative Planning and Control.*

statistical quality control, simulation, and mathematical programming. They will also include routines for constructing graphs and visual display. Specialized programs will be developed for handling recurring decisions such as inpatient scheduling and nurse staffing.

—There will be provision for both routine and specialized output. Routine outputs will be highly differentiated and oriented to the needs of individual hospitals and departments. They will stress error signals and tend to suppress normal findings. The reports will be oriented towards management action rather than data display, since the original data will be on file and special reports can draw upon the files as needed.

The health care literature indicates rapid progress in the development and installation of information systems with different levels of sophistication.*

Singer [1969] conducted a survey of 20 hospitals to study information systems using on-line and real time computer techniques. Based on the survey results, four categories of computer systems were formulated and discussed. (1) large-scale, multi-hospital systems, (2) large-scale, single hospital systems, (3) shared-service-bureau hospital systems, and (4) computer systems dedicated to servicing specialized application areas.

Needles [1969] describes how a "single" information flow system might work in a hospital to meet a wide variety of demand. Evans and Campbell [1970] provide the results of a health information system project whose aim was to develop a structured approach for the characterization and analysis of System Options and to assist in its application. The approach was utilized in choosing a time-phased health information system.

A majority of existing systems are limited to patient billing, accounts payable, payroll, and inventory. Some have developed computer applications for patient care (laboratory tests, automated master patient record files, patient logistics, etc.) and general research. For example, Siegel [1968, pp. 359–362] describes the introduction of a system called THOMIS (Total Hospital Operating and Medical Information System) at the State University of New York—Downstate Medical Center, Brooklyn. THOMIS is an integrated system consisting of three major subsystems: (1) Operations Control System (to control day-to-day operations), (2) Management Reporting System (to generate summarized management reports) and (3) Inquiry System (to yield relevant data on receiving specific inquiries). The three subsystems use the same data but their outputs are designed to meet different needs of the hospital. An example of a system at the next level of sophistication is the Connecticut Utilization and Patient Information Statistical System (CUPISS).†

---

* See References listed at the end of Chapter 8.
† See Chapter XIV of John R. Griffith's manuscript *Quantitative Techniques for Planning and Control* for a description of CUPISS.

8.6 CONCLUDING REMARKS

The concepts of information, communication, and information systems were defined and discussed. Steps for analyzing and designing a formal information system were listed and elaborated. Also outlined were the operational consequences of some major elements of an information system for hospital management. The discussion in this chapter is supplemented by two articles related to health information systems.

Schwartz (Selection 17) describes the salient items included in what can be called "techniques and applications of hospital information systems." A hospital information system (HIS) is defined and its basics listed. Benefits of HIS systems are enumerated; and a brief account of their growth is provided. The author also reviews different types* of hospital information systems, and lists the names of hospitals where they have been installed. Applications of the business office and patient care subsystems are described and their benefits to the hospital administrator are detailed. Finally, the author presents an overview of the potential HIS applications in an appendix.

Barnett's article (Selection 18) was selected because it touches on an important aspect of interface between the physician and the hospital administrator. The potential of the computer in assisting the physician for delivering improved medical care must be appreciated by the hospital administrator. Barnett provides a succinct review of seven major areas of computer applications in medicine: (1) medical diagnosis; (2) clinical laboratory; (3) screening; (4) patient monitoring; (5) medical record; (6) automated medical history; and (7) hospital information systems.

REFERENCES

Carroll, D. C., "Implications of On-Line, Real-Time Systems for Managerial
1967   Decision-Making," in C. A. Myers (ed.), *The Impact of Computers on Management,* Cambridge, Mass.: The M.I.T. Press, pp. 140–165.

Dearden, J., and F. W. McFarlan, *Management Information Systems: Text*
1966   *and Cases,* Homewood, Ill.: Richard D. Irwin.

Evans, J. A., and R. V. D. Campbell, "The Structuring of Health Information
1970   System Options: Summary and Assessment of Methodology," *Socio-Econ. Planning Sciences,* vol. 4, June, pp. 291–309.

Jackson, G. G., "The Role of Administrators and Physicians in the Develop-
1970   ment of Hospital Information Systems," *Computers and Automation,* June.

McDonough, A. M., *Information Economics and Management Systems,* New
1963   York: McGraw-Hill.

---

* The four categories reviewed by Schwartz are similar to Singer's classification [1969]. See section 8.5.

Moravec, A. J., "Basic Concepts for Designing a Fundamental Information
1965   System," *Management Services,* vol. II, no. 4, July-August, pp.
37–45.

Myers, C. A. (ed.), *The Impact of Computers on Management,* Cambridge,
1967   Mass.: M.I.T. Press.

Needles, B., Jr., "A Single Information Flow System for Hospital Data Process-
1969   ing," *Management Services,* September-October, pp. 27–37.

Prince, T. R., *Information Systems for Management Planning and Control,*
1970   Homewood, Ill.: Richard D. Irwin.

Siegel, S. J., "Developing an Information System for a Hospital," *Public Health*
1968   *Reports,* vol. 83, no. 5, May, pp. 359–362.

Singer, J. P., "Computer Based Hospital Information Systems," *Datamation,*
1969   May, pp. 38–45.

Toffler, A., *Future Shock,* New York: Random House.
1970

Wilson, I. G., and M. E. Wilson, *Information, Computers, and System Design,*
1965   New York: John Wiley & Sons.

Withington, F. G., *The Use of Computers in Business Organizations,* Reading,
1966   Mass.: Addison-Wesley.

SELECTION 17

Status of Hospital Information Systems*

Morton D. Schwartz

Medical services are now the fastest-rising item on the consumer index. They have soared by nearly eight per cent in 1969, while the consumer index rose only a little over three per cent. Hospital costs have been rising at nearly 16 per cent per year for the past few years. The cost of a hospital room averaged $68 a day in 1969. By 1975 it will reach $100 a day. The nation's total health bill for 1969 is estimated at $50 to $60 billion, or approximately six per cent of the Gross National Product. By 1975, the bill will be well over $100 billion and eight per cent of the projected GNP. In 1969, the federal government alone spent approximately $16 billion on medical care. The health care industry now employs more than 300,000 doctors, 640,000 nurses and 2 million hospital workers. By 1975, it will employ 1.5 million doctors and nurses and 4.5 million hospital workers. As the absolute and proportionate costs of medical care rise, new hospital management techniques must be developed to provide the highest standard of health care at the lowest possible cost.

Potential Source of New Management Techniques

Computer-based hospital information systems (HIS)[1] can provide new hospital management techniques. More than 10 per cent of the hospitals in the U.S. are currently using some form of electronic data processing equipment. This percentage is rapidly growing, and a definite trend has been established. The use of HIS systems is also expanding rapidly. For example, one HIS supplier plans to install fully operational HIS systems in 47 hospitals within the next 18 months. Other HIS suppliers are in the process of developing similar systems and anticipate a large market for their products. This means that a hospital, which plans on "keeping up" with the advanced state of the art and wishes to be noted for its excellence in patient care and utilization of advanced technological equipment, must plan on eventually using an HIS system.

In order to assess the impact of the new management techniques afforded

* *Hospital Progress,* June, 1970.

by HIS on the spiraling costs of health care delivery systems, a course entitled, "Hospital Information Systems: Techniques and Applications," was held in 1969 at the University of Southern California.* The results of this course are summarized in the following discussion and indicate trends for the utilization of HIS systems in automating the information flow and generating management tools for the hospital.

HIS System Basics

An HIS system is defined as a high-speed, computer-controlled, multi-station, authorized access information flow network for the hospital. It has business office and patient care subsystems, and its function is to speed and simplify administrative and medical information handling. The HIS system interfaces with the hospital staff through the use of data terminals located at the nurses' stations and at strategic points in the departments and service areas. As a result, administrative and medical personnel have instantaneous access to the electronic data banks for entry or retrieval of patient data.

The HIS system stores, retrieves, routes, sorts and verifies the information flow. It can be designed to provide patient medical histories, current medical records, statistical summaries, and legal records. It can schedule medical tests and maintain inventory control of beds and supplies. It can provide current status of meal orders and accounting/billing records. The computer makes it possible to automate the information flow in the hospital and can undertake many tasks. A brief description of potential HIS system tasks can be found in the appendix.

Data entries and retrievals of computer-stored forms or records are made from data terminals, except for accounts payable records which are accumulated and then processed. English language should be used in communicating information to the HIS data terminal system by means of touch entry devices, in order to simplify the training of hospital personnel who will use the system. Touch entry devices include lightpens, keyboards, programable keyboards, and selection buttons. Hospital personnel should identify themselves when using data terminals to ensure that only authorized personnel have access to the patient's file. Identification and access authorization are accomplished by inserting ID cards or sequences of coded numbers into the data terminal.

The most flexible data terminals consist of displays with television screens—cathode ray tubes (CRTs). Information is retrieved by computer-generation of data in bright letters and numbers on the screen. The touch entry device is used to select data and/or "action words" which appear on

---

* Revised for this article by the author in April, 1970.

the display screen. Hospital personnel can select specific data and categories for display or can complete displayed forms or documents. When "action words" are selected on the screen, the action selected is performed. This action can range from calling up additional data displays to printing out hard copies of data, to dispatching a message generated on the screen to some department or service area.

Benefits of HIS Systems

The objectives of an HIS system are improved medical information handling and more effective utilization of hospital personnel, equipment, and facilities. Examples of HIS systems currently in operation that satisfy these objectives are the Baptist Hospital in Beaumont, Tex., and the St. Francis Hospital in Peoria, Ill. These HIS systems are currently collecting and evaluating operational data to ascertain the cost-effectiveness of HIS systems.

Some of the potential benefits which may be identified when the operational data mentioned above becomes available are as follows:

1. Reduction in average length of stay through improved interdepartmental communications and availability of up-to-date medical records.

2. Reduction in clerical workload, which allows the professional staff to devote more time to patient contact and care.

3. Provision of care-oriented, computer-generated patient reports which interrelate and correlate pertinent data, such as a cumulative clinical laboratory report. Such a report would present all laboratory results to date in a summary format for the doctor.

4. Provision of hospital operations-oriented, computer-generated reports which indicate to administration and management the current operating statistics for the hospital. These statistics include information on accounting, budgeting, financial data, bed census and occupancy data, medical records, abstracting and coding, and various medico-legal documents.

Growth of HIS Systems

Most HIS systems currently under development will probably be directed toward both the business office and patient care data processing. The initial emphasis of some systems has been directed toward business office and accounting applications, but current and projected developments indicate a plan to supply a complete range of business office and patient care applications. Progress has been slow; some HIS systems have been under development fo five years and are still not ready for full hospital implementation. However, considerable progress has been made recently. Baptist

Hospital, Beaumont, Tex., is an example of a leased HIS system in operation. By 1972, there will be at least six suppliers of leased HIS systems
in the U.S.

The anticipated patient-day costs for leased HIS services will range
from $2 to $8 for hospitals with more than 200 beds. The leased rates
for smaller hospitals will probably be prohibitively high for some time.
For $2 a patient-day, the hospital would obtain interdepartmental com-
munications, billing, and records for those items and services ordered
through the HIS system. However, the data terminals would not provide
touch entry devices; pre-coded data entry cards would have to be used. At
the other end of the cost-spectrum ($8 a patient-day), a full range of in-
formation handling services would be provided, and CRT data terminals
with touch entry devices would be provided, producing a considerable
degree of flexibility. The $2 and $8 per patient-day figures include costs
for both inpatient and outpatient activities.

HIS System Review

For the purpose of this review, the various HIS systems surveyed can be
separated into the following four basic categories:

1. *Comprehensive, multi-hospital HIS systems,* such as those at El
Camino Hospital, Mountain View, Calif., and St. Francis Hospital in
Peoria, Ill. These systems are large computer information systems. They
have only recently been developed to provide data storage and retrieval
capabilities and interdepartmental communications between admitting,
business office, nursing stations, and medical services. They are designed
to offer economies by time-sharing their computer equipment among several
hospitals. The potential advantages of time-shared systems are the sharing
of hardware costs, software development costs, and common data banks
for patient care and medical research.

2. *Comprehensive, single-hospital HIS systems,* such as those at Los
Angeles-USC Medical Center, Los Angeles; St. Francis Hospital, Miami,
Fla.; Kaiser Foundation Hospital, Oakland, Calif.; St. John's Medical
Center, Joplin, Mo.; and Baptist Hospital, Beaumont, Tex. These systems
are similar to time-shared systems, except that they are used by a single
hospital as a "dedicated system" rather than being shared by several
hospitals.

3. *Business office, multi-hospital HIS subsystems,* such as those using
the Minnesota Blue Cross Computer Center and those at Chester Hospital
and Clinic, Dallas, Tex. and Glenview Hospital, Forth Worth, Tex. These
systems provide computerized office services to subscriber hospitals in the
areas of patient billing, accounts receivable, general ledger, and payroll.

Some time-shared computer centers supply a greater range of services than do others.

4. *Special purpose, single-hospital HIS systems,* such as those at Downstate Medical Center, New York City; Akron (Ohio) Children's Hospital; Texas Institute for Rehabilitation and Research, Houston; and Manchester (Conn.) Memorial Hospital. These special purpose systems will not be discussed any further in this review since they are not designed for general use.

The above categories comprise both business office and patient care subsystems of an HIS system. Examples of such subsystems are presented below.

Business Office Subsystem

Business office information is largely numeric and concentrated geographically, and automated results can be readily measured and compared with results of pre-existing techniques. Since business office personnel are well-acquainted with quantitative methods and careful control, business office functions may be used as a starting point for converting manual operations to HIS system operations. Implementation of this subsystem will acquaint the hospital's administration and part of its personnel with the advantages and the constraints of electronic data processing. It offers an opportunity to train personnel in computer systems and has the potential to provide new management techniques in improved operations reporting and improved financial management. For these reasons, several suppliers have begun to develop business office HIS subsystems.

An example of a business office subsystem that has five basic areas of application is the one under evaluation at El Camino Hospital, Mountain View, Calif. This subsystem has been under development for two and one-half years and is now fully operational. In addition to the business office subsystem, El Camino Hospital is also in the process of evaluating a preliminary patient care subsystem on a limited number of CRT data terminals. The five business office applications are as follows:

Five Applications

1. *Patient billing and accounts receivable.* The patient billing/accounts receivable application provides a patient accounting service in a batched[2] processing environment. Transaction records in the form of keypunched cards are prepared for each patient and for each charged item accrued by that patient. These transaction records may be prepared from keypunch layout transmittal forms or from source documents themselves. They are

generated by the hospital and delivered to a central computer facility upon conclusion of the hospital's working day or other daily cycle cutoff time. Included within these transactions are update and/or correction cards to fixed tables in the computer programs. These tables contain such data as room/patient type, physicians authorized/specialty, charge allocation/ charge descriptions, name, address, hospital number, and billing cycle. The tables are updated against each patient's master record. In addition to the patient's statement and accounting breakdown of receivables, the subsystem also generates both inpatient and outpatient Medicare billing forms.

This application is designed to operate on a medium-sized computer[3] with 64K core, tape drives, disk drives, and high speed printer. It is designed to interface with the general ledger program (application 4) for allocation of charges to the proper chart of accounts' summary and detail accumulations. The application will also interface with the HIS system under development in that data transactions will be accepted in a batch processing mode.

2. *Payroll application.* This application provides a payroll service in a batch processing environment. Time cards in the form of keypunched cards or their equivalent are prepared for each employe. These cards are processed against the employe's master record, which contains the necessary data to extend gross pay and to compute deductions. The end result is the creation of payroll checks and various supporting documents, both of which enable the hospital to maintain effective control of the system. A few of the features that are included in this system are automatic accrual of employe benefits (i.e., sick, holiday, vacation); acceptance of prewritten checks (interim); eligibility checking for employe benefits; handling of pay rates different from employe's established rate; labor analysis reporting to the department that the employe actually worked; confidential payroll processing; and personnel statistical reporting by department of head counts and turnover rates. Besides the time cards, the hospital submits punched cards, using various transaction codes, to establish new employes on the master file, to set up or revise constant information on the employe (i.e., rate, department assigned, address, deductions, etc.), and to show status changes. This application is designed to interface with the general ledger program (application 4), passing to it the dollar values accumulated by the various liabilities and expense accounts.

3. *Accounts payable.* This application provides an accounts payable service in a batch data processing environment. A vendor name and address file is established, and the file controls the issuance of payment checks against valid due invoices. In addition to invoice register maintenance, the application interfaces with the general ledger in that input records are prepared as a result of accounts payable activity for accumulation and posting to their associated general ledger accounts. The application can

process interim payments to vendors which are written external to the checkwriting program and incorporate these balances against the proper invoice register. The system also contains both internal and external balancing features and rejection and acceptance transaction listings.

4. *General ledger application.* This application provides a general ledger service in a batch processing mode. Five types of transactions are entered into the general ledger system. They are: establish new accounts; update revenue budgets; update expense budgets; update allocation rates; and generate journal or adjusting entries. The hospital prepares journal and adjusting entries in the form of keypunched cards. These cards along with computer-generated journal entries from other business office applications, are processed against the general ledger master account records. Trial balance reports are created and once they are balanced, the hospital's financial management reports are generated. The management reports consist of the balance sheet, various income and expense statements, and department cost accounting reports.

5. *Inventory control application.* The inventory control application provides an accounting technique for all inventory items. Direct issue items can be entered and displayed on an inventory status report and department supplies expense report.

Provisions have been made for automatic inventory price adjustments and backorder carry. A purchasing action report is keyed to a quarterly stores inventory catalog and shows all items below minimum or above maximum, along with last issue dates and total issues to date.

Patient Care Subsystem

The Baptist Hospital in Beaumont, Tex., has installed both business office and patient care subsystems at the same time. The functions of the business office subsystem are similar to those described above. The patient care subsystem uses electronic equipment to store, process, and display the patient care information that a hospital needs in its daily operation. Computer program applications have been developed for patient records, bed census list, drug files, employe records, purchase order forms, patients' medical records, and other hospital records. The resulting information can be displayed in printed form on any of the data terminals. These printed forms on the television screens are displayed in sequence by pushing the appropriate touch entry devices. Once the information is displayed on the screen, hospital personnel can update records, order supplies, and perform other routine functions by using lightpen devices or keys on the data terminal keyboard to key-in information.

In implementing the patient care subsystem, all hospital personnel are assigned special identification entry codes or badges that resemble a plastic card. If badges are used, they are inserted into the badge reader to turn the television screen on and to display a list of functions. These badges are color- and function-coded according to the duties and responsibilities of the hospital personnel. When a badge is inserted into the badge reader, the initial display corresponding to that badge function is shown. The initial display lists those tasks or functions for which a hospital department is responsible. Nurses' badges display a nurse's initial display, etc. No person can display records for which he has no need or job responsibility. Nurses can work only with nursing functions, pharmacy can work only with pharmacy functions, etc. The individual badges protect and guarantee the confidential nature of all information within the HIS system.

The data terminals are located at duty stations throughout the hospital as required. Some duty stations, such as dietary, may have only printers. The data terminal is the only piece of equipment which hospital personnel use to enter data when communicating with the HIS system. By inserting the badge into the badge reader, the data terminal is automatically turned on, the badge holder is identified, and an initial display is shown on the television screen. The initial display lists the tasks that can be done. Viewing records to see if they are complete, ordering a medication or a central supply item, and charting patient data are examples of the three main tasks that can be done. A task usually involves a sequence of screen displays.

To the side of the television screen is a lightpen device or selection buttons. The lightpen is used, or the selection button is pushed, to select a particular task. The display will show all of the information that has been added to the many different hospital records. Information is stored into the HIS system by either selecting a series of words to form a message or using the keys on the keyboard to enter the information on the screens. The keyboard is similar to that of a standard typewriter. The information is displayed in capital letters as it is keyed-in on the screen, and corrections or changes can be made before storing it into the system. The new information is immediately available for display at any of the data terminals throughout the hospital. After each task is completed, the initial display is shown again in case the person operating the equipment wishes to do additional tasks. When a task is completed, the nurse, technician, or doctor uses the appropriate codes or pushes the badge release lever to remove the badge from the badge reader. The terminal is then automatically turned off.

The patient care and business office subsystems provide the hospital administrator with the following management tools and administrative control:

1. An invoice cannot be paid more than once.

2. Patient service charges cannot vary among patients, since all charges are obtained from a computer-based file approved by the administrator.

3. A patient's account cannot be lost.

4. Through the use of computer-based inventory control, inventories cannot reach undesirable high or low levels.

5. Orders cannot be lost by service departments since the HIS system "reminds" personnel of any unfilled orders.

6. Authorized signatures are obtained whenever entries or retrievals are made on the data terminal.

7. Cash flow can be monitored on a current basis.

8. Dollar value for each test and treatment can be obtained on a monthly basis.

Cost-Benefit Trade-Offs

A hospital must be willing to increase its patient-day cost by $2 to $8 for a full HIS system and $.50 to $1 for the business office subsystem only. The resulting benefits may include reducing the length of patient stay, increasing bed occupancy, providing better management reports and tools, improving interdepartmental communications, reducing the possibility of transcription errors, and establishing a data bank for teaching and research purposes. An HIS system has the additional potential of uncovering lost or erroneous charges. This benefit alone could possibly constitute one of the major savings.

Most of these benefits will produce savings to offset the HIS system costs. However, no measure of cost-effectiveness can be made at this time since the extent to which hospitals can employ HIS systems to take advantage of labor and material cost offsetting when changing from a manual to a HIS system has not been fully assessed at this time. However, considerable data obtained over many months of operation should be shortly available from the HIS systems at Baptist Hospital, Beaumont, Tex., and St. Francis Hospital, Peoria, Ill. The resulting trade-off of manual system costs against HIS system costs will, in the end, determine the resulting economics and cost-effectiveness. The problem is further compounded by the many intangibles involved, such as the cost of computer-generated management reports for hospital administrators, which have no direct dollar return but are of benefit to the over-all operation of the hospital.

APPENDIX

This appendix[4] presents an overview of the potential HIS applications that are under consideration by various suppliers developing HIS systems.

The objective in providing such a list is to indicate the direction which such efforts are taking.

Before the HIS tasks can be defined, a set of files must be established to store the data for entry or retrieval purposes. The following set of files is extensive in scope and allows a comprehensive HIS system to be developed: Ancillary services, accounting, inventory, pending, non-completed, drug index, medical records, outpatient records, doctors' orders, reservations and bed-available, result collector, registry, blood donor registry, inpatient records (may contain patient charts), personnel, poison index, pre-admission, and glossary of terms used in HIS system.

The above files are then used in the following HIS application areas to store data entries for later retrieval. Each HIS task is an application area which provides billing and accounting, laboratory data processing, registry and indexing, administrative controls, or patient care reports.

HIS Tasks

Business Office Subsystem

BILLING & ACCOUNTING

Hospital billing function. Contains a list of the accounting files of all charges applied to a patient's account and produces detailed bills at specific intervals, with a summary and pro-rated third-party bill on discharge.

Admission/discharge. Used for inpatient and outpatient admission and discharge and includes:

1. Updating of reservations and bed-available files.

2. Establishment of inpatient and outpatient records, both in abbreviated form and in a complete form.

3. Medical record file, patient accounting file, and doctors' orders file.

Cost accounting function. Provides for the analysis and accumulation of actual costs incurred. The supporting data is used for gained reimbursement from Medicare and for adjusting charges in the following year to reflect actual costs. The system produces reports at department levels for financial control and operating control.

Payroll function. Provides all payroll and associated accounting transactions and services for hospital personnel.

Open accounts receivable. Provides inquiry capability at detail level; updates bill at detail level; periodically updates open accounts; transfers record to closed A/R on zero balance.

Purchasing function. Obtains products and services needed in the hospital and updates department records to reflect expenditures. It provides for two kinds of purchasing: emergency orders and routine orders (to be accumulated by the vendor and processed on a 24-hour basis). In addition, it updates inventory files to reflect items on order and prices and records the inventory file.

Accounts payable function. Produces checks for vendors, check register, and list by vendors of items purchased along with payment record. Updates departmental financial records to show all activity on a daily basis, thereby making it possible to generate real-time status reports of any account. Input and output is on a batch and random basis for status report of any account.

Outpatient accounting function. Provides accounts receivable function for outpatients.

General ledger function. Produces general ledger reports as follows:

1. Detail level for departmental heads.
2. Summary level for administration.
3. Detail income report showing all actual income for month and year-to-date figures.
4. Detail expense report, similar to income report.

Patient Care Subsystem

LABORATORY DATA PROCESSING

EKG analysis. Automates collection, analysis, and reporting of EKG results. EKGs can be processed in real time (monitoring or other high priority); in real time accession with batch processing; or with automated or non-automated off-line accession and batch processing.

Laboratory analysis function. Provides computer-assisted analysis of test results. (Was the test valid? Should it be rescheduled? Did the test show a critical condition?) Updates patient records showing results. Posts completion in doctors' orders file and accounting files.

Service (labs) report function. Checks results of tests when reported directly into "result collector" file, and produces reports from "result collector" file for the medical record (by patient) at intervals, adjusting to system, terminal, and ward-clerk/office staff schedules. Prints or displays report at nursing station when test is reported, and posts entries to patient medical records and in billing accounting file.

REGISTRY & INDEXING

Registry function. Maintains separate registry files by medical subject such as psychiatric, retardation, alcoholism, birth defects, crippled children and adults, tuberculosis, stroke, heart, and tumor. These files contain basic medical data, diagnosis, treatment record, and results of treatment.

Blood donor registry. Maintains current files on donors, including their location, types, and donating groups. Lists of last year's donors are prepared for collection groups, and notices of dates and times for each donating group are produced and mailed to the participants.

Poison index. Maintains up-to-date poison control index for random retrieval from hospital wards, emergency rooms, physicians' offices, or poison control center. The index lists poisons by their brand names, chemical names, industrial usage types, and toxic effects. The file also contains currently recommended treatments.

Departmental indexing function. Provides the individual departments with a tool for collecting and cataloging data that is pertinent to their particular interest. These indexes can be used for diagnostic tools and quality control.

Produces updated monthly report showing one or more of the following for new additions: Alphabetical listing, hospital number listing, diagnostic breakdown, departmental accession number listing, and frequency distribution of diagnosis. The following indexes are also available: Surgical pathology, cytology, clinical pathology, autopsy lab, radiology, EKG, and EEG.

Drug index. Maintains information concerning drugs, indexed in a fashion similar to the *Physician's Desk Reference.*

ADMINISTRATIVE CONTROLS

Patient transfer. Updates patient record for transfer from one bed location to another and possibly from one nursing station to another. Pending doctors' orders must be reprinted at the new nurses' station. When transfer occurs, the service departments must be informed of the new bed location.

Service scheduling. Prints a list of work to be done in each of the service departments for a shift of personnel.

Nursing scheduling. Prints or displays a list in the chief nurse's office and the administration office of the names and types of nurses required for each floor for each shift. This schedule is developed by examining patient status, type of service required, bed status, personnel files, and pending doctors' orders.

Maintenance scheduling function. Provides printout of routine plan maintenance procedures to be carried out by in-house maintenance staff and outside vendors. Maintains records of completed work, showing date completed, materials used, man-hours needed, and actual costs. Makes it possible to alter schedules when the need arises, when new procedures are initiated, when current practices are inadequate, etc.

Schedules maintenance of in-house medical instruments, such as recalibration of electronic metering devices, scales, etc.

Dietary function. Provides daily printout of each patient's menu, along with a list and summary report used for meal production planning. Provides for individual menu selection via the nurses' station. The food usage and services required are reported at the department level.

Terminology and procedures definition and inquiry function. Develops and maintains a glossary of terms to be used within the entire HIS system. Displays, upon request, the definition of any medical term or procedural term utilized in the system.

Inventory control function. Provides for control of consumable and non-consumable items, either patient-care directed or non-patient-care directed. Provides accurate and timely reports on existing store items, including usage analysis reports which show the necessity of either increasing or deleting items. Provides both hospital-wide and departmental level reports that contribute to cost accounting and property control. Provides departmental reports showing estimated reordering times and quantities.

Census function. Provides clocked or demand inquiry printout of census by nursing station and type of service.

Bed availability function. Provides, on request, a list of available beds by service type.

PATIENT CARE RECORDS

Nurses' notes function. Provides a means for incorporating nurses' notes and physicians' notes into the medical record file for the purpose of reporting patient condition to the physician and subsequent nursing shifts. The notes may be coded or in English form, as required, and are reported via remote terminal to the patient record.

Pre-admission. Provides for collection of data from the patient and the physician concerning type of service, credit, insurance, medical data, basic vital statistics, and pre-admission physician orders. All this information is held in a pre-admission file, pending actual admission.

Physicians' orders function. Provides a means of entering physicians' orders for patient care into the system. The orders are verified and distributed to various active ancillary services files, to the appropriate nurses' station, to accounting files for billing purposes, and to inventory files for posting. The orders are maintained in a "pending" file and, if treatment or care is not completed, a separate entry is made into a "not-completed" file for review by the medical staff.

Orders for medications are checked against the drug index file for dosage range, pharmacologic antagonism, and contra-indications. In addition, if special instructions for administration or observation of side effects are necessary, these are communicated to the nursing station and/or physicians' office.

The application ultimately includes PRN orders to be carried out, only if specific criteria (e.g., a test result in a certain range or a given change or lack of change in a patient's condition) are met.

Medical records maintenance. Provides for the manual and automated review of existing medical records for the hospital and practitioner and also includes:

1. Removal of records of deceased patients into deactivated records file, six months to one year after death.

2. Scanning of records for incompleteness or lack of diagnosis.

3. Routine file additions for result reporting and notes.

Outpatient result reporting. Provides for clinical and ancillary service reports, originated by physicians' orders, to be reported to the data management system and incorporated into the patient's medical record.

Case history and physical. This application area represents one of the most difficult and urgent of all application areas. Three basic alternatives exist with regard to entering case history and physical information:

1. Entry of material in narrative form only.

2. Entry of historical and physical data in narrative form, with diagnostic information entered in a coded or machine readable form.

3. Entry of all historical and physical information in coded or machine readable form.

By means of central dictation systems doctors may narrate history and physical data into a central stenographic "pool." The "stenographers" will "type" the information directly into the computerized medical record in an on-line, real-time mode. Dictation technique will include verbal delimiters such as "chief complaints," "history of present illness," "past history," "family history," and similar categories for the physical examination data.

Physician display function. Provides the physician with direct access to his patients' medical records, including hospital status; to his own records; and to various files in the data management system. Access is achieved by remote terminal on the nursing floor or at the physician's office in a doctors' office building.

REFERENCES

[1] The abbreviation HIS for hospital information system is used throughout this article in a generic sense.
[2] Batch refers to "batch at a time processing." Several computer programs can be batch-processed at the same time on one computer.
[3] This computer system is designed to be shared by many hospitals so that the total number of beds serviced can be about 3,000.
[4] Summarizes, in part, a presentation made by Dr. William T. Blessum, director of the Medical Computer Facility, University of California at Irvine, to the Summer Course on Hospital Information Systems, University of Southern California, Los Angeles, July, 1969.

SELECTION 18

Computers in Patient Care*

G. Octo Barnett, M.D.

In most areas of medical care, adaptations in practice have kept pace with advances in knowledge about diseases and therapeutic procedures. However, one vital area of medical practice, information processing, has been badly neglected, and little progress has been made. The technology of data processing in dozens of other fields has been revolutionized by the computer in the last two or three decades. Yet few of these changes have made their way into the medical world—in particular into the hospital. Most information used by hospitals in patient care is written, often in illegible script on multipart forms. The same information is delivered to different areas in the hospital by multiple slips of paper or a number of telephone calls. One can retrieve most information only by shuffling through the medical record—a disorganized collection of doctors' and nurses' observations, test results and records of therapeutic procedures. A recent study[1] of hospital costs has shown that over 25 per cent of the hospital budget is spent on information processing.

Early interest in bringing the revolution in computer technology to bear on medical practice was plagued with overenthusiasm, naïveté and unrealistic expectations. The use of computers would, it was held, allow rapid and accurate collection and retrieval of *all* clinical information, perform automatic diagnosis, collect, monitor and analyze a variety of physiologic signals, perform and interpret all laboratory tests automatically, and replace the telephone and the medical record by fulfilling their functions. In fact, however, attempts to apply computer technology to medicine have had only limited success, with numerous failures. The growing pains encountered in applying computer technology are not unique to medicine; the same types of experiences have been realized in all other areas of computer application. Indeed, one of the benefits of the computer revolution is that it stimulates and requires an intensity of thinking, a level of sophistication and a strictness of semantic behavior that are needed badly in the development of improved methods of delivering health care.

This review covers seven of the major areas of computer applications in medicine: medical diagnosis; clinical laboratory; screening; patient monitoring; medical record; automated medical history; and hospital infor-

* New England Journal of Medicine, December, vol. 279, 1968.

mation systems. The emphasis of the review is on functional areas of medical practice and the impact of the technology on these areas rather than on specific computer systems or programs.

Medical Diagnosis

Diagnosis is a central factor in medical science not only in the naming and classifying of diseases but, more importantly, in the choice of therapeutic regimens and the development of prognoses.[2-4] An essential part of diagnosis consists of sifting out relevant from irrelevant information (selecting a probable diagnosis from many possible diagnoses) and developing hypotheses from the available, incomplete data presented by the patient. The computer's ability to store vast amounts of data, to perform complex logical operations and to enumerate possibilities is not sufficient for the purpose of aiding in diagnosis. Precise procedures must be formulated to describe the logical operations required to deduce the clinical state of the patient from his observed signs and symptoms.

Two general approaches are possible in developing detailed descriptions of diagnostic behavior. With the first, one can attempt to capture the processes used by physicians in a manner precise enough to simulate physician behavior with a computer program. There are several drawbacks to this approach. The most obvious is the current lack of understanding of the processes employed by doctors. How a physician interprets clues from a patient is difficult to describe with the precision required if the information is to be used by a computer. Even if no such difficulty existed, the simulation of human diagnostic processes on a computer may fail to exploit the capabilities of the machine. It is unlikely that the diagnostic processes doctors use will prove to be those best suited for the computer. For this reason, most studies of computer-aided diagnosis have focused on a second approach: development of strategies particularly suited to the functions of the computer without the restriction that they be suited also to human beings.

The strategy that has received most attention is a statistical technic based on probabilities as formulated in Bayes's theorem. Bayes's theorem makes use of the probability that each disease will occur in the population and the probability of occurrence of each symptom given each disease to determine the probability of all possible diseases given the patient's symptom complex. Since Ledley and Lusted[5] properly assessed it in 1959, the Bayesian model has been applied in several studies, including the diagnosis of congenital heart disease,[6,7] thyroid disease[8] and the detection of bone tumors.[9] In each study, the computer produced results comparable to those of an expert in the clinical specialty. The relevance of these studies must be qualified by the fact that only a small part of the clinician's total task was mimicked in a limited clinical field. The same model has been expanded to include sequential diagnosis so that the computer program also determines the appropriate sequence of diagnostic tests to be performed on the patient.[10]

Bayes's decision rule is a particularly attractive strategy for medical diagnosis since a particular attribute is rarely pathognomonic. Rather, many diseases give rise to the same attributes, and it is therefore impossible to design an efficient branching tree structure to eliminate all but the correct category for a given pattern of signs and symptoms. The Bayes theorem provides a very good model for situations in which the frequency with which an attribute occurs in a given disease is known. The weakness of applications of this model is not implicit in the Bayes rule itself, but in two simplifying assumptions (a mutually exclusive and exhaustive set of diagnoses and an independent set of signs and symbols) that are not fully met in practice.[11] The error introduced by the assumption that there are no correlations or interactions among the attributes cannot be arbitrarily stated and seems to vary widely among application areas. An additional error may be introduced by the assumption that the patient with the unknown disease comes from the same population as the group on which the statistics were based.

Other statistical models of the diagnostic process that have been used in medical applications include Neyman's method,[12] relative likelihood[13] and numerical taxonomy.[14] Neyman's method requires the measurement of the relative frequency of sets of symptoms in diseased and nondiseased patients. Its principal usefulness is limited to situations in which there are only a few important symptoms. The relative-likelihood model is very similar to the Bayes decision rule except that no consideration is given to the prevalence of the entity in the population of concern. Numerical taxonomy is concerned with the systematic classification of patients into diagnostic clusters with similar characteristics; this classification is done with the use of numerical technics to express the degree of similarity between different patients and depends on deriving quantitative representation of the signs and symptoms. Numerical taxonomy has proved very useful in the classification of insects and plants and offers considerable potential as a research technic in clinical medicine, particularly when quantitative measurements are possible.

The computer's potential usefulness to manipulate clinical information and present various possibilities of disease has been universally acclaimed; however, there has been a considerable controversy over its applicability in the actual diagnostic process—particularly in determining the numerical probability of the presence of a specific disease. In addition, Sterling[15] has questioned the use of the computer in selecting initial observations and in making the inductive jumps or sequential hypotheses that an experienced clinician makes.

More fundamental criticisms of the application of computer technology to medical diagnosis have been concerned with the lack of a logical definition of "disease"[2,16] and the fact that the physician may use a varying set of criteria in determining the diagnosis depending on the total clinical situation (that is, different decisions could be made on the basis of the same information[15]). Eden's[17] summary of these criticisms is that ". . . the major problems in medical diagnosis, in the methodology of medical diagnosis, are problems for physicians and until the physician is willing to investigate his own discipline, investigate his own terminology and his own methodology, all the computer engineer, physical scientist or mathematician can do is to stand in the wings and help out in very minor ways."

Clinical Laboratory

The most widely implemented application of computers to patient care is the electronic processing of clinical laboratory data. Use of computers in this field has been stimulated by the rapidly increasing workload of laboratories (doubling every five to seven years), and the fact that data processing has become the bottleneck in the laboratory. Scarce laboratory staff members now spend up to 50 per cent of their time in paperwork—accessioning, recording, transcribing and reporting.

The challenge of data processing in the clinical laboratory is more than a problem of simple automation or mechanization of physical instruments. An optimal data-handling system should provide both rapid processing of laboratory procedures, with minimal error and minimal delay, and legible reporting of interim and final reports for the physician and for the patient's chart. A summary report should correlate, interpret and flag the results that indicate abnormalities. For future clinical care, research and quality control, the system should permit rapid retrieval and analysis of data according to patient and to type of analysis performed.

Limiting laboratory tests to those indicated by other information is as absurd as limiting the medical history and physical examination to areas indicated by the patient's complaints,[18,19] and an increasing trend is developing toward the use of batteries of tests. The introduction of automation in the clinical laboratory will facilitate this trend. In one study[19] a profile of 11 commonly requested determinations indicated that in one of 10 patients, the physician was helped directly in patient care by the reporting of abnormalities detected by the battery. Computer technics are also useful in detecting unusual patterns of clinical laboratory data in which the presence of an abnormality may be signified by a combination of several different test results rather than by a change in a single test.[20]

Different types of computer systems and technics are in use in the clinical laboratory. The most common system uses punch cards, a central computer facility and manual distribution of test reports.[21,22] Baird[23] has presented a refreshingly candid and explicit account of such a system that was discontinued because of errors of input, excessive time requirements on the medical residency staff, unacceptable time lags in reporting and, above all, a cost much higher than originally estimated. Because of these problems and the difficulty of using the computer to check errors and control quality, this type of system will probably be modified.

A number of laboratories[24,25] are using small, dedicated (single-purpose) computer systems, which are relatively low in cost and have great flexibility. However, most of these systems have been developed on an ad hoc basis to meet the needs of a specific laboratory and have only a limited generality. In addition there has been little effort to make systems commercially available that can be operated and modified by a novice in computer technology. Only one of these commercial systems has been concerned with the automatic identification of the specimen.[26]

Other medical facilities have rejected the concept of the computer dedicated to the laboratory data-processing activities in favor of using a larger central computer facility that also carries out other hospital information-processing functions.[27,28] The advantage of this approach is that it facilitates the merging of laboratory data with other information in the patient's medical record. The disadvantage is that there is often a severe conflict in the needs of the laboratory and the desire to have a multiterminal central data-processing system.

Automation and electronic data processing will be of great importance to the clinical laboratory's operation and will probably be the first computer application to affect patient care noticeably. The reasons for this are varied: the needs are well defined; the data are not ambiguous; and the personnel concerned are technologically oriented.

Screening

The concept of screening[29] has received attention in the past several years as a means of detecting diseases early and of saving the highly trained professional's time by the use of less trained personnel to administer the screening tests.

Collen,[30] of the Permanente Clinic, is the acknowledged leader in the development of automated, multitest laboratories where automatic electronic equipment and computers are used as an integral part of routine health examinations. A majority of the data generated in the Permanente Laboratory are recorded so that they can be introduced immediately into the data-processing system. The computer processes the information through a program containing various test limits and decision rules and prints out "advice" about any additional procedures that might be performed before the next patient visit. Rules for the use of this "advice" have previously been established by the internists who use the system, and the receptionist is instructed to arrange these additional procedures for the patient before the physician performs the physical examination. If a serious abnormality is detected, the computer suggests that an earlier appointment be made with the physician.

Screening places heavy demands on information-processing activities by requiring both simple, reliable and rapid data-collection technics and a processing system capable of rapid analysis and display of results.

Although there are a number of different forms of screening (selective screening, mass public-health screening, surveillance, screening of hospital patients and screening in industrial or closed populations), there is no universal agreement about the validity, yield, cost benefit and importance to medical care of this technic.

Patient Monitoring

Continuous monitoring of the physiologic functions of the major organ systems (cardiovascular, respiratory, renal, cerebral, electrolyte control and so forth) is believed to improve patient care for the critically ill. The objectives of such continuous monitoring are to measure critical physiologic variables to enable immediate detection of complications in the patient's course, and to provide a readily available, organized, legible and continuously updated record of the different variables.

Electronic data processing and automated technics are being used increasingly for patient monitoring,[31-33] because many of the tasks are repetitive and monotonous and because the computer can collect, store and display vast quantities of data at a fast rate. The computer can also derive additional physiologic information from the primary data, sort through the data for values indicating significant changes in the patient's state and provide clinical interpretations of physiologic observations. Computers may eventually be included in the closed-loop control of therapy to assure optimal administration of drugs. Accumulation of large quantities of accurately and continuously measured data on particular diseases may make it possible to formulate more accurate models of the disease and select optimal therapy more efficiently.

Development of automatic monitoring systems has proved to be much more difficult than was expected a decade ago. This is related, in part, to the lack of efficient and reliable measuring devices for clinical use and in part to the expense of the engineering and technical design of the total monitoring system.[34] Even the successful efforts are still relatively primitive and monitor only a few primary variables (such as blood pressure, heart rate, respiratory rate, respiratory volume and urine flow). The computer is also used to detect the occurrence of abnormal values, both from these primary variables and from secondary variables such as cardiac output and stroke volume. Perhaps the most valuable feature of these systems is the display of a time history of these variables, improving the attending staff's ability to visualize the course of the disease.

Medical Record

Once, when a single clinician or a small group managed a patient's care, the individual medical record was of minor importance. Now, however, it is vital. Criticisms of both the form and the format of the medical record have been numerous:

> The usual case-history form often represents a device for recording and reinforcing the interests and prejudices of the individual physician or clinical investigator reflecting current fashions in diagnoses. It is frequently no more than an essay by the physician of doubtful literary or scientific merit. Certainly this information is more or less useless in terms of being retrievable by computer methods.[35]
>
> The value of data . . . must be measured in terms of quality, completeness, and availability. Data which are difficult to retrieve on a timely basis tend to have limited value irrespective of their excellence.[36]

One of the earliest uses of computers for patient care was to store and analyze well defined, standardized abstracts of medical-record information. The most widespread applications of this approach are the Professional Activity Study (PAS) and the Medical Audit Program.[37] It has also been used quite successfully in co-operative research projects such as the Human Kidney Transplant Registry[38] and the Cancer End Results Evaluation.[39] The inflexibility of a record that must be coded entirely has led various investigators to develop experimental technics that allow the entry of a limited amount of English text in a noncoded fashion.[40-43] Most of these applications have required the development of a predefined, rather rigid classification and coding of data, frequently causing distortion or loss of information. In addition, the person doing the coding must have a solid knowledge of the subject matter.

These limitations have stimulated attempts to emulate on the computer system the natural-language-processing capability and pattern-recognition skills of the human being by accepting unmodified, free English text as input. A variety of strategies have been used to identify and retrieve pertinent data. The simplest strategy involves retrieval based on the occurrence of specific words.[44,45] Two assumptions are made in this approach: the words used in the text have relatively well defined, unique meanings, and the meaning is conveyed completely by individual words and not by the manner in which these words are connected to form sentences. There are only very limited areas of application (such as pathological diagnoses) in which these assumptions are met. Pratt[36] has described a system that uses a lexicon of specific terms and a rudimentary syntactic analysis. Currently, this is being tested on pathological data by means of the "Systematized Nomenclature of Pathology."

Wider applications for this strategy may be possible in the near future, since the American Medical Association is developing a simplified and standard vocabulary of medicine (*Current Medical Terminology*) to try to eliminate the conflicting terms, jargon and the long, involved clauses in favor of precise, specific and meaningful terminology.[46]

Some parts of the medical record are not really unconstrained, free text, but rather patterned statements that the physician usually prefers to describe particular ideas. Data from radiologic and physical examination are examples. A promising approach for the entry of this type of information is to use the computer in direct interaction with the physician, nurse, technician or clerk. Information is transferred as the user engages in a branching question-answer dialogue through a highly interactive terminal device.[47-49]

Computer processing of medical-record information can be divided into three areas: input (or the initial capture of the information); storage; and output (or the retrieval and display of that information).

In most applications the chief limiting factor is inadequate input technics. Given that the information can be captured, a number of different retrieval and display technics can be used for output. The most significant advances in this area will therefore result from innovations in methods of capturing medical-record information.

Automated Medical History

In the activities described in other sections of this review, the computer's primary role is either communications or storage, analysis and retrieval of patient-care information. Collecting medical-history data directly from the patient illustrates a different potential for computer technology. In this procedure the interface of man and machine and the computer's ability to respond rapidly and appropriately are of great importance.

Three principal motives lie behind the current interest in developing automated technics for acquiring medical histories. The first is to increase efficiency in the delivery of patient care. Obtaining and recording a patient's history now takes a significant portion of a physician's time. In addition, what he records is sometimes illegible and occasionally incomplete. Automatic technics for collecting adequate histories and producing useful abstracts would result in a great saving of the physician's time that might be put to effective use in other activities.

The second motive for developing computer aids in taking medical histories centers on the history's use as a screening device in early detection of disease. Employing the computer to acquire histories and to select diagnostic studies based on their results without the use of critical physician resources could offer a valuable adjunct to present screening technics. Questions designed to elicit early symptoms of disease would be particularly useful. The *Cornell Medical Index,* the first questionnaire to be developed as a screening tool, is reported[50] as a valuable aid in the detection of a number of common diseases.

Interest in automatic history taking is also related to the fact that this technic will give impetus to the generation of efficient procedures, standardized terminology and coded information that will be useful for epidemiologic studies and for extension to computer-aided diagnosis. The *Cornell Medical Index* has been found to have fair validity as a predictor of a physician's appraisals of emotional and overall health.[51] Collen[12] has shown that a simple, six-part questionnaire could be used to distinguish between patients with a clinical diagnosis of asthma and those known to be free of asthma. Measurements of the reliability and validity of this questionnaire indicate a sensitivity (probability of correctly diagnosing a positive case) of 90 per cent and a specificity (probability of correctly diagnosing a negative case) of 94 per cent. A questionnaire for the diagnosis of angina pectoris and intermittent claudication has been evaluated in field surveys; the result of a limited validation effort is that the questionnaire showed a reasonable sensitivity (83 per cent) and a high specificity (95 per cent) as compared with the diagnosis by physicians.[52] The presence or absence of symptoms is an important element in the diagnostic decision-making process. Present history technics do not obtain these elements in the reproducible or retrievable form required for applying statistical measures to the diagnostic problem. Considerable effort will be required before an agreement can be reached not merely on the diagnostic criteria but also on the standardized questionnaire technic.

The first attempts at standardized histories were in the form of self-administered, patient questionnaires limited to 150 to 200 questions. Results were available to the physician only if he scanned the questionnaire in its entirety. Electronic data processing has made it possible to preprocess questionnaire answers for the physician's use and has resulted in more extensive and complex questionnaires. The expansion in scope is limited, however, by the patient's willingness to answer a large number of questions.

As the physician interviews a patient and obtains a medical history, he draws his questions from an almost infinite set of potential questions. He chooses the appropriate set of questions by using each of the patient's responses as a branch point to eliminate large classes of irrelevant questions. The development of interactive computer technics has made it feasible to use such content-dependent questioning procedures in automated history collection.[48,53,54] The questioning patterns developed for the computer incorporate some of the branching criteria that a physician uses, but they include additional questions that are more detailed or quantitative to compensate for the loss of nonverbal inputs employed by the physician in his traditional questioning.

This application of computer technology offers the greatest immediate potential for physicians practicing in small hospitals or in the community. Service bureaus will soon provide remote computer terminal service in a fashion similar to the telephone company. With the use of these agencies, automated medical histories should be available to every physician and health-care facility within the next five years.

Hospital Information Systems

The application of computers to patient care that has been of greatest interest to commercial computer firms has been labeled "Hospital Information Systems" (HIS) or a similar acronym. To the physician, this means a system that will provide rapid, accurate, and legible communication of reports, better scheduling procedures and timely and precise implementation of activities ordered for patient care. To the nurse, HIS implies an operation to lighten the clerical load of communication functions, preparing requisitions and transcribing and charting. To the administrator, HIS is a means for using resources more effectively, for gathering the data necessary for appropriate management decisions and for ensuring that information necessary for the patient billing process is readily available and accurate. To the medical research investigator, HIS offers the potential for a data base of patient-care activities that is not only accurate but also organized and easily retrieved and analyzed.

The major emphasis in the development of an HIS has been in the use of a real-time, on-line, computer system with multiple input-output terminals located in patient-care units and in all service areas. "Real-time" implies that the user of the terminal is in direct communication with different areas of the hospital, and that the computer receives data, processes transactions and returns results so as to affect patient care and administrative decisions. "On-line" means that when someone uses the system, he deals directly with the computer through a terminal such as a teletypewriter.[55,56]

A number of major developmental projects are concerned with HIS.[57-59] Documentation of these projects is limited, however, and most of the information available is contained in privately published progress reports. Research in the application of computer technology to medicine is quite different from most classic medical research, and it has been difficult to use the common technics of planning, hypothesis-testing and scientific evaluation. The major initial problem is that information on objectives and procedures now in use is meager. It is therefore exceedingly difficult to specify the tasks that the computer should perform.

Most hospital computer systems are now oriented toward administrative functions. These systems provide effective communication within the hospital and a central data base of patient information that can be accessed instantaneously from many locations in the hospital. Most advanced research and developmental efforts are concerned with communication and control functions initiated by each doctor's order.

The initial wave of optimism and enthusiasm generated by beguiling promises of an immediately available total hospital computer system has passed. Now, efforts are directed toward the painful, slow, evolutionary process of developing and implementing modules or building blocks for individual functions. There is now a keen appreciation of the wide gap separating a demonstration project, however impressive, and an operational service system to daily use. Stringent reliability requirements and the difficulties attendant when nontechnical personnel (with a high turn-over rate) use a computer system on a round-the-clock basis have been two of the key limiting factors in HIS development. In addition, the very high initial costs often stagger hospital administrators; demonstration of cost-benefit savings is difficult. If the experience of other industries is repeated in hospitals, the use of computers in hospitals will not reduce total medical-care costs, but will lead to more effective use of the resources at hand and to improved patient care.

Conclusions

Computer science has introduced new dimensions into human thought and activity, and has made possible enterprises inconceivable only a few years ago. Computer applications in patient care have thus far been more dreams than reality. Now we are on the threshold of an exciting potential. Realization of this potential will require intense and continuing methodologic and technologic development.

I am indebted to the staff of the Laboratory of Computer Science for contributions to the content and philosophy of this article.

REFERENCES

1. Jydstrup, R. A., and Gross, M. J. Cost of information handling in hospitals. *Health Serv. Research* **1**:235–271, Winter, 1966. HealthServ.Research
2. Peinstein, A. R. *Clinical Judgment*. Baltimore: Williams & Wilkins, 1967.
3. Engle, R. L., Jr. Medical diagnosis: present, past, and future, Ill. Diagnosis in future, including critique on use of electronic computers as diagnostic aids to physician. *Arch. Int. Med.* **112**:520–529, 1963.
4. *Idem*. Medical diagnosis: present, past, and future. 11. Philosophical foundations and historical development of our concepts of health, disease, and diagnosis. *Arch. Int. Med.* **112**:520–529, 1963.
5. Ledley, R. S., and Lusted, L. B. Reasoning foundations of medical diagnosis: symbolic logic, probability, and value theory aid our understanding of how physicians reason. *Science*. **130**:9–21, 1959.
6. Warner, H. R., Toronto, A. F., Veasy, L. G., and Stephenson, R. Mathematical approach to medical diagnosis: application to congenital heart disease. *J.A.M.A.* **177**:177–183, 1961.
7. Toronto, A. F., Veasy, L. G., and Warner, H. R. Evaluation of computer program for diagnosis of congenital heart disease. *Prog. in Cardiovasc. Dis.* **5**:362–377, 1963.
8. Overall, J. E., and Williams, C. M. Conditional probability program for diagnosis of thyroid function. *J.A.M.A.* **183**:307–313, 1963.
9. Lodwick, G. S., Haun, C. L., Smith, W. E., Keller, R. F., and Robertson, E. D. Computer diagnosis of primary bone tumors preliminary report. *Radiology* **80**: 273–275, 1963.
10. Gorry, G. A., and Barnett, G. O. Experience with model of sequential diagnosis. *Comput. & Biomed. Research* **1**:490–507, May, 1968.
11. Bruce, R. A., and Yarnall, S. R. Computer-aided diagnosis of cardiovascular disorders, *J. Chronic Dis.* **19**:473–484, 1966.
12. Collen, F. F., et al. Automated multiphasic screening and diagnosis. *Am. J. Pub. Health* **54**:741–750, 1964.
13. Boyle, J. A., et al. Construction of model for computer-assisted diagnosis: application to problem of non-toxic goitre. *Quart. J. Med.* **35**:565–588, 1966.
14. Manning, R. T., and Watson, L. Signs, symptoms, and systematics. *J.A.M.A.* **198**:1180–1184, 1966.
15. Sterling, T. D., Nickson, J., and Pollack, S. V. Is medical diagnosis general computer problem? *J.A.M.A.* **198**:281–286, 1966.
16. Scadding, J. G. Diagnosis: clinician and computer. *Lancet* **2**:877–882, 1967.
17. *The Diagnostic Process*. Edited by J. A. Jacquez. Ann Arbor, Michigan: Malloy Lithographing, Inc., 1964. P. 47.
18. Williams, G. Z. Use of data processing and automation in clinical pathology. *Mil. Med.* **129**:502–509, 1964.
19. Bryan, D. J., et al. Profile of admission chemical data by multi-channel automation: evaluative experiment. *Clin. Chem.* **12**:137–143, 1966.
20. Lindberg, D. A., Van Peenen, H. J., and Couch, R. D. Patterns in clinical chemistry: low serum sodium and chloride in hospitalized patients. *Am. J. Clin. Path.* **44**:315–321, 1965.
21. Lamson, B. G., et al. Hospitalwide system for handling medical data. *Hospitals* **41**:67, May 1, 1967.
22. Straumfjord, J. V., Jr., Spraberry, M. N., Biggs, H. G., and Noto, T. A. Electronic data processing system for clinical laboratories system used for all laboratory sections. *Am. J. Clin. Path.* **47**:661–676, 1967.

23. Baird, H. W., and Garfunkel, J. M. Electronic data processing of medical records. *New Eng. J. Med.* **272**:1211–1215, 1965.
24. Hicks, G. P., Gieschen, M. M., Slack, W. V., and Larson, F. C. Routine use of small digital computer in clinical laboratory *J.A.M.A.* **196**:973–978, 1966.
25. Pribor, H. C., Kirkham, W. R., and Hoyt, R. S. Small computer does big job in this hospital laboratory. *Mod. Hosp.* **110**(4): 104–107, April, 1968.
26. Rappoport, A. E., Gennaro, W. D., and Constandse, W. J. Computer-laboratory link is base of hospital information system *Mod. Hosp.* **110**(4):94–102, April, 1968.
27. Lindberg, D. A. B. Collection, evaluation, and transmission of hospital laboratory data. *Methods of Inform. in Med.* **6**:97–107, 1967.
28. Davis, L. S., Collen, M. F., Rubin, L., and Van Brunt, E. E. Computer-stored medical record. *Comput. & Biomed. Research* **1**:452–469, May 1968.
29. Wilson, J. M., and Jungner, G. *Principles and Practice of Screening for Disease.* New York: Columbia Univ. Press, 1968.
30. Collen, M. F. Periodic health examination using automated multi-test laboratory. *J.A.M.A.* **195**:830–833, 1966.
31. Weil, M. H., Shubin, H., and Rand, W. Experience with digital computer for study and improved management of critically ill. *J.A.M.A.* **198**:1011–1016, 1966.
32. Warner, H. R., Gardner, R. M., and Toronto, A. P. Computer based monitoring of cardiovascular functions in post-operative patients. *Circulation* 37:(supp. 2) 68–74, 1968.
33. Vallbona, C., Spencer, W. A., Geddes, L. A., Blose, W. F., and Canzoneri, J., III. Experience with on-line monitoring in critical illness. *IEEE Spectrum* 3:136–140, 1966.
34. Wilber, S. A., and Derrick, W. S. Patient monitoring and anesthetic management: physiological communications network. *J.A.M.A.,* **191**:893–898, 1965.
35. Berkley, C. Case histories—untapped medical information resource. *Am. J. M. Electronics* (Supp.) **4**:4, 1965.
36. Pratt, A. W., and Thomas, L. B. Information processing system for pathology data. *Pathology Annual, 1966.* Series editor: S. C. Sommers. New York: Appleton, 1966.
37. Slee, V. N. Information systems and measurement tools. *J.A.M.A.* **196**:1063–1065, 1966.
38. Murray, J. E., and Barnes, B. A. Introductory remarks on kidney transplantation with observations on kidney transplant registry. *Transplantation* **5**(4):824–830. Part 2, July, 1967.
39. Haenszel, W., and Lourie, W. I., Jr. Quality control of data in large-scale cancer register program. *Meth. of Inform. in Med.* **5**:67–74, 1966.
40. Yoder, R. D. Preparing medical record data for computer processing. *Hospitals* **40**:75, 1966.
41. Allen, S. I., Barnett, G. O., and Castleman, P. A. Use of time-shared general purpose file-handling system in hospital research. *Proc. IEEE* **54**:1641–1648, 1966.
42. Levy, R. P., Cammarn, M. R., and Smith, M. J. Computer handling of ambulatory clinic records. *J.A.M.A.* **190**:1033–1037, 1964.
43. Hall, P., Mellner, Ch., and Danielsson, T. J5–data processing system for medical information. *Meth. of Inform. in Med.* **6**:1–6, 1967.
44. Korein, J., Bender, A. L., Rothenberg, D., and Tick, L. J. Computer processing of medical data by variable-field-length format. III. Statistical analysis of narrative content. *J.A.M.A.* **196**:957–963, 1966.
45. Jacobs, H. Natural language information retrieval system. *Meth. of Inform. in Med.* **7**:8–16, 1968.
46. Gordon, B. L., Biomedical language and format for manual and computer applications. *Dis. of Chest* **53**:38–42, 1968.
47. Slack, W. V., Peckham, B. M., Van Cura, L. J., et al. Computer-based physical examination system. *J.A.M.A.* **200**:224–228, 1967.
48. Barnett, G. O., and Greenes, R. A. Hospital information systems: interface prob-

lem. Conf. Proc. on "use of data mechanization and computer in medicine." *Ann. New York Acad. Sc.* (in press).

49. Templeton, A. W., Lodwick, G. S., and Turner, A. H., Jr. RADIATE: new concept for computer coding, transmitting, storing, and retrieving radiological data. *Radiology* **85**:811–817, 1965.

50. Brodman, K., Erdmann, A. J., Jr., Lorge, I., and Wolff, H. G. Cornell Medical Index: adjunct to medical interview. *J.A.M.A.* **140**:530–534, 1949.

51. Abramson, J. H., Terespolsky, L., Brook, J. G., and Kark, S. L. Cornell Medical Index as health measure in epidemiological studies: test of validity of health questionnaire. *Brit. J. Prev. & Social Med.* **19**:103–110, 1965.

52. Rose, G. A. Diagnosis of ischaemic heart pain and intermittent claudication in field surveys. *Bull. World Health Organ.* **27**:645–658, 1962.

53. Slack, W. V., Hicks, G. P., Reed, C. E., and Van Cura, L. J. Computer-based medical-history system. *New Eng. J. Med.* **274**:194–198, 1966.

54. Mayne, J. G., Weksel, W., and Sholtz, P. N. Toward automating medical history. *Mayo Clin. Proc.* **43**:1–25, 1968.

55. Rikli, A. E., Allen, S. I., and Alexander, S. N. Study suggests value of shared computers. *Mod. Hosp.* **106**:100–108, 1966.

56. Barnett, G. O., and Castleman, P. A. Time-sharing computer system for patient-care activities. *Comput. & Biomed. Research* **1**:41–51, March 1967.

57. Siler, W., and Korn, H. Working total information system is at least year away. *Hospitals* **41**:99–104, May 1, 1967.

58. Jacobus, G. C. Sorting sense from nonsense in hospital ADP programs. *Hospitals* **41**:32–36, May 1, 1967.

59. Hofman, P. B., and Barnett, G. O. Time-sharing increases benefits of computer use. *Hospitals* **42**:62–67, June 16, 1968.

Part IV

Evaluation and Control

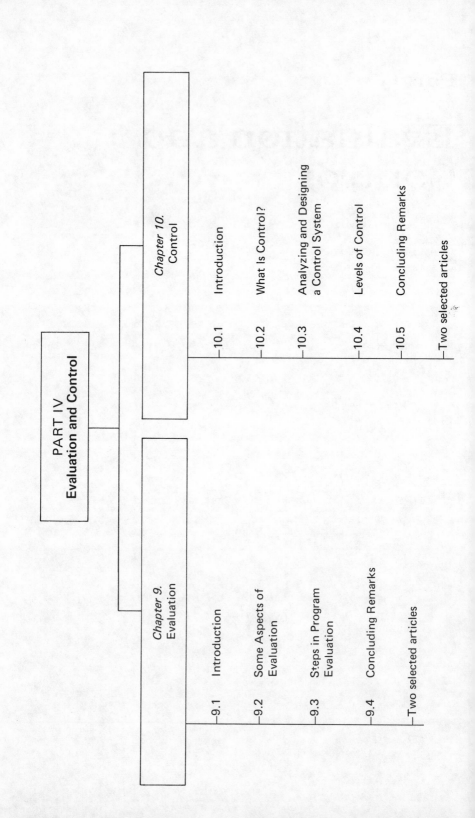

PART IV
Evaluation and Control

Chapter 9.
Evaluation

9.1 — Introduction

9.2 — Some Aspects of Evaluation

9.3 — Steps in Program Evaluation

9.4 — Concluding Remarks

— Two selected articles

Chapter 10.
Control

10.1 — Introduction

10.2 — What Is Control?

10.3 — Analyzing and Designing a Control System

10.4 — Levels of Control

10.5 — Concluding Remarks

— Two selected articles

Chapter 9

Evaluation

9.1 INTRODUCTION

The ideal state of a system or an organization is one in which management is able to exercise effective control so that organizational objectives can be fully met. By definition, the ideal state is not achievable, but it is only through striving towards such a state that organizational performance is improved [Ackoff, 1971, p. 667]. This requires that the administrator understand such management concepts and techniques as planning, programming, resource allocation, scheduling, measurement, evaluation, feedback and control. Planning, program budgeting, cost-effectiveness analysis, and information systems required to implement these management techniques were examined in Part III. In this chapter we will describe some aspects of evaluation; discuss different formats of necessary steps in the evaluation process; and mention the focus of recent research in evaluation.

9.2 SOME ASPECTS OF EVALUATION

To evaluate is to make a value judgment. It involves comparing something with another and then making either *choice* or *action* decisions. Evaluation leading to choice decisions refers to activities performed in the intitiation, exploration, and planning phases of health programs. The choice of a specific program (or a course of action) from among a set of feasible programs is the result of this type of evaluation. It operates in the planning phase (choice decision)—*before* the plans are put into effect. A second type of evaluation refers to activities performed during the operations phase (action decision). Here, evaluation is directed towards two ends:* (1) to measure the *progress* of plans, and programs, and (2) to measure the

---

* This corresponds to the classification of evaluatory studies, advanced by MacMahon et al. One category consists of studies designed to test the hypothesis that a certain program will in fact produce measurable beneficial outcomes. The second category, in which cause and effect are not at issue, is referred to as "evaluation of technics." See MacMahon et al. [in Schulberg et al., 1969, p. 51].

achievement of the plans and programs. Evaluation made during the operations phase triggers action decisions in order to effect control.

Planning, evaluation, and control are in a sense inseparable concepts. Even the best-developed plans are worthless if they cannot be successfully implemented. As we discussed in Chapter 6, the process of planning results in a system or hierarchy of plans which are then translated into specific programs and activities. *Before* plans are finalized and budget authorizations made, administrators can utilize modern management techniques, such as PPB and cost-effectiveness analysis, to make resource commitment decisions. The evaluation and control phase starts *after* the plans (and programs) are set in motion. Thus, planning, evaluation, and control are different parts of the same job; they are not separate jobs. Although we can discuss them separately for the purpose of gaining an in-depth knowledge, in the real world they are interdependent parts of a unified system of management.

The process of evaluation (or program evaluation)* consists of all necessary steps to determine the extent to which predetermined objectives are being met by a set of programs. The boundaries of program evaluation are drawn arbitrarily depending upon the scope of research and the interest of the researcher. The purpose of evaluation is to examine the effectiveness of organization plans. Evaluation is the link which connects planning with control. Evaluation requires measurement of results (in terms of agreed upon measures of performance) and their comparison with stated goals. The variance between measured results and the goals then becomes the basis for control decisions.

Evaluation is as important to the managerial process as are the functions of planning, organizing, staffing, and control. Yet, in the business management literature evaluation has received considerably less emphasis than in the health field. The reason for this is that business and industrial programs can usually be evaluated by commonly accepted measures (e.g., ROI, P/E ratios, turnover ratios) both in the planning and the operations phases. Hence, it is under the umbrella of planning and control, rather than as a separate area of study, that various aspects of evaluation are usually discussed in the management literature. The topics of Job Evaluation† and Program Evaluation and Review Techniques (PERT)‡ are the two major

---

* The terms "evaluation" and "program evaluation" will be used synonymously in this book.

† See, for example, Belcher [1958], Patton, et al., [1964], Burgess [1968], Dunn and Rachel [1971]. The purpose of job evaluation is to establish an equitable wage and salary structure. Jobs can be evaluated in several ways. One method, for example, identifies characteristics necessary for accomplishing jobs, assigns relative weights to these characteristics and then sets a level of compensation depending upon the amount of these characteristics needed to perform a job.

‡ See, for example, Lockyer [1967], Moder and Phillips [1964], and Levin and Kirkpatrick [1966], and Miller [1963].

exceptions where the word "evaluation" appears in the main title and in which formal evaluation techniques have been developed and utilized. In both job evaluation and PERT, the term evaluation operates in either the planning or progress evaluation sense.

The situation in the health field is entirely different. Evaluation constitutes an important area in and of itself, and we find a relatively large volume of published literature on this subject.* A measure of the increasing importance being attached to evaluation in the health field is indicated by the fact that a special conference on the topic was held in 1969.†

In the health care literature, discussion of evaluation touches a very broad range of elements—covering concepts, general issues, principles, techniques, indices, and specific evaluation studies. In terms of practical impact, evaluation in the health field has been conducted in the sense of comparing achievements with goals established in the planning phase (i.e., in the action-decision sense).

There is a high level of interest in the topic of program evaluation in the health area. This is because, firstly, the health sector has already become the largest segment of our economy and its sheer size demands formal evaluation of various health programs. Secondly, the ultimate objectives of health (e.g., optimum community health) are so complex that they pose serious measurement problems for administrators. Yet, in order to make intelligent resource commitment decisions, programs designed to achieve these objectives must be evaluated. The very ill-defined, ill-structured, value-laden nature of health problems makes evaluation a very important function for the health administrator.

9.3 STEPS IN PROGRAM EVALUATION

A number of authors have proposed various formats of describing the necessary steps in the process of evaluation. MacMahon et al. have suggested the following steps in the evaluation process as "principles" of program evaluation: ‡

1. The determination of what type of evaluation is required before designing the evaluatory plan.
2. The definition of the program, the population to be served, and the effects desired.

---

* See, Klein [1969] in *Evaluating Outcomes for Health Care: An Annotated Bibliography*, cited in *Outcomes Conference 1–11*, Dept. of HEW, 1969, p. 30. Also, see our Selection 26 [Roemer, 1971].
† *Outcome Conference 1–11* (Methodology of identifying, measuring and evaluating outcomes of health service programs, systems and subsystems) Department of Health, Education, and Welfare, 1969.
‡ MacMahon et al. [in Schulberg et al., 1969, p. 51].

3. The choice of comparison groups which will permit the inferences required by the type of evaluation selected.

These "principles" serve as guidelines for determining the specific steps that must be followed in designing an evaluation procedure. The essence of this procedure is contained in the three steps* of program evaluation given by Knutson.†

1. First, it is essential to have a precise statement of the program objectives and the specific, agreed-upon criteria that will be used to determine whether or not these objectives have been achieved.
2. Secondly, it is essential to have a baseline measurement of the status of the situation at the time the objectives are established; or if that should be impossible, some other agreed-upon and appropriate programs for comparison. Data obtained concerning the status of the program should relate directly to these specific objectives.
3. Thirdly, it is essential to know the status of the program relative to objectives at some point sufficiently advanced in time so that changes as a result of the program effort can reasonably be expected. Usually the methods of measurement employed to obtain baseline data may also be used to obtain follow-up data. We need to be aware, however, that the process of interviewing or collecting data is in itself an educational process. In evaluating programs, therefore, it may be necessary to use matched samples or control groups to obtain valid and reliable follow-up data.

Knutson points out that "if the principles of [program] evaluation have been applied, the first two steps will have been taken and the third already planned."

In our view, the following steps are inherent in the evaluation process and must be carefully adhered to:

1. formulation of the objectives,
2. specification of measures of performance,
3. development of the model, plans, and programs,
4. measurement of results.
5. determination and explanation of the degree of success, and
6. recommendations for appropriate actions in view of the variance between predetermined objectives and actual results.

In the operational sense, program evaluation comprises steps 4, 5, and 6. The process of planning consists of steps 1, 2, and 3; while control covers steps 3 through 6 (plus the additional step of instituting action to restore a balance between plans and performance). As mentioned earlier,

---

* As mentioned earlier, the boundaries of program evaluation are drawn arbitrarily. For a four-step procedure (which includes control), see MacMahon et al. [in Schulberg et al., 1969].
† See Knutson [in Schulberg et al., 1969, pp. 49–50].

we consider planning, evaluation, and control as separate parts of the same job, not isolated tasks divorced from each other. Our evaluation philosophy, therefore, is one that has been labelled as the systems model.

9.4 CONCLUDING REMARKS

There is evidence of significant research in the area of program evaluation in health fields.* The focus of research has been on: (1) the type of questions to be asked; (2) the type of models to be used; and (3) the improvement of programs in view of research findings. At the operational level, Deniston et al. [1968, pp. 323–324] list four categories into which evaluative questions can be grouped. These categories are *appropriateness, adequacy, effectiveness,* and *efficiency.* Questions on appropriateness focus on the relative impact of the programs; while adequacy refers to the degree by which programs will eliminate certain health problems. Effectiveness is a measure of the extent by which programs attain pre-established objectives, and efficiency is defined as "the ratio between output (net attainment of program objectives) and input (program resources expended)" [Deniston et al., 1968, p. 604]. The model described by Deniston et al. [1968, p. 324] answers two questions: "(a) to what extent were objectives attained as the result of activities (program effectiveness) and (b) at what cost (program efficiency)."

Schulberg et al. [1969, pp. 17–20] classify program evaluation models in two categories: (1) the goal attainment model and (2) the systems model. They distinguish between these models in these words: "In contrast to the goal-attainment approach which directs evaluation efforts at measuring how well a specific organizational goal was achieved, the systems model contends that such an approach is unproductive and even misleading, since an organization constantly functions at a variety of levels." This classification of program evaluation models is questionable, and it appears that the issue has been unnecessarily confused in this case. The category entitled systems model is descriptive of what is known in the literature as the systems approach to management. Its major importance is in the stage of developing objectives, resolving (to the extent possible) conflicts between objectives, choosing measures of performance, developing one or more models to represent organizational systems, and developing plans. What will be evaluated (programs and goals), how the process of evaluation will work (research design and evaluation indices), when and at what points evaluation will be made (timing and the point of entry) are all important questions which need to be considered during the planning stages. Once the plans and programs are put in effect, the process of formal (or informal)

---

* Schulberg et al. [1969].

evaluation takes place in the "goal-attainment" model sense. Thus, we think that a classification of program evaluation models into the artificial categories of goal-attainment models and systems models is not appropriate. The real issues of evaluation we feel have been addressed by the late Dr. George James [1962, p. 1151] who suggested four categories for evaluating programs in public health: *effort, performance, adequacy of performance,* and *efficiency.** Schulberg et al. summarize the contents of these four categories:

1. Evaluation of effort: how do the practices of the program under study compare with local or national standards? The use of such yardsticks as patient-staff ratios provides a simple but limited assessment of the program's functioning.
2. Evaluation of performance: what outcomes have the program's efforts produced? This approach assumes that services were provided correctly to the individuals that were helped.
3. Adequacy of performance: to what extent has the community's total problem been solved by this program? Services directed to a minority of individuals are less adequate than those focused upon the total population.
4. Evaluation of efficiency: can the same end result be achieved at lower cost? Screening programs frequently are evaluated in this manner by considering the number of false positives and false negatives produced by them.

James [1962, p. 1153] suggested that:

In addition to the four categories, every evaluation exercise should also analyze the processes involved in the program. What is it that has made the program succeed or fail? What changes in technics or methods could have improved program effectiveness? Which recipient of the program benefited the most and which the least? What did the program accomplish in terms of originally unforeseen objectives? Each program is a potential target for numerous research questions. The findings of the evaluation study, aimed though they may be at determining progress toward a specific objective, should be analyzed closely to see which additional questions might also be answered.

We selected two articles for this chapter. Roemer's article (Selection 19) presents a survey of the literature addressed to the various problems encountered in evaluating health service programs. He suggests "a framework for analysis of the relative values (evaluation) of various systems or subsystems of health organization (health service programs)." The framework is based on the premises that a system or program can be evaluated in the context of different planning horizons (short, intermediate, or long-term) and that several phenomena within each level may be defined and

---

* See Selection 20 for a discussion of efficiency and effectiveness. Also, see our last footnote on page 230.

measured. The author identifies six levels at which program evaluation can be conducted: (1) health status outcomes, (2) estimated quality of service, (3) quantity of services performed, (4) attitudes of recipients, (5) resources made available, and (6) costs of the program. Examples of evaluation at each level are provided. Finally, the author presents a matrix with six rows (corresponding to the six levels of evaluation) and two columns showing (1) eligible (or target) population, and (2) patients actually served. Within each cell of the matrix, "evaluation requires the comparison of measurements of at least two entities, defined either across time (before and after) or across space (the model of test or control group)." A rational planning of health service will benefit from program evaluation studies (dealing with systems of varying degrees of complexity) conducted within any of the matrix cells.

Deniston et al. (Selection 20) differentiates between program effectiveness and program efficiency in evaluating the performance of a program. A program consists of three components: objectives, activities, and resources. The definitions of these components are provided to prepare the reader for grasping the difference between evaluation of effectiveness and evaluation of efficiency. A measure of program effectiveness is the extent to which planned objectives have been attained as a result of undertaking activities in support of the program. Three measures of effectiveness are suggested— one overall measure and two subordinate measures. The overall measure of program effectiveness is denoted as the ratio AO:PO; that is the ratio of "attained level of objectives" to the "planned level of objectives."* The first subordinate measure is at the activity level; the ratio AA:PA (ratio of "actual level of activity performed" to the "planned level of activity"). The second subordinate measure of effectiveness is the ratio AR:PR (ratio of "actual resources expended" to "planned level of resources to be expended"). The same three measures can be applied at the sub-objective level.† The authors give a list of choices available to the administrator when program effectiveness is lower than desired. Program efficiency is defined as AO:AR (ratio of "attained level of objectives" to "actual resources expended"). The authors suggest two additional efficiency ratios. One relates "attained level of objectives" to "actual level of activity performed"—AO:AA. The other ratio is AA:AR (ratio of "actual level of activity performed" to "actual resources expended"). Problems relating to measurement and questions of quality considerations are discussed.

Efficiency measures are then discussed in terms of their limitations and

---

* The reader is cautioned here to consider the complex problem of multiple-objectives. Deniston et al. do not explicitly discuss the implications of multiple-objective decision problems. See Chapter 5.

† Objectives are hierarchical in nature—they include ultimate objectives, overall program objectives, and sub-objectives. See Chapter 7.

potential applications. Finally, the authors give the characteristics of programs for which effectiveness and efficiency measures are most useful.

REFERENCES

Ackoff, R. L., "Towards A System of Systems Concepts," *Management Science,*
1971   vol. 17, no. 11, July, pp. 661–671.

Belcher, D. W., *Wage and Salary Administration,* Englewood Cliffs, N.J.:
1958   Prentice-Hall.

Burgess, L. R., *Wage and Salary Administration in a Dynamic Economy,* New
1968   York: Harcourt, Brace, and World.

Connors, E. J., "Measuring Hospital Effectiveness: Management Patterns,"
1969   *University of Michigan Medical Center Journal,* vol. 35, no. 2, pp.
116–118.

Deniston, O. L., et al., *a,* "Evaluation of Program Effectiveness," *Public Health*
1968   *Reports,* Public Health Service, U.S. Department Health, Education,
and Welfare, vol. 83, no. 4, April.

Deniston, O. L., et al., *b,* "Evaluation of Program Efficiency," *Public Health*
1968   *Reports,* Public Health Service, U.S. Department Health, Education
and Welfare, vol. 83, no. 7, July.

Dunn, J. D., and F. M. Rachel, *Wage and Salary Administration, Total Com-*
1971   *pensation Systems,* New York: McGraw-Hill.

Hopkins, C. E. (ed.), *Conference Series: Outcomes Conference 1–11* Depart-
1969   ment of Health, Education and Welfare.

James, G., "Evaluation in Public Health Practice," *American Journal of Public*
1962   *Health,* vol. 52, pp. 1145–1154.

Klein, B., "Evaluating Outcomes for Health Care: An Annotated Bibliography"
1969   cited in *Outcomes Conference 1–11,* Department of Health, Education and Welfare, p. 30.

Knutson, A. L., "Evaluation for What?" in H. C. Schulberg, et al., *Program*
1969   *Evaluation in the Health Fields,* New York: Behavioral Publications.

Levin, R., and C. Kirkpatrick, *Planning and Control with PERT/CPM,* New
1966   York: McGraw-Hill.

Lockyer, K. G., *An Introduction to Critical Path Analysis,* 2nd Edition, New
1967   York: Pitman Publishing Corp.

MacMahon, B., et al., "Principles in the Evaluation of Community Mental
1969   Health Programs," in H. C. Schulberg, et al., *Program Evaluation
in the Health Fields,* New York: Behavioral Publications.

Malcolm, D. G., et al., "Application of a Technique for Research and De-
1959   velopment Program Evaluation," *Operations Research,* vol. 7, no. 5,
September-October, pp. 646-669.

Miller, R. W., "How to Plan and Control with PERT," *Harvard Business*
1962   *Review,* March-April, pp. 93–104.

Miller, R. W., *Schedule, Cost, and Profit Control with PERT,* New York:
1963   McGraw-Hill.

Moder, J. J., and C. R. Phillips, *Project Management with CPM and PERT,*
1964   New York: Reinhold Publishing Corp.

Patton, J. A., C. L. Littlefield, and S. A. Self, *Job Evaluation,* Homewood,
1964   Ill.: Richard D. Irwin, Chapters 6, 7, 8.

Schulberg, H. C., A. Sheldon, and F. Baker, *Program Evaluation in the Health*
1969   *Fields,* New York: Behavioral Publications.

SELECTION 19

Evaluation of Health Service Programs and Levels of Measurement*

Milton I. Roemer, M.D.

For a hundred years or more clinical medicine has applied, with varying degrees of sophistication and rigor, the method of the controlled clinical trial to test the effectiveness or value of proposed new theories for individual patients (*1*). Only in the last decade or two has serious attention been given to evaluation of the various forms of organization of health services. The problems of this type of evaluation are complicated by an admixture of variables, especially involving differences between the test and control, or comparison, groups with respect to the characteristics of the persons served, the medical technology applied, or other factors outside of the form or pattern of health service organization per se.

Need for Clarification

Because of the complexities of evaluating methods of health service organization, there has been a great deal of confusion in even deciding what should be evaluated, let alone how to go about doing it (*2*). Many different meanings have been attributed to "evaluation," and wide disparity exists in the terminology applied to the goals of a program, its end results, its quality, its effectiveness, its outcomes, and so on (*3*). The purpose of this paper is to suggest a framework for analysis of the relative values (evaluation) of various systems or subsystems of health organization (health service programs), to help clear the air and promote uniformity of terms and concepts so as to facilitate communication among investigators.

Many extensive reviews and annotated bibliographies on the problems of evaluation of health service programs have been issued in recent years. Altman and Anderson, in 1962, prepared an annotated bibliography on the evaluation of medical care (*4*). Suchman produced a book in 1967 on evaluative research in the social sciences (*5*). In 1966 the Health Services Research Study Section of the Public Health Service commissioned a series

---

* *Public Health Reports*, vol. 82, July, 1968.

of review papers on health services research. Most relevant to the issue posed here are the comprehensive accounts by Donabedian on "Evaluating the Quality of Medical Care" (*6*) and by Weinerman on "Research into the Organization of Medical Practice" (*7*). In 1967 Shapiro wrote an excellent summary on "End Result Measurements of Quality of Medical Care" (*8*). In August 1969 the California Center for Health Services Research issued an annotated bibliography, "Evaluating Outcomes of Health Care" (*9*). The World Health Organization's selected bibliography, "Methodology in Public Health Studies" (1968), also contains many references on evaluation (*10*). In 1969 volume 2 of "A Guide to Medical Care Administration," from the American Public Health Association's program area committee on medical care administration, appeared under the title of "Medical Care Appraised—Quality and Utilization," prepared by Donabedian (*11*). A very useful compilation of readings, "Program Evaluation in the Health Fields" was also assembled in 1969 by Schulberg, Sheldon, and Barker (*12*).

With this wealth of reviews on the literature of health program evaluation —and there are more papers and volumes than those noted, Mactavish's bibliography (*13*), for example—I do not intend to add another overview, but rather offer a framework that will attempt to integrate the several approaches used into a relatively simple schema.

As organization theorists have pointed out, every system or subsystem has a set of short-term ends, which in turn become means toward more long-term ends (*14*). A health service program may have as its immediate end or goal the provision of certain services (for example, prenatal examinations or intensive care of patients with coronary attacks) but the long-term goal is to advance health status. There are several more links in the chain of causation, but the basic point to be recognized is that the system or program can be evaluated on various levels: short term, intermediate, and long term. Several phenomena within each level may be defined and measured.

Donabedian speaks cogently of evaluation or appraisal of the (*a*) structure, (*b*) process, and (*c*) outcome of a medical care program (*11*). This entry to the problem is useful, especially his emphasis on importance of examining the process even though the ultimate outcome may be difficult or impossible to measure. My attempt, in a sense, is to refine this typology somewhat further, in order to build a framework into which the whole spectrum of evaluation methodologies may logically be fitted.

If the focus is on evaluation of health service programs (that is, mechanisms of organization of health services in their many aspects) it may be helpful to think of all the consequences as a chain of effects at different levels of depth. Regardless of the immediate short-term ends or goals of a health program, it must ultimately be judged or evaluated by its success in saving lives or reducing disability or advancing health status in some way. Only when the attainment of that ultimate goal becomes difficult to measure or to attribute to a specific programmatic cause, which is frequently true, must we take recourse to evaluation based on less ultimate effects (15).

Levels of Evaluation

Health status outcomes. Ideally, health planners would like to know the effect of any pattern of organization of health services, whether old, new, or projected, in terms of health status changes in the target population. Many studies have used this type of outcome measure with varying degrees of sophistication in ruling out secondary variables.

On the crudest level of a total population, for example, one may compare a large system like the British National Health Service with the U.S. health scene. Observing a higher life expectancy in Great Britain than in the United States, one might conclude that the net outcome of the British National Health Service is superior to that of the pluralistic U.S. system, or "nonsystem" (16). But such a conclusion would be unwarranted without considering the effects of diverse living conditions, genetic factors, and scores of epidemiologic variables that can influence death rates and life expectancy in the two nations, quite aside from their health service systems. Nevertheless, even this crude comparison provides a clue for more searching types of measurement of the effects of the two systems of health service at the deepest level of evaluation; namely, the outcome in health status.

More sophisticated evaluative studies are illustrated by comparisons of the membership of the Health Insurance Plan of Greater New York with the rest of the New York population, matched for sociodemographic characteristics. In the early 1950's an important study showed lower perinatal mortality in a population eligible for this prepaid group practice program (17), and in the 1960's a study showed a lower death rate among indigent aged (old-age assistance recipients) enrolled in the plan (18), compared in both instances with matched populations entitled to traditional medical care. The elaborate tasks of sampling, randomization, data analysis, and so on in studies of this type need not be reviewed here.

Health status outcomes have also been applied in comparative studies of populations actually served in varying medical settings, most frequently in hospitals of different types. Lipworth and co-workers found lower disease-specific case fatality rates in British teaching hospitals compared with non-teaching ones (19). John Thompson and colleagues compared perinatal mortality as an indicator of obstetrical care in two U.S. Air Force hospitals (20). I found lower postoperative deaths for certain surgical procedures in large, compared with small, hospitals in Saskatchewan (21).

In all such hospital-based studies, one must make adjustments for the varying severity of cases, and hence risk of death, in different hospitals; and in a 1968 paper two colleagues and I offered a statistical approach to the solution of this problem (22). If such a statistical adjustment can be perfected, we will have a much firmer basis for judging a hospital's overall effectiveness than the brief inspections of input (hospital resources, policies, practices) on which the Joint Commission on Accreditation of Hospitals or the State hospital licensure authorities now depend.

Beyond mortality data are many other measures of the ultimate outcome of a health service program, in terms of health status, that may be applied, either to total populations eligible or to persons definitely served by the program. Life expectancies, based on modified life table techniques, have been applied to measure the effect of a county public health program. This method corrects for the problem of higher morbidity rates among older persons with chronic disease who are kept alive by active medical care (23). More sensitive than this are various measures of recovery from illness or days of disability, such as absenteeism from work or school, restricted activity days, or days in bed, of persons eligible for one program as compared with another (24).

Formulated more positively, health status outcomes may be reflected in measurements of the capacities of persons to function, as applied by Sidney Katz and his colleagues in studies of rehabilitation of the aged sick (25,26). The effectiveness of family planning programs may be evaluated in terms of subsequent birth rates. There are scores of specific measurements of recovery from certain diseases, improved physical or mental functioning, and other phenomena that may be and have been applied in outcome evaluation of specialized programs (27). Sanazaro and Williamson have delineated a set of six patient end-results for judging the outcome of cases reaching the attention of specialists in internal medicine (28).

This type of health status outcome is the usual end point in clinical trials of new drug therapies or new preventive services, like the Salk antipoliomyelitis vaccine or the fluoridation of water supplies to reduce the rate of dental caries. Its application to evaluation of health service programs, however, is complicated by so many variables in the characteristics of the populations eligible or served, the diseases involved, and numerous environmental divergencies that, in practice, it is difficult and costly to apply. To adjust properly for all these confounding influences requires very large or highly selected samples, long periods of observation, and elaborate methodologies. As a practical matter, therefore, evaluation of health service programs must often resort to measurements of effect that are less ultimate in the chain of influences. Next to health status would be the level that may be described as the estimated quality of service.

Estimated quality of service. This level of program evaluation is a component of Donabedian's "process." It can be applied, by definition, only to examination of services actually rendered rather than to the experience of a total population, some members of which may receive no services at all. The measurement rests on the assumption that at any time and place there is a scientific consensus among widely acknowledged experts on what constitutes good or high-quality health service. The consensus typically, though not always, rests on a body of empirical data. The task then is to call upon an expert observer to examine, directly or indirectly, the services actually provided in a program and make judgments on the degree to which the services coincide with these accepted standards of merit. The judgment may be scaled from high to low, may be given a numerical score, or may be subdivided along different dimensions of service.

The most common application of this level of evaluation has been to hospital services through study of patient records. Known generally as the medical audit technique, it has been applied extensively by Lembcke (*29*) and Rosenfeld (*30*) as well as others with methodological variations that need not be reviewed here. Numerous investigations have been made of such outcomes as rates of appendectomy (for a physician or for a hospital) associated with nonpathological findings or the proportions of post mortem findings that did not confirm the original diagnosis. The widely publicized study of the quality of medical care received by members of the Teamsters Union under a health insurance plan was based on this audit technique (*31*). With somewhat greater difficulty, the study of written records as a basis for evaluation has been applied also to services for ambulatory patients (*32*).

Because of the many possible inadequacies of the written record as a reflection of what was actually done (that is, errors of commission or omission in the record), the quality of services may be judged also by visual observation. This technique was used in the well-known studies of general medical practice by Peterson and his colleagues in North Carolina (*33*) and by Clute in Canada (*34*). Visual observations of patients' mouths have likewise been applied in evaluative studies of dental service programs. Prescribing practices of physicians have also been examined as indicators of their quality of performance (*35*).

There are endless ramifications to the types of judgmental observations that may be made at this level of evaluation. Instead of applying a standard of excellence, the performance in a particular program may be compared with an average of many such programs, as is the strategy of the Commission on Professional and Hospital Activities (*36*). The old appraisal schedule of local public health programs used by the American Public Health Association was applied largely in this way (37).

Apart from the fallibilities in judgment of any "expert," this whole level of measuring results is often difficult to apply because of the inaccessibility of records or other objects of observation, because of the expense involved, or for other reasons. Therefore, program evaluation of results must often take recourse to a third level of measurement: the quantity of services provided. This is another facet of Donabedian's concept of process.

Quantity of services provided. The basic assumption of this evaluative level is that certain types of health service (not all types) may be regarded as generally beneficial for people, so that a higher rate of providing these services to a population is deemed more favorable than a lower rate. One can immediately think of exceptions to this generalization, but the argument for its usual validity rests on the entire literature and knowledge of the field of scientific clinical medicine. In general, other things being equal, it is assumed that a health service program which yields a high rate of contact between patients and physicians is better than one which yields a lower rate. (This view has been widely held since about 1912; Dr. Reginald Fitz of Boston set that year as the date after which an encounter between a patient and a doctor yielded a better than 50–50 chance of benefit for the patient.) The whole extension of health insurance programs, for example, has been advocated on the basis of the statistical demonstration that insured persons (of given age, sex, and socioeconomic status) get more health services per year than noninsured persons with the same characteristics (38).

The quantity of health services provided to a population by a program, or the utilization rates if viewed from the standpoint of the recipients, may be of many different categories and subcategories. Most elementary is the determination of the percentage of a stated population reached (that is, provided one or more units of service by the program) during a year. For physician contacts this is often between 50 and 75 percent, even when costs are covered by an insurance or public program (39).

Beyond this, one may determine the rate of receipt by the eligible population of ambulatory medical services, hospitalizations, prescribed drugs. dental services, and so on. Within ambulatory medical services, one may measure preventively oriented services, like physical examinations or immunizations, or many types of diagnostic or treatment procedures. Dental services may include rates of prophylaxes, fillings, extractions, prostheses, and others. Hospitalization may be measured by cases or admissions, by days of care, by diagnostic category, and so on. All these measurements, of course, depend on minimally adequate medical records and a clear definition of terms (40).

Such data on the quantity of various types of service received by an eligible population are clearly a program consequence although their appraisal as good, fair, or poor requires further interpretation. When rates of service provided are markedly different from certain well-known experiences, the judgment is easier; for example, we know that the U.S. population as a whole utilizes hospital services at the rate of about 1,100 days per 1,000 persons per year and sees physicians at the rate of about five contacts per person per year. If we then observe that the annual utilization rates in, let us say, the State of West Bengal, India, are 200 days per 1,000 persons and one physician contact per person, we need not hesitate to conclude that the West Bengal health service system has serious deficiencies. When the differentials are slight, however, we cannot usually make value judgments; yet we can draw simple conclusions on the quantitative effects of a program that can be useful for planning purposes.

When certain medical procedures have been clinically demonstrated to be of dubious benefit (for example, tonsillectomies or uterine suspensions), a high rate of their performance can reflect low programmatic quality. On the other hand, certain procedures may be deemed of generally high value, such as immunizations for the young or proctoscopic examinations of aged persons, and these rates therefore have other meaning. Rates of hospitalization as a whole under different types of insurance plans have been extensively studied as an outcome reflecting possible abuse or overuse of expensive facilities, as well as the compensatory value of out-of-hospital services to the ambulatory patient (*41*).

Focusing only on the persons actually receiving services within a program, one may undertake other measurements useful for evaluation. The time spent per patient, or the number of patients seen per physician-hour, is a useful measurement. Within a physician's practice, the proportion of patients given injections or subjected to certain diagnostic tests may be an evaluative index. In a dental program, the ratio of fillings to extractions is widely regarded as reflecting a preventive orientation. The ratio of prescribed to nonprescribed drugs consumed by a population is another index reflecting quality. The rate of noncompliance with medical orders or advice is a special form of program measurement that also has obvious qualitative implications. While interpretations of the meaning of these various quantitative rates, for specified types of health service, must obviously be made with caution, such measurements constitute a level of evaluation that permits interprogram comparisons (*42*).

Such relatively simple counts as these may not even be possible, however, if proper records are not kept in a health service program. A common difficulty is the lack of knowledge of the size of the eligible population so that, with no clear denominator, basic rates cannot be calculated at all, and only proportions of patients getting certain services can be measured. Evaluation of a health program may be most feasible, therefore, at still another level: the attitudes of the persons whom the program is intended to serve.

Attitudes of recipients. Combining quantity and quality, in a sense, is the measurement of a health service outcome that is based on the attitudes of persons entitled to or actually receiving the service. Without knowing the quantitative rates of services provided or their estimated quality (as judged by professional experts), one can ask people how they feel about the program. Many evaluative studies have been based on this type of survey measurement. The impact of diverse types of health insurance plans on persons enrolled has been studied in this way among State government employees in California (43), among insured persons in New York City (44), and in other settings. Opinion surveys of the attitudes of British people before and after the National Health Service have been used to evaluate that large program (45).

Although the judgment of a program member or patient may often be superficial and faulty, this method assumes that such judgment has some validity and will certainly reflect gross problems in a program. For the humanistic and personal aspects of health service, this level of evaluative measure is probably more cogent than any other. Moreover, this type of measurement is probably the best approach to quantification of such frequently espoused criteria for good medical care as accessibility, acceptability, continuity, comprehensiveness, sensitivity, and the like.

Within the population actually receiving services, a quantification of grievances may also be a tool of evaluation. Hospitals and health insurance plans often invite patients to comment in writing on the services they have received, using the rate of specific complaints as a key to program improvement. In more extreme form, a study of the rate of malpractice suits in a series of California hospitals found this measure to reflect the degree of rigor in the organization of the medical staff (46).

As democratic concepts become more embodied in the provision of health service and as the sophistication of people about medical science broadens, this level of evaluation can become increasingly important. Witness the ferment in the nationwide Medicaid program, associated not only with rising costs but also with documented complaints of poor people about the nature of the service they get (47). This type of measurement need not require medical records nor the other elaborate forms of data necessary for the three previous levels, but it usually requires population surveys through interviews, questionnaires, or other means, which must be done with care and may be quite costly. On a level still further from the goal of improvement in health status, therefore, one may draw inferences about the operation of a program by measuring the various attributes of the personnel and physical resources made available in it. These are equivalent to Donabedian's concept of structure.

Resources made available. While human and physical resources are ordinarily thought of as inputs rather than outputs of a system, these resources require much effort for production and distribution, so that they may also be viewed as consequences. This concept may be seen clearly in an underdeveloped country, where the results of a national program of rural health improvement may be measured by the simple ratio to population of physicians, nurses, hospital beds, and so on, achieved in rural areas (*48*). In the United States an immediate result of the national Hill-Burton program is the number or ratio of hospital beds established in regions formerly undersupplied, and similar measures may be used for personnel trained and working as an achievement of various health manpower development programs (*49*). These ratios, it may be noted, apply theoretically to total population rather than to patients reached.

The assumption, of course, is that personnel and physical resources result in services, just as the services, in turn, are presumed generally to yield benefits for health. Anyone can spot the possible fallacies in these assumptions, and yet they are more likely to be valid than not. For years the local public health promotional program of the Public Health Service reported its progress in terms of the number of counties (among the 3,070 in the nation) served each year by full-time health departments (*50*). The assumption was that these structural resources led to certain services which, in turn, reduced communicable diseases, infant mortality, and so on. There was enough independent scientific evidence of the benefits of immunizations, sterilization of baby formulas, early detection of tuberculosis, and so on, to justify these assumptions in a broad sense. More ultimate measures of the results of local health department programs are sought, naturally, but even at this fifth level certain probabilistic conclusions are warranted. In some situations, no more satisfactory evaluative data may be obtainable.

Within this evaluative level of resources made available, measurements may be further refined along qualitative lines. One may count the kinds of physicians available, for example, distinguishing general practitioners and qualified specialists (*51*). One may define the range of equipment and the scope of services offered in hospitals and health centers. The whole literature of clinical medicine justifies the assumption, if other data are lacking, that a fully trained surgeon is likely to achieve better surgical results for his patient than a general practitioner. While exceptions may occur, in a complex medical situation it is probable that a professional nurse will be more helpful to a patient than a vocational nurse. Broadly speaking, a health program may be subjected to an administrative audit in which all its resources are defined and their manner of functioning is described; certain operating procedures imply superior or inferior service.

Beyond this fifth level of evaluation of health service programs, there is still another type of question to be asked: What are the costs of the program? All five levels discussed are measures of benefits but they tell us nothing about the costs and hence of the cost-benefit ratios. Since health service resources are always limited, it is reasonable to attempt to achieve a stated outcome at the lowest possible cost, and the measurement of this cost may therefore be regarded as another type of evaluation.

Costs of the Program

If a stated health objective at any of the five levels can be reached by one method at a lower cost than by another method, there is greater efficiency and higher value in the first method. It means that more money or resources would then be left for meeting other needs or demands (52).

The costs of a program, while a type of evaluation, are along a dimension different from that of the five levels of benefits discussed. For any quantity of benefits at any of the five levels, there may be a range of costs. The difficulty is to be certain that comparative cost measurements are being applied to health service programs that do, indeed, reach the same results. If not, there must at least be some uniform units of measurement of results, such as days of disability incurred or number of dental services provided, under alternative systems, so that cost-benefit analyses and comparisons can be made (53). How much should be spent for gaining a stated objective is a matter for social policy decision, and choices must always be made among large sectors like health, military affairs, education, housing, and so on. Within the health sector alone, the choices are difficult enough, but between these large sectors the cost-benefit calculations are so formidable that they are seldom even attempted, and the decisions are usually left to political judgment.

Within the health services, costs can be calculated in several ways. As at the other levels of evaluation, the cost measurement may be applied to the total population eligible or to the population actually served. The first dimension requires calculation of the cost over time per person eligible for service; the second dimension requires only determination of the cost of services actually rendered, such as a physician visit or a hospital day. By either type of measure, comparisons of cost may be made between different methods of seeking to achieve the same goal; for example, water fluoridation versus periodic topical fluoride applications to children's teeth or group medical practice with salaried physicians in contrast to solo practice with fee-for-service remuneration (54).

These fiscal measurements are complex because hidden costs must not be overlooked. If the cost of an organized home care program is to be compared with equivalent long-term hospital care, one must not ignore the expenses incurred by a family in keeping a sick member at home (*55*). One must also not overlook administrative costs in a program's operation; for example, a high rate of personnel turnover in a clinic creates hidden costs for training new employees or reduced efficiency until new personnel learn their tasks. In hospital cost calculations, the shares of professional education and research costs that are properly accountable to patient care are perennially debated. If the laboratory in a hospital is understaffed, a bottleneck may be caused in the flow of patient care, leading to longer durations of stay; this administrative problem might not be reflected in per diem costs but only in costs per hospital case (*56*).

In any event, cost figures are a far cry from health status as measurements of the ultimate outcome of a health service program, but they are nevertheless relevant to many larger questions of social policy.

Comment

In this review of five levels of benefit evaluation for health service programs, and a sixth level of cost evaluation, each level is presented along a gradient of depth or ultimacy. In the logic of the means-and-ends chain, this is believed to be generally valid, but as a practical matter there are circumstances in which a less ultimate level of evaluation may actually be more desirable than a more ultimate one. Thus, for example, the secondary variables, outside of the health service program, influencing death rates (level 1) may be so numerous and so difficult to adjust for, that the estimated quality (level 2) or even the simple quantity (level 3) of services provided by the program may be more reliable measures of its effects. For another example, the medical records of services in a program may be so inadequate that an interview with recipients on their attitudes (level 4) toward it, despite all the fallacies of the layman's judgment, may be more reliable than estimates of quality by expert review of written charts.

Because of these difficulties, many efforts to evaluate health service programs properly seek to measure two or more different levels of results at the same time. The studies of old-age assistance clients served by the Health Insurance Plan of Greater New York, compared with the traditional patterns (*18*), obtained data on the quantity of different services provided as well as on health status (mortality rates). Our research on diverse health insurance plans in California is determining the quantity of services provided, the attitudes of recipients, and the costs or expenditures under each plan, although we are not getting health status measurements (*57*).

The most useful strategy for evaluation would be to determine the effects of health service programs at all five levels plus their costs. Until that can be achieved, we should realize that measurements at any one or more of the six evaluation levels contribute something to our understanding of health service systems and are far more useful than evaluations based on intuition or speculation.

There are endless methodological problems in sampling, data collection, analysis, and so on that I have not discussed in this paper. It should be pointed out, however, that the health service program to be studied may have varying degrees of complexity, and the problems of evaluation are corresponding. Evaluation may be attempted of an entire national health service system or, for example, of a particular prenatal clinic, or of a large series of program complexities in between. Intermediate complexities might be illustrated by a regional network of hospitals, a health insurance plan, or an air pollution control program.

The more complex the program examined, the more numerous generally are the secondary variables that must be adjusted for. The microsystem questions can usually be answered more rapidly and less expensively than the macrosystem questions. Ease of solution, however, seldom corresponds to the social importance of a question, and we should avoid tackling certain evaluative problems just because they are easily soluble, unless at the same time they are socially salient.

Level of evaluation		Eligible population	Patients served
1	Health status		
2	Estimated quality	▓▓▓	
3	Quantity of service		
4	Attitudes		
5	Resources		▓▓▓
6	Costs		

FIG. 1

In summary, then, one can conceptualize a matrix of evaluation of health service programs. Along one axis would be the six levels of results that may be measured, and along the other axis the applicability of the measurement to a total eligible population or to only the patients actually served. Within each dimension there would be programs of varying degrees of complexity that may be summarized as macro or micro systems. This matrix could be schematized as shown in Figure 1.

Within each of these conceptual cells, evaluation requires the comparison of measurements of at least two entities, defined either across time (before and after) or across space (the model of test and control groups). Studies within any of these conceptual cells can be useful for program evaluation, which can facilitate a rational planning of health services.

REFERENCES

1. Shryock, R. H.: American medical research past and present. Commonwealth Fund, New York, 1947.
2. B'tesch, S.: International research in the organization of medical care. Med Care 4: 41–46, January–March 1966.
3. Kerr, M., and Trantow, D. J.: Defining, measuring, and assessing the quality of health services. Perspectives and a suggested framework. Public Health Rep 84: 415–424, May 1969.
4. Altman, I., and Anderson, A. J.: Methodology in evaluating the quality of medical care: An annotated selected bibliography, 1955–61. University of Pittsburgh Press, Pittsburgh, Pa., 1962.
5. Suchman, E.: Evaluative research: Principles and practice in public service and social action programs. Russell Sage Foundation, New York, 1967.
6. Donabedian, A.: Evaluating the quality of medical care. Milbank Mem Fund Q 44: 104–145, October 1966.
8. Shapiro, S.: End result measurements of quality of medical care. Milbank Mem Fund Q 45: 7–30, April 1967.
9. Klein, B.: Evaluating outcomes of health care: An annotated bibliography. California Center for Health Services Research, Los Angeles, August 1969.
10. World Health Organization: Methodology in public health studies: A selected bibliography. OMC/RES/68.5. Geneva, December 1968.
11. Donabedian, A.: Medical care appraisal—quality and utilization: A guide to medical care administration. Vol. 2. American Public Health Association, New York, 1969.
12. Schulberg, H. C., Sheldon, A., and Baker, F., editors: Program evaluation in the health fields. Behavioral Publications, New York, 1969.
13. MacTavish, C. F.: Assessment of the quality of medical care: An annotated bibliography. American Rehabilitation Foundation, Minneapolis, Minn., February 1968.
14. Simon, H. A.: Administrative behavior. Macmillan Co., New York, 1961, pp. 62–66.
15. Hilleboe, H. E., and Schaefer, M.: Evaluation in community health: Relating results to goals. Bull NY Acad Med 44: 140–158, February 1968.
16. World Health Organization: Vital statistics and causes of death: World health statistics annual. Vol. 1. Geneva, 1968.
17. Shapiro, S., Jacobziner, H., Densen, P., and Weiner, L.: Further observations on prematurity and perinatal mortality in a general population and in the population of a prepaid group practice medical care plan. Am J Public Health 50: 1304–1317, September 1960.

18. Shapiro, S., et al.: Patterns of medical use by the indigent aged under two systems of medical care. Am J Public Health 57: 784–790, May 1967.
19. Lipworth, L., Lee, H., and Morris, J. N.: Case fatality in teaching and non-teaching hospitals, 1956–1959. Med Care 1: 71–76, April 1963.
20. Thompson, J. D., Marquis, D. B., Woodward, R. L., and Yeomans, R. C.: End-result measurements of the quality of obstetrical care in two U.S. Air Force hospitals. Med Care 6: 131–143, March–April 1968.
21. Roemer, M. I.: Is surgery safer in larger hospitals? Hosp Manage 87: 35–37, 50, 77, 101, (1959).
22. Roemer, M. I., Moustafa, A. T., and Hopkins, C. E.: A proposed hospital quality index: Hospital death rates adjusted for case severity. Health Serv Res 3: 96–118, Summer 1968.
23. Sanders, B.: Measuring community health levels. Am J Public Health 54: 1063–1070, July 1964.
24. Sullivan, D.: Conceptual problems in developing an index of health: Vital and health statistics. PHS Publication No. 1000, Ser. 2, No. 17. U.S. Government Printing Office, Washington, D.C., May 1966.
25. Katz, S., et al.: Studies of illness in the aged: The index of ADL, a standardized measure of biological and psychosocial function. JAMA 185: 914–919, Sept. 21, 1963.
26. Katz, S.: Practical experience in evaluating a health service program. *In* Synopsis of proceedings, outcomes meeting I, California Center for Health Services Research, Los Angeles, May 1969.
27. Hagner, S., LoCicero, V., and Steiger, W.: Patient outcomes in a comprehensive medicine clinic. Med Care 6: 144–156, March–April 1968.
28. Sanazaro, P. J., and Williamson, J. W.: End results of patient care: A provisional classification based on reports by internists. Med Care 6: 123–130, March–April 1968.
29. Lembcke, P. A.: Evaluation of the medical audit. JAMA 199: 543–550, Feb. 20, 1967.
30. Rosenfeld, L. S.: Quality of medical care in hospitals. Am J Public Health 47: 856–865, July 1957.
31. Ehrlich, J., Morehead, M. A., and Trussell, R. E.: The quantity, quality and costs of medical and hospital care secured by a sample of teamsters families in the New York area. Columbia University, New York, 1962.
32. Kroeger, H. H., et al.: The office practice of internists: The feasibility of evaluating quality of care. JAMA 193: 371–376, Aug. 2, 1965.
33. Peterson, O. L., et al.: An analytical study of North Carolina general practice. J Med Educ 31: 1–165, December 1965.
34. Clute, K. F.: The general practitioner: A study of medical education and practice in Ontario and Nova Scotia. University of Toronto Press, Toronto, 1963.
35. Furstenberg, F. F., et al.: Prescribing as an index to quality of medical care. Am J Public Health 43: 1299–1309, October 1953.
36. Slee, V. N.: Uniform methods of measuring utilization. *In* Utilization review: A handbook for the medical staff. American Medical Association, Chicago, 1965.
37. Hiscock, I. V.: Community health organization. Ed. 4, Commonwealth Fund, New York, 1950, p. 242.
38. Anderson, O. W., and Feldman, J. J.: Family medical costs and voluntary health insurance: A nationwide survey. McGraw-Hill Book Co., New York, 1956.
39. Darsky, B. J., Sinai, N., and Axelrod, S. J.: Comprehensive medical services under voluntary health insurance: A study of Windsor medical services. Harvard University Press, Cambridge, Mass., 1958, p. 62.
40. Densen, P.: Some practical and conceptual problems in appraising the outcome of health care services and programs. Paper presented at Health Services Outcomes Conference, Los Angeles, Dec. 1, 1969.
41. Klarman, H. E.: Controlling hospital use through organization of medical ser-

vices. *In* Where is hospital use headed? Paper presented at the Fifth Annual Symposium on Hospital Affairs, University of Chicago, 1962, pp. 55–63.

42. Roemer, M. I.: Research in administrative medicine: Comparative analysis of systems of health service organization. *In* Research in social welfare administration. National Association of Social Workers, New York, 1962, pp. 72–81.

43. Watts, M., et al.: A special report of the medical and hospital advisory committee to the board of administration. State Employees Retirement System, Sacramento, Calif., June 1964.

44. Anderson, O. W., and Sheatsley, P. B.: Comprehensive medical insurance: A study of costs, use, and attitudes under two plans. Health Information Foundation, Chicago, 1959.

45. Gemmill, P. F.: An American report on the National Health Service. Br Med J (supp.) 5: 17–21, July 1958.

46. Blum, R. H.: Hospitals and patient dissatisfaction. Technical Report. California Medical Association, San Francisco, 1958.

47. U.S. Department of Health, Education, and Welfare: Recommendations of the task force on Medicaid and related programs. U.S. Government Printing Office, Washington, D.C., November 1969.

48. Roemer, M. I.: The rural health services scheme in Malaysia. World Health Organization, Western Pacific Regional Office, Manila, February 1969.

49. National Commission on Community Health Services: Health manpower: Action to meet community needs. Public Affairs Press, Washington, D.C., 1967.

50. U.S. Public Health Service: Directory of local health units, 1966. PHS Publication No. 118. U.S. Government Printing Office, Washington, D.C., 1966.

51. Mott, F. D., and Roemer, M. I.: Rural health and medical care. McGraw Hill Book Co., New York, 1948.

52. McCaffree, K.: The cost of mental health care under changing treatment methods. Am J Public Health 56: 1013–1025, July 1966.

53. Klarman, H.: Present status of cost-benefit analysis in the health field. Am J Public Health 57: 1948–1954, November 1967.

54. Williams, J. J., et al.: Family medical care under three types of health insurance. Foundation on Employee Health, Medical Care, and Welfare, New York, 1962.

55. Rogatz, P., et al.: Organized home medical care in New York City. Harvard University Press, Cambridge, Mass., 1956.

56. Lave, J.: A review of the methods used to study hospital costs. Inquiry 3: 57–81 (1966).

57. Sasuly, R., and Roemer, M. I.: Health insurance plans: A conceptualization from the California scene. J Health Hum Behav 7: 36–44, spring 1966.

SELECTION 20

Evaluation of Program Efficiency*

O. L. Deniston, I. M. Rosenstock, W. Welch, and *V. A. Getting, M.D.*

An earlier paper (1) showed the logic of a consistent approach to evaluating program effectiveness. This paper builds upon that logic to provide an approach to measuring program efficiency. The measurement of effectiveness and efficiency provides an evaluation of program performance.

Program Components

Programs include three components—objectives, activities, and resources, which were defined in the earlier paper as follows:

1. Objective. A situation or condition of people or of the environment which responsible program personnel consider desirable to attain. (Objectives themselves include ultimate objectives, and sub-objectives.)

2. Activity. Work performed by program personnel and equipment in the service of an objective.

3. Resource. Personnel, funds, materials, and facilities available to support the performance of activity.

A program objective is distinct from a program activity; the term "objective" refers to a state of affairs that is expected to exist at a point in the future at a given place. Unlike activities, objectives consume neither program time nor resources.

Whatever mechanisms or approaches are used in planning a program, the administrator needs to make three major kinds of decisions after specifying the problem toward which the program is to be directed. These decisions comprise (*a*) a determination of the program objectives and sub-objectives deemed necessary and sufficient for attaining the program objective, (*b*) a selection of one or more activities believed to have a high probability of resulting in attainment of each sub-objective, and (*c*) a determination of the kind and amount of resources needed to support the performance of the planned activities. In attempting to implement a program plan, an ideal plan will frequently have to be modified on the basis of extant constraints. Resources may not be sufficient to support all desired activities, or limitations of personnel may make it impossible to under-

* *Public Health Reports,* vol. 83, no. 7, July, 1968.

take certain desired activities. In such instances, modifications must be introduced to restrict the level of activities and perhaps the scope or breadth of the program objective. The logic of program operation is to expend resources to support the performance of activities and thereby to attain sub-objectives and the program objective.

Evaluation of Effectiveness

In general, questions concerning effectiveness are directed toward assessing the extent to which a planned or intended objective has been attained as a result of program activity. An analysis is thus suggested in which the proportion of attainment of the program objective that is attributable to program activity (AO) is compared with the desired level which, during the planning process, the planners had proposed would result from the program activity (PO). The earlier paper describes methods for discounting any apparent attainment that actually results from events other than program activity (1).

Program effectiveness is denoted as the ratio AO:PO, and this ratio is the only legitimate measure of program effectiveness. However, to interpret results properly—that is, determine the soundness of the assumptions on which the program is based—two subordinate measures of effectiveness need also to be considered. The first is the extent to which an activity has been performed as planned as a result of utilization of resources, in other words, the ratio of the actual activities performed to the planned activities scheduled to be performed—AA:PA. The second measure is the extent to which the resources have been expended as planned, that is, the ratio of the actual expenditure of resources to the planned expenditure, or AR:PR.

These two subsidiary measures are important since the program logic holds (*a*) that program objectives will be attained only if the activities have been performed both in the amount and quality planned, and (*b*) that activities will be performed only if the resources have actually been used as planned. Comparisons among the three ratios AR:PR, AA:PA, and AO:PO may show that the resources and activities that it was anticipated would be needed were either overestimated or underestimated. At any rate, the important point is that the measure of program effectiveness, AO:PO, as well as the subordinate measures of attainment of planned resources and activities, requires a comparison of the actual attained status of any one program variable with the planned status of the same variable.

What has been said about evaluating the attainment of objectives applies also to evaluating the attainment of sub-objectives. Effectiveness in achieving each sub-objective can be assessed by computing the ratio AOsub: POsub. By considering the activities and resources allocated to each particular sub-objective, one can also compute AAsub:PAsub and ARsub:PRsub and thus obtain measures of the effectiveness of the activities and resources associated with a particular sub-objective.

The earlier paper provides details and examples of evaluations of program effectiveness.

Evaluation of Efficiency

If the attainment of objectives were considered desirable regardless of cost and if unlimited resources were available for health programs, efficiency would not be of great concern to administrators. Since neither of these conditions obtains, however, efficiency must be a concern in program operation.

A definition of efficiency in public health programs may be formulated by referring to the classical definition of physical efficiency—the ratio between the energy output of a machine and the energy input supplied to it. In public health programs, efficiency may be defined as the ratio between an output (net attainment of program objectives) and an input (program resources expended), or AO:AR. *The inverse of this ratio, which would be AR:AO, yields a measure of average cost.* Clearly it matters little in public health programing whether one examines efficiency or average costs, since the same relationship will emerge. However, it is sometimes more meaningful to look at one than the other. For example, it is easier to understand that it costs $10,000 to locate and cure one case of a particular disease than that 1/10,000 of a case was located and cured for $1. (This situation is not true in physics since the units of comparison—energy—are the same in both the numerator and the denominator, and maximum efficiency cannot exceed 100 percent because of the law of the conservation of energy. In instances, however, in which the numerator and denominator consist of different units, for example, of objectives and resources, there is no theoretical basis for estimating maximum possible efficiency, and the terms can be either numerator or denominator.)

Key to Abbreviations

AO—Attainment of objectives that can be attributed to the program activity
PO—Proposed objectives for attainment through the program activity
AA—Actual activities performed
PA—Planned activities to be performed
AR—Actual resource expenditure
PR—Planned resource expenditure

The measure of overall program efficiency AO:AR or AR:AO may be interpreted by examining two intermediate efficiency measures, namely, the relationship of activities to objectives and resources. Specifically, efficiency studies may answer questions about the relationship (*a*) between the extent of attainment of objectives and the resources expended, (*b*) between the extent of attainment of objectives and the number and kind of activities conducted, and (*c*) between the number and kind of activities conducted and the resources expended.

The ratio of program effectiveness, as indicated earlier, reflects the relationship between two estimates of the attainment of program objectives —the planned attainment and the actual attainment. And each of the two subordinate ratios of effectiveness involves similar comparisons of activities and resources. Program efficiency, on the other hand, reflects the relationship between two different variables—objectives and resources. Two subordinate efficiency measures also compare combinations of different variables. Three efficiency, or average-cost ratios can thus be stated as follows, one for each of the foregoing questions:

1. Objectives attained to resources expended = AO:AR or AR:AO.
2. Activities performed to resources expended = AA:AR or AR:AA.
3. Objectives attained to activities performed = AO:AA or AA:AO.

Of course, each ratio may also be computed for the portions of the program related to each sub-objective. As is true for effectiveness, consideration, as the program progresses, of the efficiency with which the plan is being carried out may demonstrate a need for modification of the original plan.

Relation of Effectiveness to Efficiency

In the typical program setting, the administrator attempts to obtain an acceptably high level of attainment of objectives at minimum cost (that is, to maximize attainment at a fixed level of resource input or to minimize resource input at a fixed level of attainment). However, a proper interpretation of efficiency requires a measurement of activity so that two subordinate efficiency ratios, AO:AA and AA:AR can be computed. Consequently, as a comprehensive evaluation of performance, data should be obtained on all three components—use of resources, performance of activity, and attainment of objectives (including sub-objectives). Measures of effectiveness must be obtained before measures of program efficiency can be interpreted meaningfully since, from the definition of efficiency, knowledge is required of effectiveness as well as of resources.

Unless the administrator is satisfied with effectiveness, studies of efficiency will be uninterpretable or misleading. A person cannot decide that a program with an efficiency ratio of two units of attainment per unit of resource is superior to a program with a ratio of one unit of attainment per unit of resource unless he has knowledge of the effectiveness of each program. For example, suppose that two programs have the same objective. Program A attains all of the objective at a given cost, whereas program B attains half of the objective at a quarter of the cost. Program A is thus twice as effective as program B, but only half as efficient. Which program is superior? A rational answer can only be based on knowledge of both the effectiveness and efficiency of each program.

The attainment of sub-objectives and of the program objective cannot be measured, of course, until some time after a program has been in operation, but other valuable information can be collected earlier. It is always desirable to collect data periodically on progress to insure that a program is being carried out as planned. If it is not, adjustments can be made in the course of operating the program.

Typically, continuous evaluative measures can be obtained in the following sequence:

1. The extent to which resources are being expended as planned (AR:PR).

2. The extent to which activities are being performed in the quantity and quality planned (AA:PA) and the efficiency of resource expenditures (AA:AR).

3. The net attainment of selected sub-objectives (AOsub:POsub) and the efficiency of sub-objective attainment (Osub:Rsub) and (Osub:Asub).

4. Program effectiveness (AO:PO), program efficiency (AO:AR), and activity efficiency (AO:AA).

If data on the first three of these evaluative measures are obtained early in the program operation, these data can provide a rational basis for changes in the program that may materially improve its effectiveness and efficiency. The only true measure of the effectiveness of a program, however, is the ratio of attained objectives to planned objectives, and the only true measure of efficiency is the ratio of attained objectives to expended resources. Therefore, for a comprehensive evaluation, the fourth evaluative measure must be applied.

Special Measurement Problems

We gave considerable attention to the measurement of objectives and sub-objectives in the earlier paper. Little was said about the measurement of activities and resources.

Since any program variable includes quantitative and qualitative components, we believe that measures of variables must reflect both dimensions. In most instances quantitative measures alone do not provide a sufficient basis for judging how adequately a program component has been implemented. Rarely are there no qualitative differences among a class of objects or actions. The dollar seems to be an exception since any one is equal to another in terms of a program's buying power at a single point in time.

Similarly, constancy of quality is probably fairly closely approached by many standardized medications and vaccines, although mishaps occasionally occur. Few problems of measurement arise when we deal with highly standardized variables.

Generally, however, an assessment of quality as well as of quantity is desirable in program evaluation. When resources are described in terms of a given number of "qualified" physicians, nurses, or sanitarians or a given number of "adequate" clinic facilities, the extent to which the resources actually fulfilled the qualitative as well as quantitative requirements has to be determined. How many physicians, nurses, sanitarians, or clinics were provided and how qualified or adequate was each? When activities are described in terms of numbers of nursing visits, sanitation inspections, physical examinations, or educational efforts, the qualitative as well as the quantitative aspects must be specified and subsequently measured. We have to measure not only the number of activities but the extent to which each was performed on the desired level of expertness.

At present no ready procedures are available for developing and applying qualitative measures; we can only point out that qualitative measures are necessary. It is desirable for program personnel to bear in mind that effectiveness and efficiency are influenced as much by the quality of resources and activities as by the quantity. In some circumstances, the program administrator and his staff will be able to work out their own systematic measures of the quality of selected factors and will thus be in a better position to evaluate overall program performance.

Use of Data on Efficiency

The major concern of the administrator obviously is to attain a desired (usually high) level of accomplishment of objectives at a minimum cost. As indicated throughout this paper, a concern with program effectiveness logically precedes a concern with program efficiency. After the desired levels of accomplishment of objectives are attained or maintained, an assessment of the program's efficiency then becomes of prime concern. The administrator who knows how effective and efficient his program is can then judge where its results are worth the cost.

We have implied that evaluation always entails comparison with a standard. In evaluations of program effectiveness, the standard for comparison most frequently selected is the attainment level that had been planned before program implementation began. A similar standard may be used for determining efficiency. One may ask whether the actual level of efficiency or the average costs are similar to what had been planned. It may have been planned that each unit of attainment would cost, say, $100.

An evaluation of efficiency may show that, in fact, each unit of attainment cost $104. A program operator might then decide that the actual efficiency was so close to what had been planned that extra attention was not warranted. On the other hand, he might conclude that the disparity between the planned and the actual efficiency was great enough to require additional analysis. The operator could then ask whether the planned efficiency of the resources or of the activities had been in error, and he would then attempt to revise the program planning accordingly.

Frequently, no sound basis for estimating planned efficiency is available, for example, in instances in which little or no evidence can be obtained about how many resources are required to support an activity or about the number and kinds of activities that will be required to attain an objective. In this situation, another standard for comparison needs to be selected. One that is frequently used, but a dangerous one, is the operation of the same program in an earlier year. Costs and circumstances may vary so from year to year that conclusions drawn from efficiency ratios obtained in two different years may be invalid. Nevertheless, with a knowledge of local circumstances and the costs of living, a person may be able to estimate from data obtained periodically whether efficiency is increasing or decreasing. The important point is that a comparison of the actual operation of a program with a reasonable standard permits a judgment as to whether the efficiency attained is satisfactory or unsatisfactory.

An administrator may be satisfied with the effectiveness of a program and still believe that its efficiency is unsatisfactory. Attempts to improve program efficiency require consideration of the subordinate efficiency measures A:R and O:A for each sub-objective and for the program objective. For example, studies may be made of ways to improve resource efficiency (A:R) by obtaining more or better activity, or both, from a given expenditure of resources. This ratio is the one being considered in speaking about the cost of a nursing visit or a sanitation inspection.

Use of a multiple-antigen immunization material in a broad communicable disease control program may be an example of improving the efficiency of an activity (O:A). In this instance, an equal or greater attainment of objectives may be accomplished as a result of a given amount of activity (thus, immunity to several diseases may be brought about from one series of inoculations). Of course, in such circumstances, resource efficiency may increase.

When program effectiveness is lower than desired, the administrator has four choices. One possibility is to reduce the desired level of accomplishment to the level actually attained. This choice might be suggested by the belief, perhaps bolstered by new data, that the observed attainment, although less than that desired, is the most which can reasonably be achieved given existing constraints. When new program objectives are set at current levels of attainment, studies of efficiency will be more useful in planning for subsequent program operations.

A second choice available to the administrator who is dissatisfied with his attainment is to decide, on the basis of his evaluative data, that he needs to increase the number or improve the quality of the activities directed toward subobjectives and objectives. Any such change will have implications for resource allocation and may thus be planned more rationally with the help of information on efficiency, namely, on the current ratios between activity and cost and between objectives and activities.

A third possibility is that the administrator will maintain the original program objective but, on the basis of evaluative data, decide to make substantial revisions in his program theory, that is, he will specify, and work toward, some new sub-objectives. In such an event, study of the efficiencies associated with the achievement of each sub-objective to be retained in the new program will aid in planning the subsequent operation of the program.

A final choice might be to abandon the program, especially if evaluation shows that it is low in efficiency and if pressures are being generated internally or externally to allocate the existing resources to other programs.

Limitations of Measures of Efficiency

One limitation on the usefulness of efficiency studies is that efficiency may not be constant at different levels of program operation. Consider a program objective to eliminate all of a given community problem. If a given input of resources and activities has eliminated 60 percent of the problem, it is not certain what returns could be expected from different levels of input. At the upper limit, doubling the resources and activities could not eliminate more than 100 percent of the problem. On the other hand, allocating exactly half of the resources and activities probably would not eliminate exactly 30 percent of the problem, but rather might eliminate 20 or 40 percent. It seems reasonable, on the basis of experience, that the expenditure of very limited resources will have little impact (low efficiency); increasing the resources will have a proportionately greater impact (higher efficiency); and finally, greatly increasing the resources will result in only a little more gain (reduced efficiency). This notion is illustrated in figure 1.

A leveling off in efficiency can be expected to occur when a program approaches complete attainment of its objective or when the greatest effectiveness possible from the types of activities performed has been attained. If the curve shown in figure 1 were known for a particular program, then an efficiency curve such as the one in figure 2 could be constructed.

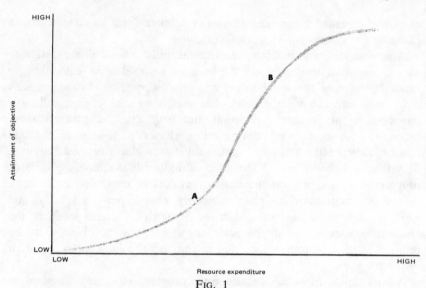

FIG. 1

HYPOTHESIZED PROGRAM EFFECTIVENESS AT VARIOUS LEVELS OF
RESOURCE EXPENDITURE

Thus, we would expect increasing efficiency with increased expenditures, but only up to a point; thereafter, the efficiency level would fall.

A single evaluation of program performance will not tell the administrator at what point on these curves his program lies. But, if the point could be determined, such knowledge would have important implications for the planning of subsequent programs. If an administrator knew what the correct shape of the curve in figure 1 would be for a given program, he would know what proportion of the objectives could be attained with varying amounts of resource expenditures. If the current level of program attainment were at point B on the curve, obviously increased expenditures would not increase the attainment markedly; whereas increased expenditures for programs that begin at point A would have a great impact on the attainment of objectives. On the other hand, if the amount of resources that could be directed toward the program objectives were fixed, the administrator would know what proportion of the objectives might be attained and thus could judge whether the program was likely to be worth the effort. For example, if only enough appropriations were available to accomplish the objectives at point A in figure 2, the administrator might decide to invest his resources in a different program in which the same financial allocation would permit greater attainment, or he might decide to go ahead with the original program if the problem being attacked was deemed to be worthy. In any event, knowledge of the efficiency curve would permit greater rationality in program planning.

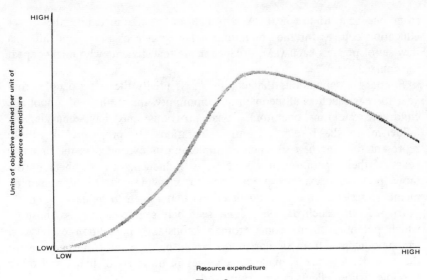

FIG. 2

HYPOTHESIZED PROGRAM EFFICIENCY AT VARIOUS LEVELS OF
RESOURCE EXPENDITURE

Constructing Efficiency Curves

One way of constructing an efficiency curve would be for the administrator
to subdivide the jurisdiction of the program and operate it at different
levels of resource input in each subdistrict. (Controls to assure that the
subdistricts were similar would be essential.)

A second way of constructing efficiency curves would be for a State
or the Federal Government to arrange to operate, in similar communities,
programs whose levels of operation are systematically varied. In such
experiments, effects of previous program operation on the subsequent
operation would be overcome. We would still be left, however, with the
question of how far this knowledge would be applicable to future programs
operating in constantly changing contexts.

How precise the prediction of future outcomes that will probably result
from various resource inputs into a program will be depends in part on the
composition of the target audience for the program. In some programs, the
target audience changes from planning period to planning period; in others,
it remains essentially the same. For example, consider a program directed
toward increasing the proportion of seat belt users among the entire population of a community. The members of this population will change somewhat from year to year; all will age, some will migrate, some will die, new
drivers will be added, but in large measure it will contain the same people

from one year to the next. A seat belt program directed to the driver education courses for the community's 10th grade classes would affect a new set of persons each year, except for the few students who might repeat the course.

For target populations that comprise essentially the same people from year to year (such as all people in a community, the mothers of school age children, restaurant operators), past programs may have considerable influence on the results of future operations. In programs like those represented in the first seat belt example, efforts expended in the first few years of their operation may succeed in influencing all members of the target population who are predisposed to act while most of the remaining members resist all the subsequent efforts undertaken to influence them.

In programs such as the second seat belt example, that is, those in which potential clients come from a "constant" population each year, similar outcomes from similar inputs would be expected from one year to the next if allowance is made for changes in the costs of living and other variables whose effects can be estimated.

Application of Methods

Application of the methods described here to real program situations will be fairly simple in programs in which resources, activities, and outcomes can be readily quantified in reasonably meaningful terms and in which the measure of attainment is consequently fairly straightforward. For example, the meaning of regular use of a seat belt is conceptually clear, although ascertaining actual achievement might require considerable ingenuity.

Such simple situations, however, are not common; more often program objectives are lacking in conceptual clarity. When a program director thinks in terms of raising the level of health in a group, he is dealing with ideas that may have no common meaning among a group of experts. One director may think of the absence of certain symptoms, a second thinks of certain physical signs, a third of emotional stability, a fourth of physical vigor, and a fifth of individual productivity. Others will think in combinations of several or all of these ideas. Before the program director can prepare an index of accomplishment, he has to specify the objectives he is going to try to measure, and this task proves most difficult in many health programs.

Similarly, in most settings, the conceptual meaning of the performance of an activity as planned is unclear. What is really meant by a "nursing visit" or an "inspection"? How, specifically, is the nurse or sanitarian expected to behave? When a person's role is termed "educational," what precisely is meant by education? Until one can specify, first in terms of concepts and then in terms of measures of quantity and quality, how the professional should behave in a particular situation, evaluation cannot be comprehensive, and programs cannot be systematically improved.

Conclusions

The tools described in these papers for evaluating effectiveness and efficiency are most useful for programs in which (*a*) the objectives have been specified qualitatively and quantitatively and have been fixed in time to particular geographic areas and to particular target audiences, (*b*) the programs are described in sufficient detail to permit reliable observations of performance of planned activity, and (*c*) all the resources that are directed toward program activity are identified.

Thus, the first step in evaluating effectiveness and efficiency appears to be to attain conceptual clarity about what the program is and what it contains. Then evaluation becomes straightforward.

REFERENCE

1. Deniston, O. L., Rosenstock, I. M., and Getting, V. A.: Evaluation of program effectiveness. Public Health Rep 83:323–335, April 1968.

Chapter 10

Control

10.1 INTRODUCTION

The function of control is so critical in management that Beer has called management the "profession of control" [1966, p. 254]. The subject of control is of far-reaching importance because it permeates all types of organizations; it exists at all levels within an organization; it affects each and every aspect of organizational life; and it is the vehicle for managing any system (man, machine, or man-machine system). We are familiar with control topics such as disease control, inventory control, quality control, profit control, pollution control, traffic control, population control, and so on. There is virtually no end to the application of the concept of control—at the operational as well as philosophical level. Nor can we conceive of any organized activity which can be managed without exercising either formal or informal control. The literature on the subject of control is enormous;* concentrating on its various aspects: functional, behavioral, scientific,† hierarchical, philosophical, operational, and structural. It is very difficult even to scratch the surface of this vast literature at an introductory level. In this chapter we will discuss the term control and its related aspects; provide a list of required elements in analyzing and designing a control system; and give a classification of "levels" of control.

---

* References are too numerous to list here. We recommend [Beer, 1966], [Anthony, 1965], [Ashby, 1956].

† The study of control as a science was pioneered by the late Norbert Wiener who gave it the name of Cybernetics. Cybernetics, which means steersman in Greek, is an interdisciplinary science. It is "the study of human control functions and of mechanical and electric systems designed to replace them." Random House Dictionary [1967]. Beer explains cybernetics as follows [1966, p. 254]:

It (cybernetics) is the science of communication and control in the animal and the machine. That is to say that cybernetics studies the flow of information round a system, and the way that information is used by the system as a means of controlling itself; it does this for animate and inanimate systems indifferently.

10.2 WHAT IS CONTROL?

The term "control" can be defined in a variety of ways,* depending upon its purpose, focus, and the hierarchical level at which the attempt to exercise control is directed. Goetz [1949, p. 3] describes control as the process of securing conformity to plans. Anthony [1965, p. 29] objects to this definition by pointing out that, because of the dynamics of time, conformity to plans does not necessarily result in best decisions. Anthony's emphasis is on effective and efficient utilization of resources, rather than conformance to plans. Tannenbaum [1968] emphasizes the behavioral aspects of control, and defines control as "any process in which a person or group of persons or organization of persons determines, that is, intentionally affects, the behavior of another person, group, or organization." This definition can be extended to embrace two additional elements, namely, the existence of predetermined goals and the domain of nonhuman or man-machine systems. We will, therefore, define control *as the process, device, or mechanism employed to influence the behavior of a system† in pursuit of predetermined goals.* What needs to be emphasized is that control is an *attempt* to influence the behavior of a system; the attempt may or may not succeed. This influence attempt has the purpose of moving the system towards a set of predetermined goals. These goals (determined by formal or informal planning) guide the actions of the initiators of control as well as of the overall organization and its diverse parts. Planning and control, therefore, are intimately connected; the former being a prerequisite for the latter.

The influence attempt (i.e., control) is implemented either through a formal control system or through informal, interpersonal channels. Informal control plays an important role even when an organization relies on a formal system of control. Beer [1966, p. 258] emphasizes the importance of informal control in these words:

> Fortunately, the formal control is usually backed up by an informal one. It is important to recognize two things about this. First, this is not necessarily inefficient and intolerable; nor is it simply a demonstration of team spirit— a good thing in itself; it is a necessary method for maintaining viability. Second, without it (and orthodox thinking about automatic control techniques for complex systems *is* without it) the organism will die.

The central task in control is to create an environment in which the motivation to *accept* control is born as a result of the nature of control

---

* The relationship of control to concepts such as power, authority, influence, and leadership has been explored in the social sciences literature. See, for example, Cartwright [1965] and the bibliography cited in that chapter.
† The system can be a person, group, organization, machine, or any defined entity of interest which is the object of control.

processes and control system.* For it is only through human beings that plans can be implemented, controlled, and brought to fruition. This is why the concept of control is intertwined with influence, leadership, and motivation.

Like planning, control is one of *the* basic managerial functions. It is inherent in the job of the manager, and *its purpose is to obtain a viable†* *system which builds correspondence between original plans and organiza-* *tional activities scheduled in support of the plans.* Since organizations are dynamic systems, their plans must be designed in such a way that they can give an 'adaptive response' to the system's changing requirements. Such a design requires the development and implementation of a control system in which, as we discussed earlier, the process of evaluation plays an important role.

One interpretation of control is that there is a fixed quantity of control within an organizational unit and people vie for obtaining relatively greater share of the fixed pie. This view casts various groups in the organization in the form of an n-person zero-sum game. That is, the gain of control by one group necessarily results in the loss (by exactly the same amount) of control by other groups. Recently, social scientists have opposed this interpretation of control and have suggested instead that control should be viewed as a variable quantity. Tannenbaum [1968] presents this idea by employing the device of what is known as "control graph" representing the hierarchical distribution of control in an organization. The horizontal axis of the graph shows various hierarchical echelons in an organization, while the vertical axis plots the amount of control exercised by these levels over organizational policies and practices. The average height of the graph represents the "total amount" of control, while its slope indicates the relative amount of control exercised by various hierarchical echelons. The control graph emphasizes the idea that the amount of control in an organization is not a fixed quantity, and that through appropriate measures we can change both the height as well as the slope of the control graph. In a majority of organizations studied by social scientists, there is "a

---

* Anthony [1965, p. 5] distinguishes between a process and a system in these words: "In brief, a system facilitates a process; it is the means by which the process occurs. The distinction is similar to that between anatomy and physiology. Anatomy deals with the structure—what it is; whereas physiology deals with process—how it functions."

† Beer [1966, p. 256] explains viable systems: "Viable systems have the ability to make a response to a stimulus which was not included in the list of anticipated stimuli when the system was designed. They can learn from repeated experience what is the optimal response to that stimulus. Viable systems grow. They renew themselves—by, for example, self-reproduction. They are robust against internal breakdown and error. Above all, they continuously adapt to a changing environment, and by this means survive—quite possibly in conditions which had not been entirely foreseen by their designer."

positive correlation between the amount of total control (i.e., the average height of the curve) and effective organizational performance" [Cartwright 1965, p. 3].

10.3 ANALYZING AND DESIGNING A CONTROL SYSTEM

The design of an effective control system requires an understanding of: (1) the nature and purpose of control, (2) the structure of control, and (3) the processes of control. Koontz [1959] has contributed to this task by classifying principles of control in the aforementioned categories. Anthony [1965] has suggested a very useful framework for analyzing (and designing) planning and control systems.* His model is shown in Fig. 10.1.

FIG. 10.1
PLANNING AND CONTROL PROCESSES IN ORGANIZATIONS

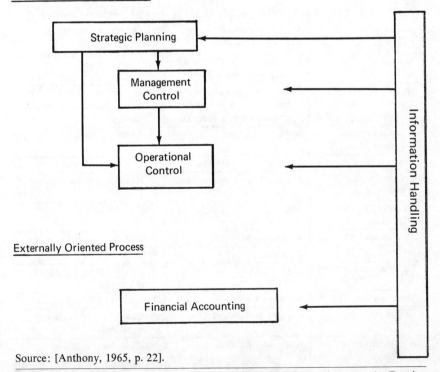

Internally Oriented Processes

Externally Oriented Process

Source: [Anthony, 1965, p. 22].

---

* Anthony's model was tested by Deming [1968]. Based on his research, Deming came to the conclusion that "the framework suggested by Professor Anthony not only is useful in thinking about planning and control systems, but sets forth distinctions which are critical to the effective design of such systems."

The main elements in Anthony's model (relating to internally oriented processes) are strategic planning, management control, and operational control. He defines strategic planning as "the process of deciding on objectives of the organization, on changes in these objectives, on the resources used to attain these objectives, and on the policies that are to govern the acquisition, use, and disposition of these resources." Management control is "the process by which managers assure that resources are obtained and used effectively and efficiently in the accomplishment of the organization's objectives." Operational control is the process of assuring that specific tasks are carried out effectively and efficiently. [Anthony 1965, p. 69] We reproduce in Figure 10.2 the distinctions made by Anthony between strategic planning and management control.*

In order to analyze, design, and implement control, the following elements must be present:

FIG. 10.2
SOME DISTINCTIONS BETWEEN STRATEGIC PLANNING AND
MANAGEMENT CONTROL

Characteristic	Strategic Planning	Management Control
Focus of plans.	On one aspect at a time.	On whole organization.
Complexities.	Many variables.	Less complex.
Degree of structure.	Unstructured and irregular; each problem different.	Rhythmic, prescribed procedures.
Nature of information.	Tailor-made for the problem; more external and predictive; less accurate.	Integrated; more internal and historical; more accurate.
Communication of information.	Relatively simple.	Relatively difficult.
Purpose of estimates.	Show expected results.	Lead to desired results.
Persons primarily involved.	Staff and top management.	Line and top management.
Number of persons involved.	Small.	Large.
Mental activity.	Creative; analytical.	Administrative; persuasive.
Source discipline.	Economics.	Social psychology.
Planning and control.	Planning dominant, but some control.	Emphasis on both planning and control.
Time horizon.	Tends to be long.	Tends to be short.
End result.	Policies and precedents.	Action within policies and precedents.
Appraisal of the job done.	Extremely difficult.	Much less difficult.

Source: [Anthony 1965, p. 67].

* See, also, Exhibit 1 in Anthony [1965, p. 19] for examples of activities in strategic planning, managerial control, and operational control.

1. *An ongoing organization or a system.* (This implies that we are able to determine organizational objectives and goals; identify individual parts of the organization and their respective goals; and specify control responsibility at various points and levels of the organization.)
2. *A standard of performance for each part of the system* (specified either as a target to be achieved during a period of time or stated in terms of an acceptable level of quality).
3. *The ability to measure actual performance and compare it with standard performance.* (This will indicate whether there are any deviations between actual performance and predetermined standards.)
4. *If necessary, the ability to take corrective action by activating the control mechanism.* (This implies that the system is left undisturbed if deviations are tolerable—that is, between prescribed limits. Otherwise, the corrective action calls for introducing necessary changes in organizational activities, plans, or both.)

10.4   LEVELS OF CONTROL

As mentioned earlier, control involves comparing actual performance with some standard performance and taking corrective actions, if necessary. This involves *feedback* of information so that inputs to the system can be modified. The feedback can be negative or positive, and periodic or continuous (without or with lag). The design of feedback determines, to a large extent, the properties of a control system.* Control system hierarchies can be arranged by the "order" of feedback and organized memory employed. Van Court Hare [1967, Ch. 5] has summarized various "levels" of prediction and control:

1. *The Simple Machine or Transformation.* The so-called open-end system or simple operation is of "zero" order, because it has no memory and no feedback.
2. *The Simple Machine with Feedback.* This is the first-order system because direct feedback is present for control. No selective memory is present.
3. *The System with Conditional Selection of Plans and Predictive Feedback.* Here error correction is based on extensive memory facilities, careful memory organization, and the ability to evaluate and act on a wide range of different input conditions, often by predicting the requirements for immediate actions based on future needs.

---

* Three major factors in any feedback system are: [Van Court Hare, 1967, p. 50].
1. The gain or amplification of the transformation to be controlled, i.e., the sensitivity of the system to input without feedback.
2. The amount of feedback that will be used for correction; and
3. The sign of the feedback correction, which, in systems with lag, is determined by a *combination* of the series of inputs to the system and the resulting lag required in the transformation and correction operations.

4. *The System That Learns.* At this level the system can also develop new plans, new decision rules, or new predictions, or change the value of plans and methods to handle new conditions. The learning system may be thought of as a higher-order system, because it must learn while performing its lower-order functions.

5. *The Goal-Changing System.* This is the "fourth-order" feedback system "which corrects methods of learning, develops new problems to solve, innovates, and controls goal-changing itself." It operates at a higher level of autonomy. Such a system "can learn and, as a result of what it has learned, consciously develop, select, and implement new and improved goals."

10.5 CONCLUDING REMARKS

In this chapter we discussed some aspects of control and control systems. We present two selections which touch on the conceptual (Selection 21), and operational (Selection 22) aspects of control. Anthony (Selection 21) provides a general description of *management control*. The reader is referred again to Figure 10.1 in which Anthony relates strategic planning, management control, operational control, financial accounting to information inputs. The concept of control is reviewed and the interpretation of control as "conformance to plans" is rejected. Anthony describes the main characteristics of the strategic planning process and the management control process. These are summarized in Figure 10.2. Anthony establishes a conceptual framework for analyzing the role of management control.

Hill's article (Selection 22) focuses on the operational implications of cost control. He discusses the use of financial incentives through the reimburse system as a method of controlling hospital costs. Having recognized that financial incentives constitute only one aspect of administrative cost control, Hill formulates "cost per unit of output" as the goal of the system. However, the pursuit of this goal might threaten several established relationships among "the establishment" leading to conflict and additional problems for the administrator. This deterrent to cost control can be countered by introducing the corporate model into hospital management. This model prescribes that the administrator, if he is to manage significant changes, must join the governing board structure in a policy-making role —as opposed to the "triad" arrangement where he is "servant" to the board and the medical staff. Two methods of incentive reimbursments are described. One is the *process method;* whereby the rewards are tied not so much to the results but to some desired target in terms of the existence and efficiency of the elements of the process. The process method is least disturbing to the existing system, and its assumption is that given certain acceptable elements, the *probability* is that the system will produce an output of satisfactory quality at a reasonable price. The other method, which corresponds more closely to the corporate model, would tie incentives to actual results and, hence, call for more freedom of action, on the part of management, in *determining* the process. The author then examines some implications of using the corporate model in controlling hospital costs.

REFERENCES

Anthony, R. N., *Planning and Control Systems,* Boston: Graduate School of
1965 Business Administration, Harvard University.

Ashby, W. R., *An Introduction to Cybernetics,* New York: John Wiley & Sons.
1956

Beer, S., *Decision and Control,* New York: John Wiley & Sons.
1966

Cartwright, D., "Influence, Leadership, Control," in J. G. March (ed.),
1965 *Handbook of Organizations,* Chicago: Rand McNally & Co.

Deming, R. H., *Characteristics of an Effective Management Control System in*
1968 *an Industrial Organization,* Boston: Graduate School of Business
Administration, Harvard University.

Goetz, B. E., *Management Planning & Control,* New York: McGraw-Hill.
1949

Hare, Van C., Jr., *Systems Analysis: A Diagnostic Approach,* New York:
1967 Harcourt, Brace and World.

Koontz, H., "Management Control: A Suggested Formulation of Principles,"
1959 *California Management Review* Winter, pp. 47–55.

Random House Dictionary of the English Language, New York: Random
1967 House.

Tannenbaum, A. S., *Control in Organizations,* New York: McGraw-Hill.
1968

SELECTION 21

Planning and Control Systems*

Robert N. Anthony

Our definition of strategic planning combines two types of planning that often are viewed as quite distinct from each other: (1) *choosing objectives* and (2) *planning how to achieve these objectives*. For some purposes, it is desirable to draw a distinction between these types and to classify them as principal subtopics under strategic planning. This is not necessary for the present purpose, however, as here our objective is only to identify the main characteristics of the strategic planning process for the purpose of distinguishing it from the management control process.

Long-Range Planning

Strategic planning does *not* correspond to what some call long-range planning. Strategic decisions do have long-range consequences, and often, but not always, a relatively long time is required to put a strategic decision into effect. However, the distinction between long-range and short-range, insofar as this refers to the time period required to formulate and implement the plan, is not crucial to the distinction between strategic planning and management control. Not uncommonly, the acquisition of an important subsidiary may be completed within a year of the time when the possibility was first conceived; yet the acquisition decision certainly is a strategic decision. More important, the differences in the principles that are relevant to the respective processes are only incidentally related to the time dimension. In 1965 General Motors is well advanced on planning its 1968 Chevrolet, but the mechanism used in this type of planning is in no essential respect different from the process of budgeting 1965's factory overhead; it is part of the management control process. But in 1965 General Motors also is thinking about introducing a turbine-powered vehicle, and this involves a rather different planning process.

The long-range, short-range distinction has more validity in relation to the duration of the consequences of decisions. Strategic decisions tend to have long-term effects; often they are irreversible in the short run. But even this distinction can be stretched too far. The addition of one employee also,

---

* *Planning and Control Systems,* Boston, Harvard University, Graduate School of Business Administration, 1965, pp. 26–47.

as a practical matter, has long-run consequences, and the reversal of such a decision is not always easy. A series of such decisions can have, in total, significant consequences.

Analogy with Military Strategy

The word strategic suggests a correspondence between the process we are describing and strategy as used in military parlance. The relationship seems to be quite close. This is fortunate for our purposes, for military leaders and researchers have done more thinking about strategic principles relevant to their profession than business leaders and researchers have done about theirs. Thus, business management should be able to profit from what the military has already learned and published. As an indication of the possibilities, see the brief summary of some of the principles of military strategy given in Appendix B. Even more important, the way in which the military does strategic planning, especially the functions of the staff, should be carefully explored, and indeed has been explored by some who are interested in possible business applications.

MANAGEMENT CONTROL, GENERAL DESCRIPTION

Management control is the process by which managers assure that resources are obtained and used effectively and efficiently in the accomplishment of the organization's objectives.

"Effectiveness" is used here in Barnard's sense:[2] "Effectiveness relates to the accomplishment of the coöperative purpose. . . . When a specific desired end is attained we shall say that the action is 'effective.' "

"Efficiency," however, is used not in the sense of Barnard ("Efficiency relates to the satisfaction of individual motives . . ."), but rather in its more usual engineering sense: the optimum relationship between input and output. The more units of outputs are obtained from a given input, the more efficient is the machine or process. Koontz, Simon, and others also use Barnard's definition of effectiveness, but not that of efficiency.

The term management control is not entirely satisfactory, inasmuch as it is used to identify not only control activities (as control is defined in the dictionary) but also a type of planning. "Management cybernetics" is a possible alternative, but cybernetics is a strange word to most people in organizations, and also it is fast becoming meaningless. There is, for example, a "science" called "psychocybernetics," which has to do with the psychological effects of plastic surgery. Programming has been suggested as another alternative, but it connotes, we believe, a different type of activity; it is described in Chapter 3 under the heading Operational Control.

The word control in its ordinary sense has unfortunate connotations. As Beckett points out,[3] it often is used in the sense of "boss, curb, dominate, enforce, forestall, hinder, inhibit, manipulate, prevail, restrain, shackle, and watch," and these connotations are not at all realistic as descriptions of what actually goes on in a well-managed organization.

The word "controller" likewise has many meanings, some of them unfortunate, for our purposes. It implies, for example, that the *controller* should exercise control, which is not so; *he should construct and operate a system through which management exercises control.* In practice, people with the title of controller have functions that are, at one extreme, little more than bookkeeping and, at the other extreme, *de facto* general management.

The Conformance Fallacy

Several authors state that the aim of control is to assure that the results of operations conform as closely as possible to plans. We emphasize that such a concept of control is basically inconsistent with the concept used in this study. To the extent that middle management can make decisions that are better than those implied in the plans, top management wishes it to do so. And the middle managers can in fact make better decisions under certain circumstances; to deny this possibility is implicitly to assume that top management is either clairvoyant, or omniscient, or both, which is not so.

Since no one can foretell the future precisely—that is, since people are not clairvoyant—it follows that in some respects actual events will differ from the assumed events that the plans were designed to meet. Even if plans are revised frequently, the preparation and communication of revisions take time, and the revised plans therefore cannot be up-to-date in the literal sense of this term. Top management wants middle management to react to the events that actually occur, not to those that might have occurred had the real world been kind enough to conform to the planning assumptions. Therefore top management does *not* necessarily want operations to conform to plans.

Furthermore, since people are not omniscient, their plans do not necessarily show the best course of action; they merely show what was thought of as best when the plan was made. Subsequently, someone may think of a way to improve on the plan; indeed, it is quite likely that he will do so as the facts and alternatives become clearer. If he does, he should act accordingly. *For this reason, also, top management does not necessarily want operations to conform to plans.*

The practical implication of the foregoing statements is that conformance to plans is *not* the standard against which performance should be measured. "The closer the better" is *not* necessarily the best rule. *That is why our definition of management control is worded in terms of the effective and efficient utilization of resources, rather than conformance to plans.* Of course, the plans do provide a starting point for the appraisal of performance, and there can be a presumption that plans should be followed in the absence of contrary evidence. But this presumption should be rebuttable, and the rebuttal process should not be made too difficult. To do otherwise is to run the great risk of stifling initiative and encouraging unthinking mediocrity.

Acceptance in Practice

Despite the semantic problems, *management control* does seem to be a meaningful term to people in organizations, and the fact that it includes planning as well as control elements does not, as a practical matter, bother people, except some of those who try to describe the relevant concepts in articles or books. Then confusion arises, as was pointed out in Chapter 1. This confusion, however, comes from the fact that the writers try to separate the planning and control aspects of the management control process, and although this can be done conceptually, such a neat separation does not exist in practice.

Although management control does involve two types of mental activity —planning and controlling—in actual operation these two are not easily distinguished. They do not serve as fruitful topics for a classification framework.

DISTINGUISHING CHARACTERISTICS

This section describes what seem to us to be the main characteristics of the strategic planning process and of the management control process. The two processes are discussed together in order to focus on the distinctions between them. The purpose is not to define, but rather to show that the differences are so significant that the systems designed for the two processes have substantially different characteristics. Some of the mistakes that are made when these differences are not recognized will be described in the succeeding section.

Since we shall emphasize differences, the reader may get the impression that we view strategic planning and management control as discrete entities. This is not so. *The planning and control process is in fact a continuum, and we imply a discrete dichotomy only because we believe that this is the best way to explain the distinction.* A corresponding approach is necessary to describe the differences between research and development, or between management and labor, or between slavery and freedom.

Management control is a process carried on within guidelines established by strategic planning. Objectives, facilities, organization, and financial factors are more or less accepted as givens. Decisions about next year's budget, for example, are constrained within prescribed policies and guidelines. The management control process is intended to make possible the achievement of planned objectives as effectively and efficiently as possible within these givens.

The management control process involves making decisions about what to do in the future, and this is planning in the ordinary meaning of the term. But the planning decisions made in the management control process are of a somewhat different character from those made in the strategic planning process. The captain of a ship is invloved in management control. His job is to take the ship to its destination as effectively and efficiently as possible. The architect who designs a new ship, the person who evolves a new concept of shipping, or the person who works out new shipping routes, is involved in strategic planning. The president of a shipping line is involved in both.

As is often the case in attempts to define basic concepts, the line dividing strategic planning from management control is fuzzy. Ford's decision to acquire Philco and thus enter new markets was a clear example of strategic planning; the decision to introduce a 1,000-pound automobile and the subsequent reversal of this decision were probably also in the strategic category. At the other extreme, clearly in the area of management control, were decisions such as the one to arrange the twin tail-lights on next year's Ford Fairlane horizontally rather than vertically. In between these extremes are product decisions that could be placed in either category: the addition to the line of the four-door Thunderbird, for example.

A more general reason for the shading of one process into the other is that there are important interactions between them. Although budgets are prepared within guidelines that emerge from the strategic planning process, the first draft of a new budget may reveal some unforeseen relationships that cast doubt on the wisdom of the guidelines and thus result in changes in strategy.

Even though the distinction may be difficult to state, it is in most instances reasonably clear-cut in practice. A food manufacturer may introduce a half-dozen or so new cake mixes in the course of a year, and all the decisions about these are made more or less routinely by people in the operating divisions acting in accordance with a set of policies governing the cake mix line; whereas the decision to introduce a new product line, such as dogfood, involves quite different considerations and is studied by quite different people. Decisions on cake mixes are part of the management control process; the dogfood decision is strategic.

Management control relates to current operations. Objectives, policies, organization structure, product lines, plant location and capacity, and so on, all are decided in the strategic planning process. Operating people make plans, but they make them within these constraints. It follows that the designer of a management control system also accepts these same constraints. For example, he accepts and adapts to whatever organization structure the strategic planners have decided is best. He designs the system to fit the organization structure, rather than insisting that the organization structure be changed to fit the management control system.

Since the management control process takes place within the guidelines of specified objectives and policies, and since these vary from one organization to another, it is inconceivable that a single management control system ever can be developed that will fit all organizations. Some authors evidently do not accept this conclusion. For example, the literature contains many articles arguing that direct costing is a universally desirable practice, and other articles arguing that direct costing has no merit. Both sets of arguments are too sweeping. Direct costing is useful in certain types of companies, for example, those that have made a policy decision to price certain products on a marginal income basis. It is not useful, at least for pricing purposes, in companies that have decided to price on the basis of full-cost recovery. Thus, a discussion of the pros and cons of direct costing should take into account differences in companies' objectives and policies.

Relation to Other Terms

The distinction between strategic planning and management control corresponds approximately to the distinction that some authors make between "administration" and "management." For example, Ordway Tead says:[4] "*Administration* is the process and agency which is responsible for the determination of the aims for which an organization and its management are to strive, which establishes the broad policies under which they are to operate, and which gives general oversight to the continuing effectiveness of the total operation in reaching the objectives sought." And he goes on to say that "*Management* is the process and agency which directs and guides the operations of an organization in the realizing of established aims." In these terms, strategic planning is a process used in administration, and management control is a process used in management.

Chandler and Redlich,[5] although using different terminology, make a similar distinction. They quote a General Motors annual report that uses administration to refer to "the daily conduct of the Corporation's affairs," and "formation of policies," for the broader types of activities. Note that General Motors uses administration to refer to the opposite process from Tead's. They, themselves, make a distinction between "operational functions" and "strategy determination," corresponding to our terms, management control and strategic planning.

In *Executive Control—The Catalyst,*[6] Jerome uses executive control for approximately the same concept that we label management control.

Goetz divides the management function into the *design* of an enterprise and the *operation* of an enterprise.[7] These terms correspond to the distinction made here between strategic planning and management control.

In public administration, a distinction is often made between "politics" and "administration."[8] This fits our distinction between strategic planning and management control.

Simon[9] makes a distinction between decisions based on value judgments and decisions based on facts. If the distinction is taken as a relative one, this also fits our classification, since strategic planning decisions involve a preponderance of value judgments, and management control decisions, a preponderance of facts.

But Malcolm[10] defines a management control system as "a set of policies, procedures, and information processing which is designed to give direction to activities by clearly establishing goals, by measuring progress toward these goals, and by indicating or initiating corrective action." He apparently lumps together the central ideas of both strategic planning and management control in this definition.

Scope of Process

Ordinarily, the system that is used in the management control process is a *total* system in the sense that it embraces all aspects of the company's operations. It needs to be a total system because an important management function is to assure that all parts of the operation are in balance with one another; and in order to examine balance, management needs information about each of the parts.

The strategic planning process is much less likely to relate to the totality of the organization; rather, with rare exceptions, a given strategic plan relates to some parts of the operation, but not all of it. For example, when the strategic planners are trying to decide whether to enter overseas markets, they must consider the ramifications of this decision throughout the organization, to the extent that there are ramifications, but only to this extent. If the domestic sales force, or the research laboratory, or the operation of a certain factory is unaffected by the decision, management needs to give no attention to these parts of the organization in making the decision. Similarly, a proposed reorganization may affect a great many people, but have no effect on financial policies, product policies, and so on.

Several people have questioned the validity of the distinction that is made above. They cite two reasons. The first is that the strategic planners, more than any other group, should be seeking to optimize the effectiveness of the whole organization; to do anything less is to "suboptimize," which is bad. We agree that conceptually it would be a fine thing to optimize the whole organization, but we doubt that people in the real world find it feasible to optimize. *A strategic plan is made within the context of an ongoing organization.* The process starts when someone gets an idea for doing something new, or when someone initiates a search for a better way because he is dissatisfied with the way a part of the enterprise is going. In either case the focus is on the new idea, or the part that is in trouble, not on the totality. As Steiner says:[11]

> ... It should be recognized that life is so complicated that it is impossible to tie together all plans into a complete coordinated set of relationships. The further out in time, the less detail is appropriate and the looser are the relationships among parts of the planning program. In developing current operational plans, tighter relationships are possible and desirable.

In exceptional situations the operations, and even the objectives, of the whole enterprise may be subjected to a basic re-examination, but these are rare; they occur perhaps once or twice during the tenure of a given management team. Also, in certain types of companies it is possible to plan for the totality, or almost the totality, of the organization. An electric utility, serving a defined geographical area, with no plans for expanding into other areas or other types of business, is perhaps the best example. In this situation, it is both feasible and desirable to make over-all plans—covering production, distribution, finance, and personnel—for many years ahead, and to optimize, at least roughly, the whole operation. But few organizations are simple enough and operate in a sufficiently predictable environment to permit this.

The second criticism made with respect to the generalization that strategic plans tend to be partial is that such a statement may encourage planners to perpetuate a mistake that is already too common; namely, it may lead them to overlook important ramifications of a proposed plan. It is a fact that the analysis of a proposed plan should take into account all the significant consequences that the proposal will have throughout the organization; it is a fact that visualizing and assessing these changes are difficult jobs; and it is also a fact that there are many examples of plans that turned out to be poor because some important consequence was overlooked. These facts, however, relate to the adequacy of the planning process in a specific situation. They do not weaken the validity of the generalization. To say that a given strategic plan relates to less than the totality of the operation is quite different from saying that it focuses on only one narrow aspect. The latter statement is just as invalid as the former, as a description of what goes on.

Complexities and Constraints

Although not usually total, the strategic planning process is often *complex.* Several aspects of the organization are involved, there are many relevant considerations, and these may involve social and political factors as well as economic matters. *The plan sets precedent, and setting precedents is invariably more complicated than working within precedents.*

The management control process is less complex. *Management control takes place within a framework of policies and plans already decided upon.* These constraints greatly simplify the task of preparing an operating plan and of operating in accordance with that plan.

Consider, for example, the problems of managing a chain of hotels. The strategic planner must face the problem of maintaining profitable operations in the face of changing travel habits, increasing competition from motels, increasing operating costs, changing tax regulations on entertainment, and so on. He seeks to answer such questions as these: Shall we acquire additional properties? Should they be city hotels, city motels, or motels on the periphery of the city? In what part of the country? Should we build them, or acquire them from someone else? But the manager of one hotel in the chain has a rather different, and much narrower, set of choices. The hotel exists; it has a certain location and a certain size, which he cannot change at all; and a certain clientele, staff, decor, etc., which he can change only with considerable effort and then only within rather narrow limits. His job is to do the best he can within these constraints. This is a strikingly different job from that of the strategic planner.

Degree of Structure

The management control process tends to be rhythmic; it follows a definite pattern and timetable, which are repeated. In budgetary control, which is an important part of the management control process, certain steps are taken in a prescribed sequence and at certain dates each year: the dissemination of guidelines, the preparation of original estimates, the transmission of these estimates up through the several echelons in the organization, the review of these estimates, final approval by top management, dissemination back through the organization, and the reporting and appraisal of performance. The procedure to be followed at each step in this process, the dates when the steps are to be completed, and even the forms that are to be used can be, and often are, set forth in a manual.

Although the general process of management control is a rhythmic, recurring one, specific actions are taken as the occasion warrants. The fact that each of these actions—promotion of a foreman, change of the price of a product, rearrangement of machinery, and so on—is a discrete event does not invalidate the generalization that the whole process should be viewed as a recurring flow. We can make generalizations about the over-all behavior of a gas, even though the individual molecules move erratically.

Strategic planning is essentially *irregular*. Problems, opportunities, and "bright ideas" do not arise according to some set timetable; they have to be dealt with whenever they happen to be perceived. The appropriate analytical techniques depend on the nature of the problem being analyzed, and currently there is no general approach (such as a mathematical model) that is of much help in the analysis of all types of strategic problems. Indeed, an attempt to introduce a systematic approach is quite likely to dampen the essential element of creativity.

Few companies have a systematic approach to strategic planning.* Most companies react to changes in their environment *after* they experience the changes; they do not have an organized means of attempting to foresee changes and to take action in anticipation of them. However, the number of companies that regard strategic planning as an important activity and one to be separated conceptually and organizationally from current operations is growing rapidly.

Failure to appreciate the distinction between regular and irregular processes can result in trouble of the following type. A company with a well-developed budgeting process decides to formalize its strategic planning. It prepares a set of forms and accompanying procedures, and has the operating units submit their long-range plans on these forms on one certain date each year. The plans are then supposed to be reviewed and approved in a meeting similar to a budget review meeting. Such a procedure does not work. For one thing, as already mentioned, new ideas do not originate according to a timetable, and it is unrealistic to assume that all new ideas can be collected on one date, and that the idea-generating process will then be shut off for a year. For another thing, there simply is not time enough in an annual review meeting for a careful consideration of a whole batch of strategic proposals.

---

* Stanford Research Institute estimates that the number of manufacturing companies with a fully developed and staffed "long-range planning program" does not exceed 25. (Stanford Research Institute, *Conference on Long-Range Planning*, 1962.) Although any attempt to count the companies that follow a given practice (out of many tens of thousands of companies in all) is suspect, there is general agreement that in this case the number is tiny.

The strategic planners work now on one problem, now on another, according to the needs and opportunities of the moment. By contrast, it is important that next year's operating budget be examined and approved as an entity so as to ensure that the several pieces are consonant with one another; and in order to do this all the pieces must be brought together on a certain date, say December 14. But there is no corresponding need to cumulate proposed strategic plans and present them all at one time. They are presented for decision whenever they are ready. *Except for very general checklists of essential considerations, the strategic planning process follows no prescribed format or timetable.* Each problem is sufficiently different from other problems so that each must be approached differently. If there is a manual of strategic planning procedures, it should contain only broad, general statements, not a specific list of steps to take. In most companies, such a manual does not even exist. As Cyert and Dill say: [12]

> Strategic problems of this sort are by their nature complex and ill structured. For decisions about goals, for the assessment of the environment, and for the basic selection of product-market strategies, current mathematical and statistical techniques have little to contribute. In strategic planning, the task is much less one of making an optimal choice than it is one of being imaginative and systematic in formulating alternatives from which the choice will be made.

Some types of strategic planning are amendable to a certain amount of structure and regularity. *The capital budgeting mechanism is the best example.* Most proposed capital investments have certain characteristics in common; in essence they involve the commitment of funds now, in the expectation of earning an adequate return on these funds in the future. Various techniques are available for analysis of the expected financial consequences of such proposals; these can be explained in manuals and the proposals can follow a prescribed set of procedures. Moreover, these capital budgeting decisions, or at least some of them, often are made according to a prescribed timetable, and are therefore more rhythmic than are other types of strategic plans. This is because of the necessity for the strategic planners to examine, at regular intervals, the total financial implications of investment proposals, and to match these against financial resources.

The foregoing discussion is not intended to minimize the importance of regular, top management strategy meetings. At these meetings management may either discuss a specific proposal, in which case the meetings are part of the strategic planning process, or merely discuss in broad terms the question, "Where should we be heading?", in which case the meetings are often the occasion for the first step in the formulation of a strategic plan.

Nature of Information

Since the management control process encompasses the totality of the organization, management control systems, with rare exceptions, have an underlying *financial* structure; that is, plans and results are expressed in monetary units. Money is the only common denominator by means of which the heterogeneous elements of outputs and inputs (e.g., hours of labor, type of labor, quantity and quality of material, amount and kind of products produced) can be combined and compared. (The Soviets once considered adopting a system in which "equivalent units of human energy" were to be used instead of money as the common denominator. In the 1930's, the Technocrats advocated a similar common denominator for use in this country. None of these alternatives is so good as a monetary system.)

Some managers, especially those in eleemosynary institutions (e.g., ministers, college presidents, hospital directors), find the whole concept of financial measurements repugnant. If they are to function as managers, however, they really cannot avoid working with money measurements, except in those rare situations where resources are practically unlimited so that there is no need to measure the relationship between inputs and outputs. The college president may say (or feel, even if he does not choose to say it): "My job is to educate students; I don't want to be bothered about money." Nevertheless, he will have choices to make as to his educational program, and he will need a means of comparing the alternatives. For example, he must choose between, on the one hand, a large number of courses, small sections, large faculty, and low faculty salaries, and, on the other hand, a limited number of courses, large sections, a smaller number of faculty, and high faculty salaries. Educational administration also involves decisions as to the relative emphasis to be given to academic matters, athletics, alumni, scholarships, tutorials, and so on. The only way of relating all these elements for the purpose of selecting the best alternative is to reduce them to financial terms.

Although management control systems have financial underpinnings, it does not follow that money is the *only* basis of measurement, or even that it is the most important basis. Other quantitative measurements, such as enrollment, grades, market share, yields, productivity measures, tonnage of output, and so on, are useful. So are nonquantitative expressions of quality, ability, cooperation, and other attributes. We simply mean that, in most organizations, money is the only denominator that can relate the various pieces to one another and that a financial structure is therefore essential to the management control process.

Management control systems are, or should be, coordinated, integrated systems; that is, although data collected for one purpose may differ from those collected for another purpose, these data should be reconcilable with one another. In a sense, a management control system is a *single* system, but it is perhaps more accurate to think of it as a set of articulated subsystems. As an example, consider the cost information that is collected in many systems. Three types of cost are needed in many companies: (1) *costs by responsibility centers,* which are used for planning and controlling the activities of responsible supervisors; (2) *full "program" costs,* used for pricing and other operating decisions under normal circumstances; and (3) *direct program costs,* used for pricing and other operating decisions under special circumstances, such as when management wishes to utilize idle capacity. "Program" is here used for any activity in which the organization engages. In industrial companies, programs consist of products or product lines, and *product costs* can be substituted in the above statements.

Direct program costs are one element of full program costs; so these two types are easily distinguished and reconcilable. All that is needed is a record in which full costs are broken into direct and indirect elements. Responsibility costs cut across program costs; so at *lower levels of detail* the two types do not correspond to one another. They should, however, be reconcilable in the aggregate. For example, the total of a budget broken down by products should equal the total of a budget broken down by responsibility centers.

Moreover, in a management control system, nonmonetary information should be reconcilable with monetary information. Information on the *number* of personnel should be relatable to information on the *cost* of personnel, for example.

The information used in the strategic planning process is of a considerably different character from that used in management control. For one thing, *strategic planning relies more heavily on external information, that is, on data collected from outside the company, such as market analyses, estimates of costs and other factors involved in building a plant in a new locality, technological developments, and so on.* When historical, internal data are used, they often must be recast to fit the needs of the problem being analyzed. For example, the current operating costs of a plant that are collected for measuring performance and for making pricing and other operating decisions almost invariably must be restructured before they are useful to management in deciding whether to close down the plant.

Another characteristic of the information relevant for strategic planning is that much of it is imprecise. The strategic planner estimates what will happen, often over a rather long time period. His estimates are likely to have a high degree of uncertainty, and he must treat them accordingly. The estimates used in management control are not certain either. (An advertisement for a book on profit planning asserts: "it enables you to present management with a plan of action which makes a given profit figure not merely a target to aim at, but a near predictable certainty;" this statement is nonsense.) Although by no means precise, the estimates used in the management control process are likely to be much much closer to actual than the estimates used in strategic planning, however.

The data used in the management control process have the same definitions and are put together in the same way month after month. The data relevant for deciding on a proposed strategic plan are put together specifically for that plan. The need for uniform definitions of terms is therefore more important in management control than in strategic planning. For example, labor cost should have a certain prescribed, generally understood meaning in all the regular, recurring performance reports: whereas the meaning of a number that is labeled "labor cost" in the analysis of a proposed plan usually requires interpretation; it can be understood only when one knows the work elements and the method of pricing the elements that the analyst had in mind.

This does not mean that problems of definition are of no concern to strategic planners, for serious misunderstandings arise when terms are implicitly defined differently by different people, and these misunderstandings can be reduced by an agreed-to dictionary of terms whose definitions are used whenever possible. Indeed, those involved in the management control process quickly come to understand the meaning of the terms used, even if these meanings are never written down, or even if the written definition has become obsolete, which happens. In the strategic planning process, misunderstandings are more common. For example, in the TFX investigation, the Senate Committee counsel made much of the fact that Boeing submitted estimates for "cost" that were lower than those submitted by General Dynamics, as if cost had the same meaning in both sets of figures. It turned out that the figures were not at all comparable.

The data needed for strategic planning depend on the nature of the problems being studied. Not all these problems can be foreseen and, even for those that can be foreseen, data collected regularly in a form that will be useful for an occasional strategic decision are not worth the cost of collection. It is because of the varied and unpredictable nature of the data required for strategic planning that an attempt to design an all-purpose, internal information system is probably hopeless. For the same reason, the dream of some computer specialists of a gigantic data bank, from which planners can obtain all the information they wish by pressing some buttons, is probably no more than a dream.

Purpose of Estimates

These estimates used in strategic planning are intended to show the *expected* results of the plan. They are neutral and impersonal. By contrast, the management control process, and the data used in it, are intended to influence managers to take actions that will lead to *desired* results. *In more formal language, the objective of management control is goal congruence;* that is, the system should be so set up that actions that operating managers take in their perceived self interest are also in the best interests of the whole organization. This difference in purpose is subtle, but important.

The difference can be illustrated by the discussion in the literature and in practice, of how "tight" an operating budget should be. Should the goals be set so high that only an outstanding manager can achieve them, or should they be set so that they are attainable by the average manager? At what level does frustration inhibit a manager's best efforts? Does an attainable budget lead to complacency? And so on. Questions of this type are highly appropriate in deciding on the nature of data in a management control system. *They are psychological considerations.* Activities such as communicating, persuading, exhorting, inspiring, and criticizing are an important part of the process. By contrast, the data used in strategic planning are impersonal; their purpose is to communicate the best estimate that can be made. If anyone thought the data were designed so as to motivate the user toward a certain course of action, he would reject them summarily.

Organizational Relationships

Both strategic planning and management control involve top management, but strategic planning is heavily staff oriented, whereas management control is heavily line oriented.

Line managers usually are not major participants in the strategic planning process; sometimes they are not even aware of the fact that a plan is being considered. There are good reasons for this. Many operating executives are by temperament not very good at strategic planning. Also, the pressures of current activities usually do not allow them to devote the necessary time to such work. For competitive reasons, furthermore, it is often essential that the number of people who are aware of strategic plans be kept quite small.

This distinction between the role of the operating manager and the role of the strategic planner is expressed in various ways in the literature. Some examples follow; first, from Selznick:[13]

. . . The role of the institutional leader should be clearly distinguished from that of the "interpersonal" leader. The latter's task is to smooth the path of human interaction, ease communication, evoke personal devotion, and allay anxiety. His expertness has relatively little to do with content; he is more concerned with persons than with policies. His main contribution is to the efficiency of the enterprise. The institutional leader, on the other hand, *is primarily an expert in the promotion and protection of value.* . . .

And this statement by Senator Henry M. Jackson:[14]

You know the typical week in the life of a Cabinet officer—seven formal speeches, seven informal speeches, seven hearings on the Hill, seven official cocktail parties, seven command dinner engagements. It is a schedule which leaves no time for the kind of reflection essential to creative planning. What they can do, should do, must do—and all that they should be asked to do—is to pass judgment on sharply defined policy issues.

Of course Cabinet members have the obligation to encourage and back the officers in their departments who are charged with policy planning. The responsibility of the policy planner should run clearly to his departmental head. In this way staff planning can be geared into line decisions and the authority of the departmental head can support and strengthen the hand of the planner.

But I am convinced that we never will get the kind of policy planning we need if we expect the top-level officers to participate actively in the planning process. They simply do not have the time, and in any event they rarely have the out-look or the talents of the good planner. They cannot explore issues deeply and systematically. They cannot argue the advantages and disadvantages at length in the kind of give-and-take essential if one is to reach a solid understanding with others on points of agreement and disagreement.

Much investigation and analysis are needed as a basis for making a strategic decision. In some organizations, this work is done by a staff unit created for the purpose. Such a unit usually has little if anything to do with current operations and therefore is not involved in the management control process. In other organizations, one or more persons are drawn from the operating organization to work on a proposed strategic plan. During the period in which they are so engaged, their activity is quite different in character from their normal operating tasks. Generalizations as to the types of person who should engage in planning are quite different, depending on whether the reference is to strategic planning or to the planning aspect of management control. The difference is essentially that between the thinker and the doer. A generalization covering both types of activities will be either invalid or so amorphous as to be useless.

SELECTION 22

Financial Incentives: How They Could Reshape the Health Care System*

Lawrence A. Hill

Incentive reimbursement is a subject (or idea or technique) that is "in" this year. Some have faith that it can be used to help control the hospital cost spiral, while others are skeptical. Who is correct, either wholly or in part, presumably will be determined after empirical evidence is accumulated. There is, however, one mistake that is clear from the outset and therefore can be avoided: financial incentives *via* the reimbursement system should not be considered separately from other programs designed to control hospital costs. Further, as emphasized by Robert Sigmond,[1] there are a number of incentives operating in the hospital field that are not related to the reimbursement question.

This paper will concentrate on financial incentives through reimbursement; in a sense, it represents a limited approach. Even the limited approach, however, becomes broadened as one thought or assumption inexorably leads to another. A logical point of departure for a discussion that in the absence of data based on experience must be speculative is examination of the goal it is hoped incentive reimbursement might achieve; second, the paper will briefly describe some means by which that goal can be achieved; third, some factors that have served as constraints to goal achievement will be mentioned; and finally, the paper will speculate on how incentive reimbursement could help to achieve the goal.

Perhaps the goal can best be described by using a very simplified model, wherein the input is composed of resources purchased and the medical care process itself, and the output is patient care.

Cost of Care

The cost of care is reflected by the cost of resources used as input and their use within the medical care process. The efficiency† of the system can be described as a fraction:

---

* *Hospitals,* vol. 43, June 16, 1969.
† "Efficiency" is used in the economic sense rather than a physicist or engineer would use the term. "Economic efficiency of a particular productive process is the ratio of useful product output to useful input of resources," R. H. Leftwich, *The*

$$\frac{\text{Cost of input}}{\text{Units of output}} = \frac{\text{Cost per unit}}{\text{of output}}$$

Obviously this model is oversimplified. For one thing, it ignores quality of output. Given the assumption, however, that quality remains constant (or at least does not decrease), the goal sought is a reduction in the value of this fraction; that is, an increase in output relative to input or a decrease in input relative to output.

The goal is simply stated and many of the means of approaching the goal are known. Industrial engineering techniques such as work simplification can help to achieve better use of personnel, space, and equipment. Rensis Likert[2-3] has developed empirical evidence to show how management techniques can increase output relative to input. Increased use of outpatient versus inpatient services, better use of postacute facilities and home care programs, and more emphasis on preventive measures including hospital programs in health education—all could serve to achieve more effective use of the system. (Prepaid group practice should not be ignored.)

Further, external controls—both voluntary and public—are imposed on hospitals. Voluntary area-wide planning agencies and Hill-Burton groups are two examples of an approach that attempts to control costs through control of capital funds. There are many other kinds of controls that need not be discussed here except to call attention to the fact that they do exist.

Constraints to Control

If all of these (and many other) means are known, why is it that they are not more effectively used? Is it local pride, motivation to protect autonomy on the part of hospital trustees and physicians, financial motives, instinctive resistance to change? The answer, it would seem, is "all of these, and more." At the risk of appearing superficial, the answer is "the establishment." What is meant by "the establishment," however, must be explained. It is made up of hospitals; doctors; Blue Cross and Blue Shield plans; insurance companies; local, state, and national health departments; welfare departments; voluntary associations; medical societies; city councils; planning agencies (public and voluntary); Congress; the Social Security Administration; and others. Each of these "institutions" embodies a set of goals, relationships, and likes and dislikes. Each has established prerogatives, each has carved out its own sphere of influence. Each has learned something about the others and the rules of the game, and each has learned how to protect itself within the rules. Each constantly tests the others in

Price System and Resource Allocation (New York: Holt Rinehart and Winston, 1964), p. 16.

trying to expand its own sphere of influence, but within the rules. This welter of institutions, goals, relationships, and rules is "the establishment." It is not "good" nor "evil," moral or immoral; it simply *is*.

If some of the means of achieving efficiency in delivering care are carried out, some of the "rules of the game" must be changed. Widespread use of hospital-based comprehensive outpatient services or hospital franchising, for example, would entail a change in relationships among several parts of the establishment. These measures might reduce the value of the input-output fraction, but certainly they would create change attended by inevitable conflict.

It is not clear whether incentive reimbursement means major change, yet it is reasonable to think that it does for one simple reason: the principle of incentive reimbursement explicitly states that the payer considers cost control so important that he is willing to pay the provider for achieving it. Until now most reimbursement formulas specifically excluded any cost item that was not closely related to patient care. Incentive payments are dollar awards or payments for good management and not for patient care. This means a major reordering of the health system's goals. Cost control has not until this moment been a prime goal of the system; it has occasioned millions of written words and countless speeches but very little in the way of action to achieve it: other goals, including that of maintaining existing relationships within the system, have taken priority. Incentive reimbursement, therefore, changes goals directly and implies resulting changes in relationships and rules within the establishment.

Another way of saying the same thing is to state that the incentives operating in the system have motivated the health service administrator to set priorities and thus to devote his energies to factors other than cost control. Two of the most powerful incentives operating in the health system are the desire to be of service to society and to achieve professional recognition. Currently the administrator or physician can achieve maximum professional recognition by providing the most expensive care known to man and thus be of service to society. The acute hospital, with its operating suites, elaborate laboratories, and intensive care units are scenes of dramatic rescue from death. Society applauds and supports this rescue and rewards those who have participated—all in spite of rising costs.

At present, the health administrator is not rewarded for cost control efforts, so why should he endure the certain conflict that lies in those efforts? He has learned to thrive in the current system with its set of goals. He has been promoted and runs a large hospital, or a Blue Cross or Blue Shield plan, or a federal agency. He knows how to play the game and he plays it well. Change means problems. Change means new or altered relationships with health professionals and institutions. This means conflict and hard work. So why should he change? What is in it for him?

Spurs to Action

The answer can be put in several ways. There are some who moralize and who criticize the administrator and physician as antisocial. Others threaten governmental takeover as the penalty for lack of action (this is often considered an incentive in itself). Still others assume an historical point of view and observe that unless the goals of the administrator change to match those of society, administrators will become obsolete and eventually will be discarded. For most persons in the voluntary system the idea of a governmental takeover should be an incentive sufficient to create some action. The threat, however, has been used too many times to have much effect anymore. And the threat of becoming socially obsolete is too philosophical to serve as an effective spur to action.

There is, however, another proven incentive—money. Money is a strong incentive; it motivates people to act. Money also is the tool that the reimbursement mechanism has at its disposal to induce action in directions it desires. The question becomes one of whether money can be used to motivate the existing system (the establishment) to implement activities and programs to create changes that will make cost control a prime goal relative to other goals involved in delivering health services.

At this moment in time there seems an almost tacit faith that money can do it. But how? In the absence of direct empirical evidence it becomes necessary to turn to the realm of theory and speculation in seeking an answer to that stubborn question.

The classic model is the competitive private enterprise marketplace where each firm is motivated by profit. Profit accrues to the owners of the firm either in direct compensation (in the case of the single proprietor or partnership) or in dividends on money invested (in the case of the corporation stockholder). The key to the system is that profit is not only institutional, but personal.

It is argued that the incentive sought by most investors is not dividends at all, but capital gain. This is true, and it is this fact that enables the corporate directors to withhold earnings from dividend payments in order to invest them in plant expansion, product development, or diversification to further increase profits. The stockholder agrees to forgo immediate gain in hopes of greater gains in the future. This has not, however, altered his major goal. The incentive of personal financial gain still governs.

In other words, a business corporation attracts resources from the public through the incentive of personal financial gain. Aside from dividend payments, the investor stands to profit if the company gains a reputation for good management, good profits, and a good outlook for the future. In such a case, demand for ownership of that company grows relative to the supply of shares of ownership, and the price of each share rises.

The voluntary hospital obviously does not fit this model. Hospital ownership is not based on a personal profit motive. How, then, without the profit motive, without the shared but personal ownership pattern and rewards, can financial incentives be used to motivate the health system to face the many difficult problems associated with cost control?

The corporate model, however, is not complete when limited to ownership. The management segment of the model also must be examined, and the relationship of management to the enterprise managed.

When this relationship is examined some similarities between the hospital and the business corporation are found. The business manager capable of producing good profits may be rewarded in several ways: He may receive salary increases, stock options, bonuses, or all three. He may be promoted within the company or attain a better position in another firm. He may gain public recognition and prestige through membership in civic or national groups (a hospital board, for example). He may become a consultant to the national government or he may attain high political office.

Potentially a hospital administrator receives the same kinds of rewards. In practice, however, these rewards are not so pronounced. Salaries of administrators are not rising at a rate comparable to those of other managers.[4] There is, of course, no potential for stock options. Bonuses are being paid in an increasing number of hospitals—13 per cent, according to one survey[4]—but the size of these is unknown. A hospital administrator does gain prestige within his field to the same extent as business managers.

Among the reasons that rewards for hospital administrators are not as pronounced as those for business managers, two stand out. First, the hospital's success or failure is not easily measured. Second, the historic social and philosophical relationship of the administrator to the hospital's ownership is difficult to define. The texts say he is the servant of the board of trustees: The board sets policy, he executes it. Thus, he avoids responsibility for the institution's major decisions. In most business corporations, on the other hand, the top manager is an officer of the board and if he and the majority of the board disagree on policy, either he resigns or—through a proxy battle or some other mechanism—board membership changes. If the board, in fact, makes all major policy decisions and the administrator merely serves as caretaker to see that they are honored in practice, there is indeed a difference between the administrator's relationship to hospital ownership and the corporation executive's relationship to his stockholders.

If hospital management is to create change to control costs it will, in the opinion of this observer, have to assume a different relationship with hospital ownership. The concept of the trustee-administrator-physician triad must disappear, and the administrator must join the board structure so that the hospital model will more closely conform to the corporate model. If the administrator is to manage significant change, he must have more structural leverage than is possible in the "triad" arrangement where he is "servant" to the board and the medical staff.

Payer-Provider Roles

Assume that financial rewards through reimbursement are to be paid. In what form are they likely to be most effective in motivating management to face the problems and conflicts inherent in creating the changes that will control costs and earn the financial rewards?

It is at this point that the question discussed by Robert Sigmond in his paper[1] is encountered. Are incentives to be based on a process or are they to be based on results? Mr. Sigmond argues well for rewarding efficient process. If a hospital is accredited, if it subscribes to the Professional Activities Study and Hospital Administrative Services, if it actively reviews utilization, if it cooperates with its areawide planning council, if it makes use of any number of proven management practices, the *probability* is that it will produce an output of satisfactory quality at a reasonable price. Because of the extreme difficulty of measuring all inputs and outputs and because of the relationship between the two, a verification that the hospital is using all of the elements of process that are judged to be helpful is the best proof available that management is attempting to produce high-quality care and control cost.

The process method, then, lends itself to some available form of measurement. It also has the advantage of operating within the system, within the rules of the establishment. Specifically the relationship of the payer and provider is not materially changed. It is worth noting that a significant amount of monitoring of the system currently occurs. Michigan's Blue Cross qualifications program and the Philadelphia Blue Cross-provider contract are two examples. The practice of paying incentives for elements of process is the least disturbing to the system.

Problem Areas

Its major disadvantages are, first, that a hospital can practice all elements of the process and do none of them well, and second, that the process approach creates yet another set of rules for management to follow and can either stifle initiative for the ambitious or provide a comfortable *modus operandi* for the not-so-ambitious.

The goal of the incentive approach says, "we care little about your processes—it is results we wish to evaluate." Turning back, for a moment, to the business marketplace, what are the possibilities of using that model as a form of incentive reimbursement?

In most commercial transactions, the seller offers a product, describes it, and names a price. The buyer specifies what he wants and the price he is willing to pay. Negotiations take place until buyer and seller agree on product specifications and price. The method by which the seller produces and delivers the product is his own business, and provided he stays within the law and stays within product specifications, there is no further control. What it costs him to produce and deliver is his own business. In other words, the buyer does not apply a set of controls to the seller other than to specify the product to be delivered and the price.

The buyer, however, has one further control at his disposal and that is competition among sellers. The buyer usually can ask for competitive bids. In negotiating hospital rates, Blue Cross cannot do this to any appreciable degree, although some competitive forces do exist in the hospital and health field. Look, for example, at prepaid groups. Some of these have told the Social Security Administration that they can offer complete care at a rate less than that paid by the population at large. This is close to bidding on a competitive price basis.

Could payments on a competitive basis motivate hospital managements to undertake strong ambulatory programs, postacute programs, institutionally centered groups, *et al.?* Obviously this would bring management into conflict with physicians, proprietary interests, and perhaps government. But so what? If competition is a viable force, perhaps those groups would make countermoves based on price and product.

It is generally agreed that the major benefit of cost control lies not so much in stimulating more efficient production of an acute patient day (although this is important) but rather in producing efficiency in combination with substitutions of less expensive but appropriate care whenever possible. This is the way to reduce the value of the input/output fraction. If financial incentives are to be useful or causal in achieving this goal, they must be sizable and management must have freedom of action in determining the process and in spending whatever rewards accrue.

Management's freedom to regulate the process through which end results and prices are obtained and management's freedom to spend whatever rewards accrue do indeed represent a change in the relationship between the payer and the provider.

It can be argued that an incentive program need not take this form and thus need not cause change in the system. But if the classical model of financial incentives—the private enterprise market—is used as a pattern (and it seems reasonable to use it in view of its success in this country) change in the health care system seems inevitable.

Conclusions

This paper contains speculations concerning the use of financial incentives *via* reimbursement formulas as a method of controlling the continuing hospital cost spiral.

The paper hypothesizes that the private enterprise market presents a reasonable model against which to compare the health field if incentives are paid. Using a private enterprise model, speculations on the form and impact of incentive programs are made. There are four major implications involved in these speculations: first, priority given to cost control as a goal in the health system becomes primary instead of secondary. Second, the relationship of hospital management to the institution's ownership would change. Management would have to become far more powerful and be eligible for greater and swifter rewards and also be held far more closely accountable for poor results as well as good ones. Third, the relationship of the physician to the system would be altered, with a diminution of his individual decision power and a hearty increase in his participation in institutional decisions. Fourth, the relationship between buyer and seller would change. Debates over reimbursable versus nonreimbursable costs would disappear. Cost elements are the seller's business only. Audits by the buyer might disappear.

It may be judged in the final analysis that these changes are too high a price to pay for cost controls or that there are alternative means of controlling costs that are less threatening to the establishment.

This paper does not advocate any line of action at this time. Even before experiments commence, parameters and measures must be worked out. It is probable, however, that the use of financial incentives can lead to policies that could reshape the health care system. Unless this fact is recognized, there is the ever-present danger that the idea of incentives can be either adopted or damned prematurely and with unfortunate consequences.

REFERENCES

1. Sigmond, R. M. *The Notion of Hospital Incentives.* Presented at the National Forum on Hospital and Health Affairs, Duke University, Durham, N.C., May 17, 1968.
2. Likert, R. *New Patterns of Management* (New York City: McGraw-Hill, 1961).
3. Likert, R. *The Human Organization, Its Management and Value* (New York City: McGraw-Hill, 1967).
4. Witt, J. A. Executive salaries rise—but not as fast as others. *Mod. Hosp.* Aug. 1968.

Part V

Management Science Models: Evolution and Applications

PART V
Management Science Models:
Evolution and Applications

Chapter 11.
Management:
Historical Background

- 11.1 — Introduction
- 11.2 — What is "Management"?
- 11.3 — "Schools" of Management Thought
  - 11.3.1 Scientific Management
  - 11.3.2 Administrative Management
  - 11.3.3 Human Relations
  - 11.3.4 Behavioral Science
  - 11.3.5 Management Science

Chapter 12.
Analytical Models

- 12.1 — Introduction
- 12.2 — What Is a Model?
- 12.3 — Classification of Models
- 12.4 — Linear Programming
- 12.5 — Dynamic Programming
- 12.6 — Inventory Models
- 12.7 — PERT and CPM
- 12.8 — Concluding Remarks
- — Two selected articles

Chapter 13.
Simulation Models

- 13.1 — Introduction
- 13.2 — Definition, Components and Characteristics
- 13.3 — Planning a Simulation Experiment
- 13.4 — Classification of Simulation Models
- 13.5 — Concluding Remarks
- — Two selected articles

Chapter 14.
Toward a Perspective

- 14.1 — The Hospital Sector
- 14.2 — New Managerial Requisites
- 14.3 — Changing the "System"

Chapter 11

Management: Historical Background

11.1 INTRODUCTION

The thrust of this book is that the health administrator can be effective only if he views his job as a *manager*—not as an administrator. The distinction between the terms "manager" and "administrator" is one of philosophy and scope and is perhaps not fully appreciated in the health field. The manager must concern himself not only with the implementation of policies but also with their formulation. An administrator on the other hand, is perceived to be the one who implements policies, but usually does not formulate them. This view of the role of the health administrator has at least two action-implications. First, the modern student of health care must prepare himself to be a manager and, therefore, ought to familiarize himself with the philosophy, potential, and limitations of various schools of management. Secondly, he should assume leadership in creating, reshaping and improving the "organizational climate" of health institutions in order to move the field towards such an orientation. This is obviously an ambitious task and it will take time to achieve even a moderate degree of success. However, it is high time that a start be made in this direction.

It is not possible to present an in-depth description of various schools of management within the constraints of an introductory chapter. A brief but informative discussion is contained in Pugh [1966]. We will present here our version of the branches of management theory. In this chapter we will examine "management" from several different perspectives; briefly describe various "schools" of management; give important characteristics of management science; and provide an operational definition of management science. A selected set of analytical models and their applications are presented in Chapter 12, and simulation models are explained in Chapter 13.

11.2 WHAT IS "MANAGEMENT"?

Management is simultaneously the integration of effort, judicious use of resources, motivating people, providing leadership, planning and controlling, and guiding an organization or a system toward a set of goals and objectives. The term "management" has many connotations, implications, and aspects. Management is a *process,* a *profession,* an *elite* or a *class of* people. Management is an *art* as well as a *science.* Along with materials, capital, and labor, management is a *resource.* Management is multi-dimensional and its different aspects are rooted in a variety of disciplines—including philosophy, economics, mathematics, social sciences, and political science. Management is a complex phenomenon because it involves people; the totality of their interpersonal relationships; questions of motivation and morale; and an innumerable combination of social, biological, physical, and political factors.

Management is not a static concept; it is rather a dynamic process which takes place in a social and political world. Management both creates and controls "change." With the ever-increasing rate of social and technological developments that are taking place in our time, management is *the* central activity needed for human survival. Without management and the resulting order of things, the whole social structure would collapse. Management pervades all aspects of human life and the process of management takes place at all levels of human interest and cooperative systems. All activities and functions performed in a system involving two or more people require management for their effective and efficient execution. This is as true for a hospital as it is for a business firm or a government agency. Any organization, producing goods or services, must essentially perform the same basic functions: securing sufficient financial resources; recruiting, training, and developing manpower; acquiring the materials, tools, and machinery; organizing the capabilities; producing goods or services; arranging distribution channels; engaging in research and development; and in general planning for the survival and growth of the organization. All these tasks and activities must be coordinated in order to achieve predetermined objectives. In all organizations, public or private, health, political, social, national or international, and regardless of the level of organizational complexity, the central task is indeed management—and it must be performed. Obviously, the scope of management is so wide and diverse that it transcends the traditional boundaries of narrowly defined disciplines. Neither the students nor the study of management can be confined within the narrow walls of a single field. Substantial contributions to the field of management have been made from such diverse disciplines as economics, engineering, mathematics, statistics, sociology, psychology, anthropology, and social psychology. This is because the focus of management activities covers both physical and human resources—singly as well as jointly. In this sense management encompasses the totality of human environments and deals with all of its phases. In view of its extremely broad scope and complex nature, we can coin several useful definitions of the term management. Each will have a special significance as it relates to a particular management situation or to a specific approach of solving management problems.

As a *process** management consists of a series of sequential or overlapping activities directed towards achieving organizational objectives. *Management is the process of effectively integrating the efforts of a purposeful group whose members have at least one common goal.* According to this view, the process of management is universal and takes place in performing managerial functions in all types of organizations, and at all levels within the organization. The process of management is the vehicle through which managerial functions are performed. The skills involved in the designing, instituting, and controlling of this process are teachable, learnable, and transferable; hence the evolution of the profession of management.† The role of management science concepts and models is to make this process more efficient and effective.

Management, like law and medicine, is a recognized *profession.* Management courses constitute the central core of all degree programs in business administration and in many health administration curricula. All major colleges and universities now offer professional degrees in management—with an increasing percentage offering specialized programs in management science and operations research. Several professional societies have been formed for the purpose of interchanging information and encouraging professional development in different branches of management.‡ The Institute of Management Sciences (TIMS), Operations Research Society of America (ORSA), and American Institute of Decision Sciences (AIDS), for example, are just three of the professional societies in the area of management science. All have journals in which persons from educational, business, health, and governmental organizations publish articles on the theory and applications of management science. Similar professional societies have been organized in Europe, Asia, South America, and other parts of the globe. In addition, private business firms and management consulting firms offer frequent management science training seminars. Even

---

* Ackoff [1971, p. 666] has defined "process" as a "sequence of behavior that constitutes a system and has a goal producing function."

† See, Simon [1960, p. 4].

‡ Important branches of management are: management science, behavioral science, labor relations, personnel management, and general management (i.e., interaction between business and society).

recruiting firms, which cater only to management scientists and operations researchers, have been organized in the United States. Thus, not only does management meet all the tests of being a profession, it is already entering an advanced stage of specialization of its various components. This is all the more remarkable when we realize that the phenomenon of the separation of ownership from management, which marks the beginning of professional management is hardly a century old. Indeed, the field of management science, as we know it today, has its foundations in the developments which took place as late as the 1950's.

As stated earlier, management also refers to an *elite* or *class of people*. In this sense, management is the group of people directing the affairs of a business firm, or for that matter, of any organization. The management is that group in an organization which has the legal authority to direct and control the organization. Typically we refer to the dichotomy of "labor" and "management"; but as most of us know such a dichotomy does not have any general validity—except perhaps when labor unions are engaged in contract negotiations.

A very general definition of management views it as an *art* of getting things done with and through people. It is an art because individual variances in approaching, and successfully solving, the same type of managerial problems can be observed in actual business practice. It is an art because management problems are often amenable to individual styles which are based on creativity, judgment, intuition, and experience rather than on the systematic methods of science. Yet, we are now in the space age. Man has already landed on the moon, and exploration of the heavenly bodies is the national goal of the two most advanced countries on earth (U.S.A. and U.S.S.R.). The National Aeronautics and Space Administration will orbit satellites in order to inventory the globe's resources.* The tremendous scope of these advanced technologically based space projects becomes obvious from the fact that, among other things, the satellites could show when and where to plant crops, when to harvest them, where forest fires threaten, where commercial fish are, where highways and urban renewal projects should be built, where oil and mineral deposits are located, where water exists in seemingly arid regions and where there are hazards to shipping. These advances in science could not possibly be either made or sustained without concurrent advances in the systems of management. Such phenomenal strides have been made possible only because the art of management has increasingly been supplemented by the *science* of management.

However, the importance of the art of management is not to be minimized. Referring to the "art" of management, Feeney writes [1971, p. 2]:

---

* *The Wall Street Journal,* Monday, June 8, 1970, p. 1.

Management, as currently practiced, is the art of forcing simple pegs into complex holes. This is a great art, essential to the survival of all institutions. . . . Thus it would be unsound to belittle the art of managing complex institutions. But we must recognize that this art is the antithesis of science. Its ingredients are intuition rather than logic, guesses rather than measurement, and group discussion rather than experimental verification.

Management as a *science* adopts the view that a substantial portion of management consists of "phenomena that can be measured, relationships that can be represented quantitatively, causal chains whose internal consistency can be logically verified, and conclusions which can be tested experimentally" [Feeney 1971, p. 1]. The objective of this approach is to bring as many management phenomena as is realistically possible into the domain of "programmed" decision-making. In this manner, knowledge and experience can be accumulated systematically, and utilized without the level of risk faced by the original researchers—thereby generating additional time for the manager to engage in creative activities. However, there are some inherent limitations in viewing management as a science because the preconditions of a truly scientific analysis are rather severe. A pragmatic synthesis of art and science appears to be the prescription for modern management.

11.3 "SCHOOLS" OF MANAGEMENT THOUGHT

Management theory* can be classified under at least five major headings: (1) scientific management, (2) administrative management, (3) human relations school, (4) behavioral science, and (5) management science. Since management, by definition, involves the integration of human effort and judicious use of scarce resources, each school of thought must in practice deal with the totality of organizational relationships. Each school of thought, however, has historically focused on different aspects of organizational behavior.

---

* Management theory has been classified by various authors in different ways. See, for example, Koontz [1964]: (1) The management process school, (2) the empirical school, (3) the human behavior school, (4) the social system school, (5) the decision theory school, and (6) the mathematical school.

Filley and House [1969]: (1) Behavioral school, (2) operations research, and (3) classical and neoclassical school and their extensions.

Starr [1971, pp. 100–103]: (1) Case-method school, (2) management science school, (3) organization theory and human behavior school, and (4) operational school.

Newman et al. [1967]: (1) Productivity approach, (2) behavioral approach, (3) rationalistic-model approach, and (4) institutional approach.

March and Simon [1958]: (1) "Classical" organization theory, (2) modern organization theory.

11.3.1 *Scientific Management*

The *scientific management**** school concentrated essentially on the basic physical activities involved in production, and this school of thought is associated with the contributions of Frederick W. Taylor, Frank Gilbreth, and Henry L. Gantt. These pioneers of scientific management built on the progress in management methods that was made during the industrial revolution and the development of the factory system of production. Taylor is known for his time study experiments and for developing the concept of "functional"† organization; Gilbreth for his work on motion study; and Gantt for developing control charts and for introducing the "task and bonus" system of wage payment. The thrust of the scientific management movement was to achieve specialization—in terms of work, the worker, and management. Scientific management neglected, for the most part, the human aspects of organizational tasks and concentrated primarily on the use of men as adjuncts to machines [March and Simon, 1958, p. 13]. The contributions of scientific management are of interest to us for the following reasons. First, they represent the first significant attempt to provide a "scientific" basis for the practice of management. Secondly, they emphasized only the functional specialization of the separate parts rather than the management system as a whole. Thirdly, for the first time, there began to emerge a body of knowledge which started to form the nucleus around which, and from which, various theories of management, including management science, were developed.

11.3.2 *Administrative Management*

The *administrative management* school, represented by the contributions of H. Fayol, R. Haldane, L. Gulick, James Mooney, Alan Reiley and Lyndall Urwick, concentrated on the questions of departmentalization, coordination, and organization. The thrust of the administrative management theory is described by March and Simon [1958, p. 22]:

> Given a general purpose for an organization, we can identify the unit tasks necessary to achieve that purpose. These tasks will normally include basic productive activities, service activities, coordinative activities, supervisory activities, etc. The problem is to group these activities into individual jobs, to group the job into administrative units, to group the units into larger

---

* For a history of the scientific management movement, see George, Jr. [1968].

† Taylor suggested that production activities be organized in terms of specialized functions to be performed and that, in each specialized area, the worker should be under the supervision of, and accountable to, a designated foreman. The present day line-and-staff, and "matrix" organization, are variants of Taylor's functional organization.

units, and finally to establish the top level departments—and to make these groupings in such a way as to minimize the total cost of carrying all the activities. In the organizing process each department is viewed as a definite collection of tasks to be allocated among, and performed by, the employees of the department.

Scientific management and administrative management theory spurred the development of several new and practical methods, tools, and techniques of management. In the functional areas, considerable progress was made in personnel work, inventory control, work sampling, waiting-line problems, forecasting, budgeting, statistical inference and so on. Immediately after World War I, business firms began to use formal personnel selection and training programs. During the 1920's, considerable progress was made in using improved methods of cost accounting, forecasting, budgeting, work simplification, advertising, and a host of other functional areas. Ronald Fisher, H. F. Dodge, and Walter Shewhart provided the industry with statistical tools for controlling quality of production at low costs. Methods of statistical quality control, work sampling, design of experiments, statistical inference, Bayesian statistics, etc. were developed, refined, and successfully applied to industrial problems during the 1930's and 1940's. These developments represented another stage in the steady march towards a scientific basis of management practice. To this day, these tools and techniques are being used—not only in the logistics area, but also in the behavioral side of business management.

11.3.3 Human Relations

The *human relations* school is associated with the names of Mary Parker Follett, and Elton Mayo and his associates. Miss Follett directed her emphasis to the need for recognizing motivating factors that exist in the individual and the group. She propounded the idea that coordination is the core of management and that effective coordination can only be achieved by promoting a cooperative organization based on education and good human relations. She identified the importance of psychology and sociology and advocated the importance of "group" thinking and the "group" process approach to management.

Elton Mayo is well known for his experimental studies in the realm of social factors and their relationships to productivity. Conducted at Western Electric's Hawthorne Works in Chicago (between 1924 and 1932), the purpose of these studies was to investigate the attitudes and reactions of workers to varying physical conditions such as changes in the degree of illumination, changes in daily working hours, shorter work weeks, different rest periods, and so on. An attempt was made to relate the effect of these physical variables to productivity by comparing the output of an experimental group (where these variables were changed) to that of a control group (where these variables were kept at a constant level). The researchers found that interaction of the worker and his participation in informal social groups had a great impact on individual behavior and productivity. Mayo observed that an organization is a social system consisting of cliques, informal groups and status systems; and that this system is a mixture of factors that are logical and economic—as well as nonlogical, emotional and human. This meant that, in addition to meeting the economic goals of the organization, management must satisfy the social and psychological needs of the workers. The importance of Mayo's contributions lies in these elements: (1) It was the first systematic and scientific exploration of group behavior in organizations. As a result, the sociological and psychological aspects of the effects of informal groups was introduced into the theoretical literature of management. (2) It gave further impetus to personnel management and labor relations; and most importantly (3) these experiments set the foundation for the behavioral science "school" of management.

Follett's writing and the results of Mayo's experimental studies produced a wave of human relation writers who began to offer advice on how companies can develop training programs to achieve maximum long-run productivity. Business managers began to introduce human relations programs in their companies based on the assumed, but not tested, premise that a "happy" worker was always a productive worker. The human relations school became popular in the 1940's and 1950's and is the precursor of the behavioral science school [Donnelly, Jr. et al., 1971, p. 116]. The human relations school introduced into the evolving theory of management the importance of human behavior. However, it soon became evident to both practitioners and scholars of management that two particular dimensions of management had thus far not received sufficient attention. The first was concerned with building a scientific basis for analyzing the sociological, psychological, and socio-psychological aspects of management; while the second pointed up the need for a "systems," as opposed to a functional, approach to management.

One dimension concerns the behavior of individuals and groups within organizations, and with the structure and functioning of organizations under various kinds of economic, political, social and technological environments. The other operates with the philosophy that objectives of the separate parts of a management system are often in conflict; that the reconciliation of these conflicting objectives is *the* executive function; and that such executive-type problems must be solved in terms of effectiveness of the *entire system* rather than its separate parts. The interest in the first dimension resulted in a series of empirical studies and theoretical publications which form the central core of what is now known as the behavioral school of management. The research conducted with the philosophy of systems approach laid the foundations of what is now called Operations Research. For our purposes, both lines of inquiry, insofar as they are based on the foundations of science, and they approach management problems in a "scientific" way, are important branches of management science.

11.3.4 Behavioral Science

The *behavioral science* school concentrates on that area of management analysis which deals with the individual behavior, group behavior, and behavior of organizations.* The attempt is to describe, explain, and predict organizational behavior and gain an insight into various patterns of leadership, motivation, morale, organizational performance—and their relationships to factors leading to organizational success. Behavioral sciences draw from such disciplines as psychology, sociology, anthropology, political science, social psychology, and other combinations of social sciences. Briefly, the behavioral science approach to management is based on the premise that actual behavior, at whatever level, must be observed, described, and then explained on a scientific (inductive) basis. Behavioral sciences have made important contributions in developing and testing several aspects of management theory. However, the predictive value of behavioral science research has been of a very small magnitude. To quote Mason Haire, a noted psychologist, [1967, p. 110]:

> . . . when I say the contributions of behavioral sciences to Management has been disappointingly small, I mean this: In the past 15 years there have been 150 books and 1500 articles written on the subject. And yet, the (practice) of management remains the same. To be sure managerial vocabulary has changed. The well-rounded manager now speaks of T groups, cognition dissonance and role conflicts, but he does just about the same things he has always done.

In another survey, conducted by Dunnette and Brown [1968], 200 industrial executives were asked to rate 33 articles and books in the behavioral sciences area in terms of several factors including "did this article or book influence how you carry out your work or how you set up systems or methods for others' work?" Only 15 percent of the responding executives said that one or more of these contributions had significantly influenced conduct of their firms' business. These figures are "surprisingly low" because, according to the surveyors, "these executive respondents were

---

* The economic aspects of organizational problems are usually not considered by behavioral scientists.

initially named because they were perceived to be persons acutely attuned to contributions by behavioral scientists."

11.3.5 Management Science

*Management science** is one of the major branches along which the theory and practice of management have evolved. Management science, as we know it today, made its start in the United Kingdom during World War II when a team of scientists was given the assignment of solving several complex military problems: selecting optimum gun sites, determination of optimum convoy size, optimum depth for detonating anti-submarine charges, optimum civil defense plans, and location of most vulnerable spots in bombers. Management science pioneers used a research methodology combining the inductive approach with the use of "analogy." That is, wherever possible, an "analogy" with previously developed and tested logical structures was utilized in the process of model building. The knowledge gained from wartime experiences was refined to arrive at a number of well-defined models (i.e., their general structure was precisely identified) dealing with problems of resource allocation, inventory control, queuing, routing, replacement, and so on. The attempt was to develop a variety of models with known properties and deductively derived solutions, which could be "matched" and applied on a routine basis to certain types of recurring problems. This was indeed done—with increasing frequency and success in the 1950's and 1960's.†

Management science is both a body of knowledge and an approach for analyzing and solving management problems. As a *body of knowledge,* management science consists of various management theories, methods, models, and specific tools and techniques that can be used to handle a wide range of management problems. Management theories range all the way from individual, group, and organization behavior to theories of planning, control, and theories dealing with inventory, maintenance, and production scheduling. Management science models cover wide areas of strategic, administrative and operational problems. Linear programming, dynamic programming, stochastic programming, Markov chains, simulation models, information models, program evaluation and review technique, critical path method, sensitivity analysis, and cost effectiveness models are only some

---

* The terms management science, operations research, systems sciences, systems analysis are often used interchangeably in the literature. We will use management science to cover the entire field of new quantitative management including behavioral sciences and econometrics.

† Important contributors to promoting the philosophy and application of management science include C. West Churchman, Russell Ackoff, George Dantzig, Richard Bellman, and many others. See Dantzig [1963, Chapter 2].

examples of the kind of topics that constitute the body of knowledge in management science.*

As an *approach,* management science refers to the attitude with which management scientists view, analyze and solve management problems. The approach is that of a man of science; grounded in the discipline of inductive as well as deductive inference, model building and theory construction. To quote Dorfman [1960, p. 577]:

> The essence of this point of view (approach) is that a phenomenon is understood when and only when it has been expressed as a formal, really mechanistic, quantitative model, and that, furthermore, all phenomena within the purview of science (which is probably all the phenomena there are) can be so expressed with sufficient persistence and ingenuity. A second characteristic of men of science, amounting to a corollary of the first, is their preference of symbolic, as opposed to verbal, modes of expression and reasoning. These characteristics I take to be the style of operations research, and I define operations research to be all research in this spirit intended to help solve practical, immediate problems in the fields of business, governmental or military administration or the like.

Management science is characterized by: (1) the systems approach, (2) interdisciplinary teamwork, and (3) the application of scientific method. Ackoff and Sasieni [1968, p. 6].

The concept of the *systems approach* is well covered in Selection 4. The practice of systems approach means that the manager makes a *conscious* attempt to understand the relationships between various parts of the organization and their role in supporting the overall performance of the organization. Before solving a problem in any functional area (production, marketing, finance, etc.), or at any organizational level (strategic, administrative, operational) or in any specific sector of the organization, and even before choosing a method of solution (or employing a specific model), the manager must understand fully how the overall system and its component parts will respond to change. In short, the systems approach is based on the conviction that before implementing any functional solution, one must examine its ultimate effect on the system. Furthermore, the process of problem formulation and definition at lower levels of the organization must, if at all possible, fit into the boundaries defined by higher level objectives. This implies comprehensiveness—both in terms of objectives and problem formulation. However, practical considerations of time, information, cost, and feasibility often force the manager to solve parts of the problem individually and in sequence. This is in contradiction to the idea of overall optimization which is the goal of management science. But, suboptimiza-

---

* In a recent survey conducted by AIDS (American Institute of Decision Science) fully 40 different subject areas were listed as being the domain of management science.

tion* is a fact of life and the thrust of management science lies in understanding when it is necessary and when it can be avoided.

The idea of *interdisciplinary teamwork* is necessary in solving complex management problems because of the state of knowledge specialization. The body of specialized knowledge has grown to a point where it is impossible for one person to be a specialist in more than one branch of a scientific discipline. And the problems of modern-day life are multi-dimensional, not single-dimensional. "There are no such things as physical problems, biological problems, psychological problems, economic problems, and so on. There are only problems; the disciplines of science represent different ways of looking at them" [Ackoff and Sasieni, 1968, p. 7]. Large and complex problems require that they be subjected to analysis by a team of specialists representing a wide range of skills. This multi-disciplinary view produces cross-fertilization of ideas, takes advantage of accumulated knowledge, and makes certain that all ramifications of the problem have been considered. Many organizational problems, for example, have economic, social, political, engineering, physical, biological and psychological aspects. While it is impossible for one person to specialize in such a range of disciplines, it is conceivable that a team can be organized so that each particular aspect of the problem could be analyzed by a specialist in that field. By pooling their specialized talents, the team can develop better and advanced solutions to old problems and new solutions to new and complex problems. The scientific mind from each discipline attempts to abstract the essence of the problem and relate it structurally to other similar problems from his own field. If there is a structural similarity between the new problem and the one familiar to the scientist, there is then the possibility of applying the old and tested solution methods for solving new problems. When the entire team is attempting to develop analogies in this manner, the possibility of finding a solution increases markedly. The use of analogy, it should be noted, is always a theoretical possibility.

> . . . the model of any one system stands in *some* sort of correspondence with the model of any other system: the question is only whether the correspondence is great or small . . . and therefore more useful or less useful. If it is useful to a sufficient extent, and useful in the right way, the scientist will solve the manager's problem. [Beer, 1966, p. 104].

Perhaps the most important feature of the management science approach is the use of *scientific method* and the building of decision models. The scientific method consists of observing, measuring, recording, refining of data; building a model which describes, explains, and predicts the behavior of the system under study; and testing and improving the model. Emshoff [1971, p. 10] describes the scientific method approach in these steps.

---

* Suboptimization occurs because of conflicting objectives or imperfect information.

1. Systematically *observe* the system whose behavior must be explained to solve the problem.
2. Use these specific observations to *construct* a generalized framework (a model) which is consistent with the specific observations and from which consequences of changing the system can be predicted. (The process of model construction is inductive; that is, specific observations are used to infer the generalized structure.)
3. Use the model to *deduce* how the system will behave under conditions which have not been observed but could be observed if the changes were made.
4. Finally, *test* the model by constructing an experiment on the actual system to see if the effects of changes predicted by using the model actually occur when the changes are made.

The three characteristics of management science (systems approach, interdisciplinary teams, and the scientific method) make it possible to define management science in a number of useful ways—operationally as well as philosophically.* Management science is that branch of the field of management which employs a rational, logical, systematic, and scientific approach in analyzing the process of management and management problems. Beer [1966, p. 92] defines O.R. (management science) as follows:

Operations Research (*management science*) is the attack of modern science on complex problems arising in the direction and management of large systems of men, machines, materials and money in industry, business, government and defence. Its distinctive approach is to develop a scientific model of the system, incorporating measurements of factors such as chance and risk, with which to predict and compare the outcomes of alternative decisions, strategies or control. The purpose is to help management determine its policy and actions simultaneously.

Management science has been effective in two ways. First, the scientific approach has yielded dividends in improving the "art" of management. Secondly, several breakthroughs have been made in isolating, and solving complex decision problems at the operational level.† However, the record is not so bright when one considers the arena of administrative and strategic decision classes.‡ It appears that further advances in the applications of management science can only be made by redefining several basic ideological premises; by finding ways to handle policy-type questions; and by accommodating relevant behavioral aspects in the formal models.§

---

* See Miller and Starr [1969, Chapter 6], Loomba [1964, p. 7].
† We refer here to problems such as: scheduling, inventory, facilities location, distribution, queuing, replacement, maintenance, design, information systems, etc. See references at the end of Chapters 12 and 13.
‡ See, for example, Gruber and Niles [1971], Ansoff [1965, Chapter 2].
§ We recommend the reader to two excellent articles on this topic: Wagner [1971], and Argyris [1971].

The various views of—and on—management are neither exhaustive nor mutually exclusive. The history of modern management is a witness to the fact that management is a multi-disciplinary field. Management science* is perhaps the most important part of management because its subject matter and approach are equally applicable to other views of management.

REFERENCES

Ackoff, R. L., "Towards a System of Systems Concepts," *Management Science,*
1971   vol. 17, no. 11, July, pp. 661–671.

Ackoff, R. L., and M. W. Sasieni, *Fundamentals of Operations Research,* New
1968   York: John Wiley & Sons.

Ansoff, H. I., *Corporate Strategy,* New York: McGraw-Hill.
1965

Argyris, C., "Management information system: The Challenge to Rationality
1971   and Emotionality," *TIMS Interfaces,* vol. 17, no. 6, February, pp.
B275–B292.

Beer, S., *Decision and Control,* New York: John Wiley & Sons.
1966

Dantzig, G. B., *Linear Programming and Extensions,* Princeton, New Jersey:
1963   Princeton University Press.

Donnelly, J. H., Jr., J. L. Gibson, and J. M. Ivancevich, *Fundamentals of*
1971   *Management,* Austin, Tex.: Business Publications, Inc.

Dorfman, R., "Operations Research," *American Economic Review,* vol. 50, no.
1960   4, September, pp. 577.

Dunnette, M., and Z. Brown, "Behavioral Science Research and the Conduct
1968   of Business," *Academy of Management Journal,* June, pp. 176–187.

Emshoff, J. R., *Analysis of Behavioral Systems,* New York: Macmillan.
1971

Feeney, G. J., "The Role of the Professional in Operations Research and
1971   Management Science," *TIMS Interfaces,* August, pp. 1–12.

Filley, A. C., and R. J. House, *Managerial Processes and Organizational Be-*
1969   *havior,* Glenview, Ill.: Scott Foresman & Co.

Flagle, C. D., "Operations Research in the Health Services," *Operations Re-*
1962   *search,* September-October, pp. 591–603.

Flagle, C. D., and J. P. Young, "Applications of O.R. and I.E. to Problems
1966   of Health Service Hospitals and Public Health," *Journal of In-*
dustrial Engineering, vol. 17, no. 11, pp. 609–613.

George, C. S., Jr., *The History of Management Thought,* Englewood Cliffs,
1968   N.J.: Prentice-Hall.

Gruber, W. H., and J. S. Niles, "Problems in the Utilization of Management
1971   Science/Operations Research," *TIMS Interfaces,* vol. 2, no. 1,
November, pp. 12–19.

Haire, M., "Coming of Age in the Social Sciences," *Industrial Management*
1967   *Review,* Spring, pp. 109–118.

Horvath, W. J., "British Experience with Operations Research in the Health
1964   Services," *Journal of Chronic Diseases,* vol. 17 pp. 779–788.

---

* For a discussion of the general role of management science (operations research) in the field of health care administration, we refer the reader to Flagle [1962], Horvath [1964], Horvath [1966], Flagle and Young [1964].

Horvath, W. J., "The Systems Approach to the National Health Problem,"
1966 *Management Science,* vol. 12, no. 10, June, pp. B391–B395.

Koontz, H., *Toward a Unified Theory of Management,* New York: McGraw-
1964 Hill.

Loomba, N. P., *Linear Programming,* New York: McGraw-Hill.
1964

March, J. G., and H. A. Simon, *Organizations,* New York: John Wiley & Sons.
1958

Miller, D. W., and M. K. Starr, *Executive Decisions and Operations Research*
1969 Englewood Cliffs, New Jersey: Prentice-Hall.

Newman, W. H., C. E. Summer, and E. Kirby Warren, *The Process of Man-*
1967 *agement,* Englewood Cliffs, N.J.: Prentice-Hall.

Pugh, D. S., "Modern Organization Theory: A Psychological and Sociological
1966 Study," *Psychological Bulletin,* vol. 66, no. 4, Oct., pp. 235–251.

Simon, H. A., *The New Science of Management Decision,* New York: Harper
1960 & Row.

Starr, M. K., *Management: A Modern Approach,* New York: Harcourt
1971 Brace Jovanovich.

Wagner, H. M., "The ABC's of OR," *Operations Research,* vol. 19, no. 6,
1971 October, pp. 1259–1281.

The Wall Street Journal, Monday, June 8, p. 1.
1970

Chapter 12

Analytical Models

12.1 INTRODUCTION

In this chapter we will describe the concept of a model; present two classifications of models; and briefly discuss a selected set of analytical* models. A general linear programming model will be described and then differentiated from integer, quadratic, and dynamic programming. The basic structures of Markovian, inventory, and queuing models will be discussed; network analysis models (PERT and CPM) will be presented; and the application potential of various analytical models to the health field will be cited.

12.2 WHAT IS A MODEL?

Management science analysis and solution of problems is based on the practice of model building and model using. *A model is a particular account of a system which, in turn, represents an object of interest or subject of inquiry in real life.* The system represents only a chosen part of the real world—that part whose behavior and characteristics we must understand. One way to understand reality is to observe it directly, experiment with it, and interact with it in real time. However, this may not be possible because of cost, time, legal and other constraints. Hence, we attempt to abstract the essence of reality by using models to represent reality. The means of representation may be physical, graphic, schematic, analog, symbolic, or a combination of these. Forrester [1961, p. 49] describes models as follows:

> Models have become widely accepted as a means for studying complex phenomena. A model is a substitute for some real equipment or system.

---

* Briefly, analytical models are those which have a specified mathematical structure and which can be "solved" by known mathematical techniques. In contrast, simulation models, although possessing a mathematical structure, cannot be "solved" by known mathematical techniques. The reader will gain additional insight into the nature, properties, and applications of analytical versus simulation models from the material covered in Chapters 12 and 13.

The value of a model arises from its improving our understanding of obscure behavior characteristics more effectively than could be done by observing the real system. A model, compared to the real system it represents, can yield information at lower cost. Knowledge can be obtained more quickly and for conditions not observable in real life.

The purpose of a model is to *describe, explain,* and *predict* the behavior of a system. If a model is a reliable predictor of the system behavior it can be used to *prescribe* preferred courses of action. Depending upon the purpose and stage of development, models can be descriptive (describe what is), explanatory (explain behavior by establishing relationships between model components), predictive (predict behavior under a variety of assumed conditions), prescriptive or normative (provide guidelines for what ought to be) or consist of a combination of characteristics that are drawn from each of these categories.*

To build models that faithfully represent the real world is not an easy task. The reality is so complex that it is often very difficult to visualize and understand it completely. Furthermore, even when we have a sufficient understanding of reality, our attempt at representing it by models may succeed only partially. First of all, the state of the art of model building may not measure up to the task (as is the case when we attempt to build models of human behavior). Second, even when a model does succeed in capturing reality in all of its complex aspects, it is usually mathematically intractable. We are therefore forced in many cases to "simplify" reality in order to build useful models of it. Thus, there are necessarily some inherent weaknesses in the idea of using models to represent reality. But this does not mean that we should reject the approach of model building and model using. On the contrary, the modeling approach is not only sound but the best available approach in analyzing and solving complex decision problems. It is much easier, more feasible, less costly, and less time-consuming to obtain relevant information (regarding the behavior of the system under various conditions) from models than from experimentation with the reality that the model represents. A model is useful when it is simple to understand, has explanatory and predictive power, and permits us to draw valid inferences regarding the behavior of the system.

The general utility of management science models can be seen by differentiating between the *form* and the *content* of models. The form refers to the structure; while the content refers to the situational context. Ackoff and Rivett [1963] have identified 8 different *classes* of problems whose *form* or structure can be mathematically described: (1) inventory, (2) allocation, (3) queuing, (4) sequencing, (5) routing, (6) replacement, (7) competitive problems, and (8) search. While the manager concerns

---

* See, for example, Horowitz [1970, Chapter 1] and Simon [1959].

himself with the *content,* the *form* of the problem is the concern of the scientist who arrives at it by testing the pattern, relevance, and coherence behind the manager's behavior [Beer, 1966, p. 73]. Once the general form (or structure) of an often repeated (and repeatable) process can be expressed in mathematical terms, we have a model. The model structure is developed either through the use of analogy or inductive inference or both. But once the model successfully captures the properties of a specific process, it can then be applied in different situational contexts. The manager's task is to provide the "content" of his strategy in relation to a *chosen* "form." For example, inventory models deal with a process in which "something is stored to meet future demands," and this class of problems is fairly general. The inventory problem exists in homes, hospitals, factories, warehouses, banks—indeed everywhere. A general inventory model, once it is tested and proved, can be used to solve a whole class of similar problems regardless of the situational context. The manager's job is to examine whether the problem at hand meets the requirement of having similar properties and structure as that of one of the tested models. If so, the general model can be used to solve the problem. If not, a specific model to solve the problem at hand must be built from scratch.*

The real issue in building a model is its utility in explaining and predicting the behavior of the system that it represents. The model should be able to explain relationships between various components of the system, between each component and the overall system, and the response of the system to changes in its components (parameters and exogenous variables). After the model has been constructed it should be tested and, if possible, elaborated and enriched. The process of alternate testing and elaboration has been described by Morris [1967].

12.3 CLASSIFICATION OF MODELS

There are various ways of classifying management science models, depending upon the purpose and criterion of classification.† One such classification, based on the degree of abstraction, is shown in Figure 12.1.

FIG. 12.1
CLASSIFICATION OF MODELS ACCORDING TO DEGREE OF ABSTRACTION

Physical Models	Graphic Models	Schematic Models	Analog Models	Mathematical Models
(⟵ Least abstract)			(Most abstract ⟶)	

---

* See Morris [1967] for an excellent discussion on the art of building management science models.

† See, for example, Montgomery and Urban [1969, p. 9], Starr [1971, pp. 37–60], Forrester [1961, p. 49], Dantzig [1963, p. 8], Ackoff and Sasieni [1968, Chapter 3], Wagner [1969], Hillier and Lieberman [1967].

Any three-dimensional model which looks like the real thing but is either reduced in size (e.g., toy airplane) or scaled up (e.g., the plastic model of the human heart) is a *physical* model. Physical models are easy to observe, build, and describe, but they are difficult to manipulate and not very useful for prediction. Three-dimensional models of plant layouts, housing developments, and city planning are often employed for improving the detail and quality of plans.

An organization chart is a graphic* (block-type) model depicting the intended system of organizational authority—responsibility relationships. The flow process chart showing what happens (operation, storage, delay, inspection, etc.) at different stages during the complete processing of a product is a *schematic* model. The main features of a computer program are often represented by a schematic description of steps that connect the start to the end of the computer program. Any PERT/CPM type model (see section 12.7) is a schematic representation of a complete project showing a network of "events" and "activities." Schematic models are extremely useful in giving a visual picture of the system under study. A picture, as they say, is worth a thousand words.

Analog models represent a system (or object of inquiry) by utilizing a set of properties different from that which the original system possesses. For example, an analog computer is the physical (mechanical or electrical) representation of the variables in a problem. Different colors on a map may represent water, desert, continents, etc.; or they may represent military alliances between nations. Graphic, schematic, and analog models are easier to manipulate and more general than physical models.

Mathematical or symbolic models represent systems (or reality) by employing mathematical symbols and relationships. Mathematical models are precise; most abstract; general rather than specific; and can be manipulated easily by utilizing the laws of mathematics. The mathematical model for *any* straight line, for example, is $y = a + bx$ where a and b are, respectively, the *intercept* and *slope* of the line. A specific straight line can be represented by assigning numerical values to the parameters a and b.

A second classification of models, developed by J. W. Forrester [1961, p. 49] is shown in Figure 12.2.

Forrester's classification is useful in understanding the nature and role of models to represent management and economic behavior of organizations.

Another classification of models results in a dichotomy (analytical and simulation models) along which we have organized Part V of this book. This is an important dichotomy because when a decision problem cannot

---

* The graphic, schematic, and analog model are of the same species—the difference is one of degree rather than kind.

FIG. 12.2
FORRESTER'S CLASSIFICATION OF MODELS

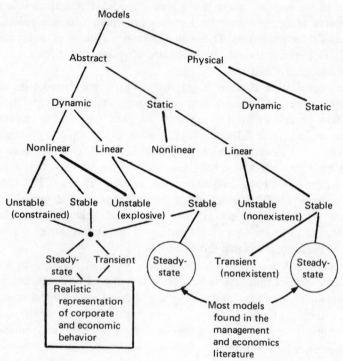

Source: [Forrester, 1961, p. 49].

be structured as, or handled by, analytical models, it is *always* possible (assuming sufficient time and financial resources) to build a simulation model for it. Analytical models are those that are mathematically tractable. This means that these models can be expressed in mathematical terms and solved by applying the laws of mathematics either directly or iteratively. Important categories of well-known analytical models of management science include linear programming,* integer programming, quadratic programming, dynamic programming, inventory models, queuing models, markovian models, and PERT and CPM. We will briefly describe these models and cite their applications to health care administration.

---

* For a classification of mathematical programming problems see Dantzig [1963, p. 8]. Dantzig first divides the set into *deterministic* and *probabilistic* subsets. Then, under the deterministic branch, programming problems are classified as either linear or nonlinear. Linear and integer programming are two important classes of linear problems, while quadratic programming is an important class under the nonlinear branch.

12.4 LINEAR PROGRAMMING

A general linear programming model is a resource allocation model under conditions of certainty. The general model consists of three parts: (1) a linear objective function, (2) a set of linear constraints, and (3) a set of non-negativity constraints. The model assumes additivity, proportionality, fixed technology, continuous variables (divisibility), pure competition, and complete information. The purpose of the model is to design an optimal program so that the objective function is either maximized or minimized without violating the given constraints. Given below is the general linear programming model.

Maximize: $c_1x_1 + c_2x_2 + \cdots + c_nx_n$
subject to

$$a_{11}x_1 + a_{12}x_2 + \cdots + a_{1n}x_n \leqslant b_1$$
$$a_{21}x_1 + a_{22}x_2 + \cdots + a_{2n}x_n \leqslant b_2$$

.

.

.

$$a_{m1}x_1 + a_{m2}x_2 + \cdots + a_{mn}x_n \leqslant b_m$$

and,

$$x_1, x_2, \cdots, x_n \geqslant 0$$

where $c_1, c_2, \cdots c_n$ are price coefficients; $x_1, x_2 \cdots, x_n$ are competing activities; $a_{11}, a_{12} \cdots, a_{mn}$ are input-output coefficients; and $b_1, b_2 \cdots, b_m$ are capacity limits.

The feasible solution space of a linear programming problem is of such a nature* that together with a linear objective function, the optimal solution can always be found at one of the corner points of the solution space. Since the number of such corner points (potential optimal solutions) is extremely large, efficient methods of locating the optimal solution must be found and applied. The regular simplex method, the revised simplex method, and the dual simplex method are examples of such efficient methods of search.† Linear programming has been applied in solving a host of problems: optimum product mix, optimum diet, facility or machine scheduling, transportation problem, assignment problem, allocating advertising dollars, fluid blending, scheduling nurses, distribution of products or services, and so on. Several health applications of linear programming have been cited by Griffith.‡ The administrator need not know the mechanics of

---

* The feasible solution space is a convex set. See Loomba [1964, p. 29].
† For a description of these methods, see Dantzig [1963], Chung [1963], Hadley [1962], and Wagner [1969].
‡ The following references are cited in John R. Griffith, *Quantitative Planning and*

linear programming (or for that matter any other mechanistic model) in order to be able to evaluate its potential. He must, however, understand its structure and properties and be able to identify "matching" situations. Commercially available computer programs can then be utilized in applying the model to solve actual problems.

Linear programming problems assume divisibility—that is, any non-negative continuous value can be assigned to the solution variables. However, in several real life situations—such as assigning nurses to operating stations or scheduling airplane flights—solution variables must be restricted to integer values. Whenever a linear programming problem is subject to the additional constraint that one or more of its solution variables be integers, we employ *integer programming* to solve the problem. Balintfy [1964] has described a special integer programming algorithm which approximates the theoretical solution to minimum cost menu planning. Various integer programming methods have been surveyed by Balinski [1965].* Quadrating programming† (one of the nonlinear programming models) deals with those problems in which a quadratic objective function is optimized subject to linear structural and non-negativity constraints. A listing of several nonlinear programming codes is given in Kuhn [1970, pp. 497–498].

12.5 DYNAMIC PROGRAMMING

Static models of mathematical programming (e.g., linear, integer, and quadratic programming), deal with single period (or stage) decision problems. In these models, the entire problem is solved with a *single* assault. Even if the problem is repetitive, the optimal solution derived by these models will hold—provided the problem parameters do not change over time. The static models do not consider those problems which require not one, but a *sequence* of independent situations, and where the parameters do change from period to period. In such time-dependent, multi-stage problems, the outcome of a decision at one stage affects the subsequent decision for the next stage, and so on. Dynamic programming was developed to determine a combination of sequential decisions for optimizing the overall measure of effectiveness. Examples of multi-stage problems that are solved by dynamic programming include: diagnostic-treatment,

---

Control (Chapter 8). Balintfy and Nebel [1966], Earickson [1968], Freeman [1967], Park and Freeman [1969], Wolfe and Young [1964], Young [1969].

* Several integer programming computer codes are available. See, for example, Balinski and Spielberg in [Aronofsky 1968], Haldi and Isaacson [1965, pp. 946–959], and Trauth and Woolsey [1969, p. 481–493].

† See Boot [1964].

hospital construction, investment decisions, production scheduling, inventory control, replacement, maintenance, and planning.

Dynamic programming is a mathematical technique for optimizing multi-period (or sequential or multi-stage) programming problems.* It produces a policy which identifies for the decision-maker an optimal decision at each stage. Dynamic programming, based on the principle of optimality,† treats problems in the following sequence: (a) starting from the last stage, proceed backward (taking in one additional stage at a time) until the problem reaches the first stage, (b) at each stage, maximize (or minimize) the sum of the *immediate return or reward* (from that stage) and the optimal return arrived at from all the previous stages. Ledley [1967] has described the use of dynamic programming as an approach to the mathematical formulation of the diagnostic-treatment cycle. Other applications of dynamic programming to management problems can be found in Bellman and Dreyfus [1962], Simone [1967], DeVries [1964], Maffei [1960], Beckman [1968], and Rosen and Souder [1965].

A Markov model is a dynamic model and is based on the concepts of Markov processes and Markov chains. A Markov process is a particular kind of stochastic‡ process. In a stochastic process the prediction of the next experiment is not affected by the knowledge of the outcomes of any preceding experiment; while in a Markov process we assume that knowledge of the immediate past will influence these predictions. The system, at any given time, is assumed to be in one of n states. As it moves from one time period to another, the transition (from one state to another) takes place according to a known set of transition probabilities. In a Markov chain, the transitional probabilities p_{ij}, are assumed to be constant§ over time. If for a given system, the probabilities for the various possible starting states and the transitional probability matrix p_{ij} are known, it is possible to determine the complete behavior of the system. It can be shown that in a Markov process with constant p_{ij} the state of a system at any future stage is completely independent of the "history" of the system. The policy

---

* Bellman [1957], Bellman and Dreyfus [1962].

† Bellman's principle of optimality states: "An optimal policy has the property that whatever the initial state and the initial decision are, the remaining decisions must constitute an optimal policy with regard to the state resulting from the first decision."

‡ Any sequence of observation that is subject to probability analysis is called a stochastic process. That is, a stochastic process is essentially a probabilistic experiment with outcomes in different stages (multi-period). For a technical definition of stochastic processes, Markov processes, and Markov chains, see Kemeny and Snell [1960].

§ Markov chains with constant (or time independent) transitional probabilities are also known as *stationary* Markov chains. Nonstationary (or time dependent) Markov chains can also be formulated, but they are difficult to solve mathematically.

implication of this property is that management efforts should be directed to changing p_{ij} for the benefit of the organization. Markov chains have been employed to analyze a number of business,* behavioral, and health related problems. Bithell [1969] has suggested the use of Markov chains for studying hospital in-patient admission. Kolesar [1970] has presented a Markovian decision model to provide optimum control of a hospital admission scheduling system.†

12.6 INVENTORY MODELS

Inventory models deal with that general class of problems in which something is stored to meet future demand. The implications of this definition are very broad and far-reaching. Almost all aspects of organized human effort can in some ways be formulated as problems in inventory management. The inventory problem persists in the setting of a hospital, a household, business firm, government, and other types of organizations. It is as common in institutions engaged in providing health care as in service or manufacturing organizations. The "things" that are stored can be perishable or non-perishable. But, in all circumstances, inventories act as connecting links between successive stages in the process of making or buying a product (or providing a service) and satisfying the demands of the patients or customers. Varying rates of demand for health care, uncertainties of services and their scheduling, rate of innovations, changes in tastes, changes in social and political values, all contribute to generate conditions which disturb the operational stability and dependence of health organizations. Inventories are necessary both as shock absorbers to cope with varying rates of demand and for the efficient operation of an organization.

The importance of inventory control cannot be overemphasized. The published literature on the subject is enormous, and inventory theory is probably the most developed aspect of operations research. An excellent summary of the status of mathematical inventory theory was published by Veinott [1966, pp. 745–777]. The first theoretical models of inventory control can be traced to 1915–22 when several inventory models, including the well known "Wilson" model, were developed. However, it was only after 1950 that an extensive development of all aspects of inventory theory and applications took place [Arrow et al., 1951, pp. 250–272] and [Arrow et al., 1958]. There is literally no end to different types of inventory models that can be built (or have been published) to correspond to myriad varieties of inventory problems. For a discussion of several of these models the reader is referred to Hanssmann [1961, pp. 65–104) and Inglehart

---

* See, for example, Harary and Lipstein [1962], Maffei [1960], Chung [1969], Draper and Nolin [1964].

† Kolesar's paper includes an excellent list of 49 references.

[1967, pp. 48–51]. In addition, many books which discuss inventory control from different points of view are available.*

Inventory models can be classified in a number of ways. In addition to the basic single product, single location models (under conditions of certainty as well as risk), several other inventory models can be identified, (e.g., multi-product, multi-level, multi-location, batch orders, price breaks, known shortage costs. fixed service level and in-process models). Inventory models are used on these building blocks:† (1) general orientation of the problem (e.g., product or service, single or multi-level, single or multi-location), (2) the nature of inventory demand and supply, (3) categories of inventory costs and their behavior, and (4) methods of information feedback. They can be solved analytically or through the use of simulation. Inventory models have also been formulated as, and solved by, such special technique models as queuing models, linear programming models and dynamic programming models [Buchan and Keonigsberg, 1965]

The inventory problem in the health field is complicated by the consideration that "stockout" costs can be prohibitive. The focus of health institutions is service—not profit. However, health institutions as their counterpart in business, must operate within the constraints of limited resources. A rational policy of inventory control must therefore be formulated in order to effectively manage health institutions. Numerous examples of successful models of inventory control in hospitals can be found in the health literature.‡ Rooke-Mathews [1966] has described the introduction of inventory control in a hospital where operations research was used to determine E.O.Q. (economic order quantity) to serve as guidelines for control. Johnson and Moore [1966] applied a computer model to maintain perpetual inventory information, write purchase orders, and to provide daily, semi-monthly, monthly, and quarterly reports for analysis of purchases and issues. Reed and Stanley [1965] have designed a model for controlling general hospital inventories. Smalley et al. [1964] have explored the inventory problem in hospitals and investigated two methods (exponential smoothing, regression analysis) for predicting usage rates of certain hospital items.§ Inventory models are usually, but not always, implemented by the use of computers.‖

---

* See, for example, Arrow et al. [1958], Buchan and Keonigsberg [1965], Brown [1967], Fetter and Dalleck [1961], Hanssmann [1962], and Magee [1962].
† For a discussion of these building blocks and some analytical models of inventory control, see Loomba [1971].
‡ See references cited at the end of Chapter 12. In 1969, Fearon [1969] conducted a survey of inventory policies of 120 hospitals located throughout the United States.
§ The total number of different items that constitute hospital inventories ranges from 1000 to 3000 units and covers a variety of departments (dietary, dispensary, x-ray, etc.) and maintenance supplies and medical equipment.
‖ See Bugby and Schwitter [1965] for an account of the conversion of a manual inventory system into a computer system.

Queuing* (or waiting-line) models deal with a class of problems in which a stream of *customers* is serviced by a set of *service facilities*, but the arrival and service times of the customers cannot be predicted with certainty. Queuing models can be considered a special category of the inventory problem because in a queuing problem also something is stored (i.e., service facilities) to meet a future demand (i.e., incoming customers). The differentiating characteristic of the queuing problem is that, because of imperfect matching between the customers and service facilities, waiting lines or queues are formed. Either the customers (or patients) wait for service or the service facilities (or doctors) remain idle; and there is a cost attached to each. The decision problem is to determine the number of service facilities and to control the arrival rate of the customers in order to minimize the sum of these two sets of costs. Management science models (analytical as well as simulation) have been utilized to solve different types of queuing problems. Young [1965] has applied a queuing model to analyze the inpatient bed occupancy problem. Thompson et al. [1960] have investigated the application of queuing theory to the delivery suite of a hospital. Queuing theory has also been considered as an aid in administrative control in hospitals.† The use of several queuing models for hospital admission scheduling has been reviewed by Kolesar [1970].

12.7 PERT AND CPM

PERT (program evaluation and review technique) and CPM (critical path method) are planning and control techniques based on network theory.‡ Both techniques, developed during the 1950's, are used for scheduling and controlling large and complex projects. In both PERT and CPM, the main objective is to identify the *critical path* through the network. The critical path is the longest path through the network and hence it equals the *minimum* time required to complete the project.§ If, for any reason, the project must be completed in less time than the critical path time, additional resources must be devoted (or overtime work authorized) to expedite the activities comprising the critical path. Paths other than the critical path offer flexibility in scheduling and transferring resources—because they take less time to complete than the critical path.

---

* For an excellent non-mathematical explanation of queuing problems, we recommend Bhatia and Garg [1963]. See, also, Miller and Starr [1969, pp. 193–197]. Morse in Ackoff [1961, pp. 273–292].

† See, for example, Balintfy [1960], Young [1962], Young [1966].

‡ See, Lockyer [1967], Moder and Phillips [1964], Levin and Kirkpatrick [1966], and Miller [1963].

§ The project can be anything: building a plant, preparing a budget, research and development, and so on.

In both PERT and CPM, the working procedure involves these steps:
1) *Analyze and breakdown the project in terms of specific activities and events.*

An activity is a well-defined amount of work that can be completed only by expending time, money or other resources. An event is a specific accomplishment occurring at a given point in time but requiring no resources or time itself. An activity is defined by its beginning and ending events.

2) *Determine the sequence of activities and produce a network.*

Sequential order of all the activities is established based on technological, administrative, and service requirements. The result is a network of activities and events which indicates the *order* of activities—that is, which activities must be completed before others can be started.

3) *Assign estimates of time, cost, or both to all the activities of the network.*

The estimates can be probabilistic (as in PERT) or deterministic (as in CPM). The estimates are obtained by pooling the judgment and experiences of all those persons who are in any way involved in the project.

4) *Identify the critical path through the network.*

In this step a complete analysis of the network is conducted. Each event is assigned two numbers—one representing the "earliest possible time" and the other "latest allowable time" for that event. These numbers are calculated by considering the "expected duration times" for the activities, and the relationship of the various paths as compared to the longest (critical) path through the network. The analysis also yields information on the *slack* available for different activities. The amount of slack in an activity is the time by which the start of that activity can be delayed without affecting the total completion time for the project.

In general two distinctions are made between PERT and CPM. The first relates to the way in which activity times are estimated and the second concerns the costs required to complete activities. The PERT activity times are probabilistic while in CPM the assumption is made that activity times are deterministic. In PERT, there are three* time estimates for each activity:

$$a = \text{optimistic estimate}$$
$$m = \text{most likely estimate}$$
$$b = \text{pessimistic estimate}$$

---

* The three different time estimates for completing the activity are based on the assumption that the Beta distribution is the probability distribution representing the various possible completion times for the activity. Thus, "a" represents the optimistic time estimate (with a probability of 1 in 100) and "b" represents the pessimistic time estimate (with a probability of 1 in 100), and "m" is the mode of the distribution as estimated by the project analyst.

The "expected duration time" of an activity t_e is then calculated as

$$t_e = \frac{a + 4m + b}{6}$$

and it is this number that is placed along the branches (i.e., activities) of the network. The branches of the CPM network also show time estimates —but these are the *single* (deterministic rather than expected values) deterministic time values.

The second usual distinction is that while in PERT the activity costs are assumed to be proportional to activity times, the CPM data gives explicit estimates of activity costs. Furthermore, in CPM, two sets of cost estimates are provided—based on "normal" as well as "crash" times. The intent of this dual estimate is to enable the management to obtain a clear picture of the costs associated with deliberate acceleration of the project completion.

PERT and CPM are valuable tools which have been employed in planning, scheduling, and controlling complex projects involving interdependent activities. The application of PERT is a basic requirement which the military imposes on all major contractors. Wahl [1964] describes how PERT has been utilized as a guide in preparing budget documents. The use of network analysis in hospital planning has been documented.* Noroian [1966] describes how CPM, when applied to a $7.5 million hospital construction project, resulted in reducing construction time by two and one-half months, provided better funding because of a more accurate schedule of cash flow, and made possible full occupancy in the existing facility based on orderly flow of building activity. Catliff [1965] has described the advantages of network analysis in hospital planning, and listed the requirements for conducting the analysis on a computer. O'Brien [1965] has explained the mechanics, potential, and limitations of CPM for hospital construction projects.

As in the case of other management science models, the computer is a necessary adjunct if the applications to real problems are to be made in any meaningful sense. Several PERT/CPM computer programs are available, and they produce three basic outputs: (1) expected time for the completion of each event and the activities that lead to it; the earliest expected time and the latest allowable time for each event; and the slack time associated with each event; (2) the identification of slack and critical areas in the programs; (3) the probability of meeting the current schedule; and (4) control information by department.

---

* See the summary of a symposium in "Network Analysis and Hospital Planning," *British Hospital Journal and Social Service Review,* June 9, 1967, pp. 1076–1077.

12.8 CONCLUDING REMARKS

We have attempted to give a brief survey of the nature, form, characteristics, properties, and application potentials of some of the major analytical models of management science. To supplement our discussion of analytical models we have selected two articles related to health care administration.

Merten's article (Selection 23) is an illustration of how PERT could be applied for planning, and controlling, health programs. The author reviews the sequential steps involved in planning; lists the main characteristics of PERT; and applies PERT in planning a multiple screening program. The reader is referred to section 12.7 for a definition of some of the PERT-related terms not defined explicitly in Merten's article.

Young's article (Selection 24) applies queuing theory in order to understand the influence of specific factors (e.g., admission rate, length of stay) on bed occupancy. It is recognized that the demand for the hospital's resources is essentially stochastic; that admissions to the hospital, lengths of stay, and discharges are to a large extent dominated by chance factors. Young describes an "adaptive control model" to investigate the effects of various bed occupancy levels (decision variable B) on the average occupancy, the expected overflow, and the size of call list required to maintain a specific B level 95 percent of the time. The investigation was conducted both analytically and via computer simulations. The objective of the model is to choose an *optimum* decision level (i.e., B level) under a given set of conditions. Young indicates how the optimum B level can be determined. The study was conducted for a specific hospital unit and we are cautioned that the application of the model to a large hospital system must consider several additional factors emanating from the practical problems of admitting and discharging, surgery scheduling, and other related activities. Young's article illustrates how some problems can be solved both by analytical and simulation models.

REFERENCES

Ackoff, R. L., and E. P. Rivett, *A Manager's Guide to Operations Research,* 1963 New York: John Wiley & Sons.

Ackoff, R. L., and M. W. Sasieni, *Fundamentals of Operations Research,* 1968 New York: John Wiley & Sons.

Aronofsky, J. S. (ed.), *Progress in Operations Research—The Relationship* 1968 *Between Operations Research and the Computer,* New York: John Wiley & Sons.

Arrow, K., T. Harris, and J. Marschak, "Optimal Inventory Policy," *Econ-* 1951 *ometrica,* vol. 19, pp. 250–272.

Arrow, K., S. Karlin, and H. Scarf, *Studies in the Mathematical Theory of*

1958 *Inventory and Production,* Stanford, California: Stanford University Press.

Balinski, M. L., "Integer Programming: Methods, Uses, Computation," *Man-*
1965 *agement Science,* vol. 12, no. 3, November, pp. 253–313.

Balinsky, M. L., and P. Spielberg, in J. D. Aronoskfy (ed.), *Progress in*
1968 *Operations Research—The Relationship Between Operations Re-search and the Computer,* John Wiley & Sons.

Balintfy, J. L., "Menu Planning by Computer," *Communications of the ACM,*
1964 vol. 7, no. 4, April, pp. 255–259.

Balintfy, J. C., and E. C. Nebel, "Experiment with Computer Assisted Menu
1966 Planning," *Hospitals,* vol. 40, no. 12, June 16.

Beckmann, M. J., *Dynamic Programming of Economic Decisions,* Berlin:
1968 Springer-Verlag.

Beer, S., *Decision and Control,* New York: John Wiley & Sons.
1966

Bellman, R., *Dynamic Programming,* Princeton, New Jersey: Princeton Uni-
1957 versity Press.

Bellman, R., and S. E. Dreyfus, *Applied Dynamic Programming,* Princeton,
1962 N.J.: Princeton University Press.

Bhatia, A., and A. Garg, "Basic Structure of Queuing Problems," *The Journal*
1963 *of Industrial Engineering,* January-February pp. 13–17.

Bithell, J. F., "A Class of Discrete-Time Models for the Study of Hospital
1969 Admission Systems," *Operations Research,* vol. 17, no. 1, January-February, pp. 48–69.

Boot, J. C. G., *Quadratic Programming,* Chicago: Rand McNally & Co.
1964

Brown, R. G., *Decision Rules for Inventory Management,* New York: Holt,
1967 Rinehart & Winston.

Buchan, J., and E. Keonigsberg, *Scientific Inventory Management,* Englewood
1965 Cliffs, N.J.: Prentice-Hall.

Bugby, D. S., and J. P. Schwitter, "Conversion to Computerized Inventory
1965 Control," *The Journal of Industrial Engineering,* September-October, pp. 328–333.

Catliff, G. C., "Use of Computers in Hospital Planning," *British Hospital*
1965 *Journal and Social Service Review,* March 19, pp. 504–505.

Chung, A., *Linear Programming,* Columbus, Ohio: Charles E. Merrill.
1963

Chung, K. H., "A Markov Chain Model of Human Needs, an Extension of
1969 Maslow's Need Theory," *Academy of Management Journal,* vol. 12, no. 2, June, pp. 223–234.

Dantzig, G. B., *Linear Programming and Extensions,* Princeton, New Jersey:
1963 Princeton University Press.

De Vries, M. G., "The Dynamic Effects of Planning Horizons on the Selection
1964 of Optimal Product Strategies," *Management Science,* vol. 10, no. 3, pp. 523–544.

Draper, J. E., and L. H. Nolin, "A Markov Chain Analysis of Brand Prefer-
1964 ences," *Advertising Research,* September, pp. 33–38.

Earickson, R., "The Case for Decentralizing Cook County Hospitals: Some
1968 Applications of Linear Optimization in Hospital Planning," available from University Microfilms, Inc., Ann Arbor, as Hospital Manage-ment Document AR 2102.

Fearon, H., "Inventory Management: Survey and Analysis of Current Practice
1969   in 55 Hospitals," *Hospital Progress,* August, pp. 84–88.

Fetter, R. B., and W. C. Dalleck, *Decision Models for Inventory Management,*
1961   Homewood, Ill.: Richard D. Irwin.

Forrester, J. W., *Industrial Dynamics,* Cambridge, Mass.: M.I.T. Press and
1961   New York: John Wiley & Sons.

Freeman, J. R., "Quantitative Criteria for Hospital Inpatient Nursing Unit
1967   Design," unpublished doctoral dissertation, Georgia Institute of
Technology.

Griffith, J. R., *Planning and Control Systems in Hospital Management* (to be
1972   published).

Hadley, G., *Linear Programming,* Reading, Mass.: Addison-Wesley.
1962

Haldi, J., and L. M. Isaacson, "A Computer Code for Integer Solutions to
1965   Linear Problems," *Operations Research,* November–December, pp.
946–959.

Hanssmann, F., "A Survey of Inventory Theory from the Operations Research
1961   Viewpoint," in *Progress in Operations,* R. Ackoff (ed.), vol. 1,
New York: John Wiley & Sons, pp. 65–104.

Hanssmann, F., *Operations Research in Production and Inventory Control,*
1962   New York: John Wiley & Sons.

Harary, F., and B. Lipstein, "The Dynamics of Brand Loyalty: A Markov
1962   Approach," *Operations Research,* vol. 10, January–February, pp.
19–40.

Hillier, F. S., and G. L. Leiberman, *Introduction to Operations Research,* San
1967   Francisco, Cal.: Holden-Day.

Horowitz, I., *Decision Making: The Theory of the Firm,* New York: Holt,
1970   Rinehart & Winston.

Inglehart, D. L., "Recent Results in Inventory Theory," *The Journal of*
1967   *Industrial Engineering,* vol. 18, no. 1, January, pp. 48–51.

Johnson, R. A., and A. N. Moore, "Inventory and Cost Control by Computer,"
1966   *Journal of the American Dietetic Association,* vol. 49, no. 11, November, pp. 413–417.

Kemeny, J. G., and J. L. Snell, *Finite Markov Chains,* Princeton, N.J.: D. Van
1959   Nostrand.

Kolesar, P., "A Markovian Model for Hospital Admission Scheduling," *Man-*
1970   *agement Science,* vol. 16, no. 6, February, pp. B384–B396.

Kuhn, H. W., *Proceedings of the Princeton Symposium on Mathematical*
1970   *Programming,* Princeton, New Jersey: Princeton University Press.

Ledley, R. S., "Computer Aids to Clinical Evaluation," *Operations Research,*
1967   vol. 15, no. 4, July–August, pp. 694–705.

Levin, R., and C. Kirkpatrick, *Planning and Control with PERT/CPM,* New
1966   York: McGraw-Hill.

Lockyer, K. G., *An Introduction to Critical Path Analysis,* 2nd Edition, New
1967   York: Pitman Publishing Corp.

Loomba, N. P., *Linear Programming,* New York: McGraw-Hill.
1964

Loomba, N. P., "Inventory Control: Basic Blocks and a Taxonomy of Selected
1971   Models," *Proceedings of the 14th Annual International Conference of
The American Production and Inventory Control Society,* November,
pp. 26–43.

Maffei, R. B., "Brand Preferences and Simple Markov Processes," *Operations*
1960 *Research,* vol. 8, no. 2, March-April.

Magee, J. F., *Production Planning and Inventory Control,* New York: Mc-
1962 Graw-Hill.

Miller, R. W., *Schedule, Cost, and Profit Control with PERT,* New York:
1963 McGraw-Hill.

Miller, D. W., and M. K. Starr, *Executive Decisions and Operations Research,*
1969 Englewood Cliffs, N.J.: Prentice-Hall.

Moder, J. J., and C. R. Phillips, *Project Management with CPM and PERT,*
1964 New York: Reinhold Publishing Corp.

Montgomery, D. B., and G. L. Urban, *Management Science in Marketing,*
1969 Englewood Cliffs, N.J.: Prentice-Hall.

Morris, W. T., "On the Art of Modeling," *Management Science,* vol. 13
1967 August, pp. 707–717.

Morse, P. M., "Dynamics of Operational Systems: Markov and Queuing
1961 Processes," in R. L. Ackoff (ed.), *Progress in Operations Research,*
New York: John Wiley & Sons.

Noroian, E. H., "Critical Path Method Saves Building Time and Dollars,"
1966 *The Modern Hospital,* vol. 106, no. 6, June, pp. 103–107.

O'Brien, J. J., "How CPM Can Expedite Your Construction Program," *Hos-*
1965 *pital Topics,* vol. 43, no. 5, May, pp. 48–53.

Park, K. S., and J. R. Freeman, "Community Health Resource Allocation with
1969 Linear Programming Methods," University of Florida Health Systems
Research Division, available from University Microfilms, Inc., Ann
Arbor, as Hospital Management Document MN 2040.

Reed, R., Jr., and W. E. Stanley, "Optimizing Control of Hospital Inventories,"
1965 *The Journal of Industrial Engineering,* January-February, pp. 48–51.

Rooke-Matthews, E. J., "Stock Control: Three Case Studies," *The Hospital,*
1966 vol. 56, no. 6, June, pp. 191–195.

Rosen, E. M., and W. E. Souder, "A Method for Allocating R. and D. Ex-
1965 penditures," *IEEE Transaction on Engineering Management,* EM-12,
no. 3, September, pp. 87–93.

Simon, H. A., "Theories of Decision-Making in Economics and Behavioral
1959 Science," *American Economic Review* June, pp. 253–281.

Simone, A. J., "A Dynamic Programming Approach to the Allocation of Pro-
1967 duction Processes of Varying Efficiencies," *Academy of Management
Journal,* vol. 10, no. 2, June, pp. 129–143.

Smalley, H. E., et al., "Hospital Supply Decisions: Inventory Policies," *Hospital*
1964 *Management,* March, pp. 92, 93, 97.

Starr, M. K., *Management: A Modern Approach,* New York: Harcourt Brace
1971 Jovanovich.

Thompson, J. B., et al., "How Queuing Theory Works for the Hospital," *The*
1960 *Modern Hospital,* vol. 94, no. 3, pp. 75–78.

Trauth, C. A., Jr., and R. E. Woolsey, "Integer Linear Programming: A Study
1969 in Computational Efficiency," *Management Science,* vol. 15, no.
9, May, pp. 481–493.

Veinott, A. F., Jr., "The Status of Mathematical Inventory Theory," *Manage-*
1966 *ment Science,* vol. 12, no. 11, July, pp. 745–777.

Wagner, H. M., *Principles of Operations Research,* Englewood Cliffs, N.J.:
1969 Prentice-Hall.

Wahl, R. P., Jr., "PERT Controls Budget Preparation," *Public Management*
1964 February, pp. 29–33.
Young, J. P., "A Queuing Theory Approach to the Control of Hospital In-
1962 patient Census," Doctoral Dissertation, Johns Hopkins University,
I.E. Dept.
Young, J. P., "Stabilization of Inpatient Bed Occupancy Through Control of
1965 Admission," *Hospitals,* vol. 39, October 1, pp. 41–48.
Young, J. P., "Administering Control of Multiple Channel Queuing Systems
1966 with Parallel Input Streams," *Operations Research,* vol. 14, no. 1, pp.
145–156.

SELECTION 23

PERT and Planning for Health Programs*

Walter Merten

As the number of community health service programs increases and their interrelationships become more complex, the public health administrator is becoming more aware of the urgency for effective health planning. PERT, an acronym for Program Evaluation and Review Technique, is suggested as a tool for mapping out interdependent program steps so that planning can follow a more rational and effective course. Prior to a discussion of PERT, a review of the planning process may be valuable.

A major assumption of all planning, including health planning, is that it is a process requiring both conscious effort and periodic surveillance (1, 2). Planning involves these sequential steps.

1. Development of goals.
2. Assessment of resources: time, money, personnel, opinion, institutionalization of individuals and groups, and other social forces.
3. Consideration of alternative ways of using resources to achieve goals.
4. Selection of an alternative.
5. Development of specific objectives to implement the plan.
6. Implementation of objectives.
7. Evaluation, not only in terms of success in meeting goals, but evaluation of the total planning sequence.

Relationships among the steps in the process are dynamic. It is imperative that the health administrator recognize this characteristic and adjust goals, resource allocations, alternatives, and specific strategies to reflect the relationships appropriate at the time between health and other community programs and interests.

What Is PERT?

PERT is an adaptation of a method long used for work flow management (3). It was developed cooperatively by government agencies and private industry to meet production difficulties arising from national defense contracts in which numerous and complex programs had to be coordinated

* *Public Health Reports,* vol 81, May, 1966.

to achieve the final objective (4). In some applications, PERT has acquired a high degree of sophistication (5–8).

Except for a few isolated instances, PERT has not been utilized by the practicing public health administrator (9, 10). Because of its ability to provide the user with a graphic representation of the components of a program, PERT has the potential to become a valuable health planning mechanism (11). In addition to serving as the basis for planning objective-oriented work, it can provide information for scheduling, costing, redirecting, and evaluating health programs. Characteristics of the technique are:

1. A work breakdown structure, beginning with a final objective subdivided into a series of smaller subobjectives. (See Figure 1.)

2. A network including all activities and events necessary to reach an objective. Activity is an effort required to move from one event to another. An activity may also indicate simply a connection or interrelationship between two events which does not require any effort. In the latter instance, estimated time for the activity would be zero. Specific and definable program accomplishments that do not require time or resources are events.

3. Identification of time estimates for various activities as well as the total process, including a critical path. The longest path, in terms of time, through the network from the beginning to the ending event is the critical path.

4. A method of network analysis that provides continuous evaluation of program status and identification of problem areas so that preventive action can be taken. The network is a diagram of activities and events necessary to reach a program objective. It shows sequences of accomplishment, interrelationships, and dependencies. Analysis of the network by the administrator at any stage of the program permits him to determine if anticipated progress is being made, and if not, specifically where the bottleneck is occurring.

Limitations

PERT is a way to plan only objective-oriented programs. Objective-oriented programs are considered here as those efforts which are designed to meet organizational goals and have specific, measurable end results. Because of this restriction, PERT cannot assist with the total health planning process. Rather, its most effective use occurs after the selection of specific objectives and during the implementation and evaluation steps (5, 6, and 7 of the planning process outlined previously).

As with any management tool, PERT has little significance by itself. In order to be effective, PERT must be thoroughly understood and used by persons with authority over broad program activities (12). Obviously, one of these persons must be the chief administrator when a program of general interest is involved. Lower level supervisors must in turn understand and use the technique as it relates to their particular areas of responsibility (13). PERT is a tool; it cannot make decisions. It will, however, assist with arriving at rational decisions on allocation of resources, by determining which program aspects will require more effort to meet the program's planned completion date and, conversely, which aspects can receive less effort without jeopardizing the timing of the entire program effort.

Illustration of Application

PERT is most advantageous when applied to a program that requires simultaneous activities and has a time limitation. We have used a multiple screening program as an illustration of the application of PERT to a typical public health program. The final objective is to have the screening program ready for the segment of the public selected as a target group.

The major steps in the construction of a PERT system after agreement on the program objective are: (*a*) compiling a work breakdown structure, (*b*) developing a network, (*c*) estimating time for each activity, (*d*) determining a critical path and slack times, and (*e*) scheduling work processes.

Work breakdown structure. The work breakdown structure is a step-by-step detail of each major component of the program. The detailed program should include program aspects, such as decisions, equipment, groups, and facilities. The extent of detail is determined by the complexity of the components and the preference of the administrator. A work breakdown structure which might be used for the hypothetical multiple screening program is given in Figure 1.

Network diagram. The work breakdown structure is the basis for the network diagram. A network for the multiple screening illustration is given in figure 2. Each event is represented by a rectangle. Activities are represented by the arrows joining events. The direction of the arrow indicates the sequence which must occur among events. The symbol t_e indicates the estimated time for an activity in weeks or fractions. Time estimates are obtained from persons most familiar with the activity. If desired, estimates can be made for the most likely, optimistic, and pessimistic times and then weighted to arrive at a single and, hopefully, more precise time estimate for the activity (14, 15).

Critical path and slack. After time estimates have been allotted to each activity, it is possible to determine the critical path and slack. The critical path is the series of activities and events that require the most time (Fig. 2). By periodically comparing actual progress of events on the critical path

Figure 1. Work breakdown structure

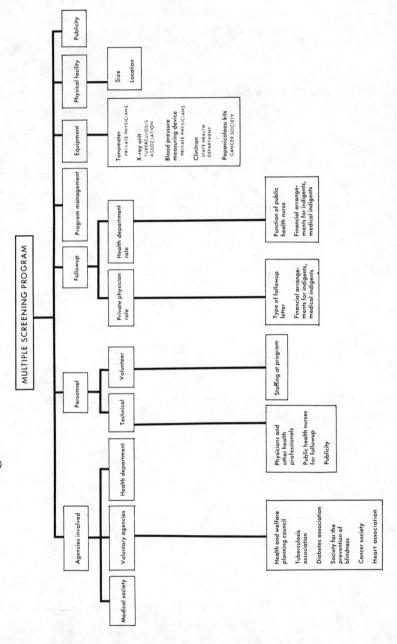

FIG. 12.2
NETWORK DIAGRAM

Figure 2. Network diagram

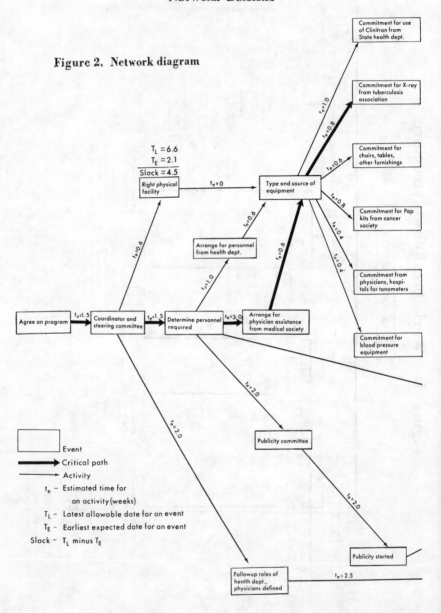

528

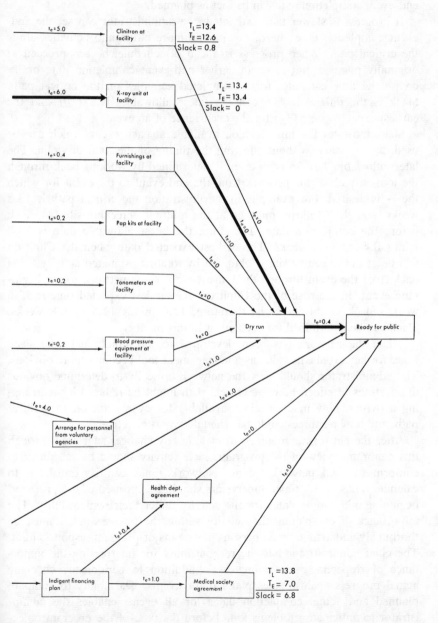

529

with their estimated completion dates, it is possible to determine if the end-event completion date can be met as planned.

If progress is slower than estimated, the administrator can set the end-event completion date ahead, or channel more effort into activities along the critical path. When progress is ahead of schedule, he can proceed as originally planned and meet an earlier end-event completion date or increase the time estimates for uncompleted activities on the critical path. Slack is the difference between the latest allowable date (T_L) and the earliest expected date (T_E) for the occurrence of an event.

Slack indicates the time cushion available at each event, which can be used, as necessary, without affecting the timing of the total program. The latest allowable date for each event is determined by working back through the longest path of the network from the end event to the event for which the T_L is desired. For example, in the illustration the critical path is 13.8 weeks, and the Clinitron must be at the multiple screening site 0.4 week before the completion date. Therefore, the latest allowable date is 13.8 minus 0.4, or 13.4 weeks. The earliest expected date when the Clinitron will be at the screening site is obtained by totaling estimated activity times back from the event through the longest path of the network to the beginning event. In the case of the Clinitron, the earliest expected time is 12.6 weeks. Slack at this event is, therefore, 13.4 minus 12.6 or 0.8 weeks. Slack can be determined for each event in this manner.

When the network has been developed to this point, including slack times for key events, its value as a management tool becomes more obvious. The administrator should view the network critically to determine obvious duplications of effort, how the critical path might be reduced by rearranging activities, how much slack is available for events not on the critical path, and how resources could be scheduled most effectively.

After the network is modified to include any changes suggested through this panoramic view of the program, each activity should be scheduled to conform to total network timing. Network times can be translated to calendar dates at this time. Supervisors should be apprised of the projected beginning and ending dates for the activity under their responsibility. The importance of completing the activity within the time estimates must be thoroughly understood by all persons having major program responsibilities. The chief administrator has the responsibility for interpreting the importance of respecting time estimates, in addition to periodically checking actual progress against times planned for events. The ability to compare planned and actual completion dates for all events enables the administrator to anticipate problems long before the time of the program objective is near. Consequently, preventive action can be taken in the appropriate place at the proper time before a major and unreconcilable problem exists.

SUMMARY

PERT can assist the public health administrator in precisely estimating program progress, coordination, rational phasing of activities, delineation of responsibility for various program components, and preliminary and final evaluation. In addition to multiple screening, PERT could be applied to other public health programs as well as budget and personnel utilization processes. Various types of large meetings, immunization programs, processing and obtaining data for vital records, and the promotion of legislation are program areas to which the technique might be profitably applied. Further experimentation could lead to an almost limitless number of complementary PERT-public health relationships.

REFERENCES

1. Webber, M. M.: Comprehensive planning and social responsibility. Amer Inst Plan J 29:232–241, November 1963.
2. Perloff, H. S., editor: Planning and the urban community. Carnegie Institute of Technology, 1961.
3. Management Research and Procedures Branch, Aeronautical Systems Division, Wright-Patterson AFB: PERT. Ohio, January 1964.
4. Malcolm, D. G., Rosebloom, J. H., and Clark, C. E.: Application of a technique for research and development program evaluation. J Oper Res Soc Amer 7:646–669, September–October 1959.
5. Fulkerson, D. R.: Expected critical path lengths in PERT networks. J Oper Res Soc Amer 10: 808–817, November–December 1962.
6. Healy, T. L.: Activity subdivisions and PERT probability statements. J Oper Soc Amer 9:341–348, May–June 1961.
7. PERT Orientation and Training Center: PERT and other management systems and techniques (bibliography). Washington, D.C., June 1963.
8. Interpretations of PERT. Harvard Business Rev 42:160–172. March–April 1964.
9. Shortcut for project planning. Business Week No. 1714, July 7, 1962, pp. 104–106.
10. Bowling, J. P.: Some aspects of mental health program planning utilizing management systems concepts. Technical Paper 26. Operations Research Inc., Silver Spring, Md., August 1963.
11. Fletcher, T. W.: A new look at budgeting. Public management. J Int City Managers Assoc 46:26–28, February 1964.
12. Pocock, J. W.: PERT as an analytical aid for program planning—its payoff and problems. J Oper Res Soc Amer 10: 893–903. November–December 1962.
13. Roman, D. D.: The PERT system: An appraisal of program evaluation review technique. J Acad Management 5: 57–65, April 1962.
14. Grubbs, F. E.: Attempts to validate certain PERT statistics or "Picking on PERT." J Oper Res Soc Amer 10:912–915, November–December 1962.
15. UNIVAC Division, Sperry Rand Corporation: PERT and CPM techniques in project management. New York, 1964.

SELECTED BASIC PERT REFERENCES

Stilian, Gabriel, et al.: PERT: A new management planning and control technique. American Management Association, New York, 1962.

Federal Electric Corporation: A programmed introduction to PERT. John Wiley & Sons, Inc., New York, 1963.

Hansen, B. J.: Practical PERT, including critical path method. America House, Washington, D.C., 1964.

SELECTION 24

Stabilization of Inpatient Bed Occupancy Through Control of Admissions*

John P. Young

To a large extent, illness and accident are events that strike the individual as a chance phenomenon. From the hospital's point of view, it can be shown, theoretically and statistically[1,2] that patients arrive at a hospital needing service according to the laws of probability. Although the hospital schedules many patients for care and can control admissions to a considerable extent, there are sufficient emergency or unscheduled arrivals each day so that the admission process may be shown to be governed by underlying natural forces similar to those in operation when rolling a pair of dice.

Because hospitalization has deep personal meaning to the individual experiencing it, this may seem to be a rather insensitive viewpoint, especially to those in the medical and nursing professions whose work brings them in constant contact with human beings in need of physiological and psychological care and comfort. But statistics do not recognize emotions, and improvements in operational effectiveness must often be based on the objective analysis of unemotional statistical data.[3]

The underlying chance phenomena in admissions introduce large amounts of variability into a hospital system. For example, one of the most frequently used administrative measures of hospital utilization is the census —a daily physical count of the number of patients occupying beds in the inpatient areas. Records are maintained of the average monthly census, and these are usually combined in an annual treasurer's report to provide an overall average daily census figure for each fiscal year. Census figures, when available, are said to give a general indication of the extent of service provided and are an approximate determinant of revenue.

But anyone who has ever plotted a time series graph of, say, average monthly census is well aware of the large random and seasonal fluctuations that can occur. Such a graph is shown in Figure 1, right. These curves compare the average monthly census figures for Johns Hopkins Hospital with comparable Baltimore hospitals and with the national averages, all normal-

* *Hospitals*, vol. 39, October 1, 1965.

ized on the basis of 1000 beds. It is seen that the curves are generally "in phase," that there are well-defined seasonal swings with superimposed random perturbations. Such fluctuations are typical and make any sort of prediction of future bed needs difficult and unreliable; as a result, the census has of necessity been used more as an historical measure than as a predictor.

Yet, the ability to predict bed occupancy accurately has long been an objective of hospital management. If one were able to anticipate bed occupancy, then one could more adequately plan for bed needs, schedule personnel, and allocate service and supply resources. As it is, one sees a great deal published about occupancy statistics and bed utilization, but the continued concern with such matters in the literature in itself reflects a sense of frustration. Hospital management intuitively realizes that most of the data are subject to too much variation to be of real value, so in most instances planning is such that some approximation of peak demand can be met with reasonable assurance.

Prediction of Bed Occupancy

In approaching this problem at the Johns Hopkins Hospital, initial concern was focused on understanding and identifying the crucial factors that influence the rises and falls in census in the various inpatient areas. It soon became apparent that demand for the hospital's services and resources is essentially stochastic, that admissions to the hospital, lengths of stay, and discharges are to a large extent dominated by chance factors. Bailey[4] recognized this fact early in his research on hospital utilization patterns in England. He proposed that the average daily census is roughly a function of the admission rate and the average length of stay; i.e.:

$$C = \lambda \bar{t}$$

where

   C = the average daily census
   λ = the average number of daily admissions
   $\bar{t}$ = the average length of stay in days

In other words, if a hospital admits an average of 10 persons per day and the average length of stay is 10 days, then it can expect an average daily census of 100. The above expression is, of course, applicable whether dealing with a single ward or an entire hospital.

Similar expressions for measuring expected occupancy have appeared recently in the literature. Many of these have been based on the observable fact that for a relatively homogeneous group of patients, the statistical

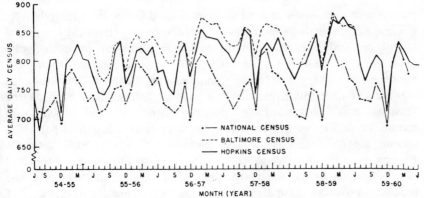

FIG. 1. Time-series graph comparing average monthly census figures of the Johns Hopkins Hospital with comparable Baltimore hospitals, and with the national averages.

frequency distribution of daily bed occupancy will follow the well known Poisson distribution of the form:

$$p(x;C) = C^x e^{-C}/x! \qquad 0 < x < \infty$$

where

  x = the number of patients occupying beds on a particular day

  C = the average daily occupancy rate

  p(x;C) = the probability of having x patients occupying beds on a particular day, given C

Investigators such as Thompson[5] and Blumberg[6] propose the use of the Poisson distribution mean as an estimate of average occupancy and the addition of one or two standard deviations to establish an acceptable risk of bed shortage. Indeed, Bailey[4] suggested that the number of admissions per day could be described by the Poisson distribution and the length of stay by the equally well known negative exponential distribution. Under these conditions, it can be shown theoretically[7] that the distribution of daily census should be Poisson, and that the formula given by Bailey becomes the mean of the Poisson distribution.

Actually, the Commission on Hospital Care[8] suggested as early as 1946, both from a theoretical point of view and on the basis of experience, that bed occupancy will rarely exceed or be less than the average daily census, plus or minus approximately four times the square root of the average daily census. Obviously, it is again assumed that the number of beds occupied daily can be predicted by the Poisson distribution.

As a rough rule of thumb, these procedures provide reasonable estimates of expected occupancy, but to a large degree the hospital still would be planning for peak needs in a manner not much different from the relatively unsophisticated methods used when merely observing statistically recorded fluctuations in daily census. A straight-edge laid across the peaks in Figure 1 will provide results not much different from those obtained when using the computation suggested by the Commission on Hospital Care. Although the Poisson distribution provides an excellent means of describing the fluctuations in daily census, little has been done about the variability in census. Predictions of bed occupancy for a particular day, or a particular season, are still imprecise if one remembers that associated with the Poisson mean is a variance as large as the mean—a plus or minus standard deviation equal to the square root of the average. If, for example, one predicts an average occupancy of 100, then approximately 67 per cent of the time the actual occupancy will range from 90 to 110.

However, the use of the Poisson formula implies[4,7] that the variation is made up of essentially two components: a variation in daily admissions and a variation in daily admissions and a variation in the length of stay. It also implies that a more precise prediction of occupancy might be achieved through a reduction in the variation of either of these. In other words, a management objective might be to establish control over admission or discharge procedures to the extent that a more stable census is obtained with all its associated benefits. Although a great deal can be accomplished through the control of discharges, efforts to date have concentrated on admission procedures.

Approach to the Problem

Initially, an extensive investigation was conducted to determine the pattern of arrivals to the hospital and to the various inpatient areas. It was found that daily arrivals to an inpatient unit, and in some cases to an entire service, could be described quite well by the Poisson frequency distribution, again reflecting and verifying the underlying stochastic nature of admissions mentioned earlier. Figure 2, right, shows histograms for four typical units of the Osler medical service. Figure 3, right, shows the frequency of occurrence of daily admissions to the entire medical service. The average admission rates to an individual unit varied between 0.5 and 2.5 patients per day. Similar data were obtained in the surgical service and other services.

In addition, over a period of three months, data were collected on approximately 600 medical ward patients, which showed that their length-of-stay pattern could be described by another familiar statistical curve known as the gamma distribution. This is illustrated in Figure 4. The bars are the measured frequencies of occurrence of a particular length of stay, and the smooth-fitted curve is the gamma curve. The average length

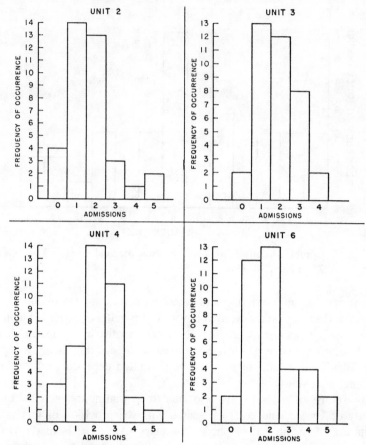

Fig. 2. Daily admission to Osler medical service in four typical units, Oct. 25 to Nov. 30, 1960.

of stay was found to be 13.5 days. Subsequently, 17,000 patient records were sampled for the fiscal year 1960–61 to verify these findings. The average length of stay and the standard deviation of length of stay were found for patients in each of the standard 27 diagnostic categories (International Classification of Diseases, Manual of International Classification of Diseases, Injuries and Cause of Death, 1955 Revision, Geneva, WHO 1957), and then classified according to private, semiprivate, or ward accommodations. For all of these categories, it was possible to fit the data quite well with a gamma distribution.

Since the author's background and experience is in the conduct of operations research, these findings appeared ideal for the application of a particular operations research technique—the mathematical theory of queues.[9-12] This theory has been extremely useful in the analysis of systems

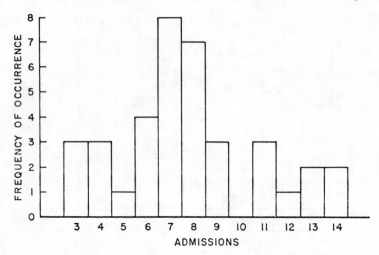

Fig. 3. Combined daily admissions to Osler medical units 2, 3, 4, 6, Oct. 25 to Nov. 30, 1960.

where one has units arriving and requiring service at one or more service channels that may be arranged in any sort of parallel or series configuration. Some obvious examples are the check-out booths in a supermarket, the toll booths on a superhighway or bridge, or the docking facilities in a harbor. Waiting lines may or may not be permitted depending on the kind of system under study.

There are, of course, costs associated with waiting, or with the unavailability of service, and costs associated with the provision of service. Such costs are often more than purely monetary. An effort is made to design and operate the service facilities to minimize the total cost of the system; this is accomplished through the manipulation of the queue discipline, the service rates, the amount of service provided, and the structure of the system itself. Generally, one is primarily interested in the state of the system at any time (i.e., the probability of having a given number of units in the service system), the average state of the system (i.e., the average number of units in the system), and the system variance. Complex mathematical derivations are often required[12] to analyze transient conditions, waiting times, idle times, overflow, and other aspects of the system.

For analytical purposes, it becomes meaningful to imbed a queuing model into a feedback control model such as those usually found in control systems engineering. Such models are becoming more and more valuable where dynamic decision making is required on the basis of instantaneous knowledge of the state of affairs in a system. Specifically, the model to be discussed here will be called the "adaptive control model." A common analogy is the household thermostat; the state of that system at any time

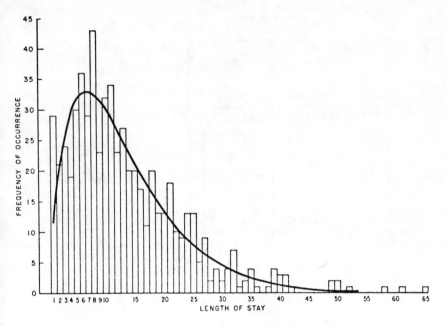

FIG. 4. Frequency distribution of length of stay for ward patients, Osler medical units 2, 3, 4, 6, Oct. 26, 1960, to Feb. 6, 1961.

is the temperature of the room. Control is maintained by a temperature setting; if the temperature drops below this level, the information is fed back to the furnace, and a heat input is initiated that restores the system to the desired state.

Model of Nursing Unit

In an analogous manner, a typical hospital ward with, say, M beds can be represented as a limited, parallel-channel queuing system with feedback control, as illustrated in Figure 5, below. Each bed represents a service channel with the service time given by the length of stay of the patient. The average length of stay is given by $\bar{t} = 1/\mu$ where μ is the average rate of discharges per day. The admissions are the input to the system. This input is essentially composed of unscheduled or emergency admissions (occurring at an average rate of λ per day,) and scheduled admissions denoted by S. The state of the system at any time is the occupancy level, N.

Since the hospital adheres to a policy of never turning away emergency cases, and since the unscheduled arrivals usually constitute urgent admission, control is maintained only over the scheduled admissions, S. This is accomplished by a feedback control mechanism similar to that of the

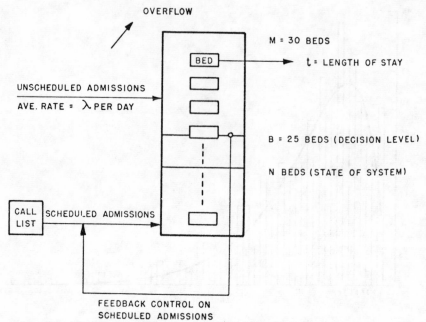

FIG. 5. Queuing model of a hospital ward with feedback control.

thermostat. One designates a particular bed-occupancy decision level, B; if occupancy drops below B, say, to N, the amount of scheduled input is equal to B minus N, or to an amount sufficient to fill beds back to the level B. If the state of the system is above B, then no patients are scheduled into the system. In any event, nonscheduled arrivals continue to come into the system. When no beds are available, an overflow results; and since no waiting lines are permitted, these patients must be taken care of on another inpatient unit.

For this kind of system, scheduled arrivals will always find beds available, since they are not called unless beds are empty. They are assumed to have arrived instantaneously if they appear within 24 hours; the beds will have been reserved and, to all intents and purposes, filled. Of course, delays in admission are possible. If a scheduled admission must be delayed, it is quite possible that the bed assigned will not be available. From an administrative point of view, reservation procedures are necessary in order to draw deferrable patients into the system in an orderly manner.

This system corresponds to the practical situation in which a physician, or an admitting officer, sets aside a percentage of beds for unscheduled admissions and accepts reservations for the remaining beds. The problem is usually to determine how many beds to set aside for emergency admissions and how many reservations to make with a reasonable degree of assurance that a bed will be available when the patient arrives. In some cases, it is found that up to 50 per cent of the beds were being saved for emergencies that never arrive, with simultaneous dismay over the low average census levels. Obviously, a high B level will result in a high average occupancy level (assuming enough patients are kept available on a call list so that scheduling to this B level can occur). But for a given average rate of unscheduled admissions, a high B level will also result in a high average overflow. On the other hand, a low B level will decrease the risk of an overflow but will also result in lower occupancy levels.

The analysis included the investigation of the effects of various B levels on the average occupancy, the expected overflow, the effects of delays in scheduled arrivals, and the size of the call list or backlog to be maintained by the admitting officer in order to make sure sufficient patients are on hand to be able to schedule to the designated B level.

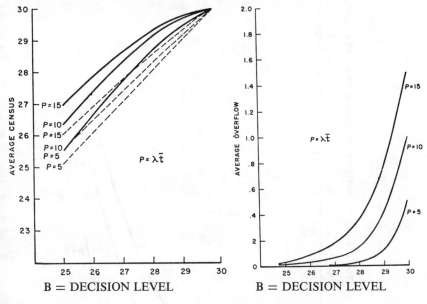

FIG. 6. Variations of average census according to bed occupancy decision levels.

FIG. 7. Variation of average overflow according to bed occupancy decision levels.

Some of the results (for practical purposes, a large portion have been obtained from computer simulation) are summarized in the figures for a hypothetical 30-bed ward. Figure 6, left, shows how average census will vary with the decision level, B. The different curves are for various combinations of average unscheduled admission rates and average lengths of stay ($\rho = \lambda \bar{t}$). The solid lines are computer simulation results and the dotted lines are theoretical, mathematical results. The difference is not great; the theoretical curves reflect an overall average occupancy, while the computer results reflect a "midnight" census with the system, so to speak, loaded up for the day. Using the solid lines, if an average occupancy level of 27 is desired, and if the seasonal unscheduled admission rate is, say, one person per day to the ward, and if the average length of stay is, say, 10 days, then one uses the curve for $\rho = 1 \times 10 = 10$ and determines the B level to be 26. Using Figure 7, page 45, for the same $\rho = 10$ curve and for a B level of 26, one can determine that the average overflow will be about 0.05 persons per day. In other words, arrangements must be made on another unit for about one patient on the average every 20 days. From Figure 8, above, it is seen that for the same B level, the probability of turn-

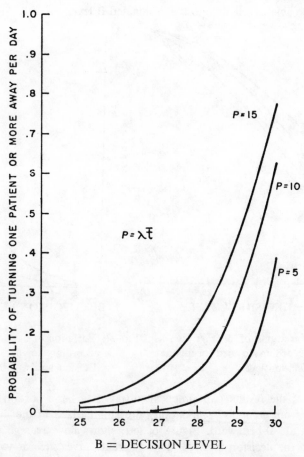

FIG. 8. Variation in the probability of turning patients away according to occupancy decision levels.

ing one or more patients away per day is only about 0.03. What this means is that although the average number of patients overflowing per day is 0.05, there will be many days when no patients overflow and a few days when as many as five patients overflow. But Figure 8 shows that overflow of any sort will have to be dealt with only one in 33 days on an average. Figure 9, right, shows that the minimum number of patients to have on a call list for an average length of stay of 10 days and for a B level of 26 is about 5.

B	λ	$\bar{t}$ = 10 DAYS
25	.5	5
	1.0	4
	1.5	4
26	.5	5
	1.0	5
	1.5	4
28	.5	5
	1.0	5
	1.5	5
29	.5	5
	1.0	5
	1.5	5

FIG. 9. Minimum number of patients on call list required to maintain the indicated B level 95 per cent of the time.

From these results, a set of decision rules has been derived for use by the admissions personnel. An administrator can periodically determine the hospital's unscheduled demand rate and the average length of stay; and by appropriately selecting a decision level, he can maintain a desired average census level on a ward of given size. This, of course, depends on the relative values he places on having idle beds as opposed to facing the risk of being caught short of beds. The selection of a decision level is a dynamic process; levels must be changed seasonally because of changes in demand. But because control is maintained at least over the scheduled admissions, it will be found that system stability is increased and average census predictions are more precise. When delays in the arrival of scheduled patients were introduced into the system, their effects on average census levels and on system variability were similar to those occurring in many control systems; instability or variability in the state of the system increased.

As delays increase from zero, the average census tends to drop, and the standard deviation in census increases to undesirable levels. What is obviously called for is a scheduling procedure, or a reservation system, that will minimize delays as much as possible. Delays of longer than seven days should be subjected to rescheduling.

In this study, the dependent variables of average daily census and average daily overflow have not been evaluated over the total possible ranges of the parameters such as average unscheduled arrival rate, λ, average length of stay, $\bar{t}$, and ward size. The possible combinations are almost limitless, and to a large extent the results of such a detailed investigation would add little to the insight already obtained on the behavior of the system. The ranges of λ, $\bar{t}$, and ward size chosen for illustration here are those which encompass the usual values encountered at Johns Hopkins Hospital. Further computations would be concerned essentially with values of these parameters that obtain in other specific situations, where a decision must be made. For a given ward size and for expected values of ρ, an administrator can readily determine for himself the consequences of a particular decision in terms of the average daily census and the average daily overflow.

This may be accomplished through the use of the analytical model or the computer. The computer is capable of providing results quickly and inexpensively; ward sizes and values of ρ do not change so rapidly that the computations need be performed frequently. If necessary and if no computer is available, tables and charts could be generated for use with reasonable values of all the parameters involved.

What is of more concern at this point is the method to be used for the selection of an *optimum* decision level under a given set of conditions. Neither a knowledge of the alternative courses of action available nor the results obtained upon the selection of one of these permits the administrator to choose an *optimal* course of action without further considerations. His primary objectives, of course, are to maintain a high average census while keeping average overflow as small as possible. Again, if the B level is raised, a higher average census will follow. This was shown in Figure 7, but at the same time the average overflow will increase as was shown in Figure 8. This presents difficulties; one cannot arbitrarily raise the B level without simultaneously increasing the amount of expected overflow. In other words, one is forced to choose between a high census level, and possibly unacceptable levels of overflow, or a lower census level to keep overflows at a minimum. Obviously, such a choice is highly dependent on the relative importance of census and overflow to the decision maker. It is also dependent on the cost or utility assigned to various amounts of these two factors.

An analysis may be conducted in terms of dollar costs alone; i.e., balancing the costs of having idle beds, C_1, with the costs of having to deal with overflow, C_2. Here C_1 is not too difficult a cost to determine, and C_2 is associated primarily with those extra costs incurred when having to take care of overflow on another nursing unit.

To a large extent, the use of costs in this manner means that one is employing a restricted form of utility function, one that considers only strictly economic values. Frequently, the administrator has no other alternative if he cannot derive a utility function that includes psychological values. Under these conditions, the total cost C_T, may be given by

$$C_T = C_1 I + C_2 O$$

where I is the average number of idle beds, and O is the average daily over-flow. If one divides this equation by C_1

$$T = C_T/C_1 = I + RO$$

where R is now the ratio of the costs, C_2/C_1. For a particular value of ρ one may determine the average number of idle beds and average overflow corresponding to a particular B level. Various values of R may then be assumed and T computed. The optimum B level is that at which T is a minimum for the value of ρ being considered. Figure 10, below, shows the optimum B level as a function of R for various values of ρ, for a 30-bed unit. With this figure, if one is willing to assume linear costs and is able to determine or estimate the relative costs, optimal B levels can be selected for a particular value of ρ. For example, it can be seen that if $\rho = 10$ and if the shortage costs are held to be 10 times that of maintaining idle beds, then the optimal B level should be set at about 28. On the other hand, if shortage costs are considered to be 100 times that of having idle beds, then the optimal B level is reduced to about 26, reflecting a more cautious attitude toward overflows.

Conclusions

This study has been, of necessity, more concerned with obtaining insight into the factors influencing bed occupancy and with the construction of appropriate decision models for controlling occupancy, than with deter-mining specific values of parameters and decision levels that would be universally applicable. The latter, of course, is clearly not practical. Each situation demands the determination of decisions and courses of action in context with the particular ward sizes, admission rates, length of stay, and other considerations that prevail. Nevertheless, the model itself is valid; to a considerable extent it reflects operating procedures that in many instances have already been adopted intuitively after long experience with admitting and discharging patterns. Together with a few simple computations, the model enables the administrator to quantify the results of whatever decisions are made, and makes possible through the reduction of variation in bed occupancy a more precise prediction of expected demand.

For many admitting personnel, the consequences of particular decisions about whether to admit or not have not been clearly foreseeable. For them, the number of beds to be set aside for random, emergency arrivals to a nursing unit should be established by the adoption of decision rules for admitting given by the model proposed here. A "B" level should be selected that takes into account the expected daily census and the expected daily overflow. This, of course, also requires an established waiting list of elective cases, under the control of the admitting officer, so that the desired B level can be maintained.

However, a caution is in order. This study has concentrated on a typical ward as a basic building block. Obviously, the translation of such a study into a set of daily operating procedures for a large system, composed of several such units with different inputs and different lengths of stay and with

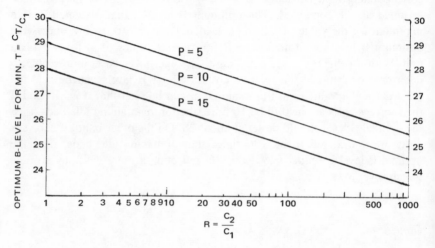

FIG. 10. Optimum B level for a 30-bed unit as function of the ratio of having idle beds to costs of handling overflow.

varying degrees of interchangeability of beds for handling overflow, cannot be accomplished without taking into account many of the practical problems of admitting and discharging, surgery scheduling, and other related activities. Further research is clearly indicated in developing suitable reservation procedures for admitting scheduled patients. From the admitting officer's viewpoint, delays in admissions are often unavoidable, but it may be possible to deal with these effectively, without decreasing system stability, by being able to predict the number of patients to admit to a selected B level.

On a broader scale, total bed needs for individual nursing units, and for entire hospitals, may be examined through the use of modified forms of the model proposed here.[7] For units where census is low and where a chosen B level cannot be maintained because of the lack of a waiting list, the total number of beds should be reduced. In effect, beds should be reassigned to those diagnostic groupings where demand is high and overflow frequent.

Although the choice of an optimum B level may be based on relative dollar costs alone, as it was in this study, the addition of subjective costs for census as compared with overflow may result in somewhat different choices of B levels. Further research is indicated to determine the nature of individual utility functions and the extent to which psychological values influence courses of action; the results would materially assist in the selection of B levels that more nearly reflect reality. It may well be that the utility functions of certain key personnel reflect attitudes that should be modified. In other words, present values may be giving rise to decisions that are hampering overall system effectiveness.

REFERENCES

1. Balintfy, J. L. A stochastic model for analysis and prediction of admissions and discharges in hospitals. *Management Sciences: Models and Techniques,* Vol. 2 (Paris, France: Pergamon Press, 1960), p. 288.
2. Flagle, C. D. The problem of organization for hospital inpatient care. *Management Sciences: Models and Techniques,* Vol. 2 (Paris, France: Pergamon Press, 1960), p. 275.
3. Flagle, C. D. Operations research in a hospital. *Operations Research and Systems Engineering* (Baltimore: Johns Hopkins University Press, 1960), p. 763.
4. Bailey, N. T. J. Statistics in hospital planning and design. *J. R. Statist. Soc. Applied Statistics* 5:146 Nov. 1956.
5. Thompson, J. B., Avant, O. W. and Spikes, E. D. How queuing theory works for the hospital. *Mod. Hosp.* 94:75 March 1960.
6. Blumberg, M. S. DPF concept helps predict bed needs. *Mod. Hosp.* 97:75 Dec. 1961.
7. Young, J. P. *A Queuing Theory Approach to the Control of Hospital In-patient Census* (doctoral dissertation. The John Hopkins University, School of Engineering Sciences, 1962.
8. Commission on Hospital Care, Hospital Care in the United States 20-1-20-6 (1946).
9. Churchman, C. W., Ackoff, R. L., and Arnoff, E. L. (eds.) *Introduction to Operations Research* (London, England: John Wiley and Sons, Inc. 1957).
10. Morse, P. M. *Queues, Inventories and Maintenance.* Publication in Operations Research, No. 1 (New York: John Wiley and Sons, Inc. 1958).
11. Flagle, C. D. Queuing theory, *Operations Research and Systems Engineering,* (Baltimore: Johns Hopkins University Press, 1960).
12. Saaty, T. C., *Elements of Queuing Theory* (New York: McGraw-Hill Book Company, 1961).

Chapter 13

Simulation Models

13.1 INTRODUCTION

In this chapter we will define and describe a simulation model; enumerate its basic components; and establish the utility of simulation models in management science. A schematic model for planning a computer simulation experiment is provided; followed by a discussion of some inherent problems in simulation modeling. A classification of simulation models is given, and some applications of simulation to health problems are cited.

13.2 DEFINITION, COMPONENTS, AND CHARACTERISTICS

To simulate is to "assume the appearance or characteristics" of something —and this is precisely the framework within which *any* model is constructed. Models of real systems can be built by employing different means; but in each case the model is supposed to either look like, or exhibit the characteristics of, the real system that it represents. In this sense, then, all models are simulation models—ranging from physical models (least abstract) to highly abstract mathematical models. However, simulation models have come to mean a special category in the taxonomy of management science models. First, simulation models are those mathematical models which are not amenable to solution by analytic (i.e., mathematical) means. Secondly, simulation models of any consequence are computer simulation models. That is, the experiments on the simulation models are performed by using the computer—rather than a hand calculator.

Simulation models do have a mathematical structure, but the structure simply describes, in terms of mathematical relationships, the sequential flow of information through a system. The underlying mathematical structure is used as the means to trace the behavior of the system through time. This is accomplished by conducting experiments* with the model in

---

* The task of designing a set of "runs" for the experiment and analyzing the resultant data requires decisions on: "(1) starting conditions of the model, (2) parameter settings to expose different system responses, (3) length of each run (the

this manner. First, the initial state of the system is described by assigning or recording the values of the parameters and relevant system variables. Next, the response of the system variables is observed as values of certain parameters are changed or different events are generated by changing various inputs to the model. This is done as provisions for advancing the clock or calendar, which are built in the model, are implemented. The results of the experiments are operational projections of the alternative decision rules or policies that are being tested.

The preceding discussion leads to the following definition of a simulation model.*

A simulation model is computer-assisted experimentation on a mathematical structure of a real-life system in order to describe and evaluate the system behavior through real time under a variety of assumptions.

The above definition implies that there are at least four distinct parts to *any* computer simulation model. First, there must be a mathematical structure representing the essential properties of the real-life system that it imitates. Secondly, experiments are conducted on the mathematical structure under a variety of assumed conditions to explore the impact of changes in inputs on a set of output variables. Thirdly, provisions are built into the model for advancing time (fixed or variable time increments). Fourth, the experimental results are evaluated in terms of identifying preferred decision rules, alternative courses of action, and contemplated policies.

There are several reasons† why simulation models are absolutely necessary for solving certain types of managerial problems and why they play an important role in management science. The most important are the following: (1) simulation models are required when, because of the high degree of complexity found in many real-life systems, it is not possible to represent them by conventional mathematical models; (2) even if we succeed in developing adequate mathematical models for some large, complex systems (e.g., economic systems, business firms) it may not be possible to "solve" them by known analytical techniques; and (3) the analytical techniques may be too costly or restricted. In all cases where one finds severe limitations (in terms of size, complexity, fidelity, time, or cost) in the application of analytical models, simulation models offer a great promise to gain an insight into systems behavior.

A number of characteristics differentiate simulation models from the category of analytical models. First, simulation models are not solvable by

---

number of simulated time periods and the amount of elapsed computer time), (4) number of runs with the same parameter settings, and (5) variables to measure and how to measure them" [Wagner 1969, p. 910].

* For other definitions, see Naylor et al. [1966, p. 3], Martin [1968, p. 5], and Ackoff and Sasieni [1968, p. 97].

† For a discussion on the rationale for computer simulation, see Naylor et al. [1966, pp. 4–9], and Morgenthaler [in Ackoff, 1961, Chap. 9].

mathematical techniques; while analytical models can be manipulated mathematically to yield optimal solutions. In this sense, simulation models, because of the complex nature of the systems they deal with, yield only near-optimal solutions—not optimal solutions. Secondly, it is often not possible to assign causality in simulation models; whereas, in analytical models there is a clear statement of causality between certain input variables and system outcomes. Thirdly, simulation models are essentially descriptive,* while analytic models are almost always prescriptive.

Simulation models have been employed to solve all types of business, economic, industry, military, health, and social problems.† Complex problems in production, inventory, scheduling, queuing, finance, and marketing have been analyzed by using simulation techniques. Models of business firms, hospitals, urban systems, population growth, and even world systems have been studied by simulation.‡ Simulation models are constructed for describing current systems, deriving solutions to problems relating to current systems, exploring ramifications of changes in the current systems, finding ways to improve current systems, and in general conducting "what-if" type of analysis.§ They can also be used for studying transitional processes, estimating values of model parameters, estimating model's functional form, evaluating courses of action that cannot be formulated into the model, initial structuring for complicated problem systems, training of decision-makers and system's operators, and analyzing human thought processes. Simulation models are particularly useful for testing and comparing decision rules for complex systems characterized by uncertainty, highly interdependent variables, and strong dynamic interactions between decisions and their consequences. Simulation is, indeed, a very powerful tool of analysis for health planners and administrators.

An idea of the wide range of problems and potentials of simulation techniques can be obtained by the following list of simulation topics.∥

1. Estimating reliability and validity in simulation experiments.
2. The use of experimental design techniques in simulation.
3. New simulation language developments.
4. Corporate and financial models.

---

* It is, however, possible to identify preferred courses of action (in prescriptive sense) from experimenting with simulation models.
† See, for example, Bonini [1967], Forrester [1961]. Also, see references at the end of this chapter.
‡ See, for example, Forrester [1961], Forrester [1971], Meadows [1972], Forrester [1971].
§ "What-if" type of analysis is aimed at finding systems response to specified changes. An illustrative question is: "What will happen to hospital inventory level if occupancy rate is increased by 25 percent?" This type of analysis, when applied to analytical models, is referred to as "sensitivity analysis." See Rappaport [1967].
∥ This is a partial list. See [Digest of the Second Conference on Applications of Simulation, 1968].

5. Transportation models.
6. Use of simulation in the design of large scale information systems.
7. Manufacturing applications.
8. Simulation of human behavior.
9. Simulation of communication systems.
10. Simulation of urban systems.
11. Gaming models.
12. Job shop models.
13. Materials handling models.
14. Marketing models.
15. The application of simulation in computer system design and optimization.
16. Facility planning models.
17. Use of simulation in ecology studies.

13.3 PLANNING A SIMULATION EXPERIMENT

In order to build a simulation model, the system must be described in terms of: (1) components of the system, (2) variables (exogeneous, status, endogenous) that relate one component to another, (3) parameters, and (4) functional relationships (describing the interaction of the components and variables).* A flow chart giving the procedure† for planning computer simulation experiments is shown in Figure 13.1.

Although simulation models offer a great promise and opportunity for handling complex managerial decisions, they present some serious problems in terms of model formulation, computer programming, search techniques, data storage, retrieval, and experimental design. Unlike the analytical models (e.g., linear programming) there are no "standard" simulation models, and each application to a large extent is tailor-made. The development of a suitable model is therefore a very important requirement in simulation. Although adequate communication and cooperation between the manager and the model builder is always a desirable ingredient of success, it is imperative in the formulation of simulation models. For, as stated earlier, the mathematical structure of a simulation model is in effect a description of "what is happening" in the real-life system. And, only the administrator who lives with the system can know its internal realities. Computer programming for simulation models also presents serious difficulties, and in many instances has proved to be a major stumbling block.‡ Attempts to overcome the computer programming problem are being made by either developing models for *specific* areas (e.g., Job Shop Simulator), or by

* Orcutt cited in Naylor et al. [1966, pp. 10–15].
† The procedure is outlined in Naylor et al. [1966, p. 23].
‡ Rowe [1966, p. 260].

FIG. 13.1
FLOW CHART FOR PLANNING SIMULATION EXPERIMENTS

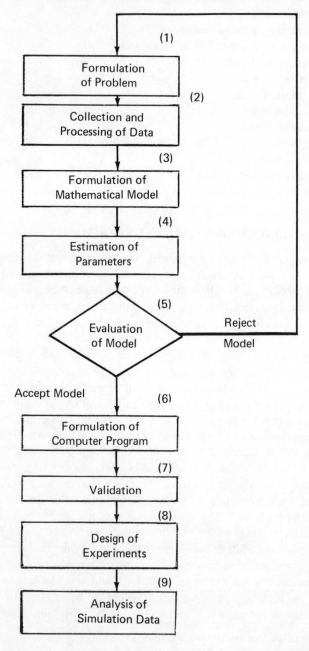

Source: [Naylor et al., 1966, p. 24].

developing special simulation languages (e.g., SIMSCRIPT, GPSS) or by making use of a Compiler (e.g., DYNAMO COMPILER).* Experimental design problems refer to the question of deciding on sufficient "runs" or "samples" so that maximum information can be obtained without violating budgetary constraints.†

13.4 CLASSIFICATION OF SIMULATION MODELS

Simulation models (or methods) can be classified into four main categories:
(1) Monte Carlo technique
(2) Heuristic programming
(3) Operational gaming, and
(4) Artificial intelligence.

Monte Carlo‡ is a technique used in simulating probabilistic or stochastic systems. In addition to simulating systems having a probabilistic or stochastic basis, Monte Carlo techniques can also be used to obtain approximate answers to certain completely deterministic problems that cannot be solved easily by strictly deterministic methods [Naylor et al., 1966, p. 4]. The basis of Monte Carlo technique is the application of random sampling to different components of the system in order to determine some probabilistic properties of the entire system. Consider, for example, a system (or machine) consisting of several components—each characterized by a probabilistic behavior. Assume that the probability distributions, representing specific properties of different components are known, but the behavior of the overall system is not known. One way to learn about the behavior of the overall system would be to observe it over a long period of time, but this is a luxury that is not always available to the manager. The alternative is to "simulate" the behavior of the system—and that is precisely what is accomplished by Monte Carlo. The rationale of Monte-Carlo is that by taking sufficient number of random samples (from a population), it is always possible to reproduce the probability distribution of individual components. If this procedure is applied to all the relevant components of the system, the results will imitate the entire system. It is then possible to infer the behavior of the overall system. Monte Carlo technique is instrumental in forecasting the future behavior of the system and in identifying preferred values of controllable variables in order to obtain the best performance from the system.

The assumptions of Monte Carlo are that the probabilistic behavior of various components of a system is known, and that the probabilistic inputs

---

* Rowe [1966], H. Markowitz et al. [1963], G. Gordon [1962], Forrester [1961].
† S. Ehrenfield and Tuvia [1962].
‡ Churchman et al. [1957, pp. 174–183].

to the system are mutually independent. The mechanics of Monte Carlo technique consists of these steps: (1) obtain probability distribution representing relevant characteristics of specific components of the system; (2) for each individual probability distribution, build a cumulative probability distribution; (3) for each cumulative probability distribution, assign Monte-Carlo numbers (random numbers) corresponding to different classes;* (4) take random samples to simulate the behavior of each component— and from these infer the relevant probabilistic property or properties of the overall system; (5) decide on a policy or course of action in view of a crierion of choice.†

Heuristic‡ programming refers to a method of problem solving based on the application of "rules of thumb" or "short cuts." A *heuristic* is an aid to discovery, or a rule of thumb to solve a particular problem; and a *heuristic program* is a computer program consisting of a set of heuristics to be applied at different stages of the solution process. Heuristic programming is useful in solving two specific types of problems. First, it is used in solving large-size, combinatorial problems because by applying *heuristics* at each decision point, one out of several possible paths is chosen—thereby considerably reducing the size of the problem as well as the computational effort.§ Secondly, it is applied for simulating decision processes that are applied in solving specific ill-structured problems.|| The purpose of simulating the decision-making activities of ill-structured decision problems is to delegate to the computer those duties that the heuristic program can effectively imitate. Heuristic programs do not yield optimal solutions (because they simply do not evaluate all the available alternatives). Instead, heuristic programs develop "good-enough" or satisfactory solutions within the cost or budgetary constraints. Herbert Simon describes heuristic programming as follows [1960, p. 30]:

> Heuristic programming represents a point of view in the design of programs for complex information processing tasks. This point of view is that the programs should not be limited to numerical processes, or even to orderly systematic non-numerical algorithms of the kinds familiar from the more traditional uses of computers, but that ideas should be borrowed also from the less systematic, more selective, processes that humans use in handling those many problems that have not been reduced to algorithm. It is a necessary point of view if the goal of the program writing is to simulate human thinking. It may turn out to be a useful point of view if the goal

---

* The procedure for assigning Monte Carlo numbers is illustrated in Selection 25. Also, see Miller and Starr [1969, pp. 178–183].
† For illustrative examples, see Mao [1967], Miller and Starr [1969, Chapt. 8].
‡ A heuristic is a rule of thumb used to solve a particular problem. See Wiest [1966, p. 130].
§ See Wiest [1966, p. 132].
|| Clarkson and Meltzer [1960].

of the program writing is to supplement natural intelligence with artificial intelligence in management decision making—to bring in the computer as a problem-solving aid to the manager.

Heuristic programs have been applied with varying degree of success to problems such as: (1) assembly line balancing, (2) facilities layout, (3) portfolio selection, (4) job shop scheduling, (5) electric motor design, (6) warehouse location, (7) inventory control, (8) resource allocation to large projects and (9) department store pricing.*

Operational gaming is the name given to simulation experiments in which humans are involved in a role-playing capacity. The two major subcategories of this branch of simulation are (1) business games, and (2) military games.† Operational gaming can be used for educational, training, experimental, and problem solving purposes—although in many cases it lacks realism.‡ In operational gaming we simulate a decision environment within which real decision-makers make decisions under competitive conditions. An observation of the decisions and their consequences sheds light on the behavior of the decision-maker as well as the decision system. Although used mainly to study and improve decision-making skills under competitive situations, operational gaming has also been applied in many functional areas under noncompetitive environment.§

The history of military games dates back to 1780 when the Prussians used war games for purposes of training their army. Since that time war games have been, and are being employed, by all major powers in order to design and test military strategies under simulated environments. Since World War II, the idea of gaming has been extended to study business systems, organizational behavior, and political problems.‖ A business game may be defined "as a *sequential* decision-making exercise structured around a model of a business operation in which participants assume the role of managing the simulated operation" [Greenlaw et al. 1962, p. 5]. Business gaming is very much akin to educational and training methods such as case study, role-playing, sensitivity training—except that a business game centers around a model to be manipulated with a set of rules. The model consists of a set of mathematical statements that simulate the decision system and define the relationships between decisions and operating results. The participants play by a set of rules which provide for *sequential* decision-making—in order to bring dynamic realism to the game.

Artificial intelligence refers to that branch of simulation models which

* Wiest [1966, p. 129].
† For another classification (according to design characteristics and purpose) see Eilon [1963, p. 138]. Also, see Greenlaw et al. [1962, p. 16].
‡ See, for example, Frank and Green [1967, pp. 100–105], and Eilon [1963, p. 144].
§ See examples in Eilon [1963].
‖ See, for example, Cohen [1960], Bloomfield and Whaley [1965], Davison [1961], Coleman [1964] and Guetzkow [1963].

attempts to imitate purposeful behavior. It is essentially an extension of heuristic programming designed to duplicate behavior patterns of individual decision-makers. It is simultaneously the boldest and most difficult branch of simulation—since it attempts to simulate human thinking. Simon [1960, pp. 30–32] cites computer programs that have been developed for proving geometrical theorems, playing checkers and playing chess. Artificial intelligence is based on the familiar components of problem solving: search, pattern recognition, inductive inference and learning. The reader is referred to Meinhart [1966], Minsky [1966], Feigenbaum and Feldman [1963] and Newell and Simon [1958] for relevant material on artificial intelligence.

13.5 CONCLUDING REMARKS

Rapid strides are being made in using simulation models in attacking several operational problems (e.g., outpatient services, obstetrical units, admission systems, facilities planning) in the health field.* Fetter and Thompson [1965] have developed simulation models to study three hospital subsystems: (1) the maternity suite, (2) an outpatient clinic, and (3) a surgical pavilion. They investigated the maternity suite model for the effect of increase in admission rate, effect of elective induction, and the results of a change in length of stay. They also reported attempts to develop a clinical laboratory model and a general model for ward design. Simulation approach has also been advanced as the means to determine the effect of introducing preoperative care unit into the surgical facility and predicting the effect of changes in several variables (e.g., demographic changes in the population, epidemiological changes, new specialities) on the operation of the system as a whole.† Barnoon and Wolfe [1968] have developed a computer simulation method (SIMSCRIPT simulation program was used) that can be used to improve the utilization of operating rooms. Computer simulation was used in New York City [Savas, 1969] to analyze the possible improvements in ambulance service that would result from proposed changes in the number and location of ambulances. Schneiderman and Muller [1972] describe how simulated medical diagnostic problems are being used to supplement traditional medical teaching. Although they are time consuming and expensive to build, simulation models offer a great potential in the planning and management of health care institutions. To supplement the discussion in this chapter, we selected two articles. The first explains the mechanics of Monte Carlo simulation, and the second discusses simulation in the context of health care administration problems.

---

* See references at the end of Chapter 13.
† Pelletier [1967].

Fogarty's article (Selection 25) presents a brief description of simulation and illustrates Monte Carlo simulation by employing an example in which arriving orders are served by machines. A classification of simulation activities is provided and conditions under which Monte Carlo simulation can be used are listed. A general procedure for conducting a Monte Carlo simulation experiment is given. The rationale of Monte Carlo is specified and by using concrete data the simulation is run for a period of five days. The role of computers and simulation languages is discussed. Finally, the advantages and limitations of Monte Carlo simulation are summarized.

Robinson et al. (Selection 26) describe a method of analyzing alternative systems of scheduling hospital admissions by computer simulation. The problem of hospital scheduling is explained, along with a set of four attributes affecting the scheduling process. An operational simulation model is developed based on a series of assumptions regarding patients, beds, and hospital operations. The simulation is divided into three programs, dealing sequentially with requests for admission, scheduling, and evaluation of costs of three basic scheduling systems and using the output of each phase of the simulation as input to the following phase. The feasibility of using the scheduling program in a real-time automated patient-scheduling system is discussed, with indications of adaptations required and additional functions that could be handled by the system.

REFERENCES

Ackoff, R. L. (ed.), *Progress in Operations Research, vol. 1,* New York: John 1961   Wiley & Sons.

Ackoff, R. L., and M. W. Sasieni, *Fundamentals of Operations Research,* New 1968   York: John Wiley & Sons.

Barnoon, S., and H. Wolfe, "Scheduling a Multiple Operating Room System: 1968   A Simulation Approach," *Health Services Research,* vol. 3, no. 4, pp. 272–285.

Bloomfield, L. P., and B. Whaley, "The Political Military Exercise: A Progress 1965   Report," *Orbis,* vol. 8, pp. 854–870.

Bonini, C. P., *Simulation of Information and Decision Systems in the Firm,* 1967   Chicago, Ill.: Markham Publishing Co.

Churchman, C. W., Russell L. Ackoff, and E. Leonard Arnoff, *Introduction to* 1957   *Operations Research,* New York: John Wiley & Sons.

Clarkson, G. P., and A. H. Meltzer, "Portfolio Selection: A Heuristic Ap- 1960   proach," *The Journal of Finance,* vol. 15, no. 4, December, pp. 465–480.

Cohen, K. J., et al., "The Carnegie Tech Management Game," *The Journal* 1960   *of Business,* vol. 23, no. 4, October, pp. 303–321.

Coleman, J. S., "Collective Decisions," *Sociological Inquiry,* vol. 34, pp. 1964   166–181.

Davison, W. P., "A Public Opinion Game," *Public Opinion Quarterly,* vol. 25, 1961   pp. 210–220.

Digest of the Second Conference on Applications of Simulation, New York,
1968   December 2-4.

Ehrenfeld, S., and S. Ben Tuvia, "The Efficiency of Statistical Simulation
1962   Procedures," *Technometrics,* May.

Eilon, S., "Management Games," *Operational Research Quarterly,* vol. 14,
1963   no. 2, June, pp. 137–149.

Feigenbaum, E., and J. Feldman, *Computers and Thought,* New York: Mc-
1963   Graw-Hill.

Fetter, R. B., and J. D. Thompson, "The Simulation of Hospital Systems,"
1965   *Operations Research,* vol. 13, no. 5, September-October, pp. 698–
        711.

Forrester, J. W., *Industrial Dynamics,* Cambridge, Mass.: M.I.T. Press.
1961

Forrester, J. W., *World Dynamics,* Cambridge, Mass.: Wright-Allen Press.
1971

Forrester, J. W., "Counterintuitive Behavior of Social Systems," *Technology*
1971   *Review,* vol. 73, no. 3, January, pp. 52–68.

Frank, R. E., and P. E. Green, *Quantitative Methods in Marketing,* Englewood
1967   Cliffs, N.J.: Prentice-Hall.

Gordon, G., "A General Purpose Systems Simulator," *IBM Systems Journal,*
1962   vol. 1, September.

Greenlaw, P. S., et al., *Business Simulation,* Englewood Cliffs, N.J.: Prentice-
1962   Hall.

Guetzkow, H., et al., *Simulation in International Relations: Developments for*
1963   *Research and Teaching,* Englewood Cliffs, N.J.: Prentice-Hall.

Mao, J. C. T., "Essentials of Computer Simulation," *Financial Executive,*
1967   October, pp. 53–57, 58, 60 and 62.

Markowitz, H., *Simscript: A Simulation Programming Language,* Englewood
1963   Cliffs, N.J.: Prentice-Hall.

Martin, F. F., *Computer Modeling and Simulation,* New York: John Wiley &
1968   Sons.

Meadows, D. H., et al., *The Limits to Growth,* New York: Universe Books.
1972

Meinhart, W. A., "Artificial Intelligence, Computer Simulation of Human
1966   Cognitive and Social Processes, and Management Thought," *Academy*
        of Management Journal, vol. 9, December, pp. 294–307.

Miller, D. W., and Martin K. Starr, *Executive Decisions and Operations Re-*
1969   *search,* 2nd edition, Englewood Cliffs, N.J.: Prentice-Hall.

Minsky, M. L., "Artificial Intelligence," *Scientific American,* vol. 215, Septem-
1966   ber, pp. 246–260.

Morgenthaler, G. W., "The Theory and Application of Simulation in Opera-
1961   tions Research," in Russell L. Ackoff (ed.), in *Progress in Opera-*
        tions Research, New York: John Wiley & Sons.

Naylor, T. H., et al., *Computer Simulation Techniques,* New York: John
1966   Wiley & Sons.

Newell, S., and H. Simon, "Chess Playing Programs and the Problem of Com-
1958   plexity," *IBM Journal of Research and Development,* vol. 2, no. 4,
        October, pp. 320–335.

Orcutt, G. H., "Simulation of Economic Systems," cited in Thomas H. Naylor,
1966   et al., *Computer Simulation Techniques,* New York: John Wiley &
        Sons.

References · 559

Pelletier, R. J., "The Future for Programming and Planning Complex Facil-
1967 ities," *Canadian Hospital,* vol. 44, no. 11, November, pp. 66–70.
Rappaport, A., "Sensitivity Analysis in Decision-Making," *The Accounting*
1967 *Review,* July, pp. 441–445.
Rowe, A. J., "Computer Simulation: A Solution Technique for Management
1966 Problems," *Proceedings of the Fall Joint Computer Conference,*
      pp. 259–267.
Savas, E. S., "Simulation and Cost-Effectiveness Analysis of New York's
1969 Emergency Ambulance Service," *Management Science,* vol. 15, no.
      12, August, pp. B 608–B 628.
Schneiderman, H., and R. L. Muller, "The Diagnosis Game: A Computer-
1972 Based Exercise in Clinical Problem-Solving," *Journal of the American
      Medical Association,* vol. 219, no. 3, January 17, pp. 333–335.
Simon, H. A., *The New Science of Management Decision,* New York: Harper
1960 & Row.
Wagner, H. M., *Principles of Operations Research,* Englewood Cliffs, N.J.:
1969 Prentice-Hall.
Wiest, J. R., "Heuristic Programs for Decision Making," *Harvard Business
1966 Review,* September-October, pp. 129–143.

SELECTION 25

Simulation: A Decision-Making Technique*

Donald W. Fogarty

INTRODUCTION

Simulation means different things to different people. And, to an extent, it should; for it is a generic term. This paper begins by noting the broad scope of simulation, examines the bases for categorization of simulation activities, and investigates Monte Carlo simulation. The investigation includes a description of the Monte Carlo technique, its rationale, different applications, some pitfalls and how to guard against them. In addition, the use of computers and special computer languages for Monte Carlo simulation is discussed.

First, what is simulation? Webster says that simulation is to assume the appearance of, without the reality. Bowman and Fetter in the book, *Analysis for Production Management,* define simulation as the taking of a real system and in some sense duplicating it.[1] Rudell Reed, Jr., in his text, *Plant Layout,* says that "Simulation is the representation of reality through the use of a model or other device, which will react in the same manner as reality under a given set of conditions."[2] James H. Greene in one of the most recent books on production control defines simulation as ". . . a model of the real system."[3]

Up to this point, none of the definitions have included any mention of computers, mathematical models, statistics or stochastic processes. But, if we look at a few definitions given in a narrower frame of reference, these terms will appear. For instance, in an *Operations Research Quarterly* article J. Harling writes, "By simulation is meant the technique of setting up a stochastic model of a real situation, and then performing sampling experiments upon the model."[4] Jay W. Forrester, author of *Industrial Dynamics,* writes, "Simulation means setting up in a digital computer the conditions that describe company operations. On the basis of the description of the company, and the assumptions made, the computer then generates the results that would occur in product movement, manpower and financial requirements, etc., when possible alternate policies are adopted."[5]

These definitions, which were selected from the many that are available,

---

* *Production and Inventory Management,* Oct. 1967.

not only reveal the general and some limited meanings of the term, but also provide an insight into the why, where and how of simulation that are discussed later. They disclose that the term covers a wide range of activities that must be subdivided and categorized in a meaningful manner for further study.

CLASSIFICATION OF SIMULATION ACTIVITIES

Simulation activities can be classified on the basis of the nature of the system being simulated or by the method of simulation being used, or into time dependent and time independent simulation models.

Classification on the basis of the nature of the system being studied renders the following categories:

1. A sociological, economic, political system, or some combination thereof.
2. A physical system.
3. An industrial system or sub-system.

Each of these categories, and some of their sub-categories, constitute a field of study in themselves. Actually, most of us are "ole" simulators from way back; the first time we played with toy soldiers, or cowboys and Indians, we were simulating in the broadest sense of the term. Speaking of war games, simulation, as well as many of the techniques which fall under the broad umbrella of operations research, received great impetus from its use in World War II.

The first of these categories includes simulated war games, national economics, etc.

The second category, simulation of physical systems, can be described in terms of the aeronautical or mechanical engineer, when unable to find mathematical expressions which predict completely or adequately the behavior of a component or system under design, falls back upon tests of a reduced scale model of that system under conditions which simulate those of the system in its environment. A whole field of knowledge concerning simularity conditions and dimensional analysis has been developed to assure the engineer that the scale model will react in the same manner as the real model. A three dimensional reduction in size will seldom accomplish this.[6]

Various types of simulation have been employed for many years by industrial engineers and business managers in understanding industrial systems and sub-systems and reaching decisions regarding the controlled variables in these systems. The two and three dimensional representations of plant and office layouts is an application of simulation with which we are all familiar. A model which represents reality is manipulated so as to study and evaluate alternate courses of action, equipment layouts in this case. Many other examples can be given. Operation process charting and flow process charting are both simulation in a sense. Most scheduling and machine loading procedures constitute simulation. A pencil is used to place the appropriate marks on a piece of paper on which, for example, rows are used to represent machines, columns are used to represent time, and colored tabs are frequently used to represent different jobs. The entire combination constitutes a simulation of a plant or a department which allows us to determine by some hueristic approach the best possible scheduling and loading combination to produce a product at the lowest cost possible and still meet our delivery date. Hueristic approach means the approach followed when working on a trial and error basis through a sequencing type problem by what appears to be sensible rules and procedures looking for the best solution. More recent developments in simulation of industrial systems and sub-systems are discussed later in this article.

Time dependent models are those models whose performance is a function of time. The status of the model, or the system itself, changes with time irrespective of the occurrence of internal events that affect the system. All queueing models are of this type. For, regardless of what happens internally to the system, inputs, whether they be customers, sales, etc., continue to enter the waiting line. Inputs are a function of time.

Time independent models are those simulation models whose performance does not depend on time, that is, the performance of the model does not depend on the length of time the model was simulated, but depends solely on the number and nature of events that affect the status of the system. Neither the performance of the system nor the creation of events is a function of time. Simulation models used to study plant location and route selection for a traveling salesman are examples of time independent models.

INDUSTRIAL APPLICATIONS

In recent years there has been virtually an explosion in the number of applications of Monte Carlo simulation to industrial system and sub-system problems. The word "industrial" is used in a very broad sense here and includes organizations such as hospitals and military units.

Many industrial situations require a system that will be able to handle developments whose occurrence is governed greatly by the laws of chance. They are stochastic in nature. For example, exactly what sales will be is frequently not known nor is the exact time when a piece of equipment will fail; but from historical data, the probabilities of various sale quantities in a period may be known as may the probability of an equipment failure after a specific number of operating hours.

Many important happenings in our daily lives are affected and at times dominated by the same laws of chance which control dice, the roulette wheel and the fall of cards. Perhaps this explains the age-old fascination of gambling to the average human. It also explains why this type of simulation has a name long-associated with a study of the laws of chance—Monte Carlo.

Frequently industrial systems can be simulated by a mathematical model which can be analytically solved to assist the manager in reaching a decision regarding a variable which he controls, e.g., the rate of production. However, many industrial systems are very complex, and do not lend themselves to analysis by a mathematical model which can be analytically "solved." A good example of this is the condition of an uncontrollable input to the system whose probability distribution is known and can be handled analytically but whose sequential pattern can't be adequately expressed for analytical solutions.

Monte Carlo simulation can be used when the following conditions exist:

1. The input is non-deterministic; exactly what the input will be is not known.
2. The sequence of inputs is not predictable and the inputs in any sequence are mutually independent. The value of any input can not be predicted; and the value of an input is not affected by the value of the preceding input and does not affect the value of the following input.
3. The probability distribution of future inputs can be determined on the basis of historical data; or a legitimate basis exists for assigning a theoretical distribution to future inputs.

Monte Carlo simulation has been applied to Air Force logistics problems,[7] different scheduling and dispatching rules,[8] steel mill furnace maintenance procedures,[9] inventory levels,[10] scheduling of barge line traffic,[11] flow of city traffic,[12] utilization of airport runways,[13] and sequencing of orders in a job shop[14]—to mention a few.

Any waiting line situation is a likely candidate for Monte Carlo simulation as both the arrival times and the service times can be simulated, assuming they are probabilistic and their distributions are known.

What are some of the advantages of Monte Carlo simulation? First, simulation is relatively inexpensive; the cost of simulating a production system and using the model to experiment with different policies (for example, different inventory reorder points) is much lower than experimenting with the system in reality. This is the cardinal virtue of simulation. Years of experience can be gained—without having to suffer the pains that usually accompany the real-life trial and error process. In addition to the cost aspects, simulation (building a model of the system, and manipulating that model, operating with different policies in effect) provides those involved with a better understanding of that system.

Monte Carlo simulation, based on the laws of probability, enables us to "run" a mathematical model of the system and by trial and error determine what controlled variable settings will generate the best operating results. That is to say, there are certain attributes of the system that management controls and Monte Carlo simulation enables us to evaluate the different possible settings of the variable attributes, or combinations of settings, in terms of how well the system operates under the different settings.

MONTE CARLO SIMULATION

Before presenting an example of how Monte Carlo simulation is applied, the general procedure for applying the technique is given. The rationale of the technique, some limitations, and safeguards are also presented in this section.

The procedure is as follows:

1. Determine the objective function—e.g., maximize profit, minimize cost, maximize service, maximize utilization of facilities.
2. Construct a model to measure the effectiveness.
3. Determine the frequency distribution of the data. Determination of more than one frequency distribution is necessary if more than one input is probabilistic.
4. Convert the frequency distribution(s) to cumulative probability distribution(s). The data may be fit to a theoretical distribution, e.g. Poisson, or to the actual distribution.
5. Generate (obtain) sets of random numbers, one set for each variable.
6. For each random number, determine the corresponding value of the data, input, of concern.
7. Insert these values in the model measuring the effectiveness and compute.
8. Repeat steps 5, 6, 7 many times, at least 100, for each of the alternatives.
9. Apply safeguard checks.
10. Select that course of action which achieves the best results on the basis of the measure and meets the safeguard check requirements.

The rationale of Monte Carlo simulation is based on two attributes of the technique. They are as follows:

1. The input values generated by simulation occur with the same relative frequency as these same values occur in the real world.

2. The numerous receptions of the procedure take into account the many possible sequential combinations and their affect on the measure of effectiveness. The probability of occurrence of each sequence is the same as it is in reality.

For example, if there is only a 5% probability that only one machine will fail during an eight-hour period, our simulated history will have one failure per eight-hour day approximately 5% of the time. In addition, an eight-hour period with only one failure can be followed by eight-hour periods with a small number of failures, a relatively large number, or an average number of failures. The more often the procedure is repeated, the more likely it is that the simulation will include each possible sequential pattern and its affect on the measure of effectiveness the same proportion of time as each pattern will occur in the real world.

Most mathematical models of real world systems greatly oversimplify; and, as the simple model is modified—expanded—to achieve greater correspondence with reality, the mathematical complexities increase at a much greater rate than the model's correspondence to reality. This limitation is applicable to Monte Carlo simulation as is the slight possibility that non-representative inputs might be generated by simulation. In one run of only 100 repetitions, there is always the possibility, slight though it may be, that the average random number, and therefore the average input, may be significantly above or below the .50 probable value. In this event the value of the measure of effectiveness would be misleading to the same extent and in the same direction as the inputs.

However, safeguards exist for minimizing these pitfalls. The latter can be handled by running the simulation four or five times thereby increasing the number of repetitions to four or five hundred. The average value of the measure of effectiveness is then used to evaluate the affect of the specific values of the controlled variables being scrutinized. In addition, the average value(s) of the simulated input(s) can be determined and compared to the average value of the probability distribution.

Concerning the extent to which the model represents reality, actual historical data (in exactly the same order in which it occurred) can be run in the model to determine the value of the measure of effectiveness with the controlled variables set at their historical values. The value of the measure of effectiveness generated by the model can then be compared to the value actually recorded to determine the accuracy of the model.

EXAMPLES

Let's take an example. Consider the case of an organization, or a department within an organization, that receives a different number of orders each day and the orders vary in the time required to process them. The company is interested in determining how many machines they should have in the department to minimize the combined cost of machine idle time and order waiting time.

The company knows the cost of machine idle time, the cost of order waiting time, the average number of orders per day, and the average number of hours per order; but the number of machines that will result in minimum total variable costs can not be analytically determined because analytical approaches do not take into account the sequential pattern of the number of orders or the sequential pattern of the number of hours to process an order. A Monte Carlo simulation will take these sequential patterns into account.

The minimization of total variable costs, idle machine time and order waiting time, is the objective function.

These costs consist of $3.00 per hour for idle machine time and $5.00 per hour for orders backordered per day. Therefore, the measure of effectiveness is as follows: total variable costs = ($3 × idle machine hours) + ($5 × hours backordered each day). (Note: The model oversimplifies reality for purposes of illustration. The cost figures are hypothetical.) The number of machines that minimizes these costs is the optimal number of machines.

The next step is to determine the frequency distribution of the inputs. There are two inputs: the number of orders per day and the number of machine hours required per order; therefore, two frequency distributions are required. The frequency distribution for these inputs, based on historical data and the cumulative probability distributions are shown in Figure 1.

For the sake of brevity, one trial of only five days is made in this example. In actual practice many more days would be run before analyzing the results to evaluate the settings of the controlled variables. Table 1 shows the random number samples which determined the number of orders per day and the number of hours per order. Table 2 shows the summarized activity of the five days simulated in the one trial of this example.

Before blindly beginning with some number of machines and determining the total variable cost, a reasonable starting point can be determined by calculating the equipment requirements for the average number of orders per day and the average number of hours per order. Both can be easily figured from their probability distributions. In the example, the average number of orders per day is 2.4 and the average number of hours per order is 26; therefore, the average number of order-hours per day is 62.4. Since eight machines operating 8 hours per day will provide 64 hours of available machine time, this is a reasonable starting point.

Total variable costs (TVC) are determined for operating with eight, nine and ten machines (See Table 2). Since the TVC of operating with

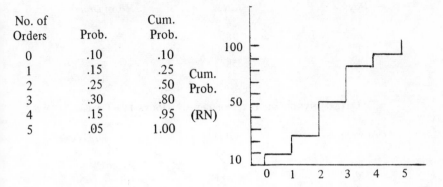

FIG. 1
Probability distribution – Number of Orders

No. of Orders	Prob.	Cum. Prob.
0	.10	.10
1	.15	.25
2	.25	.50
3	.30	.80
4	.15	.95
5	.05	1.00

Cum.
Prob.

(RN)

Probability distribution – Number of hours per order

Hours/ Order	Prob.	Cum. Prob.
5	.05	.05
10	.05	.10
15	.10	.20
20	.10	.30
25	.20	.50
30	.25	.75
35	.15	.90
40	.10	1.00

Cum.
Prob.

(RN)

Hours/order

nine machines is less expensive than operating with eight or ten machines, the cost curve is a minimum at this point and the TVC's of seven and eleven machines must be higher. Therefore, it is not necessary to calculate TVC for seven or eleven machines.

TABLE 1
DETERMINATION OF THE NUMBER OF ORDERS

Day	R.N.	No. of Orders
1	26	2
2	78	3
3	57	3
4	58	3
5	23	1

DETERMINATION OF THE NUMBER OF HOURS PER ORDER

Order No.	R.N.	Hrs./Order
1	85	35
2	75	30
3	74	30
4	28	20
5	40	25
6	69	30
7	60	30
8	11	15
9	74	30
10	15	15
11	04	5
12	21	20
13	97	40
14	66	30
15	42	25

TABLE 2
TRIAL ONE
FIVE DAYS SIMULATED ACTIVITY

Where:
Total Variable Cost = CI, Cost of Idle Time, + CW, Cost of Waiting Time
C.I. = $3.00 per hour of machine idle time
C.W. = $5.00 per hour of orders held over each day
H.B.O. — Hours backordered

Using 8 machines — 64 hours of available machine time/day

Day	Order Received	Total Order Hours to be proc.	Hrs. Idle	H.B.O.	C.I.	C.W.
1	65	65	0	1	0	5
2	75	76	0	12	0	60
3	75	87	0	23	0	115
4	50	73	0	9	0	45
5	20	29	35	0	105	0
					$105 +	$225 = $330 TVC

Using 9 machines — 72 hours of available machine time/day

1	65	65	7	0	21	0
2	75	75	0	3	0	15
3	75	78	0	6	0	30
4	50	56	16	0	48	0
5	20	20	52	0	156	0
					225 +	45 = $270 TVC

Using 10 machines — 80 hours of available time
Similar calculations render TVC = $345.

Therefore, the cost curve has bottomed out at 9 machines which is the optimum number of machines.

The following is a brief explanation of how the simulation was run for the first few days using 8 machines. All others were performed in essentially the same manner.

1. The random numbers (RN's) listed in Table 1 were obtained from a table of random numbers.[15] The table was entered at two different points, one for the RN's for the number of orders per day and another for the RN's for the number of hours per order.

2. To determine the number of orders per day the first RN, 26, is compared to the cumulative probability distribution for number of orders per day (Figure 1) and found to correspond to 2 orders, in the same manner 78 corresponds to 3 orders for the second day.

3. The number of hours per order are determined in the same manner using the second set of RN's and the cumulative distribution for the hours per order. (Figure 1.)

4. Thus, on the first day of simulation, two orders are received and they require 30 and 35 machine hours respectively which is one hour more than capacity. Thus, one order hour is backordered at a cost of $5.00. (Table 2.)

5. On the second day three orders arrive and they require 30, 20, and 25 machine hours for a total of 75 hours. Adding the one hour backordered results in a total of 76 hours, 12 more than capacity at a cost of $60. (Table 2.)

6. The simplated inputs and costs for all other days are determined in the same manner.

COMPUTERS

Although the concept of Monte Carlo Simulation has long been understood, the digital computer with its tremendous speed and accuracy has made practical the application of these concepts to industrial problems.

A technician with a desk calculator and pencil and paper can perform the same tasks that the computer does. However, a model involving five to twenty-five calculations which must be run from 100 to 200 times for each possible setting of the controlled variables will take the technician anywhere from a week to a month to carry out. The same problem can be run on a computer in five to forty-five minutes depending upon the speed of the computer, the efficiency of the program, and the nature of the program. In addition to its speed, the computer is extremely accurate, much more so than the technician with his calculator, pencil, and pad.

One thing a computer can't do is construct the model which measures the effectiveness of the alternate policies. It can't evaluate assumptions, determine to what extent the future will conform to the past, or calculate the different constants that are involved in any model, unless it has been given specific instruction how to do so. The designer still performs this function.

Much of the early use of computers in simulation was performed using standard programming languages such as FORTRAN. Though developing the FORTRAN program and running the simulation model on a digital computer was faster and more efficient than using a desk calculator, writing and debugging the program was a tedious and time consuming task. The development of special simulation languages significantly reduced this task. For example, a progressive assembly line problem utilizing a utility worker required eleven pages of FORTRAN programming but only one and a half pages of GPSS, General Purpose Systems Simulator.[16]

Dr. Liittschwager comments on simulation languages as follows:

"A general simulation language provides a variety of services, all aimed at easing the job of translating a conceptual model of a system into an operating computer program which generates useful statistical outputs. . . . Desirable services include (1) ease of programming, (2) ease of initializing the model, (3) ease of obtaining statistical output, (4) ease of altering the model and (5) efficient error checks."[17]

It is not the purpose of this paper to investigate simulation programming languages in detail. Detailed descriptions and analysis of these languages are contained in reference 18. It will suffice here to list the most commonly used simulation languages and their developers. They are:[18]

1. GPSS, General Purpose System Simulation, developed by G. Gordon and R. Efron at the Advanced Systems Development Division of IBM
2. SIMSCRIPT, developed by H. Markowitz, B. Hausner, and H. Karr at Rand Corp.
3. CSL, Control and Simulation Language, developed by J. N. Buxton, IBM United Kingdom Ltd. and J. G. Laske, Esso Petroleum Co., Ltd.

4. SIMPAC, developed by M. R. Lackner and others at the System Development Corporation
5. DYNAMO, developed by A. L. Pugh III and others at the Massachusetts Institute of Technology

Most computer service centers and computer manufacturers have packaged simulation program that can be adapted to many different simulation problems. A word of caution is appropriate here though. Not all simulation languages or "canned" programs are ideally suited to all simulation problems. Each has its own built-in assumptions, restrictions, and limitations. Before using such a language or "canned" program, its assumptions, restrictions, and limitations should be evaluated in relation to the problem at hand.

SUMMARY AND CONCLUSIONS

The advent of the digital computer with its capacity to handle a large quantity of data through many mathematical steps in a relatively short period of time with a high degree of accuracy has been a boon to the utilization of Monte Carlo simulation.

Monte Carlo simulation provides a synthetic method to dynamically represent a system over time and thereby evaluate the results of different settings and combinations of settings of controlled variables. The results can be obtained more quickly and less expensively through simulation than through trial and error in the real world.

Monte Carlo simulation can be used to advantage where the complexities of the situation prevent solution of an analytical model. It can be used as a training device as the individuals involved get a feel for the interaction of the controlled variables and their effect on the output. Similar to many techniques, it can also be used to evaluate alternate courses of action or demonstrate the benefits of a proposed plan.

Monte Carlo simulation is based on the facts that the simulated input values occur with the same relative frequency as the same values occur in the real world and that the many possible sequential combinations have the same probability of occurrence in the simulated system as they do in the real system. Numerous repetitions of the procedure guarantee that the effect of the sequential patterns will be taken into account in the value of the measure of effectiveness.

Monte Carlo is only one of many different simulation techniques that have been utilized in the business, engineering, and scientific world. It has been applied to many different problems in many different industries as evidenced by articles in technical journals in the last five to ten years.

Monte Carlo is no panacea. Many problems too complex for solution by analytical methods may also prove to be too complex for solution by Monte Carlo. If historical data is to be used, large quantities must be gathered and probability distributions determined. This can be a time consuming and expensive task.

Critical assumptions are always necessary. Will the future conform to the past? If historical data is not to be used, can a standard probability distribution be used to generate inputs? Inaccurate assumptions can generate misleading answers.

Finally, Monte Carlo simulation is just a neophyte; many further developments, refinements, should be forthcoming. The development of special simulation programming languages has significantly reduced the cost of Monte Carlo simulation.

REFERENCES

1. Bowman, Edward H., and Fetter, Robert B., *Analysis for Production Management,* Richard D. Irwin, Inc., Homewood, Illinois, 1961.
2. Read, Ruddell, Jr., *Plant Layout,* Richard D. Irwin, Inc., Homewood, Illinois, 1961.
3. Greene, James H., *Production Control,* Richard D. Irwin, Inc., Homewood, Illinois, 1965.
4. Harling, J., "Simulation Techniques in Operational Research," *Operations Research,* 6, No. 3, (May–June 1958), 307–319.
5. Forrester, Jay W., *Industrial Dynamics,* John Wiley and Sons, New York, 1961.
6. Flagle, Charles D., Higgins, William H., and Roy, Robert H., *Operations Research and Systems Engineering,* The John Hopkins Press, 1960.
7. . . . "Gentle Art of Simulation," *Business Week,* November 29, 1958.
8. Dickie, H. F., and Throndsen, E. C., "Manufacturing Systems Simulation," *Factory,* October 1960.
9. Green, P., "Solving Your Plant Problems by Simulation: How Monte Carlo Works," *Factory,* Vol. 117, (Feb. 1959), 80–85.
10. Larson, W. H., "Computer Simulation in Inventory Management," *Systems and Procedures,* May 1964.
11. O'Brien, George G., and Crane, Roger R., "Scheduling of a Barge Line," *Operations Research,* Vol. 7, No. 5, Sept. 1959, 561–570.
12. . . . , "City Traffic Simulated by a Computer," *Computers and Automation,* Volume 11, May 1962.
13. Marks, B. L., "Digital Simulation of Runway Utilization," *Operations Research Quarterly,* Vol. 15, Sept. 1964, 249–259.
14. Sisson, Roger L., "Methods of Sequencing in Job Shops," *Operations Research,* Vol. 7, No. 1, Jan. 1959, 10–29.
15. Dixon, Wilfred J., and Massey, Frank J., Jr., *Statistical Analysis,* McGraw-Hill Book Company, Inc., 1951.
16. Buffa, Elwood, S., *Models for Production and Operations Management,* John Wiley & Sons, Inc., New York, 1963.
17. Liittschwager, J. M.: "Simulation, Analytical Methods and Management Applications" presented at the AIIE Region VIII Department Heads Meeting, 15 October 1965.
18. Krasnow, Howard S., and Merikallio, Reino.: "The Past, Present and Future of General Simulation Languages," *Management Science,* Vol. 11, No. 2, Nov. 1964.

SELECTION 26

Computer Simulation of Hospital Patient Scheduling Systems*

Gordon H. Robinson, Paul Wing, and *Louis E. Davis*

By far the largest financial investment in a hospital, both in personnel and in physical plant, is directly related to the number of patients being serviced. Of critical importance to the possible economic value of a sophisticated hospital scheduling system is the fact (common among "emergency" organizations) that this plant and staff size are more a function of peak than of average utilization, thus a reduction in the variation of the census would allow either an increase in the average census or a decrease in the plant and staff. This report discusses a computer simulation currently being used to analyze scheduling systems for elective patients. The intent is to provide insight into the general framework and usefulness of this simulation technique, as well as information useful in attacking a specific scheduling problem.

Hospital Scheduling

Hospital patients are usually classified as elective or emergency; emergency patients, however, simply represent a limiting case of electives with no scheduling flexibility. Elective patients usually enter the scheduling system as the result of a telephone call from the diagnosing physician to the hospital admissions office. At this point the potential patient has four attributes of importance to scheduling: (1) desired admission day; (2) flexibility in possible admission days; (3) potential length of stay in the hospital; and (4) hospital service demands (medical or surgical patient, room type, operating room needs, special care or service needs). Information on items (1), (2), and (3) must be available if a scheduling system is to function; and scheduling cannot be effected if item (2) does not exist, as is essentially the case for the emergency patient. Demands under item (4) appear to add little to the conceptual complexity of scheduling models, although they could detract seriously from their effectiveness.

No information is available to the hospital on a potential patient prior to the physician's request for admission. Before this point the hospital

* *Health Services Research,* Summer 1968.

scheduling system can obtain and use general predictive information describing such phenomena as growth trends, seasonal fluctuations, and weekend differences. These data can be used to perform appropriate parameter adjustments on the various scheduling models. Our concern here is with the scheduling of individual patients.

One important reason why quantitative scheduling methods are not employed in hospitals is a lack of data on the patient attributes defined above. This lack applies both to the potential patient requesting admission and, perhaps surprisingly, to the patient who is actually in the hospital. Prior to his actual admission the patient must be described by all four attributes identified above. The description of items under (4), service demands, is relatively straightforward. Information on desired admission day is generated by the physician in accordance with his and his patient's needs. Information on possible flexibility of this day, however, is generated only implicitly by negotiations between the admissions office and the physician. No normative medical information is available indicating the explicit costs of deferring hospital admission for specific patient disease states. A number of other factors such as pain, discomfort, and inconvenience enter this determination, and a quantitative consideration of these would appear to be beyond any presently envisaged system. The quantification of this variable will therefore probably remain a dual effort of the physician and the admissions office. It is perhaps not unreasonable to assume, however, that this "game" will be played fairly and well by both parties if it is clear to both that effective scheduling will benefit the total hospital–medical system; that is, the game is not zero sum.

The simulation models discussed here use a highly simplified scheme for representing the desired admission day and its flexibility. It is believed that this scheme represents the quantitative nature of the results of the physician–admissions office negotiation and, furthermore, may present a framework within which the physician and the admissions office can carry out this negotiation.

Substantial progress has been made in uncovering ways to produce data on item (3), the patient's estimated length of hospital stay. It is immediately evident that whatever the status of all other information or whatever the scheduling policy devised, information must be available on patient length of stay, and it must be available at the time of scheduling. Recent studies [1–3] have shown the feasibility of using the admitting physician as an estimator, either directly or indirectly; his estimate is apparently at least as good as that available from statistical techniques using diagnostic data, and the data production cost is substantially less.

Descriptive data on the statistical nature of admission requests, time between request and actual admission, and length of stay were gathered at two general hospitals in California: Alta Bates Community Hospital,

Berkeley (152 beds), and Mount Zion Hospital and Medical Center, San Francisco (372 beds) [4].

Basic Assumptions

Several simplifying assumptions were made in order to develop an operational simulation. These arose primarily as the result of incomplete data on certain aspects of the hospitals or as programming expedients that were judged not to have a large effect on the simulation results. They were:

1. *Patients:* Only elective patients are processed by the scheduler. Emergency patients (including maternity) are admitted according to hospital policy outside the present scheduling considerations. One reasonable policy is simply to reserve a fixed block of beds for emergency admissions, the size of the block being a function of the emergency history and the hospital's policies toward emergencies.
2. *Beds:* The hospital has a fixed number of identical beds, available to any patient regardless of his description. Problems of adjusting capacity to meet varying demand and shifting patients from one bed to another are therefore ignored. This assumption can be relaxed by classifying the beds according to accommodation type (private, semiprivate, ward) and tagging patients with desired accommodations and personal characteristics (sex, medical isolation needs, and the like).
3. *Hospital operations:*
   a. The number of available, or potentially available, beds is the only scheduling criterion. This assumption can be interpreted as implying either that all other facilities are adequate or that consideration of them is incorporated in the patient demand description. (For example, restrictions on the availability of the operating room could be handled by modifying the patient's desired admission day and its flexibility).
   b. Patients actually enter the hospital once they have been scheduled. No data were available on the number of "no shows" in the hospital system. If this number is significant, an additional routine can be added to withdraw scheduled patients.
   c. Discharge of any specific patient is certain on the morning of his actual discharge. This is close to observed practice, in which the discharge decision is usually made at the attending physician's morning visit, and the patient actually leaves the hospital before a new patient arrives.
   d. Requests for admission are processed after the day's discharges have taken place and the state of the hospital has been subsequently updated.
   e. Priorities arising from social or professional status are not consid-

ered. This kind of priority can be considered as embedded in the dimensions of desired admission day and scheduling flexibility.

f. Admission requests arise from a stationary source; that is, no periodic or aperiodic changes are made in the characteristics of the admission-request generator. Consideration of this class of variation is a relatively straightforward addition to any scheduling policy and does not warrant study until basic scheduling models are investigated.

g. No changes in admission-request descriptions or scheduling policies are permitted during a single run.

Assumptions 3a and 3g are basic to the simulation model and could be relaxed only by fairly extensive modification. All the others could be relaxed relatively simply, depending, of course, on the precise policy desired.

THE SIMULATION

The simulation is run in three phases [5]. The first phase, Request Generator, produces a set of patients and their attributes for use as input to the second phase, the Scheduler program. The third phase, the Evaluator, uses the output from several runs of the Scheduler plus cost data to determine the optimal operating point of the hospital for a particular scheduling rule. The first two phases have been coded in Simscript language [6] and the third in Fortran 4. Simscript was chosen for the first two phases primarily because of its timing and its Random Table Look-up feature, which, at least in the initial stages of development of the model, made up for slower compilation and execution times. The faster Fortran 4 was selected for the relatively straight-forward third phase.

The Request Generator Program

All input parameters relating to requests for admission are produced by this program and stored on magnetic tape. This tape is then used for a series of runs of the Scheduler program, saving computation time and, more important, eliminating one source of variation in the data.

Each day of the simulation has an Exogenous Event that contains data on all patients requesting admission on that day. The number of patients requesting admission is a random variable drawn from a Poisson distribution (a reasonable fit to the descriptive data).

Each patient has a set of four parameters, plus a numerical name for reference. These parameters are based on the descriptive data [4] and the physician's estimation abilities [1, 2] and are drawn randomly from their corresponding distributions. They are:

1. Actual length of stay (ALOS), to determine the discharge day for the

patient. The distribution of ALOS was based on the descriptive data from Alta Bates Hospital [2].

2. Expected length of stay (ELOS), a parameter in two scheduling rules presented in this study. These estimates were drawn from a binomial distribution with mean equal to ALOS and variance proportional to ALOS. Unbiasedness is not critical, since the proper operating point of the hospital can be determined regardless of bias.

3. Earliest possible arrival date (EPA) and latest possible arrival date (LPA), to establish bounds on admission dates for patients. No data exist on these values, since they are generally only implicit in the scheduling process. The present program selects one EPA-LPA pair for each patient as follows: EPA is drawn from a geometric distribution approximating that portion of the Alta Bates Hospital distribution of admission intervals (time between request and actual admission) in excess of five days [4]. LPA is then selected with mean and variance increasing with EPA. For an EPA of 1 or 2, LPA is approximately 1 or 2, with a probability of about 0.1 of being as high as 4 or 5. For an EPA of 11–14, LPA is approximately 6, with a 0.1 probability of being as high as 9–12. Although this is a fairly arbitrary procedure, the resulting distribution of admission intervals gathered from the simulation compares favorably with the descriptive data.

The Scheduler Program

This phase of the simulation is essentially a bookkeeping routine that maintains complete records of the status of the hospital and of future admissions lists. It has been designed primarily as a vehicle for testing various scheduling rules that appear in a replaceable subroutine.

As requests for admission are read from the Exogenous Events tape, the system attempts to schedule each patient by using the scheduling rules residing in the system at the time. Totals for various patient parameter (e.g., ELOS) are accumulated separately for patients who are accepted and patients who are rejected. At the end of each run these totals and measures of performance such as census mean and census standard deviation, are printed out.

Provision has been made for faster transition to steady state operations by starting the system at a point near the normal operating level. The initial conditions are derived from the state-of-hospital and admission lists at the end of any previous run. Because the same Exogenous Events tape, and thus the same initial conditions, are used for a complete series of runs, it is necessary to run the system for several "days" to allow transients peculiar to the scheduling rule that is used to generate the initial conditions to die out.

A simulation day is organized as follows: (1) Each patient in the hospital is checked and discharged if necessary. In scheduling systems that are based on ELOS, each patient has his estimate updated if this is appropriate. (2) Requests for admission are accepted after all discharges and estimate revisions have taken place. Requests can be handled on a first-in first-out basis or can be batched according to some external priority code. Each request is handled in turn by the scheduling subroutine, which schedules the patient for admission on the first encountered acceptable day. (3) Patients who have been scheduled for admission on this day are admitted. (4) A daily report is generated, presenting the supplementary data: daily census, daily overflow, and daily turnaways.

Three basic scheduling systems of increasing sophistication were investigated. The simplest of the three was termed the "filled page" method and is analogous to the system that appears to be used in the hospitals observed. This method derives its name from the book used to record scheduled admissions, with one page per day and a fixed maximum number of entries per page. A patient is scheduled for admission on the first requested day that has an open entry on the corresponding page in the book.

Next in sophistication is the method termed "ELOS" scheduling, based on the estimated length of stay of the patient. This method assumes the ELOS to be correct and uses it without any direct consideration of its possible error. The system requires carrying the expected census in the hospital out to some fixed horizon. A patient is scheduled for admission on the earliest requested day on which his presence in the hospital will not cause the expected census to exceed some previously defined limit. Once a patient is scheduled, the expected census is increased by 1 for each day that the patient's ELOS indicates his presence in the hospital.

The third method is an extension of the ELOS method called the "PT" (probability table) version and includes information about the conditional probability distribution of actual length of stay, given the ELOS. Instead of increasing the expected census by 1 each day of the ELOS, the expected census is increased by the probability that the patient will still be in the hospital on that specific day. For example, on the scheduled day of admission the expected census would be increased by 1; however, for the second day after the expected discharge, the expected census might be increased by only 0.3, reflecting a 0.3 probability of the patient's being in the hospital two days longer than the ELOS. This system is somewhat complicated, in that after each day's stay the probabilities must be normalized to reflect the patient's having completed part of his stay.

The "filled page" scheduling system is, of course, the easiest to implement, as it makes no use of information on the current or projected state of the hospital. It also requires a minimum of bookkeeping and no computations. Both the ELOS and the ELOS-PT systems depend on the accuracy of the physician's estimates of length of stay; hence they cannot be designed at an optimal operating level unless the accuracy of these estimates is well specified and time-invariant. Since neither of these conditions is likely, it would probably be necessary with these systems to adjust their operating level during operation, measure the resulting costs, and thereby experimentally determine the optimal level.

The Evaluator Program

The outputs from a series of runs of the Scheduler program are used as inputs to the third phase of the simulation, which evaluates the performance of the different scheduling rules. A separate program was used for this function for economic reasons. The procedure consists in completing a series of four or five runs at internal operating levels varying by five beds; interpolating between these points to obtain a complete set of data; and then applying relative costs to empty beds, to hospital overflow, and to the turning away of prospective patients, in order to determine the "best" scheduling rule and its associated "optimal" operating level. This procedure offers substantial savings in computer time over the alternative of incorporating costs into the Scheduler program, which would require a set of runs for each set of costs under consideration. Since the rules under investigation do not functionally depend on the relative costs, there is no loss of accuracy with this approach.

As an approximation of the cost structure relevant to hospital scheduling, the average daily cost of operation is computed as follows:

Mean daily cost of operation = cost of empty bed × mean number of empty beds
+ cost of overflow × mean number of overflows
+ cost of turnaway × mean number turned away

where the mean numbers of empty beds, overflows, and turnaways are outputs of the Scheduler program. Turnaway costs have been included as indicative of various costs and relationships that can, at this time, be discussed only in subjective terms. Administrators who adopt quantitative methods in their operations are continually called upon to define equally vague quantities as their systems become more sophisticated. Attempts to grapple with these problems often lead to a better understanding of the operation of the firm: one of the hidden returns of quantitative methods. Extensions of the above cost model rapidly lead to other subjective areas.

Fidelity and Errors

The extent to which the simulation matches any particular hospital, with its specific patient-population, physician, and administrative characteristics, will depend mainly on the quality of data available on these attributes. The simulation was designed to match the general characteristics of the descriptive data available from the two cooperating hospitals. Where no data were available, educated estimates were produced if necessary, or the variable was eliminated if it seemed reasonably unrelated to the main scheduling issues. All the principal variables—patient arrival rate, ALOS, the probability distribution of ELOS/ALOS, EPA, and LPA, and of course, the scheduling rule itself—are easily adjusted to suit any particular measured or postulated situation. The scheduling rule itself can be used to effectively extend the simple EPA-LPA assumption to a more sophisticated scheme. The cost figures are completely flexible, although limited to the three types: empty beds, overflows, and turnaways. These three are sufficient to define stable operation of the hospital, and given their uncertain values at present, it would seem unreasonable to include more.

Three provisions have been made to increase the validity of output data and the statistical significance of comparisons between runs. Most important of these is the large sample size. Each run of the simulation is 200 "days," processing approximately 3200 patients in a 100-bed hospital. A major source of variation between runs is eliminated by using the same patient input data for all runs, thus assuring that the scheduling rule is the only source of variation. The hospital also is started at an initial condition with patients in bed and on a scheduled admissions list and is run for 25 days before data collection is started. Measurements indicate that any transients due to the initial conditions have died out in 25 days. If the hospital is started empty, as many as 50 days may be needed for stable operation.

RESULTS

Six scheduling systems were investigated for one set of cost ratios: 1:10:1, empty beds/overflows/turnaways. These scheduling systems were the three discussed earlier (filled page, ELOS, and ELOS-PT), with four degrees of estimate precision within the ELOS system ("poor," "normal," normal with revision after hospitalization, and perfect).

With perfect estimation, ELOS = ALOS for all estimates. The results of this system indicate the range of improvement possible with improvements in estimating techniques. The costs measured in the system reflect those resulting from patient-request variability.

The "poor" estimation system assigned ELOS values to patients according to the following scheme:

ALOS, in days	ELOS, in days
1–3	2
4–8	6
>8	10

Length of stay is thus classified in three categories, corresponding roughly to short, medium, and long stay in general hospitals. This represents possibly the least accuracy that would be expected by any reasonable estimation technique.

The "normal" estimation system was designed to represent the results of studies on the physician as an estimator of length of stay at the time an admission is requested [1, 2]. The ELOS is drawn from a Poisson distribution with mean equal to the ALOS and variance equal to 0.55 ALOS.

The normal estimation with revision selects a new value of ELOS after three days of actual hospitalization. The variance of the new estimate is 0.55 times the remaining portion of stay (ALOS–3). Data on the third day of hospitalization indicate this to be a conservative assumption. There is good reason to believe that a carefully constructed revision system can substantially reduce the ELOS variance [2, 3].

The ELOS-PT scheduling system uses the normal estimate variance for ELOS/ALOS and produces expected census values based on the probabilities of stay for each day, rather than simply assuming the precise termination of stay at ELOS, as the ELOS systems do.

The results of this study are shown in the accompanying table. The optimal operating level is simply the parameter value in the model yielding the lowest cost figure. It is the size of the "page" for the filled-page technique, and it *represents* the size of the hospital for the ELOS and ELOS-PT systems. The actual size of the hospital is 100 beds.

The performance of the scheduling systems is indicated by the census

OPERATING CHARACTERISTICS FOR SEVERAL SCHEDULING RULES
FOR A 100-BED "HOSPITAL"

Basic scheduling rule	Variance of ELOS for each ALOS	Optimal operating level	Census mean	Census standard deviation	Mean no. overflows	Mean daily operating cost
Filled page	—	16	95.0*	4.8*	0.3*	12.5*
ELOS "poor"	—	82	94.1	5.5	0.3	12.8
ELOS "normal"	0.55 × ALOS	95	95.3	4.0	0.3	11.5
ELOS normal with revisions	0.55 × ALOS and 0.55 × (ALOS–3)	95	95.5	3.4	0.2	10.3
ELOS perfect	0.0	100	98.9	2.3	0.0	4.3
ELOS-PT normal	0.55 × ALOS	105	93.4	4.2	0.1	11.5

* The probable error of these measures is somewhat less than the least significant figure. All differences shown are, with relatively high probability, indicative of true values.

mean, census standard deviation, number of overflows, and mean daily operating cost. Several interesting properties of the system are immediately evident. Looking only at the cost figures, it can be seen that (1) an ELOS system with poor estimates can be worse than a simple filled-page system; (2) the complex ELOS-PT system appears to offer no particular advantage over the ELOS system; and (3) better estimates, and the estimate-revision process, seem to offer a substantial gain over the filled-page system (about 17 percent cost reduction for the revision system, 8 percent for the normal ELOS system).

One problem brought clearly to light by the simulation is the scheduling discrimination against late requests (those having early EPA dates). The ratio of the average EPA dates for those turned away to EPA dates for those scheduled is approximately 1:10 for all three scheduling systems. To alleviate this situation, a procedure has been incorporated into the Scheduler program to reserve beds for late requests. No information is available, however, as to precisely what pattern of priorities ought to be established, presumably as a function of medical need but, at least for metropolitan hospitals, also a function of adopted service policy.

A relatively simple solution to this problem is the establishment of a monotonically decreasing (with time) "priority" function as a multiplying factor on future scheduling capacity [17]. Such a function would start with value 1 for the current day (fill all available beds, if possible) and decrease at a rate depending on the hospital's service desires. If the function remains at 1 for all days, the system is the usual first-come first-served system. If it drops immediately to 0 for the second and all succeeding days, it is a rather trivial example of a last-come first-served system. It may be argued that for hospital scheduling the latter system is closer to the reality, as can be seen by noting the emergency nature of low EPA requests often indicated by their correspondingly low LPA values. If the hospital is unable to determine a normative priority scheme, it is possible to construct a priority function that allows an approximation to the hospital's current operating data. This function could then easily be modified to reflect thoughts on "better" operation.

Analysis has shown, as one might expect, that the average cost of using a particular scheduling rule is smallest for rules yielding the smallest census standard deviation. If it were true that the scheduling rule yielding the lowest census standard deviation at a particular operating level remained the lowest at all operating levels, then the evaluation of scheduling rules could proceed without cost considerations. Such a situation is unlikely, particularly with increasingly sophisticated rules. In any event, it is, of course, necessary to take costs into account in determining the optimal operating level for any particular rule.

AN AUTOMATED SCHEDULING SYSTEM

The Scheduler program used in the simulation could form the core of a real-time automated patient-scheduling system. The economic feasibility of such a design would depend, of course, on a number of factors specific to the particular hospital, including the availability and cost of computer time. The gain suggested by sophisticated scheduling techniques (see table) seems to indicate feasibility, particularly if the data necessary to operate the system are produced at essentially zero cost and if the present manual record-keeping and scheduling function can be eliminated.

The data input to the system (EPA, LPA, ELOS, and special room and service needs) would probably be generated by the admissions office and the physician in a manner similar to present practice. With computer scheduling, however, specific values for these quantities would have to be produced, as contrasted with their implicit state in most current systems. Special EPA-LPA needs could be handled by successive scheduling attempts; for example, such a request as "Monday or Tuesday or the following Monday or Tuesday" could be handled by two successive EPA-LPA inputs, if necessary. If the hospital noted any patterns of requests not easily handled by the Scheduler program, they could be incorporated in new subroutines.

It would probably be necessary to allow both the physician and the admissions office to interrogate the Scheduler program as to why a request was not met or was filled in a particular way. This would be particularly useful during the early periods of operation, when ability to generate the data and confidence in the system were being produced. Both parties would learn the mutual advantages of the system quickly.

Given the input data, the computer could then (1) schedule or turn away prospective patients, depending on the expected load on the facilities during the expected period of hospitalization; (2) maintain complete records of expected demands on the hospital's facilities; (3) determine optimal assignment patterns for facilities to suit current and future demand;* (4) assign patients to accommodations that would minimize movement and inconvenience; (5) handle changes in estimates of length of stay, diagnoses, or projected treatments as they might affect scheduling; and (6) perform time-series analyses of data gathered by the system for use in predicting such phenomena as future trends and cyclical variations. A possible system is described by Wing [8].

Functions (1), (2) and (5) are included in the Scheduler program

---

* For example, the system could be programmed to determine which words should be reserved for a particular sex or disease and to change these assignments if better utilization would result.

described in this report; function (4) would be a simple extension; and functions (3) and (6) are presented as relatively sophisticated extensions that would enable the system to handle unusual situations and trends and optimize itself according to more sophisticated criteria than simply the costs used in the present simulation. A computer system to handle these tasks could be a small or medium-size machine equipped with a disk file for data storage, one (or several) remote stations at information-gathering points, and an "interrupt" feature to facilitate fast handling of requests.

REFERENCES

1. Robinson, G. H., L. E. Davis, and G. C. Johnson. The physician as an estimator of hospital stay. *Human Factors* 8:201, 1966.
2. Robinson, G. H., L. E. Davis, and R. P. Leifer. Prediction of hospital length of stay. *Health Serv. Res.* 1:287 Winter 1966.
3. Gustafson, D. H. Length of stay: Prediction and explanation. *Health Serv. Res.* 3:12 Spring 1968.
4. Robinson, G. H. *Statistics on Hospital Census, Admission and Discharge Rates, and Admission Intervals.* Report No. HFT-64-4, Human Factors in Technology Research Group, University of California, Berkeley, 1964.
5. Wing, P. and G. H. Robinson. *Computer Programs for Simulating Hospital Scheduling Systems.* Report No. HFT-66-1, Human Factors in Technology Research Group, University of California, Berkeley, 1966.
6. Markowitz, H. M., B. Hansner, and H. W. Carr. *SIMSCRIPT, A Simulation Programming Language,* Prentice-Hall, 1963.
7. Robinson, G. H. *Hospital Admission Scheduling Control.* Report No. FHT-65-4, Human Factors in Technology Research Group, University of California, Berkeley, 1965.
8. Wing, P. Automated system for scheduling admissions, *Hosp. Mgt.,* 104:53 October 1967.

Chapter 14

Toward a Perspective

Because of the accelerating rate of change and because of technological innovations, maintaining a balanced perspective toward the principal health care issues and problems is more imperative at this juncture than at any time previously. The existing system (frequently referred to as a nonsystem) should be carefully examined in terms of its strength and weaknesses. The weak points should be eliminated, but the strong elements should be preserved and used as foundation stones for designing new and improved systems of health care.* This will require structural and operating changes at all levels: institutional, community, regional, state, and national. The community (and its total health needs) should be considered as the basic building block in developing new health plans. Health institutions must become part of integrated community and regional networks of social services, and planning for health must be dovetailed with related programs (e.g., social welfare). This is the only way through which true responsiveness to community and individual needs can be achieved. Such an approach will have to emphasize the compatibilities and creative aspects of the private sector on the one hand, and the federal, state, and local triumvirate on the other.

Although the private sector has thus far been the primary sponsor for the development of health institutions, the federal government has become involved in virtually every aspect of health care, including research, education and training, construction of facilities, organization and delivery of services, direct and indirect hospital and medical services, and prevention and control of disease. As we have previously emphasized, the federal government already supports close to 40 percent of the total health bill, and federal expenditures for health services are certain to accelerate in the years ahead in response to rising consumer demands and expectations.

---

* See, Pomrinse [1971].

The role of government in formulating and monitoring standards for evaluation of efficiency and effectiveness of state and local programs will also be extended by the fact that more federal dollars are flowing into the system. Government, especially through the vast power that a modern state can bring to bear, can theoretically exert overwhelming influence in the organization, financing and delivery of services. However, health care managers must never lose sight of the fact that the government often finds itself paralyzed by political considerations to act promptly upon many of the recommendations that it either directly espouses, or which are proposed by external commissions or groups. Health managers will have to play an important role in achieving resolution of conflicts that are certain to develop as we move toward a greater interaction between private and public health activities.

The increasing specialization at the governmental level, and the organizational separation of several related agencies and programs, have already created the need for legislative measures to promote necessary communication between different sectors in the health field. The possible formation of a cabinet level Department of Health could exert a beneficial impact toward the integration of various subsystems, and elimination of redundancy in health-related programs and activities.* The creation of such a department would lead toward more effective formulation and implementation of federal health policies.†

14.1 THE HOSPITAL SECTOR

The 1968 report of the *Secretary's Advisory Committee on Hospital Effectiveness*‡ emphasized four foci for study and action in the hospital sector. These were: (1) ways to improve the internal efficiency of the hospital as a functioning mechanism; (2) the extent to which the hospital should serve as the organizing focus of a new and more effective system for the delivery of health care; (3) considerations of the community mix of health care facilities; and (4) the formula for reimbursement to hospitals and other health care institutions by third-party payers. Each area is crucial in terms of integrating the hospital sector with other elements of

---

* See, Editorial, "Eliminate health 'splinters' through single U.S. Agency," [The Nation's Health, April 1972, p. 1].

† In 1967, the National Advisory Commission on health manpower [Vol. II, 1968, p. 3] suggested the creation of a Council of Health Advisers, "similar to the Council of Economic Advisers," to be based in the Office of the Secretary of Health, Education, and Welfare. The scope of the Council was stated as including all health and health-related interests and setting priorities in vital areas such as facilities, manpower, financing and planning.

‡ *Secretary's Advisory Committee on Hospital Effectiveness*—Report, U.S. Department of Health, Education, and Welfare, Washington, D.C.; U.S. Government Printing Office, 1968.

the total health system; but how the total health system ought to be structured is an issue that remains to be resolved.* It is nevertheless evident that formulating realistic solutions (or responses) to various problems in each category requires broad-ranging health services research programs and invites studies regarding the viability of alternatives beyond the required policy and legislative changes.

The hospital, serving as the primary workshop for the physician, has evolved as a principal center of power and influence in the total health framework. The hospital is, and will continue to be, a key institution in the community and it affects the life of every family. In the past, the consumer of health services did not exert any significant influence in the development of programs and policy for the hospital. Recently, however, the consumer and the community have begun to influence the organization and delivery of hospital and related community services. The health manager must be sensitive to this trend and develop his institutional service plans accordingly.

14.2 NEW MANAGERIAL REQUISITES

Substantial progress has been made in implementing modern management concepts and methods in business, industry and government. However, it appears that modern management (including management science) has had a slow beginning in terms of its impact upon the resolution of health systems problems. There are many reasons for the delay involved, including a lack of knowledge of the discipline by health care administrators, and a reluctance to employ techniques that may appear to be sophisticated (theoretically) but are perceived as lacking practical application in the analysis and solution of complex decision problems. The authors anticipate that what occurred in industry will become more prevalent in the health sector. The recent trend towards incorporating quantitative methods and management science in the graduate programs in health care administration,† schools of public health and related university curricula, will extend an important momentum in this regard, and the attitude of the professional leadership is already moving toward a similar recognition.‡ The principal questions in the future will revolve not about whether or not modern management concepts will be employed—but what are the most feasible problems for attack and how to set priorities for problem-solving. In the health care setting, problems which relate directly to patient-care functions

---

* See *Secretary's Advisory Committee on Hospital Effectiveness* [1968, p. 1].
† See, for example, *The Curriculum in Quantitative Methods: A Task Force Report,* Association of University Programs in Hospital Administration, December 1970.
‡ Loomba, N. Paul and Samuel Levey, "Review of AUPHA Task Force Report," *Program Notes,* Association of University Programs in Hospital Administration, no. 42, October 1971, pp. 16–17.

frequently lend themselves to management approaches embodied in the philosophy of disciplines such as management science or operations research. The health care manager should be sufficiently knowledgeable in these areas so that the quality of patient care can be improved.

There appears to be little question that the demands and expectations of the consumer, the increased role of government in the planning process for health delivery, and the pressures for improved efficiency and effectiveness of management and administration require new knowledge, skills and attitudes. The modern health care manager will be expected to function in several newly-emerging roles that were not demanded as often of his predecessors in the forties and fifties. These are:

1. *To serve as an organizational change agent and innovator in terms of process and productivity**

2. *To serve as a systems integrator and regulator*
   (The health care manager's objective is to insure the enhanced performance of the total organization in the delivery of health services, particularly as it relates to quality of care. Each subgroup within the organization expects the manager to assist in the resolution of professional rivalries and conflicts, to integrate the specialized services provided by physicians, nurses, and allied health professionals, and to equitably allocate resources among them.)

3. *To serve as a mediator in external relationships with the community, with other providers, with third party payers, and government*
   (The external relationships of any health care organization have multiplied considerably, and the manager is expected to serve more frequently than at any time previously as a mediator in sensitive or "gray" areas.)

4. *To exhibit strong leadership*
   (The health manager will have to provide strong leadership for the purpose of maintaining a balance between diverse demands of health institutions. This is especially important in view of the increasing emphasis on organizational productivity, more demands for institutional and regional planning, greater efforts for coordination among various health units. The manager must be less autocratic and more supportive. He must practice participative management so that both personal and professional needs of the employees can be met.)

14.3 CHANGING THE "SYSTEM"

In the past, emphasis has been frequently placed on expensive technology for a few individuals while the needs of the many (particularly in poverty

---

* Where productivity is defined as the ability to increase the flow of outputs in relation to inputs.

areas) have remained untended. It could be argued that improved medical technology and increased specialization have absorbed resources that could have been better utilized in building a more equitable and effective system of health care. A change in the system is needed; based on the philosophy that health of society is a social goal—not the prerogative of a selected few.

The development of the new system cannot be obtained by a piecemeal approach. It will demand a holistic, multi-disciplinary and systems approach. Solving the issues of cost, control, shortages, access, quality, productivity, and fragmentation will require changes in attitudes, public and private financing mechanisms, public education, utilization of resources, regional planning, and medical education.*

Some argue that all we need is more financial resources. However, the mere fact of pouring more money into the system cannot be considered a sufficient condition (or guarantee) for its effective operation. First of all, there is an obvious ceiling to the rate at which inputs of health manpower, money, biomedical technology and plant and equipment to the health delivery system can be increased. Secondly, it is well to recognize that decisions to spend augmented sums in the health services in order to protect the rights of every citizen to adequate care are social value judgments.† Whether or not to significantly increase expenditures in health care as opposed to housing, education, and environmental protection, for example, largely depends upon public opinion and political forces. Greater expenditures for health will result in proportionally less for other elements or problem areas of society, and we cannot be certain that more money in additional health services will necessarily improve health status.‡

In the long-run, alterations in the role of hospitals, medical schools, neighborhood health centers, health maintenance organizations, and the development of shared services, mergers, and mega-health corporations, are certain to realize important advances in the delivery of services. However, at least in the short-run, it is highly improbable that even significantly enhanced spending will directly affect the health status of the population. What is needed is an optimal combination of organizational innovation, new management perspective, change in attitudes, and a reasonable level of financial commitment.

Managers of health care are invariably confronted with a variety of

---

* For further elaboration, see Knowles [1970].

† For a discussion of social values and health care, see Donabedian, Avedis, "Social Responsibility for Personal Health Services: An Examination of Basic Values," *Inquiry,* vol. VIII, no. 2, June 1971, pp. 3–19.

‡ "Little evidence exists that personal health services provided in any current system materially affect the health status of populations. The scientific problems of measurement and the difficulties of experimental design in medical care are constraints." Saward and Greenlick [1972].

perspectives and arguments for reconciling the incongruities and obstacles to comprehensive care which are manifested in the health services. The development of an integrated, adequate, and optimal system of health care will demand high levels of technical, human, and conceptual skills on the part of health care managers. They will have to understand how the pool of available knowledge and technology, manpower, capital, and health organizations can be utilized in developing an optimal structure of health services. The influence and outlook of pressure groups, the network of social and political forces on the regional and national level, and the future role of the state and federal government will have to be considered in making policy decisions. Health care managers must understand the nature and function of each subsystem of health services (e.g., personal and public) and appreciate the historic forces* which have played an important part in the evaluation of our pluralistic health care system. Only in this manner can an improved system of health care be evolved.

Finally, we recognize that the phenomenon of social evolution is such that social plans do not always meet their stated objectives. This is all the more reason that the questions relating to a society's health should not be left to vagaries of chance. Health planning at the national level is absolutely essential. More importantly, we need to develop operational excellence at the institutional level. For it is at the institutional level that the strengths of any social system are finally resolved into actuality. It should also be noted that where the product is patient care, the administrator has greater social-humanitarian responsibilities than in the profit-making production-marketing enterprise. Hence, although we favor the design of the reorganization of health services in terms of benefits and costs, the human needs of the patient can never be ignored.

REFERENCES

AUPHA Program Notes; *The Curriculum in Quantitative Methods: A Task*
1970   *Force Report,* December, reviewd by N. Paul Loomba and Samuel
        Levey.
Donabedian, Avedis, "Social Responsibility for Personal Health Services: An
1971   Examination of Basic Values," *Inquiry,* vol. VIII, no. 2, June, pp. 3–
        19.
Kissick, William L., "Health-Policy Directions for the 1970's" *New England*
1970   *Journal of Medicine,* June 11, vol. 282, no. 24, pp. 1343–1354.
Knowles, John H., "Where Doctors Fail," *Saturday Review,* August 22,
1970   pp. 23–25.
National Advisory Commission on Health Manpower, vol. II, Washington,
1968   D.C.: U.S. Government Printing Office.
The Nation's Health, "Eliminate health 'splinters' through single U.S. Agency,"
1972   April, p. 1.

---

* See, for example, Kissick [1970].

Pomrinse, S. David, "The Crisis in the Health Care Systems: A Contrary
1972   Opinion," presented at: the 13th Annual Institute of Hospital Finan-
        cial Management Association, April 13, pp. 1–30.
Saward, E. W., and M. R. Greenlick, "Health Policy and the HMO," *The*
1972   *Milbank Memorial Fund Quarterly,* vol. L, no. 2, April, part 1, pp.
        147–176.
Secretary's Advisory Committee on Hospital Effectiveness—Report, U.S. De-
1968   partment of Health, Education, and Welfare, Washington, D.C.:
        U.S. Government Printing Office.

Indexes

Author Index

595

Subject Index